Atlas of
Diabetes

Atlas of
Diabetes

Fourth Editon

Edited by

Jay S. Skyler, MD, MACP

Diabetes Research Institute
University of Miami Miller School of Medicine
Miami, FL, USA

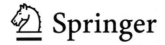 Springer

Editor
Jay S. Skyler, MD, MACP
Professor of Medicine, Pediatrics, and Psychology
University of Miami Miller School of Medicine
Deputy Director, Clinical Research & Academic Programs
Diabetes Research Institute
1450 NW 10th Avenue, Suite 3054
Miami, FL 33136, USA
JSkyler@med.miami.edu

ISBN 978-1-4614-1027-0   e-ISBN 978-1-4614-1028-7
DOI 10.1007/978-1-4614-1028-7
Springer New York Dordrecht Heidelberg London

Library of Congress Control Number: 2011941604

Printed on acid-free paper

Springer is part of Springer Science+Business Media (www.springer.com)

Preface

Diabetes mellitus is increasing in incidence, prevalence, and importance as a chronic disease throughout the world. The International Diabetes Federation projects that by 2030 there will be 552 million people with diabetes on a global scale. In the USA, the Centers for Disease Control calculates that 25.8 million people (or 8.3% of the population) have diabetes and nearly 2 million Americans develop diabetes each year. Thus, the burden of diabetes is enormous in terms of the magnitude of the population affected.

Among those under 20 years of age, the disease pattern is changing rapidly. One out of every 300–400 children and adolescents has type 1 diabetes. The incidence of type 1 diabetes is sky-rocketing, particularly in children less than 5 years of age. In addition, the incidence of type 2 diabetes among adolescents has increased 15- to 20-fold since 1982. Indeed, the average age of onset of type 2 diabetes is dropping. With more people developing the disease in their teens, 20s, and 30s, their lifetime potential for complications is dramatically increased.

Strikingly, although type 2 diabetes is increasing among the young, its burden on older patients is growing as well. The prevalence among people 60 years of age or older now is nearly 27%, with diabetes afflicting 10.9 million Americans in this age group. A recent United Health report estimated that health spending associated with diabetes is about $194 billion in 2010, and that cost is projected to rise to $500 billion by 2020. All told, the report projects that over the next decade the nation may spend almost $3.4 trillion on diabetes-related care.

There are a number of paradoxes in terms of complications. Diabetes is the leading cause of new blindness in working-age adults (20–74 years old), yet the National Eye Institute estimates that 90% of vision loss caused by diabetic retinopathy is preventable. Diabetic nephropathy is far and away the leading cause of renal failure, accounting for 44% of all new cases, yet the National Institute of Diabetes, Digestive, and Kidney Diseases estimates that most future end-stage renal disease from diabetes is probably preventable. Diabetes accounts for more than 60% of all nontraumatic lower extremity amputations, with diabetes imposing a 15- to 40-fold increased risk of amputation compared to the nondiabetic population; however, the American Diabetes Association and the Centers for Disease Control estimate that more than 85% of limb loss is preventable. The presence of type 2 diabetes imposes a risk of coronary events equal to that of a previous myocardial infarction in the nondiabetic population, yet people with diabetes are not as likely to be prescribed cardioprotective medication. Although in the USA the incidence and mortality rates from heart disease and stroke are decreasing in the nondiabetic population, patients with diabetes are two- to six-fold more likely to develop heart disease and two- to four-fold more likely to suffer a stroke.

Optimal glycemic control is critical for reducing the risk of long-term complications associated with diabetes, particularly those effecting the eyes and kidneys. The Diabetes Control and Complications Trial provided strong evidence of the importance of achieving near-normal blood glucose levels in type 1 diabetic patients by means of intensive insulin therapy programs. The United Kingdom Prospective Diabetes Study suggested similar beneficial effects of improved glycemic control in type 2 diabetes. Yet, diabetes patients still are not achieving the recommended target blood glucose values. Data from the Third National Health and Nutrition Examination Survey of 1988–1994 showed that approximately 60% of patients with type 2 diabetes had A_{1c} values greater than 7% and that 25% had A_{1c} values greater than 9%. In the 1999–2000 update, over 37% had A_{1c} values greater than 8%.

The bottom line is that neither physicians nor patients are paying enough attention to diabetes. Diabetes is under-represented in medical school curricula compared to the burden of the disease. This is particularly the case when it is appreciated that this disease impacts virtually all medical specialties. Our health care system fails to adequately meet the needs of patients with chronic diseases in general, diabetes in particular. Referrals of patients with diabetes to diabetes specialist teams (which include medical nutrition therapists and certified diabetes educators, as well as diabetologists/endocrinologists) are infrequent, and there are not enough of these teams or the specialists who constitute them.

Meanwhile, treatment options are expanding dramatically. As recently as 1995, the only classes of medications available in the USA to lower glycemia were sulfonylureas and insulins. Now, we have added biguanides, α-glucosidase inhibitors, glitazones, glinides, rapid-acting insulin analogues, long-acting basal insulin analogues, incretin mimetics, incretin enhancers, amylin mimetics, bile acid sequestrants, and dopamine agonists. Several additional classes of agents are in development. The use of insulin pumps has increased dramatically. Continuous glucose monitoring has made its appearance. Attempts to develop an artificial pancreas are underway. Pancreatic transplantation has become a routine procedure in the company of kidney transplantation.

There has been an exciting explosion of knowledge about fundamental mechanisms related to diabetes. We have gained insights into the pathogenesis both of type 1 and type 2 diabetes, and with that, the prospect of implementing prevention strategies to delay or interdict the disease processes. Great progress has been made in islet transplantation, which offers the potential of reversing diabetes, while approaches to islet replacement by regeneration or stem cell therapy are in their infancy. Whether diabetes prevention will come from advances in understanding the processes of islet neogenesis and proliferation, from genetic engineering, or from protecting xenoislets or stem cells from immunologic attack remains unclear. All are potential avenues of pursuit.

It is with this background that we have asked leading authorities to contribute their thoughts and images concerning various aspects of diabetes. Their input makes this *Atlas* possible.

Jay S. Skyler, MD, MACP

Contributors

Lloyd Paul Aiello, MD, PhD
Professor, Department of Ophthalmology,
Harvard Medical School, Boston, MA, USA;
Vice Chair, Harvard Department
of Ophthalmology, Centers of Excellence,
Boston, MA, USA;
Medical Director of Ophthalmology,
Brigham & Women's Hospital,
Boston, MA, USA;
Section Head, Eye Research;
Vice President of Ophthalmology;
and Director, Joslin Diabetes Center,
Harvard Medical School, Boston, MA, USA;
Beetham Eye Institute, Boston, MA, USA

Rodolfo Alejandro, MD
Professor of Medicine,
Diabetes Research Institute,
University of Miami, Miami, FL, USA;
Division of Endocrinology, Department
of Medicine, University of Miami Miller
School of Medicine, Miami, FL, USA

Mazen Alsahli, MD
Endocrine Fellow, Department
of Medicine, School of Medicine
and Dentistry, University of Rochester,
Rochester, NY, USA

Mark A. Atkinson, PhD
American Diabetes Association
Eminent Scholar for Diabetes Research,
Professor, Department of Pathology,
College of Medicine, The University
of Florida, Gainesville,
FL, USA;
Department of Pediatrics,
College of Medicine, The University
of Florida, Gainesville, FL, USA

Bruce W. Bode, MD, FACE
Associate Professor of Medicine,
Emory University School of Medicine,
Atlanta, GA, USA;
Atlanta Diabetes Associates,
Piedmont Hospital, Atlanta, GA, USA

Susan Bonner-Weir, PhD
Investigator/Professor of Medicine,
Islet Cell and Regenerative Biology
Department, Joslin Diabetes Center,
Harvard Medical School,
Boston, MA, USA

Michael Brownlee, MD
Anita and Jack Saltz Chair in Diabetes
Research, Associate Director for Biomedical
Sciences, Departments of Medicine
and Pathology, Diabetes Research Center,
Albert Einstein College of Medicine,
Bronx, NY, USA

John E. Gerich, MD
Emeritus Professor of Medicine;
School of Medicine, University of Rochester,
Rochester, NY, USA

Ferdinando Giacco, PhD
Postdoctoral Fellow, Diabetes Research
Center, Albert Einstein College of Medicine,
Bronx, NY, USA

Robert R. Henry, MD
Professor of Medicine/Chief,
Departments of Medicine, Endocrinology,
and Diabetes, VA San Diego Healthcare
System, San Diego, CA, USA

Irl B. Hirsch, MD
Professor of Medicine,
University of Washington, Roosevelt,
Seattle, WA, USA

Lois Jovanovič, MD
CEO and Chief Scientific Officer,
Sansum Diabetes Research Institute,
Santa Barbara, CA, USA

Francine R. Kaufman, MD
Emerita Professor of Pediatrics,
Center for Endocrinology, Diabetes,
and Metabolism, Children's Hospital
of Los Angeles, Los Angeles, CA, USA

**Abbas E. Kitabchi, PhD, MD,
FACP, FACE**
Professor of Medicine and Molecular
Sciences, Department of Medicine/
Endocrinology, University of Tennessee
Health Science Center, Memphis, TN, USA;
Department of Immunology, Metabolism,
and Biochemistry, University of Tennessee
Health Science Center, Memphis, TN, USA

Jennifer B. Marks, MD
Professor of Medicine,
Department of Medicine, Miami VA
Healthcare System, School of Medicine,
University of Miami, Miami, FL, USA

**Sunder Mudaliar, MD, FRCP,
FACP, FACE**
Clinical Professor of Medicine,
Departments of Medicine, Endocrinology,
and Diabetes, VA San Diego Healthcare
System, San Diego, CA, USA

**Mary Beth Murphy, RN, MS, CDE,
MBA, CCRP**
Research Nurse Director,
Department of Medicine/Endocrinology,
University of Tennessee Health Science
Center, Memphis, TN, USA

Antonello Pileggi, MD, PhD
Diabetes Research Institute, University of
Miami, Miami, FL, USA;
DeWitt-Daughtry Department of Surgery,
University of Miami Miller School of
Medicine, Miami, FL, USA;
Department of Microbiology and
Immunology, University of Miami Miller
School of Medicine, Miami, FL, USA;
Department of Biomedical Engineering,
University of Miami, Miami, FL, USA

Camillo Ricordi, MD
Diabetes Research Institute, University of
Miami, Miami, FL, USA;
DeWitt-Daughtry Department of Surgery,
University of Miami Miller School of
Medicine, Miami, FL, USA;
Department of Medicine, University
of Miami Miller School of Medicine,
Miami, FL, USA;
Department of Microbiology and
Immunology, University of Miami Miller
School of Medicine, Miami, FL, USA;
Department of Biomedical Engineering,
University of Miami, Miami, FL, USA;
Wake Forest Institute of Regenerative
Medicine, Wiston-Salem, NC, USA;
Karolinska Institutet, Stockholm, Sweden

Arun Sharma, PhD
Investigator/Assistant Professor of Medicine,
Islet Cell and Regenerative Biology
Department, Joslin Diabetes Center,
Harvard Medical School, Boston, MA, USA

Paolo S. Silva, MD
Instructor in Ophthalmology, Department
of Ophthalmology, Harvard Medical School,
Boston, MA, USA;
Staff Ophthalmologist and Assistant Chief
of Telemedicine, Beetham Eye Institute,
Joslin Diabetes Center, Boston, MA, USA

Jay S. Skyler, MD, MACP
Professor of Medicine, Pediatrics, and
Psychology, Deputy Director, Clinical
Research & Academic Programs, Diabetes
Research Institute, University of Miami Miller
School of Medicine, Miami, FL, USA

Steven R. Smith, MD
Scientific Director, Translational Research
Institute for Metabolism and Diabetes, Florida
Hospital and Sanford Burnham Medical
Research Institute, Winter Park, FL, USA

Robert C. Stanton, MD
Chief, Renal Section, Joslin Diabetes Center,
Boston, MA, USA;
Associate Professor of Medicine,

Department of Medicine, Harvard Medical
School, Boston, MA, USA

Jennifer K. Sun, MD, MPH
Assistant Professor of Ophthalmology,
Department of Ophthalmology,
Beetham Eye Institute and Eye Research
Section, Harvard Medical School, Boston,
MA, USA;
Assistant Investigator,
Joslin Diabetes Center, Harvard Medical
School, Boston, MA, USA

**Aaron I. Vinik, MD, PhD,
FCP, MACP**
Professor of Medicine, Pathology,
and Neurobiology, Director of Research
and the Neuroendocrine Unit,
Department of Internal Medicine,

The Strelitz Diabetes Center,
Eastern Virginia Medical School,
Norfolk, VA, USA

Gordon C. Weir, MD
Investigator/Professor of Medicine, Islet Cell
and Regenerative Biology Department,
Joslin Diabetes Center, Harvard Medical
School, Boston, MA, USA

Morris F. White, PhD
Investigator, Howard Hughes Medical
Institute, Boston, MA, USA;
Professor of Pediatrics,
Division of Endocrinology, Department
of Medicine, Children's Hospital Boston,
Harvard Medical School, Boston, MA, USA

Jamie R. Wood, MD

Assistant Professor of Pediatrics,
Center for Endocrinology, Diabetes,
and Metabolism, Children's Hospital
of Los Angeles, Los Angeles, CA, USA

Contents

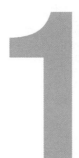

Regulation of Insulin Secretion and Islet Cell Function

Gordon C. Weir, Susan Bonner-Weir, and Arun Sharma

The β cells of the islets of Langerhans are the only cells in the body that produce a meaningful quantity of insulin, a hormone that has evolved to be essential for life, exerting critical control over carbohydrate, fat, and protein metabolism. Islets are scattered throughout the pancreas; although they vary in size, they typically contain about 1,000 cells, of which approximately 70% are β cells. A human pancreas contains about one million islets, which comprise only about 2% of the mass of the pancreas. Insulin is released into the portal vein, which means the liver is exposed to particularly high concentrations of insulin.

Insulin secretion from β cells responds very precisely to small changes in glucose concentration within the physiologic range, thereby keeping glucose levels within the range of 70–150 mg/dL in normal individuals. β cells have a unique differentiation that permits linkage of physiologic levels of glucose to the metabolic signals that control the release of insulin. Thus, there is a close correlation between the rate of glucose metabolism and insulin secretion. This is dependent on the oxidation of glucose-derived acetyl-coenzyme A (CoA) and also nicotinamide adenine dinucleotide plus hydrogen generated by glycolysis, which is shuttled to mitochondria to contribute to adenosine triphosphate production. Insulin secretion is also regulated by various other physiologic signals. During eating, insulin secretion is enhanced not only by glucose, but also by amino acids and the gut hormones glucagon-like peptide-1 (GLP-1) and gastrointestinal insulinotropic peptide. Free fatty acids can also modulate insulin secretion, particularly to help maintain insulin secretion during prolonged fasting. The parasympathetic nervous system has a stimulatory effect exerted by acetylcholine (Ach) and probably the peptidergic mediators, such as vasoactive intestinal polypeptide, these contribute to enhanced insulin secretion during the early period of a meal. Through epinephrine from the adrenal medulla and norepinephrine from nerve terminals, the sympathetic nervous system acts on α-adrenergic receptors to inhibit insulin secretion. This suppression of insulin is particularly useful during exercise. Important drugs include sulfonylureas and exendin-4, which have stimulatory effects useful for the treatment of diabetes, and diazoxide, which has an inhibitory effect useful for treating hypoglycemia caused by insulin-producing tumors.

Type 1 diabetes is caused by reduced β-cell mass resulting from autoimmune destruction of β cells, which leads to profound insulin deficiency that can progress to fatal hyperglycemia and ketoacidosis. The non-β cells of the islet are spared, and glucagon secretion is actually excessive, which accounts for some of the hyperglycemia of the diabetic state. The situation is more complicated in type 2 diabetes, which has a strong genetic basis that predisposes individuals to obesity and insulin resistance, a problem greatly magnified by our Western lifestyle with its plentiful food and lack of physical activity. Diabetes, however, only develops when β cells are no longer able to compensate for this insulin resistance. Indeed, most people with insulin resistance never develop diabetes, but as our population ages, more β-cell decompensation occurs and the prevalence of diabetes increases. Pathology studies indicate that β-cell mass in type 2 diabetes is about 50% of normal and that islets often are infiltrated with amyloid that may have a toxic effect on β cells.

In all forms of diabetes, whether type 2 diabetes, early type 1 diabetes, or failing pancreas or islet transplants, insulin secretory abnormalities are found that seem largely secondary to exposure of β cells to the diabetic milieu and that are reversible if normoglycemia

J.S. Skyler (ed.), *Atlas of Diabetes: Fourth Edition*,
DOI 10.1007/978-1-4614-1028-7_1, © Springer Science+Business Media, LLC 2012

can be restored. This appears to be due to adverse effects of chronic hyperglycemia, hence the term glucotoxicity. The most prominent abnormality is an impairment of glucose-induced insulin secretion, which is more severe for early release (first phase) than the longer second phase of secretion. In contrast, β-cell responses to such nonglucose secretagogues as arginine, GLP-1, isoproterenol, or sulfonylureas are more intact. The cause of these β-cell secretory abnormalities is not fully understood, but β cells exposed to abnormally high glucose concentrations lose the differentiation that normally equips them with the unique metabolic machinery needed for glucose-induced insulin secretion. Marked abnormalities are found at the level of gene expression that appears to have a crippling effect on the metabolic integrity of the β cell.

Abnormalities of glucagon secretion are also found in both forms of diabetes, with secretion not being appropriately suppressed by hyperglycemia or stimulated by hypoglycemia, which is problematic because glucagon is an important counterregulatory hormone for protection against hypoglycemia. This failure of glucagon to respond makes people with type 1 diabetes more vulnerable to the dangers of insulin-induced hypoglycemia.

Anatomy, Embryology, and Physiology

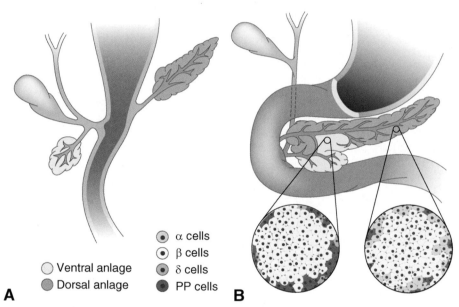

α cells
β cells
δ cells
PP cells

○ Ventral anlage
● Dorsal anlage

A

B

FIGURE 1-1. Embryologic origin of the pancreas and islet cells. A dorsal anlage and one or two ventral anlagen form from the primitive gut (**A**) and later fuse (**B**). The ventral anlage forms part of the head of the pancreas and has pancreatic polypeptide-rich islet cells with few, if any, α cells. The dorsal anlage forms the major portion of the pancreas, that being the tail, body, and part of the head; here, the islets are glucagon rich and pancreatic polypeptide (PP) poor. Roughly, the α and pancreatic polypeptide cells substitute for each other in number (15–25% of the islet cells); the percentages of β cells (70%) and δ cells (5%) remain the same.

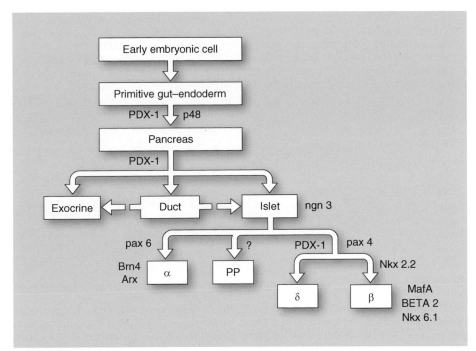

Figure 1-2. Pancreatic and islet cell differentiation. The complex control of differentiation of the pancreas and its three major components (exocrine acinar cells, ducts, and islets of Langerhans) is being elucidated by genetic analysis [1–3]. At present, only some of the transcription factors that are involved in the transition from endoderm to pancreas and then to final mature pancreatic cell types are known; several of them (BETA 2, Nkx 2.2, Nkx 6.1, and ngn 3) are also involved in the development of the nervous system. One that is clearly necessary, but not sufficient, is PDX-1 (ipf-1, stf-1, idx-1); without it, no pancreas is formed, and later it seems to be needed for β-cell differentiation. Exocrine and islets differentiate from the embryonic pancreatic progenitor tubules, but whether they arise from the same precursor pool or even whether all the islet cells share a cell lineage remains unanswered. *IAPP* islet amyloid polypeptide; *mGPDH* mitochondrial glycerol phosphate dehydrogenase, *PEPCK* phosphoenolpyruvate carboxykinase (adapted from Edlund [4]).

Unique β-Cell Differentiation	
Increased expression	**Decreased expression**
MafA	Glucose-6-phosphatase
Glucokinase	Hexokinase 1
mGPDH	Lactate dehydrogenase
Pyruvate carboxylase	PEPCK
Insulin	MCT1
IAPP	
pdx-1	
Nkx 6.1	

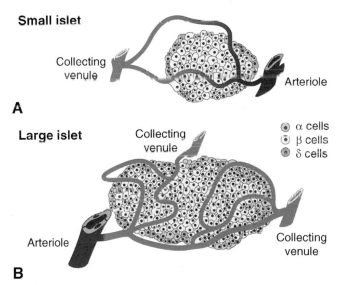

Figure 1-3. Islet vasculature and core/mantle relations. A diagrammatic summary of combined data from corrosion casts and the serial reconstructions of rat islet cells [5]. In small and large islets, β cells make up the central core and the non-β cells (α, PP, and δ cells) form the surrounding mantle. The α cells containing glucagon are found mainly in islets of the dorsal lobe of the pancreas, PP cells are found mainly in ventral lobe islets, and δ cells containing somatostatin are found in the islets of both lobes of the pancreas.

Short arterioles enter an islet at discontinuities of the non-β-cell mantle and branch into capillaries that form a glomerular-like structure. After traversing the β-cell mass, capillaries penetrate the mantle of non-β cells as the blood leaves the islet. The vascular pattern of human islets has not yet been defined but is likely to have similarities. (**A**) In small islets (<160 μm in diameter), efferent capillaries pass through exocrine tissue before coalescing into collecting venules. (**B**) In large islets (>260 μm in diameter), capillaries coalesce at the edge of the islet and run along the mantle as collecting venules.

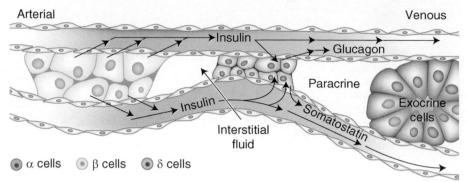

FIGURE 1-4. The relationship between islet core and mantle, indicating potential intraislet portal flow and paracrine interactions. This formulation is based on the known vascular anatomy and studies with passive immunization [5, 6]. These relationships suggest that β cells, being upstream, are unlikely to be very much influenced by the glucagon and somatostatin produced by the α cells and δ cells of the islet mantle, respectively. The downstream α cells, however, may be strongly influenced by insulin or possibly other secreted factors from the upstream β cells, which have a suppressive influence on glucagon secretion. This helps explain why glucagon secretion cannot be suppressed by the hyperglyce- mia of diabetes, which means that glucagon is secreted in excessive amounts, thus further contributing to the hyperglycemia of diabetes. This vascular pattern is known as the islet-acinar portal circulation, which means that islet hormones are released downstream directly onto exocrine cells; insulin in particular is thought to have a trophic effect on the exocrine pancreas. The relationship between β and non-β cells in human islets is more complex in that α cells can be found in the islet centers. However, there are still β-cell and non-β-cell domains that appear to maintain the physiological intraislet relationships [7].

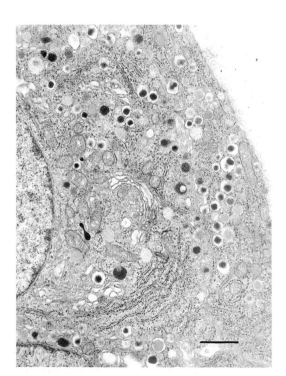

FIGURE 1-5. Electron micrograph of a β cell. The four major endocrine cell types in mammalian islet cells are the insulin-producing β cell, the glucagon-producing α cell, the somatostatin-producing δ cell, and the *PP* producing PP cell. Recently, the ε cell expressing ghrelin has been identified as a consistent small population of cells in the islet [8]. Ultrastructural and immunocytochemical techniques are used to distinguish these cell types. β cells are polyhedral, being truncated pyramids about 10×10×8 μm, and are usually well granulated with about 10,000 secretory granules. The two forms of insulin granules (250–350 nm in diameter) are (1) mature ones with an electron-dense core that is visibly crystalline in some species and a loosely fitting granule-limiting membrane giving the appearance of a spacious halo; and (2) immature granules with little or no halo and moderately electron-dense contents. Immature granules have been shown to be the major, if not the only, site of proinsulin to insulin conversion [8]. In each granule besides insulin, there are at least 100 other peptides, including islet amyloid polypeptide (amylin) [9].

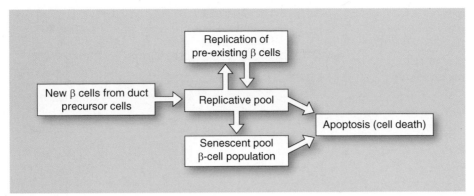

Figure 1-6. Mechanisms responsible for maintenance of β-cell mass. In normal development and in experimental studies, it has become apparent that the population of β cells within an adult pancreas is dynamic and responds to metabolic demand with changes in mass and function in an effort to maintain euglycemia. The mass of β cells can change by cell number or cell size. The cell size or volume can change markedly in moving from an atrophied to a hypertrophy state. Two mechanisms add new β cells: differentiation from precursor or stem cells in the ducts (often called *neogenesis*) and replication from preexisting β cells [10, 11]. It has been suggested that most cell types have a limited number of replications, after which the ability to respond to replication signals is lost and they are considered senescent cells. These terminally differentiated senescent cells can be long lived and maintain good function. β-cell replication rates have been found to slow in older experimental animals [12]. Additionally, as with all cell types, β cells must have a finite lifespan and die by apoptosis [13]. The turnover of β cells implies that there are differently aged β cells at any stage of development. In adult rodents, β-cell replication is the major mechanism for expansion in response to demand. In humans, the relative contributions of replication and neogenesis remain to be defined.

−360 bp   +1 bp

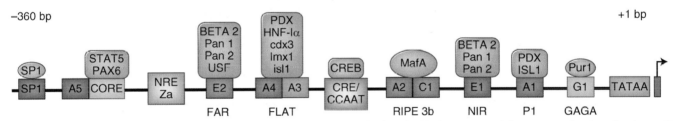

Figure 1-7. The promoter region of the insulin gene showing key enhancer elements and known binding transcription factors. Insulin gene expression is regulated by sequences at least 4 kb upstream from the transcription start site (represented by an *arrow* and designated as +1 bp) of the insulin gene. In adult mammals, insulin is selectively expressed in pancreatic β cells. A small (<400 bp) region of insulin promoter that is highly conserved in various mammalian species can regulate this selective expression and contains the major glucose control elements. This region can also recapitulate glucose responsive insulin gene expression.

In the figure, the organization of the proximal portion (−360 to +1 bp) of the insulin promoter is shown. Functionally conserved enhancer elements are illustrated as boxes. New names for these elements are shown within the boxes, and old names are shown below each box. Above the boxes are shown the names of cloned transcription factors that can bind corresponding elements. Enhancer elements E1, A2-C1, A4-A3, and E2 have been implicated in β-cell-specific expression of the insulin gene. The cell type-specific expression is mediated by the restricted cellular distribution of the transcription factors (such as BETA 2, MafA, and PDX-1) that bind these elements [3]. Furthermore, these elements, along with element Za, are also responsible for glucose-regulated insulin gene expression. Other enhancer elements, CRE/CCAAT and CORE, regulate insulin gene expression in response to other signals, such as cAMP (cyclic adenosine 3′,5′-monophosphate) by regulating cAMP response element-binding (CREB) protein and growth hormone or leptin (via signal transducer and activator of transcription [STAT] factor 5).

In addition to their role in regulating cell-specific and glucose-responsive expression, insulin gene transcription factors are involved in pancreatic development and differentiation of β cells. Lack of transcription factors, such as PDX-1, BETA 2, PAX6, hepatocyte nuclear factor (HNF)-1α, and isl1 results in the complete absence of, or abnormal, pancreatic development. Although humans with a mutant allele for PDX-1, BETA 2, or HNF-1α develop maturity-onset diabetes of youth, individuals with mutations in both PDX-1 alleles show pancreatic agenesis (adapted from Sander and German [14]).

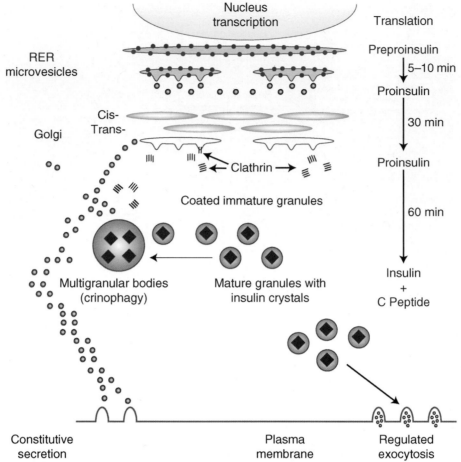

Figure 1-8. Pathways of insulin biosynthesis. Glucose stimulates the production of preproinsulin through effects on transcription and even stronger influences on translation. Shortly after its inception, preproinsulin is cleaved to proinsulin, which is then transported through the Golgi and packaged into clathrin-coated immature granules, where proinsulin is further processed to proinsulin-like peptides, insulin, and C peptide. Granules containing crystallized insulin can either remain in a storage compartment; be absorbed into multigranular bodies, where they are degraded by the process of crinophagy; or be secreted via the regulated pathway of secretion, the final event being exocytosis. Although the vast majority of insulin is secreted through the regulated pathway, a small amount can be released from microvesicles through the pathway of constitutive secretion [8, 9, 13–15].

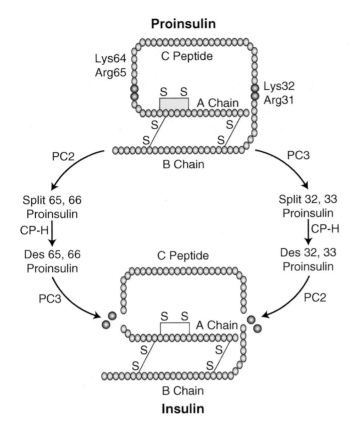

Proinsulin

Lys64
Arg65

C Peptide

Lys32
Arg31

A Chain

B Chain

PC2

PC3

Split 65, 66
Proinsulin

CP-H

Des 65, 66
Proinsulin

PC3

Split 32, 33
Proinsulin

CP-H

Des 32, 33
Proinsulin

PC2

C Peptide

A Chain

B Chain

Insulin

Figure 1-9. Proinsulin processing. Proinsulin is cleaved by endopeptidases contained in secretory granules, which act at the two dibasic sites, Arg31, Arg32 and Lys64, Arg65. PC2 also is known as type 2 proinsulin-processing endopeptidase, and PC3 is the type 1 endopeptidase. After cleavage by either PC2 or PC3, the dibasic amino acids are removed by the exopeptidase carboxypeptidase H (CP-H). Insulin and C peptide are usually released in equimolar amounts. Of the secreted insulin immunoreactivity, about 2–4% consists of proinsulin and proinsulin-related peptides. Because the clearance of these peptides in the circulation is considerably slower than that of insulin, they account for 10–40% of circulating insulin immunoreactivity. About one third of proinsulin-like immunoreactivity is accounted for by proinsulin, and most of the rest by des 32–33 split proinsulin, with only small amounts of des 65–66 split proinsulin being present. In type 2 diabetes, the ratio of proinsulin-like peptides to insulin is increased; in impaired glucose tolerance, this finding is less consistent. The increased proportion of secreted proinsulin-like peptides is thought to be caused by depletion of mature granules from the increased secretory demand by hyperglycemia, leading to the release of the incompletely processed contents of the available immature granules [13, 14] (adapted from Rhodes et al. [16]).

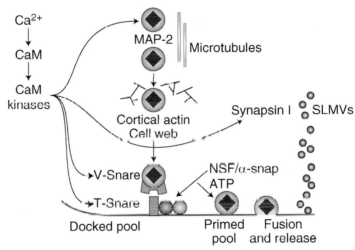

Ca^{2+}

CaM

CaM
kinases

MAP-2

Microtubules

Synapsin I

SLMVs

Cortical actin
Cell web

V-Snare

NSF/α-snap
ATP

T-Snare

Docked pool

Primed
pool

Fusion
and release

Figure 1-10. Distal steps of secretion. Insulin-containing secretory granules are associated with microtubules, and then move to the cell surface via further interactions with the microfilaments of the cortical actin web. Increased cytosolic calcium plays a key role in several distal steps. Initially, calcium binds to calmodulin (CaM), which can bind the CaM kinases. CaM kinase II has been localized to insulin secretory granules. These kinases can then phosphorylate proteins, such as microtubule-associated protein-2 (MAP-2) and synapsin I, which may be involved in the exocytosis of synaptic like microvesicles (SLMVs). They may also regulate the key proteins involved in the docking of granules, v-SNARES (synaptobrevin [VAMP] and cellubrevin) and t-SNARES (SNAP-25 and syntaxin). The docking complex binds to α-SNAP (soluble N-ethyl-maleimide-sensitive fusion protein [NSF] attachment protein) and NSF, the latter having ATPase activity, which probably allows the formation of fusion competent granules that are primed for release as the first phase of insulin secretion (adapted from Easom [17]).

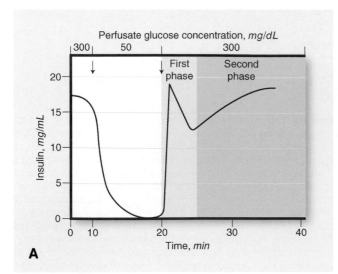

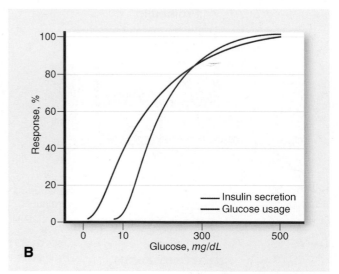

FIGURE 1-11. Glucose stimulation of insulin secretion. (**A**) Insulin secretion from the isolated perfused rat pancreas. At glucose concentrations at 50 mg/dL or below, insulin secretory rates are very low. Challenge with a high concentration of glucose provokes a biphasic pattern of insulin response [16]. (**B**) Comparative rates of insulin secretion and glucose utilization in isolated rat islets.

Glucose utilization was measured by the conversion of 5-tritiated glucose to tritiated H_2O [17]. The *curves* show the close relationship between the two except at glucose concentrations below 4 mmol. Similar relationships are found between insulin secretion and glucose oxidation as measured by conversion of labeled glucose to carbon dioxide (adapted from Leahy et al. [18]).

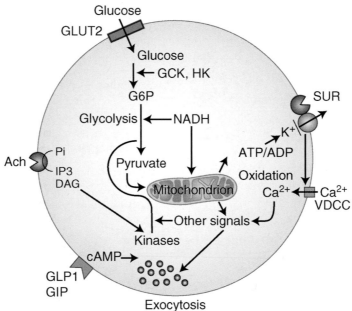

FIGURE 1-12. Mechanisms of β-cell secretion. Glucose enters the β cell through a facultative glucose transporter that allows rapid equilibration between extra- and intracellular glucose concentrations. Although glucose transporter 2 (GLUT2) is dominant in many species, glucose transporter 1 (GLUT1) appears to be more important in humans [19]. Glucose is phosphorylated mainly by glucokinase (GCK) rather than hexokinase (HK) [20]. Metabolism increases the ratio of adenosine triphosphate (ATP) to adenosine diphosphate (ADP) through oxidation via pyruvate and by nicotinamide adenine dinucleotide phosphate (NADP) that is brought by shuttles into mitochondria [21]. The increases in the ATP-to-ADP ratio inhibit the ATP-sensitive potassium channel, which leads to depolarization and opening of voltage-dependent calcium channels (VDCC), with a resultant major increase in cytosolic calcium that, in turn, triggers exocytosis. Glucose-stimulated insulin secretion is caused by two mechanisms: the triggering pathway, which is potassium channel ATP dependent, and the amplifying pathway, which is potassium channel ATP independent [22]. The molecular basis of the latter pathway is unknown. Cytosolic calcium levels can also be increased by the release of calcium from the endoplasmic reticulum. Insulin secretion can also be stimulated by agents, such as acetylcholine (Ach) that, via muscarinic receptors, work through lipid mediators, including inositol 1,4,5-triphosphate (IP3) and diacylglycerol (DAG). GLP-1 and gastric inhibitory peptide (GIP) are hormones released from the gut with meals that stimulate secretion via adenylate cyclase and cAMP [23]. Many other agents also influence insulin secretion.

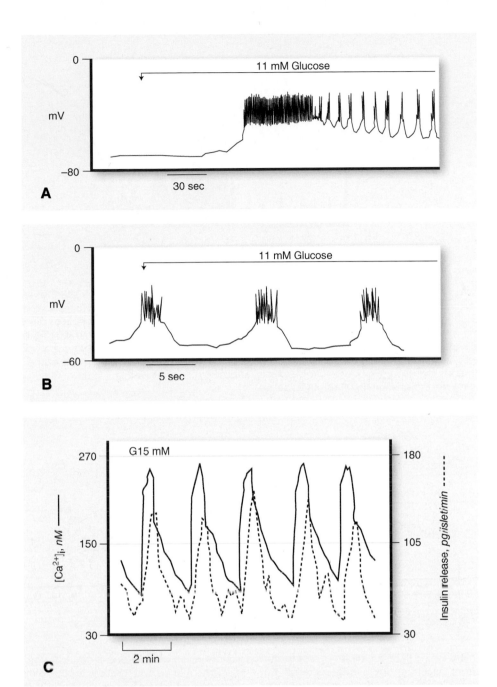

FIGURE 1-13. Glucose-induced electrical activity of the mouse β cell. (**A**) The electrical activity of a mouse β cell contained in an isolated islet induced by stimulation with 11-mM glucose. When the membrane depolarizes to about –50 mV, bursting occurs, which is periodic electrical activity. Note the biphasic pattern of electrical activity that may be related to the first phase of insulin secretion but is shorter in duration and unlikely to be the full explanation. (**B**) When depolarization reaches about –35 mV, action potentials, or spikes, occur, which are best seen in the expanded scale here. When glucose levels are very high (>22 mM), continuous spiking activity is observed. (**C**) Comparison of the oscillations of insulin release and calcium in a single pancreatic mouse islet during steady state stimulation with 15-mM glucose, suggesting a cause-and-effect relationship. Calcium was measured with fluorescence of fura-2 loaded into islets. Increased calcium spikes come mainly from the entrance of extracellular calcium through L-type voltage-gated calcium channels. The depolarization is mainly caused by the closure of adenosine triphosphate-regulated potassium channels [22] ((**A**, **B**) adapted from Mears and Atwater [24]; (**C**) adapted from Gilon et al. [25]).

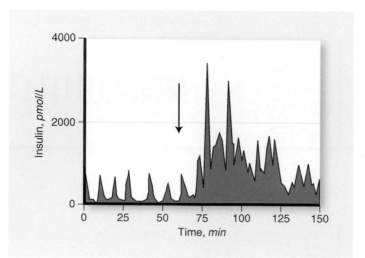

FIGURE 1-14. Pulsatile insulin secretion. Insulin is normally secreted in coordinated secretory bursts. In humans, pulses occur about every 10 min. In dogs, they occur somewhat more rapidly, at about 7-min intervals in a basal state. Although the variations in peripheral insulin levels are modest, marked variations can be found in the portal vein [26]. Basal pulsation is depicted during the 60-min period. After oral ingestion of glucose (*arrow*), which produces a glucose stimulus and an incretin effect, an increase in the amplitude of the bursts is seen, as well as an increase in frequency, with intervals decreasing from about 7 to 5 min. The mechanisms controlling the oscillations are uncertain. Metabolic oscillation of glycolysis must play a key role, but there may also be some kind of neural network that can coordinate communication between islets in different parts of the pancreas (adapted from Porksen et al. [26]).

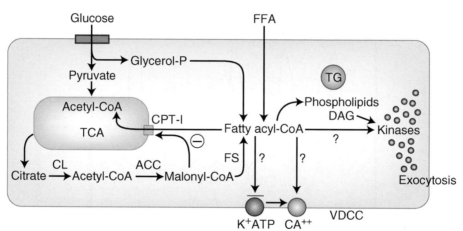

FIGURE 1-15. Fatty acid influence on β-cell function. Fat metabolism is likely to have important influences upon insulin secretion, but the mechanisms responsible for these effects are still not well understood. It appears that the modest elevations of free fatty acids (FFAs) of obesity contribute to the insulin resistance of that state. Depletion of circulating FFAs during prolonged fasting when glucose levels are low and β-cell lipid stores depleted results in impairment of insulin secretion. Excessive elevations of FFAs can have an inhibitory influence on insulin secretion when studied in vitro with isolated islets, but there is little evidence that the high FFA levels found with obesity and type 2 diabetes exert a deleterious effect upon β cells.

Some glucose-stimulated insulin secretion may be mediated not only by glucose metabolism, but also by fatty acid mediators. Thus, increases in glucose metabolism may produce increased cytosolic concentrations of citrate, which can be converted by citrate lyase (CL) to acetyl-coenzyme A (CoA), which can be turned into malonyl-CoA by acetyl-CoA carboxylase (ACC). Malonyl-CoA can inhibit carnitine palmitoyl-transferase I (CPT-I), which helps control the entrance of fatty acyl-CoA into the fatty acid oxidation pathways of mitochondria. By inhibiting the entrance of fatty acyl-CoA into mitochondria, fatty acid mediators that may influence insulin secretion may be generated in the cytoplasm.

Fatty acids that enter the β cell could be converted to fatty acid mediators, which can act upon ion channels, kinases, or through other mechanisms to stimulate the exocytosis of insulin. Some of the lipid mediators include the phospholipid IP3 and DAG, which can act via protein kinase C. Alternatively, fatty acids could be stored as triglycerides (TGs) for use during times of fuel deprivation. Under some circumstances, fatty acid oxidation may contribute to ATP formation and thus help close the ATP-sensitive potassium channel (K$^+$ ATP), resulting in depolarization and opening of the VDCC. *TCA* tricarboxylic acid cycle (adapted from McGarry and Dobbins [27] and Prentki and Corkey [28]).

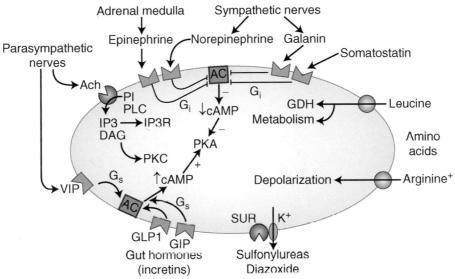

FIGURE 1-16. Effects on insulin secretion by the autonomic nervous system, gut hormones, amino acids, and drugs. The parasympathetic arm of the autonomic nervous system has a stimulatory influence upon insulin secretion exerted by acetylcholine acting mainly through phospholipase C (PLC) to generate inositol phosphate mediators and DAG. Parasympathetic stimulation also leads to the release of the peptide mediator vasoactive intestinal peptide (VIP), which enhances secretion via stimulatory G proteins (G$_s$) acting through adenylate cyclase (AC). The sympathetic nervous system inhibits insulin secretion, with epinephrine and norepinephrine having a negative effect on AC through inhibitory G proteins (G$_i$). The sympathetic peptide mediator galanin and somatostatin have inhibitory effects on insulin secretion through similar mechanisms. The gut hormones GLP-1 and GIP stimulate insulin secretion through cAMP, which acts on either protein kinase A (PKA) or cAMP-regulated guanine nucleotide exchange factors (cAMPGFFs, also known as Epac) [29]. Sulfonylureas stimulate insulin secretion by acting on the sulfonylurea receptor (SUR) to close the ATP-sensitive potassium channel, which causes depolarization. Diazoxide has an opposite effect, leading to hyperpolarization, which is inhibitory. Amino acids stimulate insulin secretion by several mechanisms. Arginine is positively charged, producing depolarization when transported into β cells, but this is not an important mechanism at physiologic concentrations of arginine. Leucine can influence insulin secretion by being oxidized via acetyl CoA or through a more complex metabolic effect mediated by glutamate dehydrogenase (GDH). *IP3R* inositol 3 phosphate receptor.

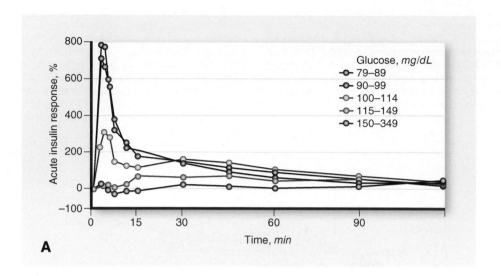

A

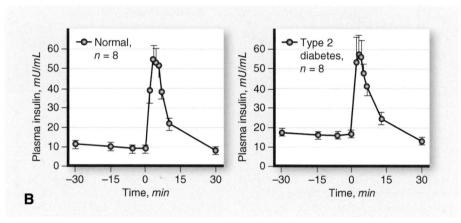

B

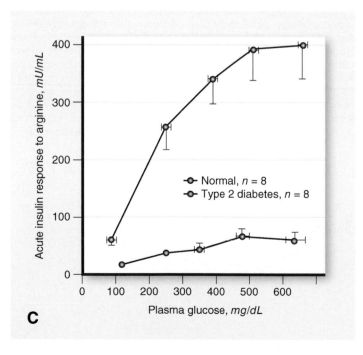

C

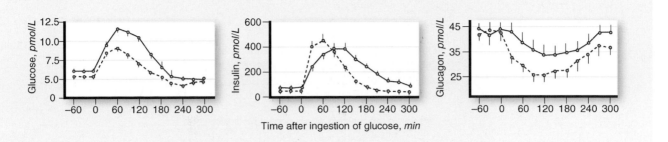

Time after ingestion of glucose, *min*

FIGURE 1-18. Insulin secretory profiles in the state of impaired glucose tolerance (IGT) (*solid line*) during an oral glucose tolerance test (OGTT). The insulin responses at 60 and 90 min may be higher than those found in control patients (*broken line*), which probably reflects the combined influence of higher glucose levels at these time points and insulin resistance. Importantly, the insulin responses at 30 min in patients with IGT are typically lower than normal, indicating the presence of a reduction in early impairment of gluca-

gon suppression, leading to an inefficient suppression of hepatic glucose output, which contributes to the higher glucose levels found in the latter stages of OGTT. The early insulin responses found after oral glucose are higher than those seen after an intravenous glucose challenge. This is thought to be attributable to the insulinotropic effects of the gut peptides GLP-1 and GIP, and possibly to some influence from activation of the parasympathetic nervous system (adapted from Mitrakou et al. [32]).

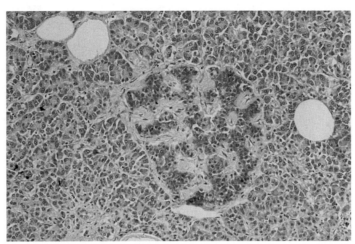

FIGURE 1-19. Amyloid deposits in islets in type 2 diabetes. In this photomicrograph of an islet, insulin containing cells are immunostained and amyloid deposition can be seen in the pericapillary space. The amyloid, found in a high proportion of the islets of people with type 2 diabetes, consists of β-pleated sheets of the islet amyloid polypeptide (IAPP, amylin), which consists of 37 amino acids. The sequence between positions 20 and 29 is important for the ability of this peptide to form amyloid. Production of IAPP is restricted to β cells and its content is only approximately 1%

that of insulin. Amyloid deposition adjacent to β cells is found in patients with diabetes and some insulinomas but neither in the normal state nor in obesity, with its insulin resistance and high rates of insulin secretion [33]. The mechanisms responsible for its deposition are not known. It is also unclear whether this amyloid formation contributes to the pathogenesis of type 2 diabetes, but it has been shown that human IAPP aggregates have a toxic effect on islet cells.

FIGURE 1-17. Insulin secretory characteristics in type 2 diabetes. (**A**) Loss of early insulin secretory response to an intravenous (IV) glucose challenge as fasting plasma glucose increases in subjects progressing from the normal state toward type 2 diabetes [30]. It should be noted that impaired insulin responses to glucose can even be seen before glucose levels increase to levels required for the diagnosis of impaired glucose tolerance (fasting glucose levels ≥110 mg/dL). (**B**) Preservation of acute insulin secretion in response to an IV pulse of arginine in type 2 diabetes [27]. The acute insulin responses to glucose were lost in these subjects. Insulin responses are also preserved for a variety of other secretagogues, including isoproterenol, sulfonylureas, and the gut hormone glucagon-like peptide 1. (**C**) Loss of glucose influence on

arginine-stimulated insulin secretion in type 2 diabetes [28]. The insulin secretory responses to a 350-mg/dL glucose concentration in subjects with type 2 diabetes were similar to the responses to an 80-mg/dL glucose concentration in control subjects. However, when the glucose concentrations in control subjects were increased with glucose infusions, the insulin responses far exceeded those of subjects with type 2 diabetes. Because individuals with type 2 diabetes have been found to have a β-cell mass approximately 50% of normal, the response in these subjects, which is only about 15% of control subjects, suggests that the secretory capacity for a given β-cell mass is severely impaired (adapted from Ward et al. [31]).

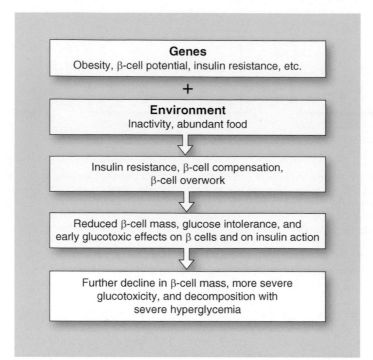

Figure 1-20. Pathogenesis of type 2 diabetes. This schema shows the various factors that contribute to the pathogenesis of type 2 diabetes. Genes are likely to determine how well β cells can function over a lifetime. For example, most of the gene defects of maturity-onset diabetes of youth ([MODY] 1, 3, and 4) and some mutations of mitochondrial DNA lead to diabetes, which often does not become manifest until middle age [34]. There are also patients with mutations of the K⁺-ATP channel with neonatal diabetes, who can be treated successfully with sulfonylureas [34]. The diabetes of MODY 2 is caused by mutations of the glucokinase gene, but rare mutations can be activating and cause hypoglycemia [35]. Genome-wide association studies have identified over 20 genes associated with type 2 diabetes [36]. Many of these have been linked to β cells, possibly influencing embryological development, susceptibility to death, and secretory capacity. Thus, genetic background seems likely to be an important determinant of loss of β-cell mass and deterioration of secretory function. Everything is made worse by the challenges of Western lifestyle, with its plentiful food and lack of exercise. After hyperglycemia develops, glucotoxicity can produce further impairment of β-cell function and worsen insulin resistance.

Stages of β-Cell Decompensation in Diabetes

Compensation for insulin resistance

β-cell hypertrophy

β-cell hyperplasia

Shift to the left of glucose dose–response curve

(Increased secretion per cell at a given glucose level)

"Normal" or increased glucose-induced insulin secretion

Decompensation: mild hyperglycemia

Loss of glucose-induced insulin secretion

Preservation of responses to nonglucose secretagogues

    (arginine and others)

Normal insulin stores

Early β-cell dedifferentiation

Decreased gene expression of GLUT2, glucokinase,

    mGPDH, pyruvate carboxylase, VDCC, SERCA3, IP3R-

    II, and transcription factors (PDX-1, HNFs, Nkx 6.1, pax-

    6, and MafA)

Increased gene expression of LDH, hexokinase 1, glucose-6-

    phosphatase, and the transcription factor c-myc

Decompensation: severe hyperglycemia

Loss of glucose-induced insulin secretion

Impairment of responses to nonglucose secretagogues

    (arginine and others)

Increased ratio of secreted proinsulin to insulin

Reduced insulin stores (degranulation)

More severe β-cell dedifferentiation

Decreased gene expression of insulin, IAPP, glucokinase, Kir

    6.2, SERCA2β, and transcription factor BETA 2

Increased gene expression of glucose-6-phosphatase, 12-

    lipoxygenase, fatty acid synthase, and the transcription

    factor C/EBPβ

FIGURE 1-21. Stages of β-cell decompensation in diabetes [37–40]. The changes in gene expression have been found in rodent models of diabetes and have not yet been confirmed in studies with human islets. However, the stages of decompensation found in humans and rodents are similar. *LDH* lactate dehydrogenase, *mGPDH* mitochondrial glycerol phosphate dehydrogenase, *SERCA* sarcoendoplasmic reticulum Ca^{2+}-ATPase.

β-Cell Glucotoxicity

Abnormal β-cell function in diabetes: β-cell function in diabetes is abnormal, whether in type 2 diabetes, early type 1 diabetes, or with an inadequate number of transplanted islets. A variety of secondary abnormalities has been identified, most notably loss of GSIS, thought to be caused by the exposure of β cells to the diabetic milieu

Definition problem: Descriptive terms include the following: glucotoxicity, exhaustion, excess demand, decreased reserve, fatigue, overwork, desensitization, stress, dysfunction, and others

Glucotoxicity

Loss of GSIS is tightly tied to even modest increases in glucose levels

Reduction of GSIS can be seen with a FPG of 100 mg/dL

Complete loss is usually when the FPG is greater than 115 mg/dL

Abnormal GSIS in a diabetic state can be seen in the absence of a FFA increase

Problems with the concept of lipotoxicity

Evidence supporting the concept that FFAs have deleterious effects on the diabetic state is not convincing

FFAs are important for β-cell function, at least as a permissive factor, and are important for maintaining insulin secretion during a prolonged fast

Increased FFAs of obesity are associated with high GSIS: a correlation between FFAs of mild or severe diabetes and the loss of GSIS is not well established. Synergy between FFAs and hyperglycemia is not yet understood. Toxic effects of FFA on islets appear to be an in vitro phenomenon

FIGURE 1-22. β-cell glucotoxicity [39]. *FPG* fasting plasma glucose, *GSIS* glucose-stimulated insulin secretion.

References

1. Habener JF, Kemp DM, Thomas MK: Minireview: transcriptional regulation in pancreatic development. *Endocrinology* 2005, 146:1025–1034.

2. Olbrot M, Rud J, Moss LG, Sharma A: Identification of beta-cell-specific insulin gene transcription factor RIPE3b1 as mammalian MafA. *Proc Natl Acad Sci U S A* 2002, 99:6737–6742.

3. Kawaguchi Y, Cooper B, Gannon M, *et al.*: The role of the transcriptional regulator Ptf1a in converting intestinal to pancreatic progenitors. *Nat Genet* 2002, 32:128–134.

4. Edlund H: Transcribing pancreas. Diabetes 1998, 47:1817–1823.

5. Bonner-Weir S, Orci L: New perspectives on the microvasculature of the islets of Langerhans in the rat. *Diabetes* 1982, 31:883–939.

6. Weir GC, Bonner-Weir S: Islets of Langerhans: the puzzle of intraislet interactions and their relevance to diabetes. *J Clin Invest* 1990, 85:983–987.

7. Bonner-Weir S, O'Brien TD: Islets in type 2 diabetes: in honor of Dr. Robert C. Turner. *Diabetes* 2008, 57:2899–2904.

8. Orci L: The insulin factory: a tour of the plant surroundings and a visit to the assembly line. *Diabetologia* 1985, 28:528–546.

9. Guest PC, Bailyes EM, Rutherford NG, Hutton JC: Insulin secretory granule biogenesis. *Biochem J* 1991, 274:73–78.

10. Inada A, Nienaber C, Katsuta H, *et al.*: Carbonic anhydrase II-positive pancreatic cells are progenitors for both endocrine and exocrine pancreas after birth. *Proc Natl Acad Sci U S A* 2008, 105:19915–19919.

11. Bonner-Weir S, Weir GC: New sources of pancreatic beta-cells. *Nat Biotechnol* 2005, 23:857–861.

12. Rankin MM, Kushner JA: Adaptive beta-cell proliferation is severely restricted with advanced age. *Diabetes* 2009, 58:1365–1372.

13. Finegood DT, Scaglia L, Bonner-Weir S: (Perspective) Dynamics of B-cell mass in the growing rat pancreas: estimation with a simple mathematical model. *Diabetes* 1995, 44:249–256

14. Sander M, German MS: The B cell transcription factors and development of the pancreas. *J Mol Med* 1997, 75:327–340.

15. Rhodes CJ, Alarcon C: What beta cell defect could lead to hyperproinsulinemia in NIDDM? *Diabetes* 1994, 43:511–517.

16. Rhodes CJ: Processing of the insulin molecule. In *Diabetes Mellitus: A Fundamental and Clinical Text*, edn 3. Edited by LeRoith D, Taylor SI, Olefsky JM. Philadelphia: Lippincott Williams & Wilkins; 2004:27–50.

17. Easom RA: CaM kinase II: a protein kinase with extraordinary talents germane to insulin exocytosis. *Diabetes* 1999, 48:675–684.

18. Leahy JL, Cooper HE, Deal DA, Weir GC: Chronic hyperglycemia is associated with impaired glucose influence on insulin secretion. A study in normal rats using chronic in vivo glucose infusions. *J Clin Invest* 1986, 77:908–915.

19. DeVos A, Heimberg H, Quartier E, *et al.*: Human and rat beta cells differ in glucose transporter but not in glucokinase gene expression. *J Clin Invest* 1995, 96:2489–2495.

20. Matschinsky FM: A lesson in metabolic regulation inspired by the glucokinase glucose sensor paradigm. *Diabetes* 1996, 45:223–241.

21. Eto K, Tsubamoto Y, Terauchi Y, *et al.*: Role of NADH shuttle system in glucose-induced activation of mitochondrial metabolism and insulin secretion. *Science* 1999, 283: 981–985.

22. Henquin JC: Triggering and amplifying pathways of regulation of insulin secretion by glucose. *Diabetes* 2000, 49:1751–1760.

23. Lovshin JA, Drucker DJ: Incretin-based therapies for type 2 diabetes mellitus. *Nat Rev Endocrinol* 2009, 5:262–269.

24. Mears D, Atwater I: Electrophysiology of the pancreatic b-cell. In *Diabetes Mellitus: A Fundamental and Clinical Text*, edn 2. Edited by LeRoith D, Taylor SI, Olefsky JM. Philadelphia: Lippincott Williams & Wilkins; 2000:47–60.

25. Gilon P, Shepherd RM, Henquin JC: Oscillations of secretion driven by oscillations of cytoplasmic Ca2 as evidenced in single pancreatic islets. *J Biol Chem* 1993, 268: 22265–22268.

26. Porksen N, Munn S, Steers J, *et al.*: Effects of glucose ingestion versus infusion on pulsatile insulin secretion. *Diabetes* 1996, 45:1317–1323.

27. McGarry JD, Dobbins RL: Fatty acids, lipotoxicity and insulin secretion. *Diabetolgia* 1999, 42:128–138.

28. Prentki M, Corkey BE: Are the beta-cell signaling molecules malonyl-CoA and cystolic long-chain acyl-CoA implicated in multiple tissue defects of obesity and NIDDM? *Diabetes* 1996, 45:273–283.

29. Holz GG, Chepurny OG, Schwede F: Epac-selective cAMP analogs: new tools with which to evaluate the signal transduction properties of cAMP-regulated guanine nucleotide exchange factors. *Cell Signal* 2008, 20:10–20.

30. Brunzell JD, Robertson RP, Lerner RL, *et al.*: Relationships between fasting plasma glucose levels and insulin secretion during intravenous glucose tolerance tests. *J Clin Endocrinol Metab* 1976, 42:222–229.

31. Ward WK, Bolgiano DC, McKnight B, *et al.*: Diminished B cell secretory capacity in patients with noninsulin-dependent diabetes mellitus. *J Clin Invest* 1984, 74:1318–1328.

32. Mitrakou A, Kelley D, Mokan M, *et al.*: Role of reduced suppression of glucose production and diminished early insulin release in impaired glucose tolerance. *N Engl J Med* 1992, 326:22–29.

33. Hull RL, Westermark GT, Westermark P, Kahn SE: Islet amyloid: a critical entity in the pathogenesis of type 2 diabetes. *J Clin Endocrinol Metab* 2004, 89:3629–3643.

34. Murphy R, Ellard S, Hattersley AT: Clinical implications of a molecular genetic classification of monogenic beta-cell diabetes. *Nat Clin Pract Endocrinol Metab* 2008, 4: 200–213.

35. Matschinsky FM: Assessing the potential of glucokinase activators in diabetes therapy. *Nat Rev Drug Discov* 2009, 8:399–416.

36. Florez JC: Newly identified loci highlight beta cell dysfunction as a key cause of type 2 diabetes: where are the insulin resistance genes? *Diabetologia* 2008, 51:1100–1110.

37. Jonas JC, Sharma A, Hasenkamp W, *et al.*: Chronic hyperglycemia triggers loss of pancreatic beta cell differentiation in an animal model of diabetes. *J Biol Chem* 1999, 274:14112–14121.

38. Weir GC, Laybutt DR, Kaneto H, *et al.*: Beta-cell adaptation and decompensation during the progression of diabetes. *Diabetes* 2001, 50(Suppl 1):S154–S159.

39. Weir GC, Bonner-Weir S: Five stages of evolving beta-cell dysfunction during progression to diabetes. *Diabetes* 2004, 53(Suppl 3):S16–S21.

40. Tabak AG, Jokela M, Akbaraly TN, *et al.*: Trajectories of glycaemia, insulin sensitivity, and insulin secretion before diagnosis of type 2 diabetes: an analysis from the Whitehall II study. *Lancet* 2009, 373:2215–2221.

2 Mechanisms of Insulin Action

Morris F. White

Insulin-like signaling integrates the storage and release of nutrients with somatic growth during development and in adult life. It is a feature of all metazoans, revealing a common mechanism used by animals to integrate metabolism and growth with environmental signals [1, 2]. Lower animals have a wide array of insulin-like peptides—seven in fruit flies and 38 in *Caenorhabditis elegans*—that bind apparently to a single insulin-like receptor tyrosine kinase to control metabolism, growth, reproduction, and longevity [3]. The human genome also encodes a superfamily of structurally related insulin-like peptides. Insulin, insulin-like growth factor 1 (IGF1), and insulin-like growth factor 2 (IGF2) activate a family of receptor tyrosine kinases [4]. However, the other structurally similar peptides, which are related to relaxin, are functionally distinct and activate G-protein-coupled receptors [5, 6].

Mammalian insulin is released from pancreatic islet β cells in response to circulating glucose concentrations. Endocrine IGF1 is secreted largely from hepatocytes stimulated by nutrients and growth hormone; however, IGF1 and IGF2 are also produced locally in many tissues and cells, including the central nervous system [7]. Although insulin has a major role in metabolic regulation, IGF1 and IGF2 can work coordinately with insulin to regulate nutrient homeostasis, insulin sensitivity, and pancreatic β-cell function [7, 8]. Owing to their mitogenic role, hyperactivated IGF1 and IGF2 signaling is thought to contribute to cancer [9]. By contrast, hyperactivated insulin signaling is rare, whereas insulin resistance is common and usually progresses to diabetes.

Diabetes is a complex disorder that arises from various causes, including impaired glucose sensing or insulin secretion (maturity onset diabetes of the young [MODY]), autoimmune-mediated β-cell destruction (type 1 diabetes), and insufficient β-cell insulin secretory capacity to compensate for peripheral insulin resistance (type 2 diabetes) [10]. MODY is caused by mutations in genes necessary for β-cell function, including hepatocyte nuclear factor 4α (HNF4α; MODY1), glucokinase (MODY2), hepatocyte nuclear factor 1α (HNF1α; MODY3), pancreatic and duodenal homeobox 1 (PDX1; MODY4), hepatocyte nuclear factor 1β (HNF1β; MODY 5), and neurogenic differentiation 1 (NEUROD1; MODY6) [11–13]. By comparison, the autoimmunity of type 1 diabetes is genetically complex and is marked by circulating autoantibodies against a variety of islet antigens. Insulin is thought to be one of the principle autoantigens in the pathogenesis of type 1 diabetes, but other antigens deserve attention [14, 15]. Because new β-cell formation occurs slowly while type 1 diabetes progresses, it might be possible to treat the disease by accelerating the rate of β-cell regeneration while attenuating the autoimmune response [16].

J.S. Skyler (ed.), *Atlas of Diabetes: Fourth Edition*,
DOI 10.1007/978-1-4614-1028-7_2, © Springer Science+Business Media, LLC 2012

Type 2 diabetes is the most prevalent form of diabetes. Although it typically manifests at middle age, type 2 diabetes in the developed world is becoming more common in children and adolescents [17]. Type 2 diabetes is an epidemic disorder that arises when insulin secretion from pancreatic β cells fails to maintain blood glucose levels in the normal range owing to peripheral insulin resistance. The underlying pathophysiology of diabetes is diverse, but pancreatic β-cell failure is the common theme [18, 19]. Physiologic stress – the response to trauma, inflammation, or excess nutrients – promotes type 2 diabetes by activating pathways that impair the post-receptor response to insulin in various tissues [20, 21]. Work during the past decade suggests that type 2 diabetes begins with skeletal muscle insulin resistance [22]; however, peripheral insulin resistance might not be enough, as transgenic mice lacking muscle insulin receptors or patients with muscle insulin resistance due to defective messenger RNA (mRNA) splicing do not ordinarily develop diabetes [23, 24]. Despite incontrovertible evidence of genetic links for type 2 diabetes, diabetes is not a mendelian disorder, so the genes responsible have been difficult to identify [25]. In a few informative cases, mutations in the insulin receptor or AKT2 explain severe forms of insulin resistance [26]. Generally, however, type 2 diabetes depends on multiple gene variants with modest effects on insulin action – including peroxisome proliferator-activated receptor-γ (PPARG), PPARG coactivator 1-α (PPARGC1A), inward rectifying K$^+$ channel Kir6.2 (KCNJ11), calpain 10 (CAPN10), transcription factor 7-like 2 (TCF7L2), adiponectin (ADIPOQ), adiponectin receptor 2 (ADIPOR2), HNF4α, uncoupling protein 2 (UCP2), sterol regulatory element-binding transcription factor 1 (SREBF1), and high plasma interleukin 6 concentrations [27]. Although the effect of each gene is small, these discoveries provide important clues to the pathogenesis of type 2 diabetes [28].

Regardless of the underlying etiology, dysregulated insulin signaling, exacerbated by chronic hyperglycemia and compensatory hyperinsulinemia, promotes a cohort of acute and chronic sequelae [29, 30]. Untreated diabetes progresses to ketoacidosis (most frequent in type 1 diabetes) or hyperglycemic osmotic stress (most frequent in type 2 diabetes), both of which are immediate causes of morbidity and mortality [31]. In the long term, diabetes is associated with chronic life-threatening complications, including reduced cardiovascular function and systemic oxidative stress that damages capillary endothelial cells in the retina, mesangial cells of the renal glomerulus, and the peripheral nerves [32, 33]. Diabetes is also associated with age-related degeneration in the central nervous system [34]. Humans beyond 85–90 years of age display less insulin resistance than expected – and centenarians are surprisingly insulin sensitive [35]. Most centenarians escape age-related diseases associated with insulin resistance, including cardiac disease, stroke, and diabetes [36, 37]. The best means to coordinate nutrient homeostasis and insulin signaling with strategies that consistently promote longevity across all metazoans remains to be established [38].

This chapter summarizes a broad array of work conducted in many laboratories over the past decade to understand the molecular basis of insulin signal transduction. Understanding the molecular basis of insulin action can reveal the pathophysiology of diabetes. It is firmly established that patients with type 2 diabetes have defects of insulin action; however, it remains difficult to understand which defects lead to functional insulin resistance in various tissues. Our approach to understanding diabetes has been based on the hypothesis that common signaling pathways might mediate both peripheral insulin action and pancreatic β-cell function. When elements of these pathways fail, owing to a combination of genetic variation and epigenetic challenge, diabetes occurs. Evidence supporting this hypothesis emerged from our work on the insulin receptor substrates (*IRS* proteins) [39]. Disruption of the gene for *Irs2* in mice causes diabetes because of peripheral insulin resistance and dysregulated hepatic gluconeogenesis exacerbated by pancreatic β-cell failure [40]. Although all the experimental evidence is not yet available, especially in humans, failure of signals transduced and regulated by the IRS1 and IRS2 branches of the insulin/IGF signaling pathway might be an important cause of diabetes. This chapter outlines how many of these signals are produced and integrated to control nutrient homeostasis throughout the organism.

Overview of Insulin Action

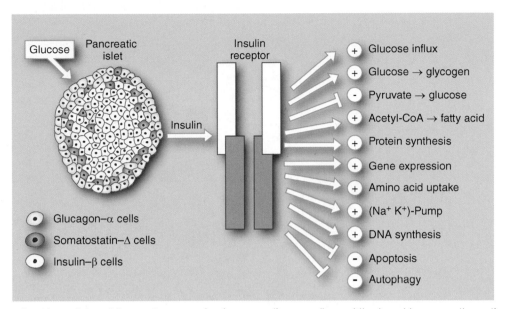

Figure 2-1. Insulin actions in peripheral tissues. Increases in circulating glucose levels lead to the secretion of insulin from pancreatic β cells found in the islets of Langerhans. Insulin action in the peripheral tissues requires the presence of the insulin receptor that initiates a cascade of intracellular protein phosphorylation upon hormone binding. The intracellular subunit of the receptor is a tyrosine-specific kinase that autophosphorylates and catalyzes the phosphorylation of several proteins that promote the multifaceted actions of insulin. Different tissues are known to respond differently to insulin. Although tissue sensitivity to the hormone correlates with the levels of insulin receptors expressed on the plasma membrane, it is clear the assembly of different components of the insulin signaling pathway also confers specificity of insulin action on target cells. Insulin stimulates glucose turnover, favoring its influx into cells, followed by oxidative metabolism to release energy or produce lipids or by nonoxidative metabolism to store glucose as glycogen. Insulin-stimulated glucose transport is observed only in skeletal muscle, adipose cells, and the heart because these tissues express the insulin-dependent glucose transporter GLUT4. In the liver and kidney, insulin inhibits gluconeogenesis because of the tissue-specific expression of hormone-sensitive metabolic enzymes involved in this process. Insulin simultaneously stimulates lipid synthesis while preventing lipolysis in adipose cells, skeletal muscle, and liver. By contrast, insulin promotes protein synthesis in almost all tissues by virtue of combined changes in gene transcription, mRNA translation, amino acid uptake, and autophagy. Autophagy, a major bulk proteolytic pathway, contributes to intracellular protein turnover and protein synthesis, which are subject to dynamic control by insulin. Insulin acts as a mitogen via increased DNA synthesis and prevention of programmed cell death or apoptosis. In addition, insulin stimulates ion transport across the plasma membrane of multiple tissues. There is increasing evidence for a direct role of insulin, acting through the insulin or IGF receptors, to regulate pancreatic β-cell growth, survival, and insulin release.

Insulin and Its Receptor

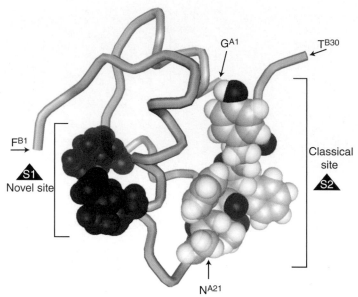

FIGURE 2-2. Insulin structure showing the position of critical amino acids that compose two asymmetric receptor-binding surfaces, designated S1 and S2. Insulin is synthesized as a single polypeptide called proinsulin, which is processed into the disulfide-linked A and B chains of mature insulin and the excised C-peptide. Referred to as the "classical site," S2 is defined by residues from the A and B chains, including Asn^{A21}, Gly^{B23}, Phe^{B24}, Phe^{B25}, and Tyr^{B26} [41]. Systematic analysis by site-directed mutagenesis reveals a distinct binding surface (S1) necessary for high-affinity receptor binding. S1 includes amino acid residues outside the classical site, especially Leu^{A13} and Leu^{B17}. Insulin-binding kinetics suggest that S1 binds to the receptor before S2 [41]. Human IGF1 and IGF2 display high-sequence similarity to both the A and B chains of insulin but retain the homologous connecting peptide; IGFs also have an extension at the C-terminus known as the D domain [42].

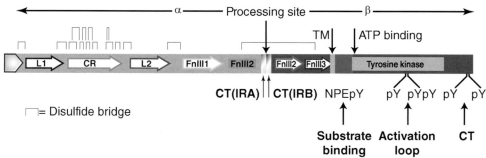

FIGURE 2-3. The human insulin proreceptor is the product of a single-copy gene located on the short arm of chromosome 19 (cytogenetic band 19p13). The proreceptor is synthesized as a single-chain polypeptide precursor with a classical signal sequence at the NH_2-terminus. The proreceptor undergoes posttranslational cleavage to form separate α- and β-subunits. The α-subunit is composed of well-defined motifs, including two leucine-rich motifs (L1 and L2) flanking a cysteine-rich (CR) region followed by three fibronectin III motifs (FnIII1, FnIII2, and FnIII3). FnIII2 is interrupted by a 120-amino acid insert domain containing the processing site that generates the α- and β-subunits of the mature receptor. The IRA/IRB splice site [CT(IRA)/(IRB)] is located immediately in front of the processing site. One hydrophobic transmembrane (TM) domain is located in the β-subunit, followed by the juxtamembrane region, which contains an NPXpY motif that binds to the phosphotyrosine-binding domain in the insulin receptor substrates. The intracellular tyrosine kinase is composed of an ATP-binding motif and kinase regulatory domains activated by tris-tyrosyl phosphorylation of the activation loop. The carboxyl terminal region also contains two tyrosine phosphorylation sites (CT).

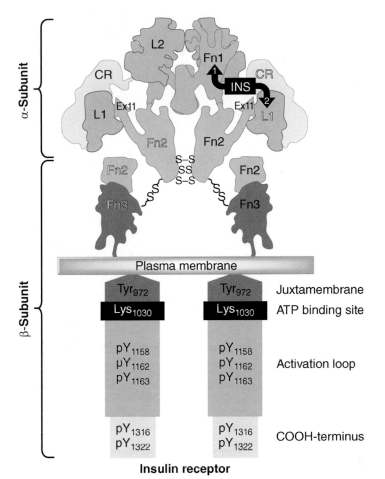

Insulin receptor

FIGURE 2-4. Insulin receptor membrane topology. During maturation, the receptor is glycosylated and acylated, and forms a heterotetramer composed of two α- and two β-subunits (α2-β2). The α-subunits are entirely extracellular and generate both high- and low-affinity binding sites for insulin (INS). Insulin binding apparently begins through interactions between the SI site on insulin and the FnIII1 (FN1) region in the α-subunit [41]. Sixteen amino acid residues at the COOH-terminus (CT) of FnIII2 (Fn2) interacts with the L1::CR region to create a composite insulin-binding site – L1::CR::CT – that interacts with the classical receptor-binding surface on insulin (S2). Although the α subunits are arranged symmetrically in the dimer, there is a sharp bend between the L2 and FnIII1 regions that juxtaposes the L1::CR::CT domain antiparallel to FnIII1 [43–45]. Owing to this arrangement of α subunits, insulin binds to the L1::CR::CT domain of one α-subunit and to FnIII1 of the adjacent α-subunit, creating the crosslink that activates the kinase. Because of space constraints, only one insulin molecule can bind with high affinity [43, 45, 46]. Inclusion of exon 11 (Ex11) in IRB lengthens the CT region by 12 amino acids, which modifies the L1::CR::CT domain to exclude IGF2 binding and increase the insulin-binding affinity. The β-subunits span the plasma membrane once and are linked to the α-subunit through disulfide bridges and noncovalent interactions. The insulin receptor is expressed as two variably spliced isoforms, resulting from exclusion (isoform IRA) or inclusion (isoform IRB) of 12 amino acids encoded by exon 11 of the insulin receptor gene. The intracellular portion of the β-subunit contains a tyrosine-specific protein kinase domain. Insulin binding to the receptor extracellular domain causes a conformational modification in the intracellular domain such that the receptor undergoes autophosphorylation and can bind ATP. Several tyrosine residues are phosphorylated – numbered according to the human IRB isoform including tyrosine 972, which promotes substrate binding and phosphorylation [47, 48]. Specific phosphorylation sites in the catalytic domain (tyrosine 1158, 1162, and 1163) are essential to promote the kinase activity of the receptor toward other protein substrates [49–51]. The role of the COOH-terminal phosphorylation sites (tyrosine 1328 and 1334) is more controversial, with certain studies suggesting that these sites play a role in stimulating the mitogenic activity of the receptor [52].

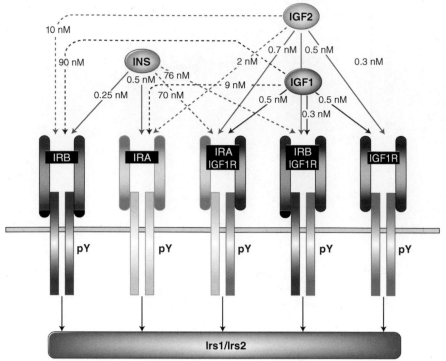

Figure 2-5. Specificity of homologous and heterologous insulin-like receptors. The insulin/IGF family consists of three peptide hormones: insulin (INS), IGF1, and IGF2. These factors bind as indicated to five distinct receptor isoforms that generate cytoplasmic signals: two insulin receptor isoforms, IRA and IRB; the IGF receptor, IGF1R; and two hybrid receptors, IRA::IGF1R and IRB::IGF1R. Insulin binds with high affinity (K_d<0.5 nM) to the homodimeric IRB, which predominates in the classical insulin target tissues – adult liver, muscle, and adipose tissues. IRB is selective for insulin as its K_d for IGF1 and IGF2 is at least 50- to 100-fold higher. Adult liver and adipose are purely insulin-responsive tissues as they express IRB but lack IGF1R [7]. By comparison, IRA predominates in fetal tissues, the adult central nervous system, and hematopoietic cells [53–56]. IRA binds insulin almost as well as IRB, but also binds IGF2 with moderate affinity. IGF1 and IGF2 bind with high affinity (K_d<1 nM) to the homodimeric IGF1R and to the hybrid receptors (IGF1R::IRA and IGF1R::IRB), whereas insulin barely binds to these proteins [57, 58]. Thus, under ordinary conditions, insulin never activates the IGF1R tyrosine kinase, whereas IGF1 and IGF2 can activate the insulin receptor tyrosine kinase, especially when it forms a hybrid with the IGF1R.

Regulation of Insulin Receptor Kinase Activity

Inactive

Active kinase

Active kinase + substrate

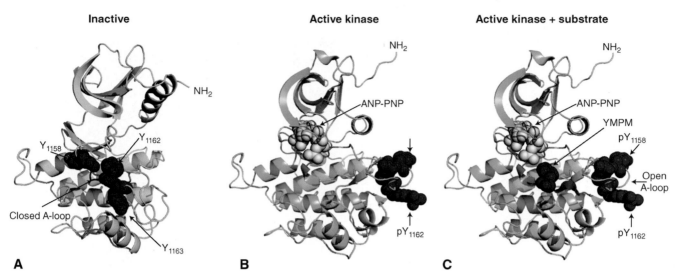

A

B

C

FIGURE 2-6. Insulin receptor autophosphorylation regulates kinase activity. The structure of the insulin receptor activation loop is shown as a series of space-filling diagrams on the surface of the insulin receptor kinase domain; the three activation loop tyrosine residues (Y_{1158}, Y_{1162}, and Y_{1163}) are shown with their side chains. In the inactive and unphosphorylated state (**A**), the activation loop blocks access by potential substrates. Following phosphorylation, the activation loop moves out of the active site (**B**), which allows substrates, such as YMXM peptides (also shown as a space-filling model) of the insulin receptor substrates or other recognized proteins to access the active site (**C**). ANP-PNP – adenylyl-imidodiphosphate.

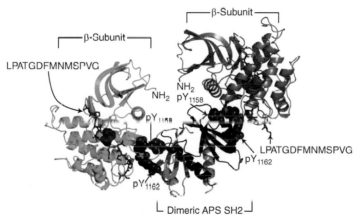

FIGURE 2-7. Structural representation of the binding of dimeric APS (adapter protein with a pleckstrin homology and Src homology 2 domain) SH2 domains to the phosphorylated A-loop of the insulin receptor. Regulation of the insulin receptor kinase is modulated by heterologous protein interactions with the phosphorylated A-loop. At least two phosphotyrosine residues in the A-loop are completely solvent exposed, creating sites that bind to various SH2 domain-containing proteins [59]. In this figure, structural analysis reveals how the dimerized SH2 domains of APS can bind to the A-loop of adjacent β-subunits to stabilize the active conformation [60–62]. Variable expression of these or other regulatory proteins – owing to genetic variation or physiologic or environmental challenge – should be expected to modulate insulin signaling and glucose tolerance [59].

Insulin Receptor Substrates

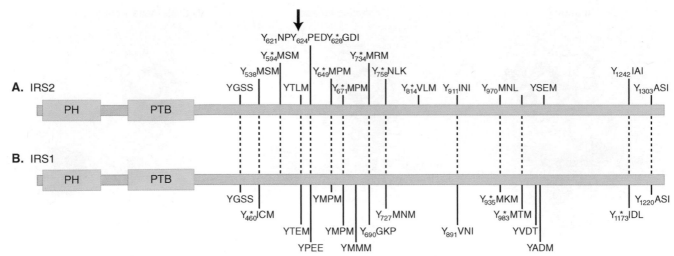

FIGURE 2-8. Insulin receptor substrate proteins IRS1 and IRS2. The figure compares IRS1 and IRS2 domains, including amino-terminal pleckstrin homology (PH) and phosphotyrosine binding (PTB) domains and numerous known or potential tyrosine phosphorylation sites. The amino acid sequences surrounding the tyrosine sites are shown, and motifs conserved between IRS1 and IRS2 are linked by *broken lines*. Phosphorylation sites revealed by MS/MS are indicated by *asterisks*. The kinase regulatory loop-binding (KRLB) motif in IRS2 is centered about Y_{624} (*arrow*); this motif is not conserved in IRS1. The structure of the activated insulin receptor β-subunit reveals a mechanism by which the activated insulin receptor kinase phosphorylates tyrosine residues within specific amino acid motifs, including the YMXM, YVNI, and YIDL motifs [61, 63–65]. These motifs are targeted as antiparallel β-strands to the COOH-terminal end of the open A-loop, allowing hydrophobic residues in the Y+1 and Y+3 positions to occupy two small hydrophobic pockets on the activated kinase. Tyrosine residues lying within amino acid motifs that contain charged or bulky side chains at the Y+1 and Y+3 positions fit poorly in this site, excluding them from phosphorylation [61].

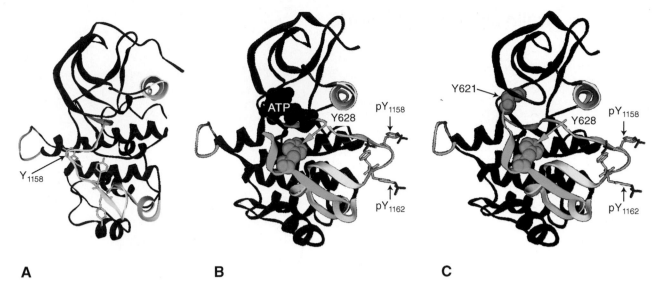

A **B** **C**

FIGURE 2-9. Unique interaction between the insulin receptor kinase domain and IRS2. In addition to the PH and PTB domains, IRS2 uses the KRLB motif located between amino acid residues 591 and 786 – especially Tyr_{624} and Tyr_{628} – to interact with the activated insulin receptor [66, 67]. This binding region in IRS2 was originally called the *kinase regulatory-loop binding domain* because tris-phosphorylation of the insulin receptor A-loop was required to observe its interaction [66]. Autophosphorylation moves the A-loop out of the catalytic site (**A**, **B**) so the functional part of the KRLB motif – residues 620 to 634 in murine IRS2 – can fit into the catalytic site (**B**, **C**) [68]. This interaction aligns Tyr_{628} of IRS2 for phosphorylation (space-filling model); however, it also inserts Tyr_{621} into the ATP binding pocket, which might attenuate signaling by blocking ATP access to the catalytic site (**C**). By contrast, this interaction might promote signaling by opening the catalytic site before insulin-stimulated tris-autophosphorylation. Interestingly, the KRLB motif does not bind to the IGF1R, which might explain some of the signaling differences between the insulin receptor and IGF1R, as well as the receptor hybrids [68].

Canonical Insulin Signaling Cascade

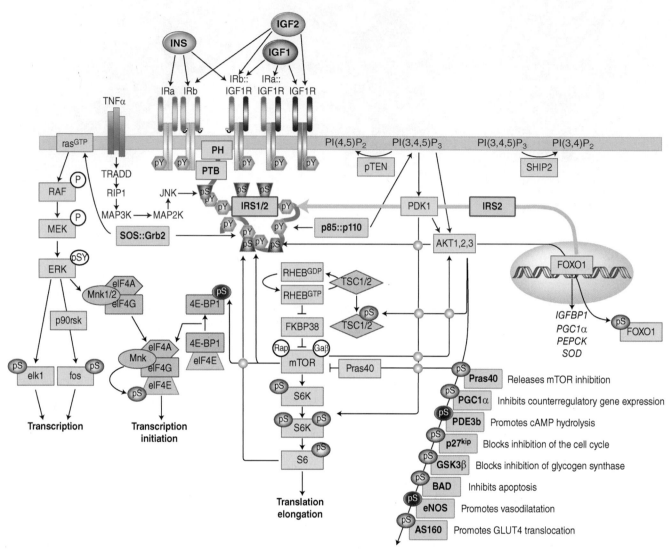

Figure 2-10. The canonical insulin-like signaling cascade. Insulin and IGF1 receptors, together with the hybrids, engage the two main branches of the signaling cascade through the IRS proteins: the phosphatidylinositol (PI) 3 kinase (PI3K)→3'-phospho-inositide-dependent protein kinase 1 (PDK1)→Akt cascade and the Grb2/SOS→ras kinase cascade. Activation of the receptors for insulin and IGF1 results in tyrosine phosphorylation of the IRS proteins, which bind PI3K (p85/p110) and Grb2/SOS. The Grb2/SOS complex promotes GDP/GTP exchange on p21ras, which activates the ras→RAF→MEK→ERK1/2 cascade [4]. Nuclear translocation of ERK1 and ERK2 is critical for both gene expression and DNA replication induced by growth factors. In the nucleus, ERK phosphorylates an array of targets, including transcription factors and the mitogen- and stress-activated protein kinases. Probably, the best-characterized transcription factor substrates of ERKs are ternary complex factors, including Ets-like gene 1 (Elk1). Ternary complex factors transcriptionally activate numerous mitogen-inducible genes, including FOS and JUN, which are indirectly phosphorylated

through ERK-activated p90rsk [69]. The ERK pathway is also linked to the regulation of protein synthesis through the activation of MAPK signal-interacting kinases 1 and 2 (MNK1/2). MNK also resides in the eukaryotic translation initiation factor 4F (eIF4F) complex, where it phosphorylates eIF4E at Ser209 [70, 71]. eIF4F mediates 40S ribosomal subunit binding to the 5'-end of capped mRNA. It contains several proteins, including eIF4E (the cap-binding subunit), eIF4A (an RNA-dependent ATPase/ATP-dependent RNA helicase), and eIF4G (a high molecular weight protein that acts as a scaffold for binding eIF4E and eIF4A) [72]. Phosphorylation of eIF4E increases the binding affinity for mRNA caps enhancing translation initiation. One of the best studied and most important signaling cascades activated by insulin involves the production of PI lipids by the class 1A PI3K. The PI3K is composed of a regulatory subunit that contains SH2 domains and a catalytic subunit that phosphorylates the D-3 position of the inositol ring [73]. The catalytic subunit is unstable and detected only in association with the regulatory subunit. The PI3K is inactive until both SH2 domains in the regulatory subunit

Figure 2-10. (continued) are occupied by phosphorylated YXXM motifs, especially those in the IRS proteins [74]. Inhibition of the PI3K by chemical or genetic means blocks almost all metabolic responses stimulated by insulin – including glucose influx, glycogen and lipid synthesis, and adipocyte differentiation – confirming that the PI3K is a critical node coordinating insulin action [75–77]. $PI(3,4,5)P_3$ produced by the activated PI3K recruits several Ser/Thr kinases to the plasma membrane, including PDK1 and AKT (v akt murine thymoma viral oncogene also known as PKB), where AKT is activated by PDK1-mediated phosphorylation of Thr_{308} in its activation loop. AKT has a central role in cell biology as it phosphorylates many proteins that control cell survival, growth, proliferation, angiogenesis, metabolism, and migration [78]. Phosphorylation of several AKT substrates is especially relevant to insulin-like signaling: GSK3αβ (blocks inhibition of glycogen synthesis), AS160 (promotes GLUT4 translocation), the BAD→BCL2 heterodimer (inhibits apoptosis), the FOXO transcription factors (regulates gene expression in liver and β cells and the hypothalamus), p21[CIP1] and p27[KIP1] (blocks cell cycle inhibition), endothelial nitric oxide synthase (eNOS; stimulates nitric oxide synthesis and vasodilatation), and PDE3b (hydrolyzes cAMP). AKT directly stimulates cell growth through the activation of mammalian target of rapamycin C1 (mTORC1) complex – composed of mTOR, mLST8, and raptor – which phosphorylates the S6 kinase and eIF4E-BP1 (also known as PHAS-1) to stimulate protein synthesis [78–80]. The regulatory mechanism involves several steps, beginning with AKT-mediated phosphorylation of at least five sites (Ser939, Ser981, Ser1130, Ser1132, and Thr1462) on TSC2 (tuberin), which in complex with TSC1 (hamartin) functions as a GTPase-activating protein for the small G protein RHEB (Ras homolog enriched in brain). RHEB accumulates in its GTP-bound form when TCS1/2 is inhibited, which activates mTORC1. In one possible regulatory mechanism, FKBP38 (FK506-binding protein 8) binds to mTORC1 and inhibits mTOR until RHEB-GTP binds to FKBP38 to disinhibit the kinase [81–83]. This complex regulatory cascade is augmented by other pathways, including the direct inhibition of the mTOR catalytic site by Pras40 (the proline-rich AKT substrate of 40 kD) until AKT-mediated phosphorylation of Pras40 reverses the inhibition [78]. The mTORC2 complex is also composed of mTOR and mLST8, but instead of raptor, this rapamycin-insensitive complex contains rictor and mSIN1 and is regulated mainly by nutrients. Downstream effectors of mTORC1 – p70[S6K] and 4E-BP1 – control protein synthesis and cell growth. The p70[S6K] occurs as two isoforms called p70[S6K1] and p70[S6K2]. Disruption of the *S6k1* gene in mice causes glucose intolerance owing to reduced size of pancreatic islet β cells; however, peripheral insulin action is enhanced, suggesting that p70[S6K1] contributes to feedback inhibition of insulin signaling [84]. p70[S6K1] is activated by multisite phosphorylation events from various kinase activities in response to insulin and other mitogens when amino acids are available [85, 86]. Nutrient sensitivity might arise when mTORC1 mediates the phosphorylation of a hydrophobic motif needed for interaction of p70[s6k] with PDK1. The mRNA cap-binding protein eIF4E is inactive during association with 4E-BP1. Insulin activates eIF4E by stimulating mTORC1-mediated phosphorylation of 4E-BP1. Phosphorylated 4E-BP1 dissociates to facilitate the interaction between eIF4E and eIF4G, the scaffold protein for the eIF4F complex [87]. The phosphorylation of 4E-BP1 has an important systemic role in insulin action, as deletion of the 4E-BP1 gene dramatically decreases white adipose tissue depots while increasing insulin sensitivity [88].

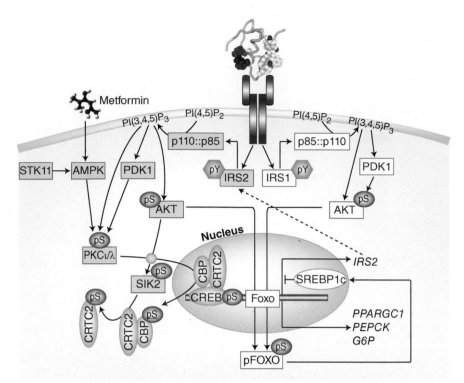

FIGURE 2-11. Partial scheme of the insulin/IRS signaling cascade in hepatocytes and the role of metformin. In the absence of insulin, nuclear FOXO strongly stimulates the expression of PPARGC1a (also known as PGC1alpha) and the gluconeogenic genes. However, the CREB:CBP:CRTC2 complex (CREB, cAMP-responsive element-binding protein; CBP, CREB-binding protein; CRTC2, CREB-regulated transcription coactivator 2) also needs to be inactivated by atypical protein kinase C (PKC)-mediated phosphorylation of CBP. During insulin stimulation, CBP phosphorylation might occur exclusively through the IRS2 branch of the pathway [89]; how this signaling specificity arises is unknown. Regardless, this specificity is probably very important because IRS2 expression is ordinarily augmented during starvation by CREB:CBP:CRTC2, FOXO1, and transcription factor E3 (TFE3), which should increase the basal insulin signaling and attenuate fasting gluconeogenesis. Moreover, this mechanism can prepare hepatocytes to shut down postprandial gluconeogenesis quickly and with minimal insulin stimulation. However, nutrient excess and compensatory hyperinsulinemia preferentially suppress hepatic IRS2 expression, at least in part, by sustained IRS1 signaling that increases the expression of SREBP1c – an important transcriptional regulator of lipid synthesis that also blocks IRS2 expression [90]. This mechanism is expected to prevent insulin-stimulated CBP phosphorylation, whereas the ensuing compensatory hyperinsulinemia stimulates the IRS1 branch of the insulin signaling cascade to sustain SREBP1c expression and promote triglyceride synthesis. Metformin might be an important insulin sensitizer because it activates atypical PKCι/λ through a different mechanism, which circumvents hepatic insulin resistance to phosphorylate CBP and inactivate the CREB:CBP:CRTC2 transcription complex, especially during hepatic insulin resistance associated with obesity and type 2 diabetes. Elements of the IRS2 branch of the insulin signaling cascade are shaded, whereas elements of the IRS1 branch of the cascade are not shaded; underscored phosphorylation sites (pS) indicate inhibitory steps.

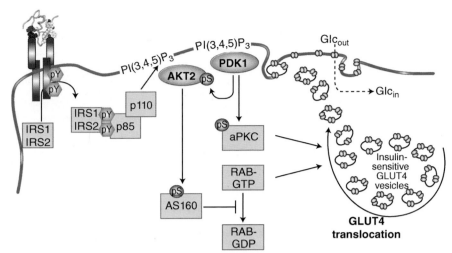

Figure 2-12. Glucose transport is the prototype insulin response. Insulin stimulates glucose influx into adipose and cardiac muscle as well as into skeletal muscle. GLUT4 is the principle insulin-responsive glucose transporter. It is glycosylated in its first exofacial loop, and it contains a phosphorylation site (Ser_{488}) and a di-leucine motif in its COOH-terminus that plays a role in endocytosis [91]. Upon synthesis, GLUT4 is unavailable to transport glucose across the plasma membrane, as it enters a continuously recycling pathway that concentrates it in intracellular membranes of unstimulated cells [92]. During insulin stimulation, GLUT4-containing vesicles move from their intracellular sequestration compartment to the cell surface through targeted exocytosis. Simultaneously, GLUT4 endocytosis is repressed, leading to an overall increase in glucose uptake [93]. It is not clear whether the effect of insulin in stimulating glucose uptake in muscle and fat can be accounted for entirely by translocation, as other factors that increase transporter activity are not ruled out. The PI3K→AKT cascade plays a key role in insulin-stimulated GLUT4 translocation to the plasma membrane [94–96]. How AKT promotes GLUT4 redistribution to the plasma membrane is an important area of investigation. Important progress came from the identification of a 160-kD AKT substrate (AS160) [97]. AS160 and the related TBC1D1 are RabGAPs (Rab GTPase-activating proteins) implicated in regulating the trafficking of GLUT4 storage vesicles to the cell surface (reviewed by Sakamoto and Holman [98]). Because Rab proteins regulate many steps in vesicle transport, AS160 might link the insulin signaling cascade to the redistribution and fusion of GLUT4-containing vesicles to the plasma membrane. AS160 contains six AKT phosphorylation sites, which can regulate the activity of the Rab GTPase-activating (GAP) domain. AKT-mediated phosphorylation might alter the subcellular location of AS160 or inactivate the Rab-GAP domain, which is needed to keep GLUT4 in the intracellular compartment [99]. Mutation of four AKT phosphorylation sites converts AS160 into a dominant negative protein that uncouples GLUT4 translocation from insulin signaling in 3T3L1 adipocytes, in L6 muscle cells, and even in mouse skeletal muscle ex vivo [98]. However, the partial nature of this uncoupling suggests that the homologous TBC1D1 protein – or another mechanism – might have an important complementary role in regulating vesicle trafficking in response to insulin. The exact target Rabs of AS160 are poorly established, but several possibilities have been proposed [100]. The atypical PKC isoforms – PKCζ and PKCλ – are also implicated in the regulation of GLUT4 translocation in adipose tissue and muscle [101–103]. PKCζ and PKCλ are downstream of the PI3K→PDK1 cascade, but independent of AKT.

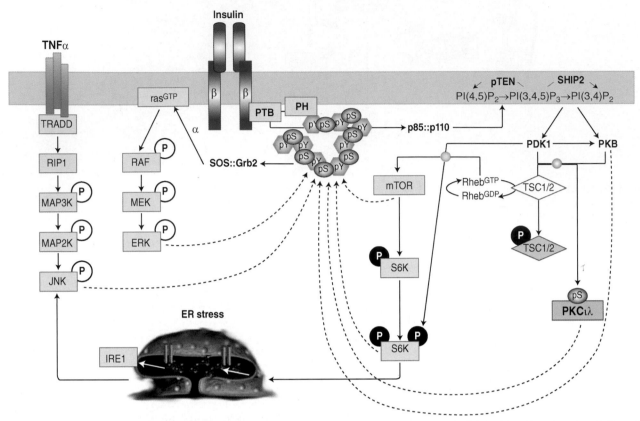

Figure 2-13. Heterologous and feedback inhibition of insulin signaling mediated by serine phosphorylation of IRS1. Heterologous signaling cascades initiated by proinflammatory cytokines or metabolic excess – including tumor necrosis factor-α (TNFα), endothelin-1, angiotensin II, excess nutrients (free fatty acids, amino acids, and glucose), and endoplasmic reticulum (ER) stress – can promote Ser/Thr phosphorylation of IRS1 and cause insulin resistance [104, 105]. Many biochemical and genetic experiments show that individual Ser/Thr phosphorylation sites throughout the structure of IRS1 can reduce its insulin-stimulated tyrosine phosphorylation by up to 50% [106]. This level of inhibition is sufficient to cause glucose intolerance that progresses to diabetes, especially if pancreatic β cells fail to provide adequate compensatory hyperinsulinemia [107]. Moreover, hyperinsulinemia itself may exacerbate Ser/Thr phosphorylation of IRS1 through the PI3K→Akt, atypical PKCι/λ, or mTORC1→p70^{s6k} cascade.

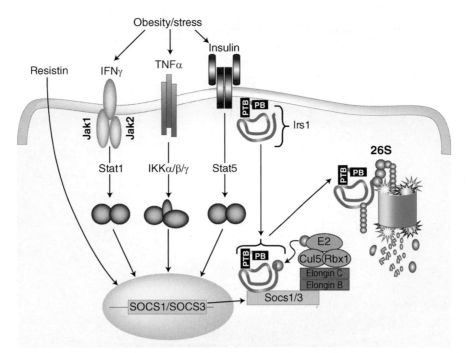

Figure 2-14. Degradation of IRS1 and IRS2. Significant regulation of IRS1 and IRS2 is thought to occur by ubiquitin-mediated degradation [108, 109]. Suppressor of cytokine signaling (SOCS) proteins participate in crosstalk with insulin-like signaling and contribute to insulin resistance. SOCS1 and SOCS3 can bind to distinct domains of the insulin receptor, which influences insulin receptor-mediated phosphorylation of IRS1 and IRS2 [110]. Overexpression of SOCS1 in the liver preferentially inhibits IRS2 tyrosine phosphorylation, whereas SOCS3 overexpression decreases tyrosine phosphorylation of both IRS1 and IRS2 [110, 111]. Resistin can increase SOCS3 in H4IIE hepatocytes, which might explain the inhibitory effect of resistin on insulin action [111, 112]. SOCS1 and SOCS3 also target IRS1 – and possibly IRS2 – for ubiquitinylation by the elongin BC-containing E3 ubiquitin–ligase complex [113]. Overexpression of SOCS1/3 in the liver causes insulin resistance and upregulation of key regulators involved in fatty acid synthesis and SREBP1c, whereas inhibition of SOCS1/3 by antisense oligonucleotides in obese and diabetic mice improves insulin sensitivity and normalizes SREBP1c expression [114]. In this manner, SOCS1 and SOCS3 can link infection, inflammation, or metabolic stress to insulin resistance and glucose intolerance. Interestingly, the core protein of hepatitis C virus upregulates SOCS3, which might explain why infected patients have increased fasting insulin levels compared with patients with other chronic liver diseases [115].

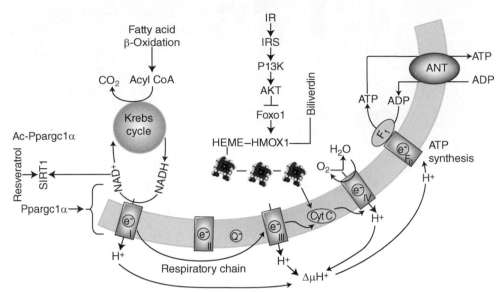

FIGURE 2-15. Putative mechanism to explain the paradoxic accumulation of free fatty acids and triglycerides in the insulin-resistant hepatocytes. Hepatic insulin resistance leads to uncontrolled gluconeogenesis, which contributes to hyperglycemia; however, β-oxidation of free fatty acids is paradoxically inhibited [116, 117]. This figure outlines a possible mechanism whereby failure of the insulin signaling cascade leads to constitutive activation of nuclear Foxo1, which promotes the expression of many genes, including heme oxygenase 1 (HMOX1). HMOX1 converts heme into biliverdin, which compromises the stability and function of essential cytochromes needed for the function and stability of complexes III and IV of the mitochon-drial electron transport chain. Reduced electron transport diminishes the capacity to oxidize NADH produced during the oxidation of glucose or fatty acids. The diminished hepatic oxidative capacity is associated with the accumulation of free fatty acids and triglycerides [118]. Moreover, the reducing environment leads to the inhibition of NAD^+-dependent deacetylase (SIRT1), resulting in the accumulation of acetylated proteins, such as the transcriptional cofactor PPARGC1α. Because acetylated PPARGC1a fails to promote the gene expression needed to increase compensatory mitochondrial biogenesis and function, the oxidative capacity of persistently insulin-resistant hepatocytes is impaired.

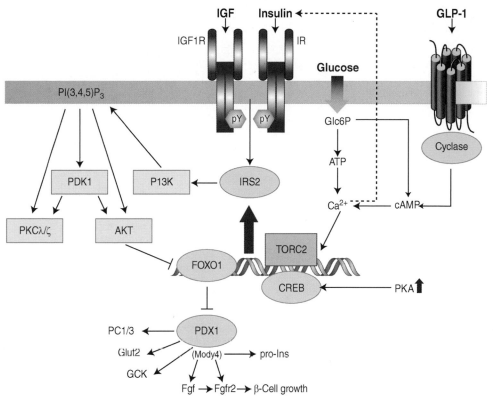

FIGURE 2-16. The integrative role of IRS2 in pancreatic β cells. The diagram shows the relation between the MODY genes, especially PDX1, and the IRS2 branch of the insulin signaling pathway [119]. Drugs that promote IRS2 signaling are expected to promote the phosphorylation of BAD and FOXO1, which enhance β-cell growth, function, and survival. Many factors are required for proper β cell function, including the homeodomain transcription factor PDX1. PDX1 regulates downstream genes needed for β-cell growth and function, and mutations in PDX1 cause autosomal forms of early-onset diabetes in people (MODY) [120, 121]. PDX1 is reduced in Irs2−/− islets, and PDX1 haploinsufficiency further diminishes the function of β cells lacking IRS2 [119]. By comparison, transgenic PDX1 expressed in Irs2−/− mice restores β-cell function and normalizes glucose tolerance, which links the insulin-like signaling cascade to the network of β-cell transcription factors [119, 122]. Transgenic upregulation of IRS2 or suppression of FOXO1 increases PDX1 concentrations in Irs2−/− mice, supporting the hypothesis that PDX1 is modulated by the IRS2→FOXO1 cascade in β cells [122, 123]. Haploinsufficiency for PTEN also prevents β-cell failure in Irs2−/− mice, owing at least in part to the simulation of the PI3K→PKB/AKT cascade that inhibits FOXO1 [124]. Glucose and glucagon-like peptide 1 (GLP1) have strong effects on β-cell growth, which depends on the IRS2 signaling cascade. In β cells, IRS2 is strongly upregulated by cAMP and Ca2+ agonists – including glucose and GLP1 – which activate CREB and CREB-regulated transcription coactivator 2 (TORC2) [125, 126]. Although many cAMP-mediated pathways oppose the action of insulin, the upregulation of IRS2 by glucose and GLP1 reveals an unexpected intersection of these important signals. Thus, hyperglycemia resulting from the daily consumption of high-caloric food promotes β-cell growth by increasing IRS2 expression [126]. Mice expressing low concentrations of glucokinase in β cells display impaired intracellular calcium responses to glucose, which suppress the phosphorylation of CREB that induces IRS2 expression. Similarly, GLP1 couples into this mechanism by directly increasing the concentration of cAMP in β cells [125]. Thus, glucose and GLP1 have no effect on β-cell growth in Irs2−/− mice [127]. Together, these results suggest that the IRS2 branch of the insulin-like signaling cascade – rather than IRS1 or the upstream receptor kinases – is the "ordinary gatekeeper" for β-cell plasticity and function.

Summary and Perspectives

The investigation of the insulin signaling cascade has revealed a broad physiologic role that extends far beyond the classical insulin target tissues – liver, muscle, and fat. It is now clear that insulin-like signaling plays a major role in pancreatic β cells and in the central nervous system. Peripheral insulin resistance is ordinarily opposed by increased insulin secretion from pancreatic β cells; however, compensatory hyperinsulinemia might have negative consequences in the brain that shorten lifespan. The tools now available to probe the insulin-like signaling cascades in healthy and diabetic tissues provide a rational platform to develop new strategies to treat insulin resistance and prevent its progression to type 2 diabetes and neurodegeneration. Understanding how the IRS proteins integrate, the conflicting signals generated during insulin and cytokine action might be a valuable starting point. Whether better management of inflammatory responses can attenuate insulin resistance and diminish its consequences is an important area of investigation. Future work must better resolve the network of insulin responses that are generated in various tissues because too much insulin action might also shorten our lives.

References

1. Conlon JM: Evolution of the insulin molecule: insights into structure-activity and phylogenetic relationships. *Peptides* 2001, 22:1183–1193.

2. Geminard C, Arquier N, Layalle S, *et al.*: Control of metabolism and growth through insulin-like peptides in drosophila. *Diabetes* 2006, 55(suppl 2):S5–S8.

3. Kenyon C: The plasticity of aging: insights from long-lived mutants. *Cell* 2005, 120:449–460.

4. Schlessinger J: Cell signaling by receptor tyrosine kinases. Cell 2000, 103:211–225.

5. Sherwood OD: Relaxin's physiological roles and other diverse actions. *Endocr Rev* 2004, 25:205–234.

6. Wilkinson TN, Speed TP, Tregear GW, Bathgate RA: Evolution of the relaxin-like peptide family. *BMC Evol Biol* 2005, 5:14.

7. Clemmons DR: Involvement of insulin-like growth factor-I in the control of glucose homeostasis. *Curr Opin Pharmacol* 2006, 6:620–625.

8. Dunger DB, Ong KK, Sandhu MS: Serum insulin-like growth factor-I levels and potential risk of type 2 diabetes. *Horm Res* 2003, 60(suppl 3):131–135.

9. Samani AA, Yakar S, LeRoith D, Brodt P: The role of the IGF system in cancer growth and metastasis: overview and recent insights. *Endocr Rev* 2007, 28:20–47.

10. Stumvoll M, Goldstein BJ, van Haeften TW: Type 2 diabetes: principles of pathogenesis and therapy. *Lancet* 2005, 365:1333–1346.

11. Fajans SS, Bell GI, Polonsky KS: Molecular mechanisms and clinical pathophysiology of maturity-onset diabetes of the young. *N Engl J Med* 2001, 345:971–980.

12. Frayling TM, Evans JC, Bulman MP, *et al.*: beta-cell genes and diabetes: molecular and clinical characterization of mutations in transcription factors. *Diabetes* 2001, 50(suppl 1):S94–S100.

13. Froguel P, Velho G: Molecular genetics of maturity-onset diabetes of the young. *Trends Endocrinol Metab* 1999, 10:142–146.

14. Nakayama M, Abiru N, Moriyama H, et al.: Prime role for an insulin epitope in the development of type 1 diabetes in NOD mice. *Nature* 2005, 435:220–223.

15. Zhang L, Nakayama M, Eisenbarth GS: Insulin as an autoantigen in NOD/human diabetes. *Curr Opin Immunol* 2008, 20:111–118.

16. Meier JJ, Bhushan A, Butler AE, *et al.*: Sustained beta cell apoptosis in patients with long-standing type 1 diabetes: indirect evidence for islet regeneration? *Diabetologia* 2005, 48:2221–2228.

17. Monzavi R, Dreimane D, Geffner ME, *et al.*: Improvement in risk factors for metabolic syndrome and insulin resistance in overweight youth who are treated with lifestyle intervention. *Pediatrics* 2006, 117:e1111–e1118.

18. Halban PA, Kahn SE, Lernmark A, Rhodes CJ: Gene and cell-replacement therapy in the treatment of type 1 diabetes: how high must the standards be set? *Diabetes* 2001, 50:2181–2191.

19. DeFronzo RA: Pathogenesis of type 2 diabetes: metabolic and molecular implications for identifying diabetes genes. *Diabetes Rev* 1997, 5:177–269.

20. Hotamisligil GS: Inflammation and metabolic disorders. *Nature* 2006, 444:860–867.

21. Petersen KF, Dufour S, Savage DB, *et al.*: The role of skeletal muscle insulin resistance in the pathogenesis of the metabolic syndrome. *Proc Natl Acad Sci U S A* 2007, 104:12587–12594.

22. Cline GW, Rothman DL, Magnusson I, *et al.*: ^{13}C-nuclear magnetic resonance spectroscopy studies of hepatic glucose metabolism in normal subjects and subjects with insulin-dependent diabetes mellitus. *J Clin Invest* 1994, 94:2369–2376.

23. Bruning JC, Michael MD, Winnay JN, *et al.*: A muscle-specific insulin receptor knockout exhibits features of the metabolic syndrome of NIDDM without altering glucose tolerance. *Mol Cell* 1998, 2:559–569.

24. Savkur RS, Philips AV, Cooper TA: Aberrant regulation of insulin receptor alternative splicing is associated with insulin resistance in myotonic dystrophy. *Nat Genet* 2001, 29:40–47.

25. Burghes AH, Vaessin HE, de La Chapelle A: Genetics. The land between Mendelian and multifactorial inheritance. *Science* 2001, 293:2213–2214.

26. Semple RK, Sleigh A, Murgatroyd PR, *et al.*: Postreceptor insulin resistance contributes to human dyslipidemia and hepatic steatosis. *J Clin Invest* 2009, 119:315–322.

27. Vaxillaire M, Veslot J, Dina C, *et al.*: Impact of common type 2 diabetes risk polymorphisms in the DESIR prospective study. *Diabetes* 2008, 57:244–254.

28. Nandi A, Kitamura T, Kahn CR, Accili D: Mouse models of insulin resistance. *Physiol Rev* 2004, 84:623–647.

29. DeFronzo RA (2004) Pathogenesis of type 2 diabetes mellitus. *Med Clin North Am*, 88:787–835, ix.

30. Reaven GM: Pathophysiology of insulin resistance in human disease. *Physiol Rev* 1995, 75:473–486.

31. Kitabchi AE, Nyenwe EA: Hyperglycemic crises in diabetes mellitus: diabetic ketoacidosis and hyperglycemic hyperosmolar state. *Endocrinol Metab Clin North Am* 2006, 35:725–751, viii.

32. Brownlee M: The pathobiology of diabetic complications: a unifying mechanism. *Diabetes* 2005, 54:1615–1625.

33. Stentz FB, Umpierrez GE, Cuervo R, Kitabchi AE: Proinflammatory cytokines, markers of cardiovascular risks, oxidative stress, and lipid peroxidation in patients with hyperglycemic crises. *Diabetes* 2004, 53:2079–2086.

34. Cole GM, Frautschy SA: The role of insulin and neurotrophic factor signaling in brain aging and Alzheimer's Disease. *Exp Gerontol* 2007, 42:10–21.

35. Barbieri M, Rizzo MR, Manzella D, *et al.*: Glucose regulation and oxidative stress in healthy centenarians. *Exp Gerontol* 2003, 38:137–143.

36. Andersen SL, Terry DF, Wilcox MA, *et al.*: Cancer in the oldest old. *Mech Ageing Dev* 2005, 126:263–267.

37. Terry DF, Wilcox MA, McCormick MA, *et al.*: Lower all-cause, cardiovascular, and cancer mortality in centenarians' offspring. *J Am Geriatr Soc* 2004, 52:2074–2076.

38. Perls TT: The different paths to 100. *Am J Clin Nutr* 2006, 83:484S–487S.

39. White MF: Regulating insulin signaling and beta-cell function through IRS proteins. *Can J Physiol Pharmacol* 2006, 84:725–737.

40. Withers DJ, Gutierrez JS, Towery H, *et al.*: Disruption of IRS-2 causes type 2 diabetes in mice. *Nature* 1998, 391:900–904.

41. De Meyts P: Insulin and its receptor: structure, function and evolution. *Bio Essays* 2004, 26:1351–1362.

42. Brzozowski AM, Dodson EJ, Dodson GG, *et al.*: Structural origins of the functional divergence of human insulin-like growth factor-I and insulin. *Biochemistry* 2002, 41:9389–9397.

43. Lawrence MC, McKern NM, Ward CW: Insulin receptor structure and its implications for the IGF-1 receptor. *Curr Opin Struct Biol* 2007, 17:699–705.

44. Ward CW, Lawrence MC, Streltsov VA, *et al.*: The insulin and EGF receptor structures: new insights into ligand-induced receptor activation. *Trends Biochem Sci* 2007, 32:129–137.

45. McKern NM, Lawrence MC, Streltsov VA, *et al.*: Structure of the insulin receptor ectodomain reveals a folded-over conformation. *Nature* 2006, 443:218–221.

46. Kiselyov VV, Versteyhe S, Gauguin L, De Meyts P: Harmonic oscillator model of the insulin and IGF1 receptors' allosteric binding and activation. *Mol Syst Biol* 2009, 5:243.

47. White MF, Livingston JN, Backer JM, *et al.*: Mutation of the insulin receptor at tyrosine 960 inhibits signal transmission but does not affect its tyrosine kinase activity. *Cell* 1988, 54:641–649.

48. Eck MJ, Dhe-Paganon S, Trub T, *et al.*: Structure of the IRS-1 PTB domain bound to the juxtamembrane region of the insulin receptor. *Cell* 1996, 85:695–705.

49. Yang Feng TL, Francke U, Ullrich A: Gene for human insulin receptor: localization to site on chromosome 19 involved in pre-B-cell leukemia. *Science* 1985, 228:728–731.

50. White MF, Shoelson SE, Keutmann H, Kahn CR: A cascade of tyrosine autophosphorylation in the beta-subunit activates the phosphotransferase of the insulin receptor. *J Biol Chem* 1988, 263:2969–2980.

51. Rajagopalan M, Neidigh JL, McClain DA: Amino acid sequences Gly-Pro-Leu-Tyr and Asn-Pro-Glu-Tyr in the submembranous domain of the insulin receptor are required for normal endocytosis. *J Biol Chem* 1991, 266:23068–23073.

52. Van Horn DJ, Myers MG Jr, Backer JM: Direct activation of the phosphatidylinositol 3'-kinase by the insulin receptor. *J Biochem* 1994, 269:29–32.

53. Mosthaf L, Grako K, Dull TJ, *et al.*: Functionally distinct insulin receptors generated by tissue-specific alternative splicing. *EMBO J* 1990, 9:2409–2413.

54. Moller DE, Yokota A, Caro JF, Flier JS: Tissue-specific expression of two alternatively spliced insulin receptor mRNAs in man. *Mol Endocrinol* 1989, 3:1263–1269.

55. Goldstein BJ, Kahn CR: Analysis of mRNA heterogeneity by ribonuclease H mapping: application to the insulin receptor. *Biochem Biophys Res Commun* 1989, 159:664–669.

56. Seino S, Bell GI: Alternative splicing of human insulin receptor messenger RNA. *Biochem Biophys Res Commun* 1989, 159:312–316.

57. Barzilai N, Wang J, Massilon D, *et al.*: Leptin selectively decreases visceral adiposity and enhances insulin action. *J Clin Invest* 1997, 100:3105–3110.

58. Benyoucef S, Surinya KH, Hadaschik D, Siddle K: Characterization of insulin/IGF hybrid receptors: contributions of the insulin receptor L2 and Fn1 domains and the alternatively spliced exon 11 sequence to ligand binding and receptor activation. *Biochem J* 2007, 403:603–613.

59. Hubbard SR, Miller WT: Receptor tyrosine kinases: mechanisms of activation and signaling. *Curr Opin Cell Biol* 2007, 19:117–123.

60. Hu J, Liu J, Ghirlando R, *et al.*: Structural basis for recruitment of the adaptor protein APS to the activated insulin receptor. *Mol Cell* 2003, 12:1379–1389.

61. Hubbard SR: Crystal structure of the activated insulin receptor tyrosine kinase in complex with peptide substrate and ATP analog. *EMBO J* 1997, 16:5572–5581.

62. Hubbard SR, Wei L, Ellis L, Hendrickson WA: Crystal structure of the tyrosine kinase domain of the human insulin receptor. *Nature* 1994, 372:746–754.

63. Songyang Z, Carraway KL 3rd, Eck MJ, *et al.*: Catalytic specificity of protein-tyrosine kinases is critical for selective signalling. *Nature* 1995, 373:536–539.

64. Songyang Z, Cantley LC: Recognition and specificity in protein tyrosine kinase-mediated signaling. *Trends Biochem Sci* 1995, 20:470–475.

65. Shoelson SE, Chatterjee S, Chaudhuri M, White MF: YMXM motifs of IRS-1 define the substrate specificity of the insulin receptor kinase. *Proc Natl Acad Sci U S A* 1992, 89:2027–2031.

66. Sawka-Verhelle D, Tartare-Deckert S, White MF, Van Obberghen E: Insulin receptor substrate-2 binds to the insulin receptor through its phosphotyrosine-binding domain and through a newly identified domain comprising amino acids 591–786. *J Biol Chem* 1996, 271:5980–5983.

67. Sawka-Verhelle D, Baron V, Mothe I, *et al.*: Tyr624 and Tyr628 in insulin receptor substrate-2 mediate its association with the insulin receptor. *J Biol Chem* 1997, 272:16414–16420.

68. Wu J, Tseng YD, Xu CF, *et al.*: Structural and biochemical characterization of the KRLB region in insulin receptor substrate-2. *Nat Struct Mol Biol* 2008, 15:251–258.

69. Rubinfeld H, Seger R: The ERK cascade: a prototype of MAPK signaling. *Mol Biotechnol* 2005, 31:151–174.

70. Waskiewicz AJ, Johnson JC, Penn B, *et al.*: Phosphorylation of the cap-binding protein eukaryotic translation initiation factor 4E by protein kinase Mnk1 in vivo. *Mol Cell Biol* 1999, 19:1871–1880.

71. Minich WB, Balasta ML, Goss DJ, Rhoads RE: Chromatographic resolution of *in vivo* phosphorylated and nonphosphorylated eukaryotic translation initiation factor eIF-4E: increased cap affinity of the phosphorylated form. *Proc Natl Acad Sci U S A* 1994, 91:7668–7672.

72. Svitkin YV, Herdy B, Costa-Mattioli M, *et al.*: Eukaryotic translation initiation factor 4E availability controls the switch between cap-dependent and internal ribosomal entry site-mediated translation. *Mol Cell Biol* 2005, 25:10556–10565.

73. Cantley LC: The phosphoinositide 3-kinase pathway. *Science* 2002, 296:1655–1657.

74. Backer JM, Myers MG Jr, Shoelson SE, *et al.*: Phosphatidylinositol 3'-kinase is activated by association with IRS-1 during insulin stimulation. *EMBO J* 1992, 11:3469–3479.

75. Farese RV, Sajan MP, Yang H, *et al.*: Muscle-specific knockout of PKC-lambda impairs glucose transport and induces metabolic and diabetic syndromes. *J Clin Invest* 2007, 117:2289–2301.

76. Taniguchi CM, Tran TT, Kondo T, *et al.*: Phosphoinositide 3-kinase regulatory subunit p85alpha suppresses insulin action via positive regulation of PTEN. *Proc Natl Acad Sci U S A* 2006, 103:12093–12097.

77. Taniguchi CM, Kondo T, Sajan M, *et al.*: Divergent regulation of hepatic glucose and lipid metabolism by phosphoinositide 3-kinase via Akt and PKClambda/zeta. *Cell Metab* 2006, 3:343–353.

78. Manning BD, Cantley LC: AKT/PKB signaling: navigating downstream. *Cell* 2007, 129:1261–1274.

79. Astrinidis A, Henske EP: Tuberous sclerosis complex: linking growth and energy signaling pathways with human disease. *Oncogene* 2005, 24:7475–7481.

80. Hu C, Pang S, Kong X, *et al.*: Molecular cloning and tissue distribution of PHAS-I, an intracellular target for insulin and growth factors. *Proc Natl Acad Sci U S A* 1994, 91:3730–3734.

81. Jaeschke A, Hartkamp J, Saitoh M, *et al.*: Tuberous sclerosis complex tumor suppressor-mediated S6 kinase inhibition by phosphatidylinositide-3-OH kinase is mTOR independent. *J Cell Biol* 2002, 159:217–224.

82. Tee AR, Fingar DC, Manning BD, *et al.*: Tuberous sclerosis complex-1 and –2 gene products function together to inhibit mammalian target of rapamycin (mTOR)-mediated downstream signaling. *Proc Natl Acad Sci U S A* 2002, 99:13571–13576.

83. Proud CG: Cell signaling. mTOR, unleashed. *Science* 2007, 318:926–927.

84. Pende M, Kozma SC, Jaquet M, *et al.*: Hypoinsulinaemia, glucose intolerance and diminished beta-cell size in S6K1-deficient mice. *Nature* 2000, 408:994–997.

85. Isotani S, Hara K, Tokunaga C, *et al.*: Immunopurified mammalian target of rapamycin phosphorylates and activates p70 S6 kinase alpha in vitro. *J Biol Chem* 1999, 274:34493–34498.

86. Jacinto E, Lorberg A: TOR regulation of AGC kinases in yeast and mammals. *Biochem J* 2008, 410:19–37.

87. Brunn GJ, Hudson CC, Sekulic A, *et al.*: Phosphorylation of the translational repressor PHAS-I by the mammalian target of rapamycin. *Science* 1997, 277:99–101.

88. Tsukiyama-Kohara K, Poulin F, Kohara M, *et al.*: Adipose tissue reduction in mice lacking the translational inhibitor 4E-BP1. *Nat Med* 2001, 7:1128–1132.

89. Farese RV, Sajan MP, Standaert ML: Atypical protein kinase C in insulin action and insulin resistance. *Biochem Soc Trans* 2005, 33:350–353.

90. Ide T, Shimano H, Yahagi N, *et al.*: SREBPs suppress IRS-2-mediated insulin signalling in the liver. *Nat Cell Biol* 2004, 6:351–357.

91. Czech MP: Molecular actions of insulin on glucose transport. *Annu Rev Nutr* 1995, 15:441–471.

92. Huang S, Czech MP: The GLUT4 glucose transporter. *Cell Metab* 2007, 5:237–252.

93. Pessin JE, Thurmond DC, Elmendorf JS, *et al.*: Molecular basis of insulin-stimulated GLUT4 vesicle trafficking. Location! Location! Location! *J Biol Chem* 1999, 274:2593–2596.

94. Khan AH, Pessin JE: Insulin regulation of glucose uptake: a complex interplay of intracellular signalling pathways. *Diabetologia* 2002, 45:1475–1483.

95. Farese RV: Function and dysfunction of aPKC isoforms for glucose transport in insulin-sensitive and insulin-resistant states. *Am J Physiol Endocrinol Metab* 2002, 283:E1–E11.

96. Bandyopadhyay G, Standaert ML, Sajan MP, *et al.*: Protein kinase C-lambda knockout in embryonic stem cells and adipocytes impairs insulin-stimulated glucose transport. *Mol Endocrinol* 2004, 18:373–383.

97. Kane S, Sano H, Liu SC, *et al.*: A method to identify serine kinase substrates. Akt phosphorylates a novel adipocyte protein with a Rab GTPase-activating protein (GAP) domain. *J Biol Chem* 2002, 277:22115–22118.

98. Sakamoto K, Holman GD: Emerging role for AS160/TBC1D4 and TBC1D1 in the regulation of GLUT4 traffic. *Am J Physiol Endocrinol Metab* 2008, 295:E29–E37.

99. Sano H, Kane S, Sano E, *et al.*: Insulin-stimulated phosphorylation of a Rab GTPase-activating protein regulates GLUT4 translocation. *J Biol Chem* 2003, 278:14599–14602.

100. Miinea CP, Sano H, Kane S, *et al.*: AS160, the Akt substrate regulating GLUT4 translocation, has a functional Rab GTPase-activating protein domain. *Biochem J* 2005, 391(pt 1):87–93.

101. Kotani K, Ogawa W, Matsumoto M, *et al.*: Requirement of atypical protein kinase clambda for insulin stimulation of glucose uptake but not for akt activation in 3T3-L1 adipocytes. *Mol Cell Biol* 1998, 18:6971–6982.

102. Hill MM, Clark SF, Tucker DF, *et al.*: A role for protein kinase Bbeta/Akt2 in insulin-stimulated GLUT4 translocation in adipocytes. *Mol Cell Biol* 1999, 19:7771–7781.

103. Bandyopadhyay G, Kanoh Y, Sajan MP, et al.: Effects of adenoviral gene transfer of wild-type, constitutively active, and kinase-defective protein kinase C-lambda on insulin-stimulated glucose transport in L6 myotubes. *Endocrinology* 2000, 141:4120–4127.

104. Zick Y: Role of Ser/Thr kinases in the uncoupling of insulin signaling. *Int J Obes Relat Metab Disord* 2003, 27(suppl 3):S56–S60.

105. Gual P, Le Marchand-Brustel Y, Tanti JF: Positive and negative regulation of insulin signaling through IRS-1 phosphorylation. *Biochimie* 2005, 87:99–109.

106. Zick Y: Ser/Thr phosphorylation of IRS proteins: a molecular basis for insulin resistance. *Sci STKE* 2005, 2005:e4.

107. Kido Y, Burks DJ, Withers D, *et al.*: Tissue-specific insulin resistance in mice with mutations in the insulin receptor, IRS-1, and IRS-2. *J Clin Invest* 2000, 105:199–205.

108. Haruta T, Uno T, Kawahara J, *et al.*: A rapamycin-sensitive pathway down-regulates insulin signaling via phosphorylation and proteasomal degradation of insulin receptor substrate-1. *Mol Endocrinol* 2000, 14:783–794.

109. Rui L, Fisher TL, Thomas J, White MF: Regulation of insulin/insulin-like growth factor-1 signaling by proteasome-mediated degradation of insulin receptor substrate-2. *J Biol Chem* 2001, 276: 40362–40367.

110. Ueki K, Kondo T, Kahn CR: Suppressor of cytokine signaling 1 (SOCS-1) and SOCS-3 cause insulin resistance through inhibition of tyrosine phosphorylation of insulin receptor substrate proteins by discrete mechanisms. *Mol Cell Biol* 2004, 24:5434–5446.

111. Liu F, Yang T, Wang B, *et al.*: Resistin induces insulin resistance, but does not affect glucose output in rat-derived hepatocytes. *Acta Pharmacol Sin* 2008, 29:98–104.

112. Palanivel R, Maida A, Liu Y, Sweeney G: Regulation of insulin signalling, glucose uptake and metabolism in rat skeletal muscle cells upon prolonged exposure to resistin. *Diabetologia* 2006, 49:183–190.

113. Rui L, Yuan M, Frantz D, et al.: SOCS-1 and SOCS-3 block insulin signaling by ubiquitin-mediated degradation of IRS1 and IRS2. *J Biol Chem* 2002, 277:42394–42398.

114. Ueki K, Kondo T, Tseng YH, Kahn CR: Central role of suppressors of cytokine signaling proteins in hepatic steatosis, insulin resistance, and the metabolic syndrome in the mouse. *Proc Natl Acad Sci U S A* 2004, 101:10422–10427.

115. Kawaguchi T, Yoshida T, Harada M, *et al.*: Hepatitis C virus down-regulates insulin receptor substrates 1 and 2 through up-regulation of suppressor of cytokine signaling 3. *Am J Pathol* 2004, 165:1499–1508.

116. Brown MS, Goldstein JL: Selective versus total insulin resistance: a pathogenic paradox. *Cell Metab* 2008, 7:95–96.

117. Postic C, Girard J: Contribution of de novo fatty acid synthesis to hepatic steatosis and insulin resistance: lessons from genetically engineered mice. *J Clin Invest* 2008, 118:829–838.

118. Cheng Z, Guo S, Copps K, *et al.*: Foxo1 integrates insulin signaling with mitochondrial function in the liver. *Nat Med* 2009, 15:1307–1311.

119. Kushner JA, Ye J, Schubert M, *et al.*: Pdx1 restores beta cell function in Irs2 knockout mice. *J Clin Invest* 2002, 109:1193–1201.

120. Jonsson J, Carlsson L, Edlund T, Edlund H: Insulin-promoter-factor 1 is required for pancreas developement in mice. *Nature* 1994, 371:606–609.

121. Stoffers DA, Zinkin NT, Stanojevic V, *et al.*: Pancreatic agenesis attributable to a single nucleotide deletion in the human IPF1 gene coding sequence. *Nat Genet* 1997, 15:106–110.

122. Kitamura T, Nakae J, Kitamura Y, *et al.*: The forkhead transcription factor Foxo1 links insulin signaling to Pdx1 regulation of pancreatic beta cell growth. *J Clin Invest* 2002, 110:1839–1847.

123. Hennige AM, Burks DJ, Ozcan U, *et al.*: Upregulation of insulin receptor substrate-2 in pancreatic beta cells prevents diabetes. *J Clin Invest* 2003 112:1521–1532.

124. Kushner JA, Simpson L, Wartschow LM, *et al.*: Phosphatase and tensin homolog regulation of islet growth and glucose homeostasis. *J Biol Chem* 2005, 280:39388–39393.

125. Weir GC, Bonner-Weir S: A dominant role for glucose in beta cell compensation of insulin resistance. *J Clin Invest* 2007, 117: 81–83.

126. Terauchi Y, Takamoto I, Kubota N, *et al.*: Glucokinase and IRS-2 are required for compensatory beta cell hyperplasia in response to high-fat diet-induced insulin resistance. *J Clin Invest* 2007, 117:246–257.

127. Park S, Dong X, Fisher TL, *et al.*: Exendin-4 uses irs2 signaling to mediate pancreatic Beta cell growth and function. *J Biol Chem* 2006, 281:1159–1168.

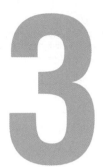

Consequences of Insulin Deficiency

Abbas E. Kitabchi and Mary Beth Murphy

Diabetes [mellitus] is a remarkable disorder, and not one very common to man. The disease is chronic in its character, and is slowly engendered, though the patient does not survive long when it is completely established for the marasmus produced is rapid, and death speedy. Life too is odious and painful, the thirst is ungovernable, and the copious potations are more than equaled by the profuse urinary discharge; for more urine flows away, and it is impossible to put any restraint to the patient's drinking or making water. For if he stop for a very brief period, and leave off drinking, the mouth becomes parched, the body dry; the bowels seem on fire, he is wretched and uneasy, and soon dies, tormented with burning thirst.

Aretaeus of Cappodocia (ea. 120 AD–200 AD) [1]

Diabetes mellitus (type 1 or type 2) is the result of an absolute or relative insulin-deficient state that, if not corrected, gives rise to the acute metabolic decompensation of hyperglycemic crises so poignantly described above by Aretaeus of Cappodocia more than 1,800 years ago. The two major hyperglycemic crises are diabetic ketoacidosis (DKA) and hyperglycemic hyperosmolar syndrome (HHS). These two syndromes are the hallmark of insulin-deficient states. These crises continue to be important causes of mortality and morbidity among patients with diabetes. The annual incidence of DKA hospital admissions ranges from 4.6 to 8 episodes per 1,000 patients with diabetes. It is estimated that DKA accounts for 4–9% of all hospital admissions for patients diagnosed with diabetes, whereas this figure for HHS is less than 1% [2, 3].

DKA is a proinflammatory state resulting in the production of reactive oxygen species indicating oxidative stress [4, 5]. Recently, it has been demonstrated that serum levels of inflammatory cytokines (interleukin [IL]-1β, IL-6, IL-8, and tumor necrosis factor-α [TNF-α]), growth hormone (GH), cortisol as well as markers of cardiovascular risk factors, plasminogen activator inhibitor-1, C-reactive protein, and lipid peroxidation markers (thiobarbituric acid) and free fatty acids (FFAs) are elevated in DKA [6]. These parameters return to normal at resolution of hyperglycemia with insulin therapy, thus demonstrating a robust anti-inflammatory effect of insulin in response to the general alarm reaction associated with the hyperglycemic ketotic state [6].

T-lymphocytes, which are usually insulin-insensitive, on activation with antigens, become insulin-sensitive and develop de novo growth factor receptors for insulin, insulin growth factor-1, and IL-2 [7]. Because DKA is a proinflammatory state, T-lymphocytes may be activated in vivo and, therefore, there may be in situ development of de novo growth factor receptors. In a recent study, T-lymphocytes (CD4+ and CD8+) were evaluated in eight patients with DKA by measuring insulin growth factor, insulin, and IL-2 receptors by flow cytometry on admission and after treatment with insulin and resolution of DKA. This study demonstrates in situ emergence of these growth factor receptors (insulin, insulin growth factor-1, and IL-2), as well as elevated levels of oxidative stress, including dichloroflourescein- and thiobarbituric acid-reacting material on admission and at resolution of DKA with insulin therapy, compared with matched control subjects [8].

The most common precipitating causes for these hyperglycemic emergencies are (a) infection; (b) undertreatment or omission of insulin; (c) previously undiagnosed diabetes; (d) illicit drug abuse; and (e) the presence of comorbid conditions [9, 10]. Contributing factors for the development of HHS include decreased intake of fluid and electrolytes, excessive use of such drugs as glucocorticoids, diuretics, β-blockers, as well as the use of immunosuppressive agents and diazoxide [10]. Although DKA is most frequently seen in type 1 diabetes and HHS is often associated with type 2 diabetes, each of these conditions can be seen in both types of diabetes because DKA and HHS have common underlying causes (i.e., ineffective insulin concentration, dehydration, and increased counterregulatory [stress] hormones, but at different levels). DKA can also occur in young, obese, previously undiagnosed blacks who demonstrate the characteristics of type 2 diabetes [11].

It is important to note that some patients may present with an overlapping metabolic picture of both DKA and HHS. The incidence of combined HHS and DKA in some series has been noted to be as high as 30% [11]. HHS and DKA can also occur in relatively pure form. Generally, in DKA, insulin levels are deficient, whereas in HHS, the insulin may be insufficient relative to the excessive levels of stress hormones (cortisol, glucagon, catecholamines, and GH).

With better understanding of the pathogenesis of insulin-deficient states, the use of more physiologic doses of insulin, and frequent monitoring of such patients in the hospital, the mortality rate has been reduced to 0.41% for DKA and less than 15% for HHS with a higher death rate among black males and the lowest rate among white females [3, 9, 12–15]. Interestingly, data as of 2009 have shown that those ≤45 years old had a higher DKA mortality rate (25.2 per 100,000 diabetic population) than those 65–74 years old (8 per 100,000 diabetic population) [13].

Indications for hospitalization include loss of more than 5% body weight at presentation, respiration rate greater than 35 per minute, intractable blood glucose elevation, changes in mental status, uncontrolled fever, and/or unresolved nausea and vomiting [9,10]. Poor prognostic signs for DKA and HHS include advanced age, decreased mental state, and lower blood pressure [15]. The cost of DKA in one study was estimated to be $17,559 per episode, with annual costs exceeding 2.4 billion dollars [13].

Prevention of these metabolic emergencies poses important medical and social challenges. Preventive actions should include extensive diabetes educational programs that review steps to be taken during sick days, including frequent blood glucose and urine ketone monitoring, ingestion of a liquid diet containing salt and carbohydrates, close contact with health care providers, and above all the proper use of rapid/short-acting insulin during the illness. Finally, improved access to a health care delivery system and the availability of affordable medication in less affluent segments of society are some of the most effective methods for prevention of these crises.

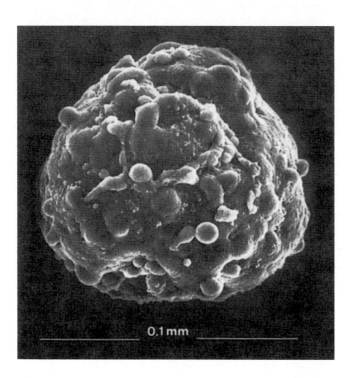

FIGURE 3-1. Surface topography of the periphery of the islet cell (×900) (from Orci [16], with permission).

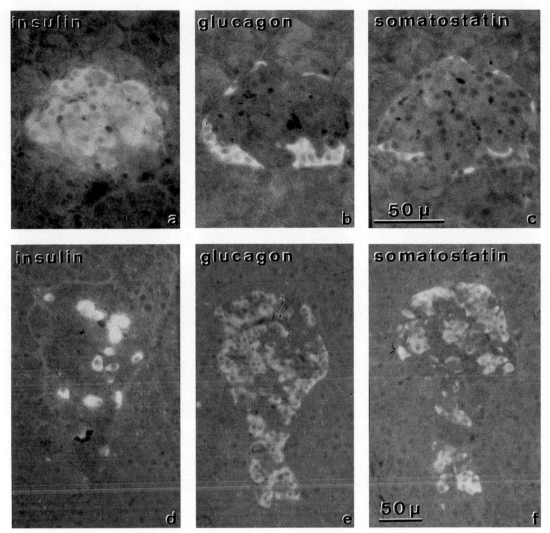

Figure 3-2. Consecutive serial sections of islets of Langerhans processed for indirect immunofluorescence. (**A–C**) The location of insulin-, glucagon-, and somatostatin-containing cells, respectively, in the islet of a control rat. (**D–F**) The profound perturbation of this normal distribution in the islet of a rat rendered experimentally diabetic for 17 months after a single intravenous injection of streptozotocin, 45 mg/kg. Note that the number of insulin-containing cells is strikingly reduced while that of glucagon- and somatostatin-containing cells is greatly increased (from Orci et al. [17], with permission).

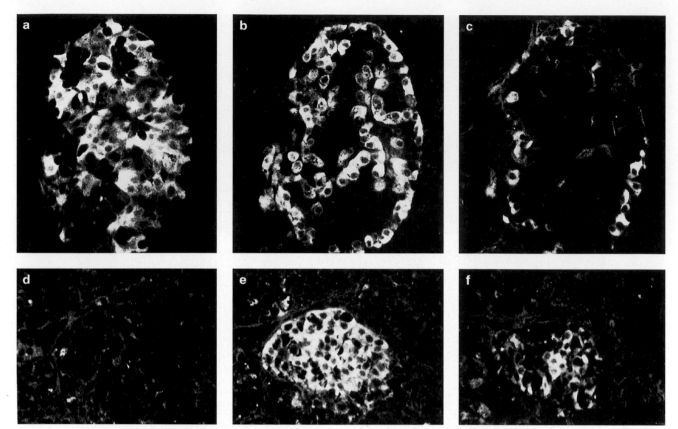

Figure 3-3. Distribution of β-, α-, and Δ-cells on serial sections of an islet from an adult nondiabetic subject. The indirect immunofluorescent technique demonstrates insulin (**A**), glucagon (**B**), and somatostatin cells (**C**). (**D–F**) Serial sections of the islet of Langerhans in a patient with type 1 diabetes treated with the indirect immunofluorescent technique against insulin, glucagon, and somatostatin, respectively. The only detectable immunofluorescent cells within the islet are the numerous glucagon- and somatostatin-containing cells (×200) (from Orci et al. [17], with permission).

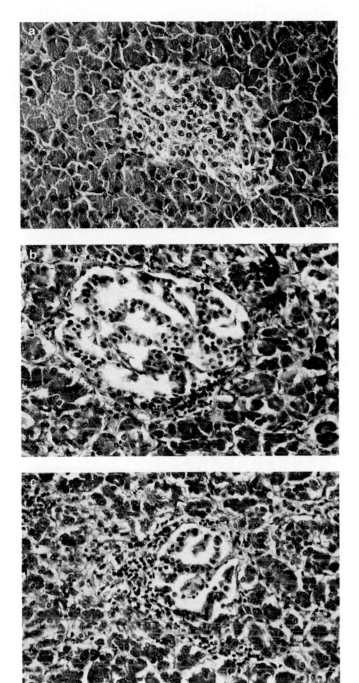

FIGURE 3-4. Islet cell necrosis and lymphocyte infiltration. **(A)** Pancreatic islet section from normal, nondiabetic control patient. **(B)** Pancreatic islet section from patient with type 1 diabetes. Lymphocytic infiltration can be seen throughout the pancreatic islets with residual islet cells, **(C)** Pancreatic islet section from patient with type 1 diabetes showing lymphocytic infiltration in the pancreatic islets, particularly the peripheral islets [18].

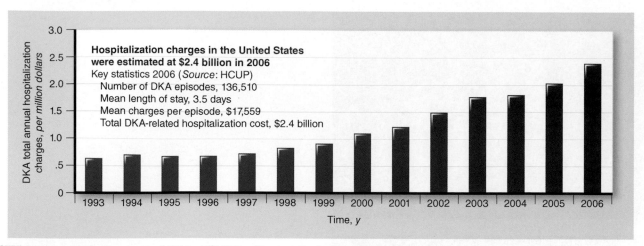

FIGURE 3-5. Hospitalization cost of DKA. *HCUP* Healthcare Cost and Utilization Project (from Centers for Disease Control and Prevention [13]).

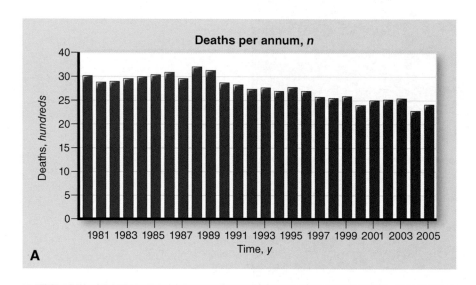

A

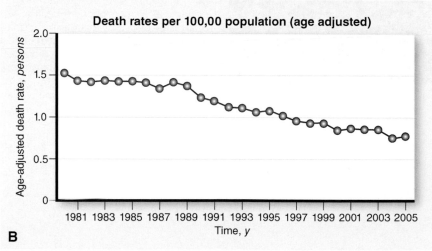

B

Figure 3-6. Mortality rates for hyperglycemic crises as underlying cause in the general population. (**A**) Number of deaths per year and (**B**) age-adjusted death rate per 100,000 people.

However, in 2006 the overall mortality rate for DKA alone was 0.41% (from Centers for Disease Control and Prevention [13]).

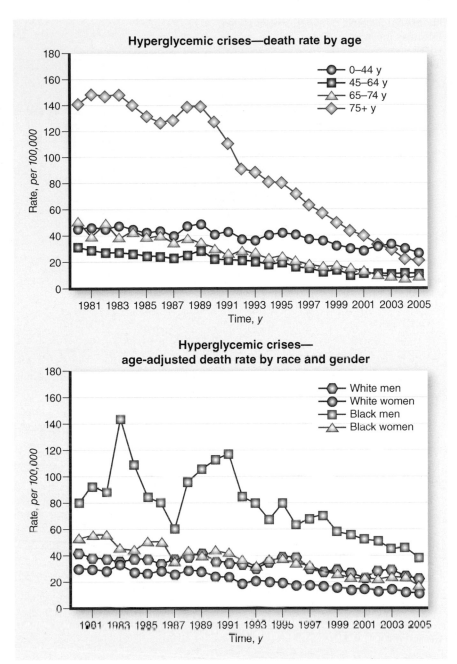

Figure 3-7. Death rates by age, race, and gender for hyperglycemic crises as underlying causes per 100,000 in the diabetic population. However, in 2006, the overall mortality rate for DKA alone was 0.41% [13] (from Centers for Disease Control and Prevention [13]).

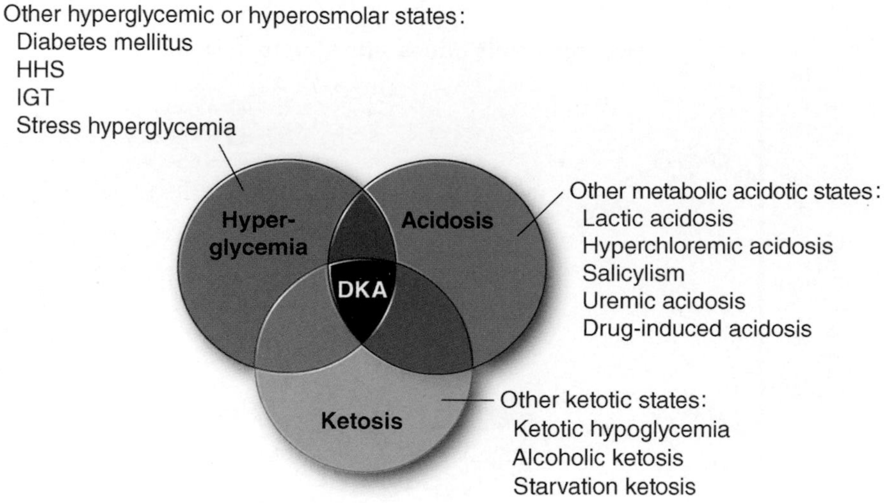

Other hyperglycemic or hyperosmolar states:
   Diabetes mellitus
   HHS
   IGT
   Stress hyperglycemia

Other metabolic acidotic states:
   Lactic acidosis
   Hyperchloremic acidosis
   Salicylism
   Uremic acidosis
   Drug-induced acidosis

Other ketotic states:
   Ketotic hypoglycemia
   Alcoholic ketosis
   Starvation ketosis

Hyper-glycemia **Acidosis** **DKA** **Ketosis**

FIGURE 3-8. Other conditions in which the components of the diagnostic triad for DKA (hyperglycemia, ketosis, and acidosis) may be found (adapted from Kitabchi and Wall [19]).

Diagnostic Criteria and Typical Total Body Deficits in DKA and HHS

Diagnostic criteria and classification	DKA			HHS
	Mild	Moderate	Severe	
Plasma glucose, mg/dL*	> 250	> 250	> 250	> 600
Arterial pH	7.25–7.30	7.00 < 7.24	< 7.00	> 7.30
Serum bicarbonate, mEq/L	15–18	10– < 15	< 10	> 18
Urine ketone[†]	Positive	Positive	Positive	Small
Serum ketone[†]	Positive	Positive	Positive	Small
Effective serum osmolality[‡]	Variable	Variable	Variable	> 320
Anion gap[§]	> 10	> 12	> 12	Variable
Mental status	Alert	Alert/drowsy	Stupor/coma	Variable

Typical deficits	DKA	HHS
Total water, L	6	9
Water, mL/kg[¶]	100	100–200
Na+, mEq/kgl[¶]	7–10	5–13
Cl−, mEq/kg[¶]	3–5	5–15
K+, mEq/kg[¶]	3–5	4–6
PO4, mmol/kg[¶]	5–7	3–7
MG++, mEq/kg[¶]	1–2	1–2
CA++, mEq/kg[¶]	1–2	1–2

*Euglycemic DKA has been reported [22, 23].
[†]Nitroprusside reaction method.
[‡]Effective serum osmolality calculation: $2[\text{measured Na}^+ (\text{mEq/L})] + \text{glucose (mg/dL)}/18 [\text{mOsm/kg}]$.
[§]Anion gap calculation: $(\text{Na}^+) - (\text{CL}^- + \text{HCO}_3^- (\text{mEq/L})$ [normal = 12 ± 2].
[¶]Per kilogram of body weight.

Figure 3-9. Diagnostic criteria and typical total body deficits of water and electrolytes in DKA and HHS [10, 20, 21].

Laboratory Evaluation of Metabolic Causes of Acidosis and Coma

Factor studied	Starvation or high fat intake	DKA	Lactic acidosis	Uremic acidosis	Alcoholic ketosis (starvation)	Salicylate intoxication	Methanol or ethylene glycol intoxication	Hyperosmolar coma	Hypoglycemic coma	Rhabdomyolysis
pH	Normal	↓	↓	Mild ↓	↑↓	↑↓[†]	↓	Normal	Normal	Mild ↓ may be ↓
Plasma glucose	Normal	↑	Normal	Normal	↓ or normal	Normal or ↓	Normal	↑↑ > 500 mg/dL	↓↓ < 30 mg/dL	Normal
Glycosuria	Negative	++	Negative	Negative	Negative	Negative[‡]	Negative	++	Negative	Negative
Total plasma ketones[*]	Slight ↑	↑↑	Normal	Normal	Slight to moderate ↑	Normal	Normal	Normal or slight ↑	Normal	Normal
Anion gap	Slight ↑	↑	↑	Slight ↑	↑	↑	↑	Normal	Normal	↑↑
Osmolality	Normal	↑	Normal	↑ or normal	Normal	Normal	↑↑	↑↑ > 330 mOsm/kg	Normal	Normal or slight ↑
Uric acid	Mild ↑ (starvation)	↑	Normal	Normal or ↑	↑	Normal	Normal	Normal	Normal	↑
Miscellaneous			Serum lactate > 7 mM	BUN > 200 mg/dL		Serum salicylate +	Serum levels positive			Myoglobinuria, hemoglobinuria

BUN—blood urea nitrogen.

* Acetest and Ketostix (Bayer; Leverkusen, Germany) measure acetoacetic acid only; thus, misleadingly low values may be obtained because the majority of "ketone bodies" are β-hydroxybutyrate.

† Respiratory alkalosis/metabolic acidosis.

‡ May get a false-positive or false-negative urinary glucose caused by the presence of salicylate or its metabolites [21].

Figure 3-10. Laboratory evaluation of metabolic causes of acidosis and coma (adapted from Morris and Kitabchi [24]).

Fed state　　　　　　　　　**DKA**

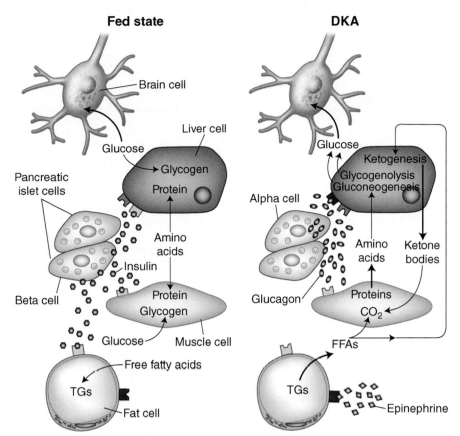

Figure 3-11. Mechanisms of glucose regulation. Glucose supply to the brain can be maintained for days and even weeks when the body has been deprived of caloric intake. In the fed state (*left*), assimilation of metabolic fuels and substrates is promoted by insulin in tissues sensitive to the hormone. In DKA (*right*), counterregulatory hormones (notably glucagon and epinephrine) reverse these processes, promoting glycogenolysis and creating substrates for ketogenesis and gluconeogenesis [25–28]. Denial of glucose to insulin-sensitive tissues preserves it for the brain. The insulin receptor is depicted as a *dark-notched square*; the glucagon receptor depicted as a *light-notched square*. *TGs* triglycerides (adapted from Kitabchi and Rumbak [28]).

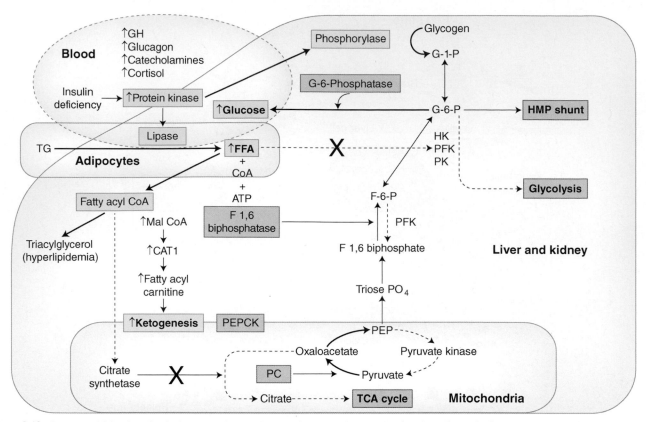

Figure 3-12. Proposed biochemical changes that occur during DKA. These alterations lead to increased gluconeogenesis, lipolysis, ketogenesis, and decreased glycolysis. *Note*: Lipolysis occurs mainly in adipose tissue. Other events occur primarily in the liver (except some gluconeogenesis in the kidney) [29]. *Thick arrows* indicate stimulated pathways in DKA, which consist of rate-limiting enzymes of gluconeogenesis, whereas *thin arrows* indicate inhibitory pathway in glycolysis. *X* indicates an inhibitor effect of the compound on the particular enzyme system. The tricarboxylic acid (TCA) cycle is inhibited by fatty and acyl coenzyme A (CoA)-induced inhibition of citrate synthesis, a rate-limiting enzyme in the TCA cycle. *ATP* adenosine triphosphate, *CAT1* carnitine acyltransferase-1, *F-6-P* fructose-6-phosphate, *G-1-P* glucose-1-phosphate, *G-6-P* glucose-6-phosphate, *HK* hexokinase, *HMP* hexose monophosphate, *PC* pyruvate carboxylase, *PEP* phosphoenolpyruvate, *PEPCK* phosphoenolpyruvate carboxykinase, *PFK* phosphofructokinase, *PK* pyruvate kinase (adapted from Kitabchi et al. [15]).

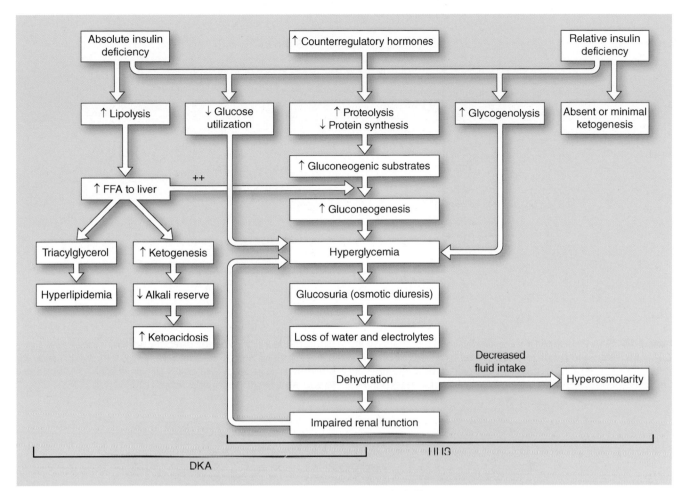

FIGURE 3-13. Pathogenesis of DKA and HHS. Alteration of fat, protein, and carbohydrate metabolism leads to metabolic changes toward catabolic states and symptoms of polyuria, polydipsia, polyphagia, osmotic diuresis, severe dehydration, and, if not treated, coma and death. The hallmark of these events is the insulin-deficient state and increased counterregulatory hormones. In HHS, in addition to the relative insulin deficiency and greater dehydration, there is also a greater amount of hyperglycemia (secondary to lower intake of fluid) than in DKA. Although the mechanism for the lack of a significant amount of ketosis and acidemia in HHS (compared with DKA) is not entirely clear, in one study the level of C-peptide (as an indication of pancreatic insulin reserve) was shown to be five- to tenfold lower in DKA than in HHS [30]. This has been offered as a partial explanation for the lack of ketonemia in HHS. Because the required amount of insulin for its antilipolytic action is about five- to tenfold lower than for the glucose transport action [31], it follows that the larger amount of residual insulin (C-peptide) in HHS is sufficient to prevent lipolysis (thus no ketogenesis in HHS). This amount of insulin is not enough to promote glucose transport and its metabolism, thus the resultant hyperglycemia is noted in HHS without severe ketonemia (adapted from Kitabchi et al. [20])

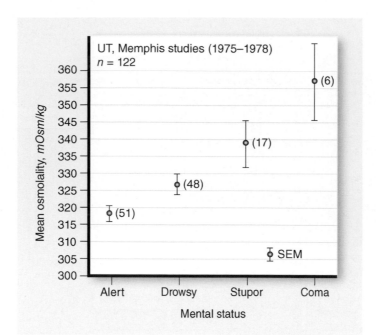

FIGURE 3-14. Calculated serum osmolality in 122 patients with DKA with relation to mental status. About one third of patients with hyperglycemic crises may present with altered mental status. This can be correlated to serum osmolality but needs to be differentiated from various clinical conditions associated with altered mental status or coma (see Fig. 3.8), which may be present in diabetic patients. *UT* University of Tennessee (adapted from Kitabchi and Fisher [12]).

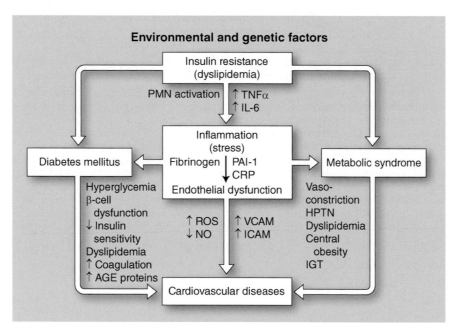

FIGURE 3-15. Environmental and genetic factors of insulin resistance, diabetes mellitus, metabolic syndrome, and aberrant pathways in the development of cardiovascular diseases. *AGE* advanced glycation end products, *CRP* C-reactive protein, *HPTN* hypertension, *ICAM* intercellular adhesion molecule-1, *IGT* impaired glucose tolerance, *NO* nitric oxide, *PAI-1* plasma plasminogen activator inhibitor type 1, *PMN* polymorphonuclear cells, *ROS* reactive oxygen species, *VCAM* vascular cellular adhesion molecules (adapted from Kitabchi [32]).

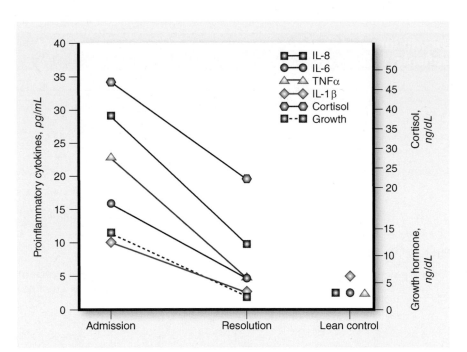

FIGURE 3-16. Serum levels of proinflammatory cytokines, cortisol, and GH in lean patients with DKA on admission and after resolution of DKA with insulin therapy [6].

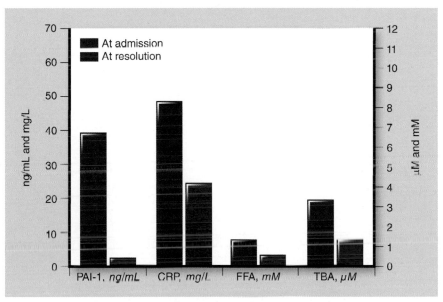

FIGURE 3-17. Serum levels of cardiovascular risk factors (PAI-1 and CRP), FFA, and lipid peroxidation (thiobarbituric acid [TBA]) in lean DKA patients on admission and after resolution of DKA with insulin therapy [6].

Growth factor receptors' expression on T-lymphocytes in DKA patients

Receptor	DKA admission		DKA resolution	
	CD4, %	CD8, %	CD4, %	CD8, %
CD69	68±6	74±9	46±5	49±6
Insulin (IR)	18±6	24±7	39±7	41±7
IGF-I (IGFR)	23±5	29±8	48±6	52±5
IL-2 (IL2R)	39±4	43±5	62±6	64±6
Markers of oxidative stress				
	DKA admission		DKA resolution	
DCF (µM)	8.7±0.8		3.4±0.6	
TBA (µM; as malonaldehyde)	3.9±0.4		1.7±0.3	

Figure 3-18. Growth factor receptor expression on T-lymphocytes and markers of oxidative stress in eight patients with DKA [8]. *DCF* dichlorofluorescein, *IGF* insulin growth factor, *IGFR* insulin growth factor receptor, *IL2R* interleukin-2 receptor.

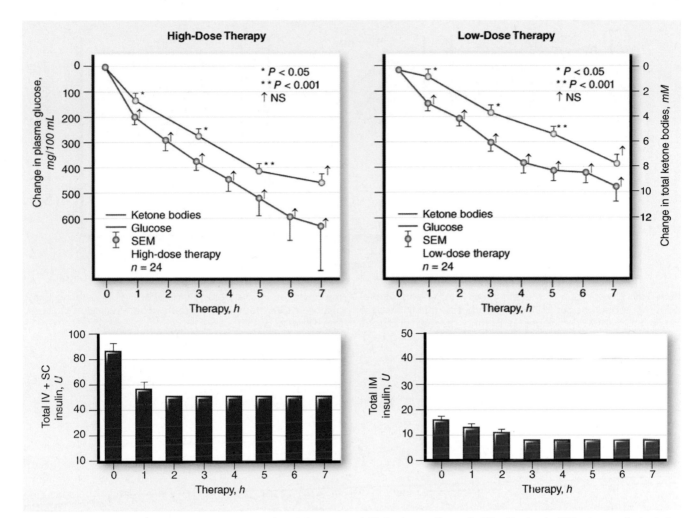

Figure 3-19. Efficacy of low-dose versus conventional therapy of insulin for the treatment of DKA. Treatment of hyperglycemic crises has undergone numerous modifications since the discovery of insulin. In the early decades after the discovery of insulin, low-dose therapy was the norm due to the limited availability of insulin, but In subsequent decades, doses of insulin were modified from physiologic to pharmacologic and even suprapharmacologic doses until the mid-1970s. The initial observation of Alberti et al. [33] demonstrated the effectiveness of low-dose insulin and gave impetus to the first prospective randomized study, which is summarized here [34]. This study confirms the similarity of the responses to low-dose and high-dose insulin in DKA without the disadvantages of greater hypoglycemia and hypokalemia associated with high-dose insulin therapy. *NS* not significant (adapted from Kitabchi et al. [34]).

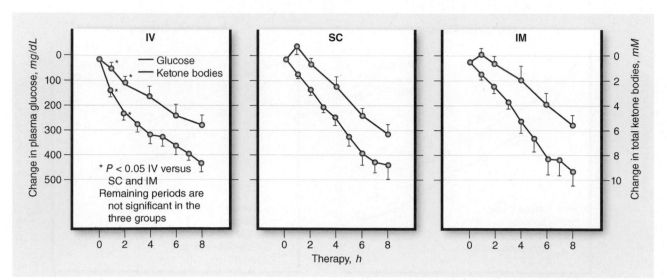

Figure 3-20. Comparison of the effects of randomized intravenous (IV), subcutaneous (SC), and intramuscular (IM) low-dose insulin regimens on changes in plasma glucose and total ketone bodies in patients with DKA (15 patients in each group). The low-dose insulin therapy was effective in lowering blood glucose in DKA therapy by any route of administration (adapted from Fisher et al. [35]).

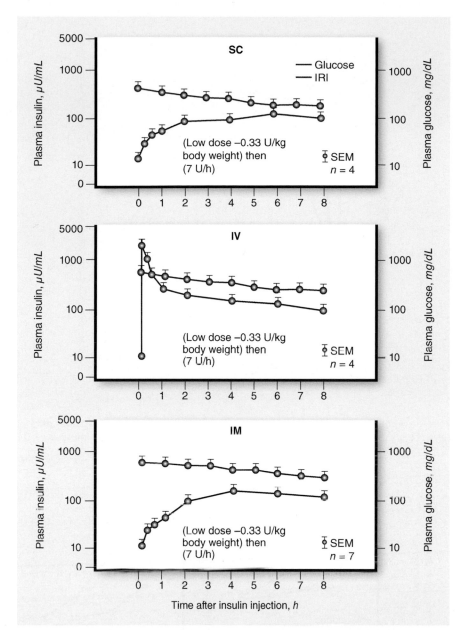

Figure 3-21. Comparison of the effect of low-dose insulin regimen (7 U/h) administered by SC, IV, and IM injections on plasma immunoreactive insulin (IRI) levels (*blue line*) and plasma glucose decrements (*pink line*) in three groups of DKA patients who had not previously been treated with insulin. In these patients, IV insulin caused serum insulin to rise immediately to supraphysiologic levels, whereas SC and IM injections of the same amount of insulin resulted in lower serum insulin concentrations, which reached near physiologic concentrations (postprandially) only after 2–3 h. This low level of insulin may be the reason for the slow clearance of ketone bodies noted in Fig. 3.20 for the IM and SC routes compared with the IV route of the same amount of insulin injection (7 U/h) (adapted from Kitabchi et al. [36]).

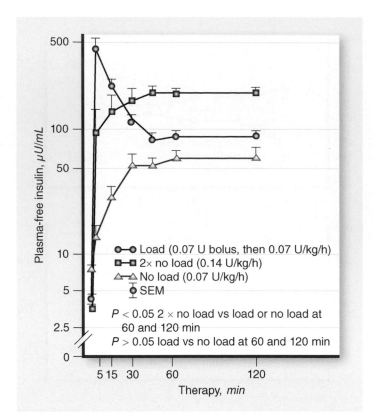

Figure 3-22. Kinetics of three doses of low-dose insulin in patients with DKA. This study demonstrated that the use of a bolus or priming dose of insulin is not needed when an adequate insulin infusion of 0.14 unit/kg/h (10 units per hour in a 70-kg patient) is used compared with an infusion of 0.07 unit/h with a bolus dose of 0.07 unit/kg [37].

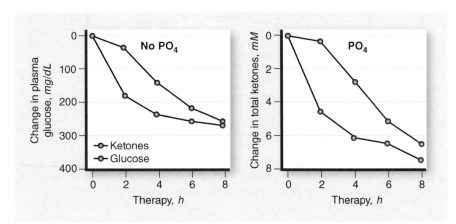

Figure 3-23. Use of phosphate (PO_4) in DKA. Another controversial issue in the management of DKA prompted study on the use of phosphate replacement in DKA. This study shows that phosphate therapy does not affect the clinical and biochemical outcomes (plasma glucose and ketone bodies) of low-dose insulin therapy. However, the use of phosphate in DKA was associated with a certain degree of hypocalcemia (adapted from Fisher and Kitabchi [38]).

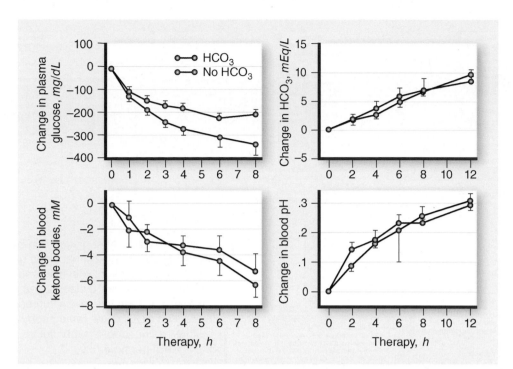

Figure 3-24. The role of bicarbonate therapy in the treatment of DKA. This prospective randomized study shows the effect of bicarbonate (HCO₃) therapy on various recovery parameters of DKA, indicating that bicarbonate did not alter outcomes of DKA therapy on hours of recovery from hyperglycemia, acidosis, or hypocapnia [40]. There is, therefore, very little reason for the use of bicarbonate therapy in DKA, particularly when the pH level is greater than 7 [39] (adapted from Morris et al. [40]).

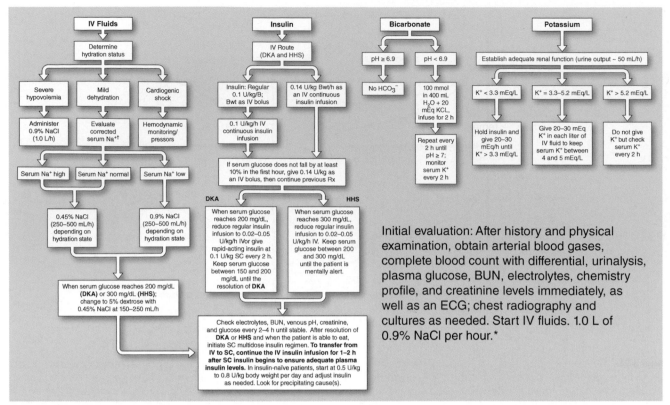

FIGURE 3-25. Protocol for management of adult patients with DKA or HHS. DKA diagnostic criteria: blood glucose 250 mg/dL, arterial pH less than 7.3, bicarbonate less than 15 mEq/L, and moderate ketonuria or ketonemia. HHS diagnostic criteria: serum glucose 600 mg/dL, arterial pH greater than 7.3, serum bicarbonate greater than 18 mEq/L, and minimal ketonuria and ketonemia. The *asterisk* indicates 15–20 mL/kg/h and the *dagger* indicates serum Na should be corrected for hyperglycemia (for each 100 mg/dL glucose above 100 mg/dL, add 1.6 mEq to sodium value for corrected serum value). *Bwt* body weight, *ECG* electrocardiography, *Rx* therapy (adapted from Kitabchi et al. [20]).

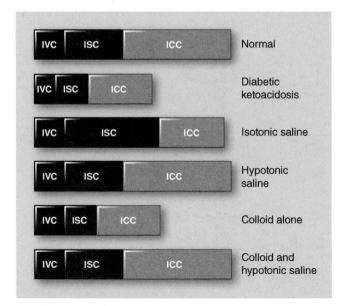

FIGURE 3-26. Use of hypotonic versus isotonic saline and plasma expanders. This figure demonstrates the effect of these solutions in various cellular compartments. The diagram depicts the decreased intravascular (IVC), interstitial (ISC), and intracellular (ICC) compartments present in patients with DKA, compared with control patients. Subsequent panels show the effects of fluid resuscitation of DKA with different solutions. Isotonic solutions replete only IVC and ISC compartments, whereas hypotonic solutions replete all compartments. However, larger volumes of hypotonic solutions are required to produce equivalent increases in IVC. Colloid alone is restricted to the IVC; therefore, combined use of colloid plus hypotonic solution can lead to a rapid increase in IVC, followed by more gradual replacement of the other compartments. It is also important to remember that hydration in DKA and hyperglycemic hyperosmolar syndrome dilutes concentrations of the stress hormones and thus makes peripheral tissues more sensitive to lower doses of insulin [41] (adapted from Hillman [42]).

Suggested DKA/HHS Flowsheet Weight:

0°_____

24°_____

Date															
Mental status*															
Temperature															
Pulse															
Respiration/depth[†]															
Blood pressure															
Serum glucose, *mg/dL*															
Serum "ketones"															
Urine "ketones"															

Electrolytes

Serum Na^+, *mEq/L*															
Serum K^+, *mEq/L*															
Serum Cl^-, *mEq/L*															
Serum HCO_3^-, *mEq/L*															
Serum BUN, *mg/dL*															
Effective osmolality 2 [measured Na mEq/L] + glucose mg/dL/18															
Anion gap															

ABG

pH venous (V) arterial (A)															
pO_2															
pCO_2															
O^2 SAT															

Insulin

Units past h															
Route															

Intake — Fluid/metabolites

0.45% NaCl (mL) past h															
0.9% NaCl (mL) past h															
5% dextrose (mL) past h															
KCL (mEq) past h															
PO_4 (mmol) past h															
Other															

Output

Urine, *ml*															
Other															

*A–Alert D–Drowsy S–Stuporous C–Comatose

[†]D–Deep S–Shallow N–Normal

FIGURE 3-27. Flow sheet to document serial changes in laboratory/clinical values and supplementary measures during recovery from DKA. *ABG* arterial blood gases, *KCl* potassium chloride, *SAT* saturation (adapted from Kitabchi et al. [15]).

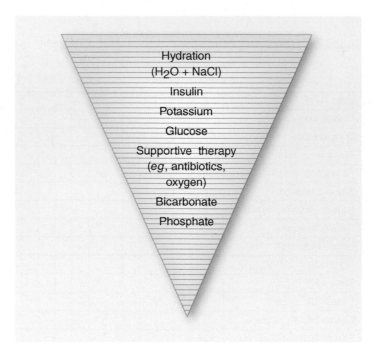

FIGURE 3-28. Treatment of hyperglycemic crisis. This figure summarizes the relative importance of various modalities of therapy. The importance of frequent monitoring of patients by health care providers cannot be overemphasized. Precipitating causes of these crises must be sought while the patient is being managed, and the patient should be referred to an educational program for prevention of future recurrence of such events. A detailed description of these works is highlighted in our recent publication summarizing 30 years of research in the pathophysiology and treatment of DKA [43] (adapted from Kitabchi et al. [44]).

References

1. Turnebum A: Of the causes and signs of acute and chronic disease, 1554. Reynolds TF, translator. London: William Pickering; 1837.

2. Faich GA, Fishbein HA, Ellis SE: The epidemiology of diabetic acidosis: a population-based study. *Am J Epidemiol* 1983, 117:551.

3. Fishbein HA, Palumbo PJ: *Acute Metabolic Complications in Diabetes.* Diabetes in America (National Diabetes Data Group). Bethesda, MD: National Institutes of Health; 1995. NIH Publication 95–1468.

4. Jain SK, McVie R, Jackson R, et al.: Effect of hyperketonemia on plasma lipid peroxidation levels in diabetic patients. *Diabetes Care* 1999, 22:1171–1175.

5. Jain SK, Kannan K, Lim G, et al.: Elevated blood interleukin-6 levels in hyperketonemic type 1 diabetic patients and secretion by acetoacetate-treated cultured U937 monocytes. *Diabetes Care* 2003, 26:2139–2143.

6. Stentz FB, Umpierrez GE, Cuervo R, Kitabchi AE: Proinflammatory cytokines, markers of cardiovascular risks, oxidative stress, and lipid peroxidation in patients with hyperglycemic crises. *Diabetes* 2004, 53:2079–2086.

7. Stentz FB, Kitabchi AE: De novo emergence of growth factor receptors in activated human CD4+ and CD8+ T-lymphocytes. *Metabolism* 2004, 53:117–122.

8. Kitabchi AE, Stentz FB, Umpierrez GE: Diabetic ketoacidosis induces in vivo activation of human T-lymphocytes. *Biochem Biophys Res Commun* 2004, 315:404–407.

9. Nyenwe EA, Loganathan RS, Blum S, et al.: Active use of cocaine: an independent risk factor for recurrent diabetic ketoacidosis in a city hospital. *Endocr Pract* 2007, 13:22–29.

10. Kitabchi AE, Umpierrez GE, Murphy MB, et al.: Management of hyperglycemic crises in patients with diabetes. *Diabetes Care* 2001, 24:131–153.

11. Umpierrez GE, Kelly JP, Navarrete JE, et al.: Hyperglycemic crises in urban blacks. *Arch Int Med* 1997, 157:669–675.

12. Kitabchi AE, Fisher JN: Insulin therapy of diabetic ketoacidosis: physiologic versus pharmacologic doses of insulin and their routes of administration. In *Handbook of Diabetes Mellitus*, vol 5. Brownlee M, ed. New York: Garland ATPM; 1981:95–149.

13. Centers for Disease Control and Prevention: Diabetes data and trends. Available at http://www.cdc.gov/diabetes/statistics/complications_national.htm. Accessed September 2009.

14. Carroll P, Matz R: Uncontrolled diabetes mellitus in adults: experience in treating diabetic ketoacidosis and hyperosmolar coma with low-dose insulin and uniform treatment regimen. *Diabetes Care* 1983, 6:579–585.

15. Kitabchi AE, Fisher JN, Murphy MB, Rumbak MJ: Diabetic ketoacidosis and the hyperglycemic hyperosmolar nonketotic state. In *Joslin's Diabetes Mellitus*, edn 13. Kahn CR, Weir GC, eds. Philadelphia: Lea & Febiger; 1994:738–770.

16. Orci L: A fresh look at the interrelationships within the islets of Langerhans. *Diabetes Research Today.* Stuttgart, Germany: Meeting of the Minkowski Prizewinners. Symposium Capri, FK Schattauer, Verlag; 1976.

17. Orci L, Baetens D, Rufener C, *et al.*: Hypertrophy and hyperplasia of somatostatin-containing D-cells in diabetes. *Proc Natl Acad Sci USA* 1976, 73:1338–1342.

18. Yoon JW, Huang SW, MacLaren NK, *et al.*: Antibody to encephalomyocarditis virus in juvenile diabetes. *N Engl J Med* 1977, 297:1235–1236.

19. Kitabchi AE, Wall BM: Diabetic ketoacidosis. *Med Clin North Am* 1995, 79:9–37.

20. Kitabchi AE, Umpierrez GE, Miles JM, Fisher JN: Hyperglycemic Crises in Adult Patients With Diabetes. American Diabetes Association position statement. *Diabetes Care* 2009, 32:1335–1343.

21. Ennis ED, Stahl EJVB, Kreisburgh RA: The hyperosmolar hyperglycemic syndrome. *Diabetes Rev* 1994, 2:115–126.

22. Munro JF, Campbell IW, McCush AC, Duncan LJ: Euglycaemic diabetic ketoacidosis. *Br Med J* 1973, 2:578–580.

23. Burge MR, Hardy KJ, Schade DS: Short-term fasting is a mechanism for the development of euglycemic ketoacidosis during periods of insulin deficiency. *J Clin Endocrinol Metab* 1993, 76:1192–1198.

24. Morris LE, Kitabchi AE: Coma in the diabetic. In *Diabetes Mellitus: Problems in Management.* Schnatz JD, ed. Menlo Park, CA: Addison-Wesley; 1982:234–251.

25. DeFronzo RA, Matsuda M, Barrett E: Diabetic ketoacidosis. A combined metabolic-nephrologic approach to therapy. *Diabetes Review* 1994, 2:209–238.

26. Miles JM, Rizza RA, Haymond MW, Gerich JE: Effects of acute insulin deficiency on glucose and ketone body turnover in man: evidence for the primacy overproduction of glucose and ketone bodies in the genesis of diabetic ketoacidosis. *Diabetes* 1980, 29:926–930.

27. McGarry JD, Woeltje KF, Kuwajima M, Foster DW: Regulation of ketogenesis and the renaissance of carnitine palmitoyl transferase. *Diab Metab Rev* 1989, 5:271–284.

28. Kitabchi AE, Rumbak MJ: Management of diabetic emergencies. *Hosp Pract* 1989, 24.129–160.

29. Myer C, Stumvolle M, Nadkarni V, *et al.*: Abnormal renal and hepatic glucose metabolism in type 2 diabetes mellitus. *J Clin Invest* 1998, 102:619–624.

30. Chupin M, Charbonnel B, Chupin F: C-peptide levels in ketoacidosis and in hyperosmolar non-ketotic diabetic coma. *Acta Diabet* 1981, 18:123–128.

31. Schade DS, Eaton RP: Dose response to insulin in man: differential effects on glucose and ketone body regulation. *J Clin Endocrinol Metab* 1977, 44:1038–1053.

32. Kitabchi AE: The escalating pandemics of obesity and sedentary lifestyle. *IAMA Bulletin* 2006, 10:27–28; 50–52.

33. Alberti KGMM, Hockaday TDR, Turner RC: Small doses of intramuscular insulin in the treatment of diabetic coma. *Lancet* 1973, 5:515–522.

34. Kitabchi AE, Ayyagari V, Guerra SMO, Medical House Staff: The efficacy of low dose versus conventional therapy of insulin for treatment of diabetic ketoacidosis. *Ann Intern Med* 1976, 84:633–638.

35. Fisher JN, Shahshahani MN, Kitabchi AE: Diabetic ketoacidosis: low-dose insulin therapy by various routes. *N Engl J Med* 1977, 297:238–247.

36. Kitabchi AE, Young RT, Sacks HS, Morris L: Diabetic ketoacidosis: reappraisal of therapeutic approach. *Ann Rev Med* 1979, 30:339–357.

37. Kitabchi AE, Murphy MB, Spencer J, *et al.*: Is a priming dose necessary in a low-dose insulin protocol for the treatment of diabetic ketoacidosis? *Diabetes Care* 2008, 31:2081–2085.

38. Fisher JN, Kitabchi AE: A randomized study of phosphate therapy in the treatment of diabetic ketoacidosis. *J Clin Endocrinol Metab* 1983, 57:177–180.

39. Matz R: Diabetic acidosis: rationale for not using bicarbonate. *NY State J Med* 1977, 76:1299–1303.

40. Morris LR, Murphy MB, Kitabchi AE: Bicarbonate therapy in severe diabetic ketoacidosis. *Ann Intern Med* 1986, 105:836–840.

41. Waldhausl W, Kleinberger G, Korn A, *et al.*: Severe hyperglycemia: effects of hydration on endocrine derangements and blood glucose concentration. *Diabetes* 1979, 28:594–5102.

42. Hillman K: Fluid resuscitation in diabetic emergencies: a reappraisal. *Intensive Care Med* 1987, 13:4–8.

43. Kitabchi AE, Umpierrez GE, Fisher JN, *et al.*: Thirty years of personal experience in hyperglycemic crises: diabetic ketoacidosis and hyperglycemic hyperosmolar coma. *J Clin Endocrinol Metab* 2008, 93:1541–1552.

44. Kitabchi AE, Matteri R, Murphy MB: Optimum insulin delivery in diabetic ketoacidosis and hyperglycemic hyperosmolar nonketotic coma. *Diabetes Care* 1982, 5:78–87.

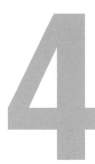

Type 1 Diabetes

Mark A. Atkinson and Jay S. Skyler

Type 1 diabetes is a chronic disorder resulting from autoimmune destruction of the insulin-producing pancreatic β cells. The epidemiologic features of type 1 diabetes are described and the possible contributions of genetics and environment to its development are illustrated. In addition, based on improved knowledge of the immunopathogenesis of this disorder, we report on work that holds promise for future interventions aimed at disease prevention and reversal.

The exact cause or causes of type 1 diabetes remain unclear [1]. It occurs most frequently in whites descended from northern Europe, with more than a 100-fold difference (or greater) observed in disease incidence rates based on geographic location. Environmental factors, such as diet, stress, and viruses, have been proposed to play a modifying, and perhaps even a primary, role in the development of type 1 diabetes. Thus, these factors may contribute to its varying prevalence. The disorder was once termed *juvenile diabetes* and was thought to occur predominantly in people under 18 years of age. However, more recent evidence suggests that the number of new cases in those over and under 30 years of age may be equal.

Susceptibility to type 1 diabetes is inherited and increased risk is associated with being a first-degree relative to a person with a diabetic proband. However, approximately 85% of new cases show no such familial lineage. The major genetic region associated with predisposition to the disease is the one that encodes genes for the highly polymorphic human leukocyte antigens (HLAs). However, over 40 other loci have been proposed as contributing from 50 to 70% of the total genetic susceptibility.

Multiple lines of evidence support the theory that type 1 diabetes has an autoimmune nature, which include: the aforementioned association with HLA; the presence of a lymphocytic infiltrate within the pancreatic islet cells, termed *insulitis*; and the expression of islet-reactive autoantibodies. Although once viewed as an acutely developing illness, today it is known that the natural history of type 1 diabetes is that of a chronic autoimmune process. In most patients, the disease exists for months to years in a preclinical, asymptomatic phase. Many improvements in our knowledge of the pathogenesis of type 1 diabetes derive from investigations of spontaneous animal models for the disease, most notably the nonobese diabetic (NOD) mouse.

Although it remains unclear which immune system component or mechanism plays the major role in β-cell destruction, most studies point toward the cellular immune system as providing a key role. Furthermore, multiple interrelated flaws in immunoregulation may underlie the failure to form a tolerance to self-antigens that results in type 1 diabetes. A large number of islet cell antigens have been associated with type 1 diabetes. Their biochemical identification has led to improved markers for predicting future cases and to the potential to design antigen-specific therapies geared toward prevention. Numerous intervention studies have been directed toward patients with new-onset type 1 diabetes (predominantly involving immunosuppression), with varying degrees of success in terms of disease reversal. Improvements have been made in the ability to predict future cases of type 1 diabetes and to assess metabolic activity. Therefore, some more recent clinical trials have sought to use alternatives, such as vitamin D, omega-3 fatty acids, and insulin, which are much less likely than immunosuppressive agents to have serious side effects, thus potentially providing a safe and effective means of disease prevention. Unfortunately, these trials have not, as yet, proven successful. However, hope exists that continuing gains in knowledge regarding the immunologic, genetic, and environmental features of this disease (described within this chapter) will eventually lead to a means to prevent as well as reverse the disorder.

Comparison of Clinical, Genetic, and Immunologic Features of Type 1 and Type 2 Diabetes		
Characteristics	Type 1	Type 2
Onset	Abrupt	Progressive
Endogenous insulin	Low to absent	Normal, elevated, or depressed
Ketosis	Common	Rare
Age at onset	Any age	Vast majority of adults
Body mass	Usually nonobese	Obese or nonobese
Treatment	Insulin	Diet, oral hypoglycemics, insulin
Family history	10%–15%	30%
Twin concordance	30%–50%	70%–90%
HLA association	HLA-DR, HLA-DQ	Unrelated
Autoantibodies	Present in most (> 85%)	Absent, except in patients with coincident type 1 diabetes

FIGURE 4-1. Comparisons of clinical, genetic, and immunologic features of types 1 and 2 diabetes. The terms applied to the subgroup of disorders known collectively as *diabetes mellitus* are useful. However, they often break down in practice owing either to confusion regarding the age at diagnosis or to an overlap or absence of the indicated features normally associated with the specific disorder. In many instances, the terms *type 1 diabetes* and *insulin-dependent diabetes* are used interchangeably, as are the terms *type 2 diabetes* and *non-insulin-dependent diabetes*. However, enthusiasm has grown for the terms *type 1 diabetes, immune-mediated diabetes* and *type 1a diabetes* to identify the forms of diabetes involving an autoimmune destruction of the insulin-producing pancreatic β cells.

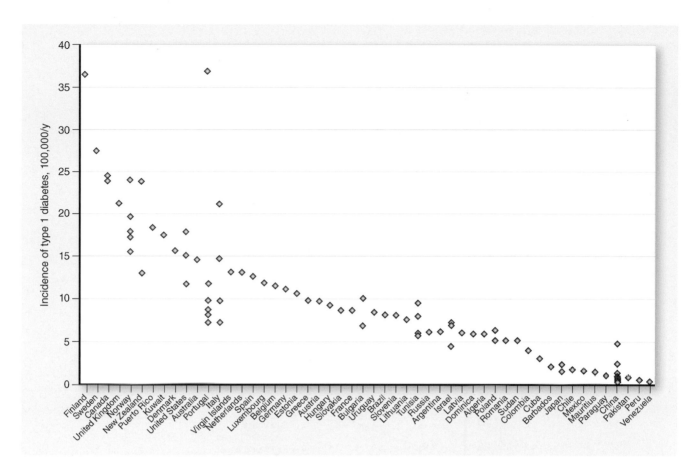

Figure 4-2. Variations in the Incidence of type 1 diabetes based on geographic location. This disease predominantly affects populations with a substantial white genetic admixture. Based on data available in the most recent time period with widespread representation among countries (i.e., 1990–1994), in Finland the incidence rate approaches 40 cases per 100,000 people per year, whereas in Korea and Mexico the rate is ~0.6 per 100,000 per year. In Europe, the incidence is highest in the northern regions and generally declines in countries that lie in the south. Exceptions do exist, especially in the case of Sardinia, Italy, where the incidence rate approximates that of Finland. Furthermore, the disease incidence in Iceland is only one-third of that of Finland. Multiple studies suggest a continuing increase in the incidence of the disease, reporting regional increases of 6–20% per decade (adapted from Karvonen et al. [2]).

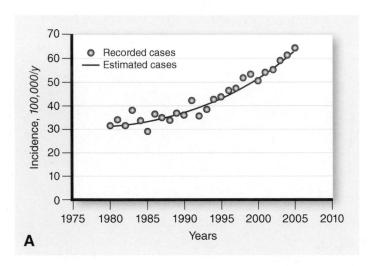

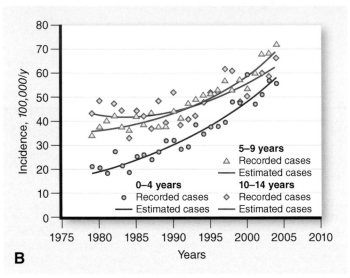

FIGURE 4-3. Striking increase in type 1 diabetes in Finland. Finland has the highest incidence of type 1 diabetes worldwide. Children with newly diagnosed type 1 diabetes in Finland who were listed on the National Public Health Institute diabetes register, Central Drug Register, and Hospital Discharge Register in 1980–2005 were included in a cohort study. (**A**) The incidence rate of type 1 diabetes diagnosed at or before 14 years of age in Finland is shown. The incidence of type 1 diabetes in Finnish children is increasing even faster than previously thought. (**B**) Time trends in age-specific incidence rates of type 1 diabetes are shown. Based on this information, the number of new cases diagnosed at or before 14 years of age will double in the next 15 years and the age of onset will be younger in children aged 0–4 years (adapted from Harjutsalo et al. [3]).

FIGURE 4-4. Seasonality of type 1 diabetes. Over the years, there have been many efforts, on a worldwide basis, to determine if there is a seasonal pattern in the clinical onset of type 1 diabetes. To address this, an analysis of the seasonality in diagnosis of type 1 diabetes was determined based on the incidence data in infants to 14-year-old children collected by the World Health Organization Diabetes Mondiale project over the period of 1990–1999. A total of 105 centers from 53 countries worldwide provided enough data for the seasonality analysis. (**A**) The geographical situation of contributing centers is shown. Only 42 centers exhibited significant seasonality ($P<0.05$) in the incidence of type 1 diabetes when the data were pooled for age and sex. These are marked by *black dots*, whereas those without significant seasonality are marked by *gray dots*. (**B**) The estimated seasonality patterns for the type 1 incidence in the centers with significant seasonality are shown, arranged by latitude. The shades of gray reflect the difference between the percentage of annual incident cases estimated to occur in each month and the percentage expected under the completely uniform month distribution, i.e., 100%/12 months=8.33% per month. *Darker shades* of *gray* correspond to annual peaks and *lighter shades* correspond to troughs. Hence, the seasonality of the incidence of type 1 diabetes in children under 15 years of age is a real phenomenon. The seasonality pattern appears to be dependent on the geographical position, at least as far as the northern/southern hemisphere dichotomy is concerned (adapted from Moltchanova et al. [4]).

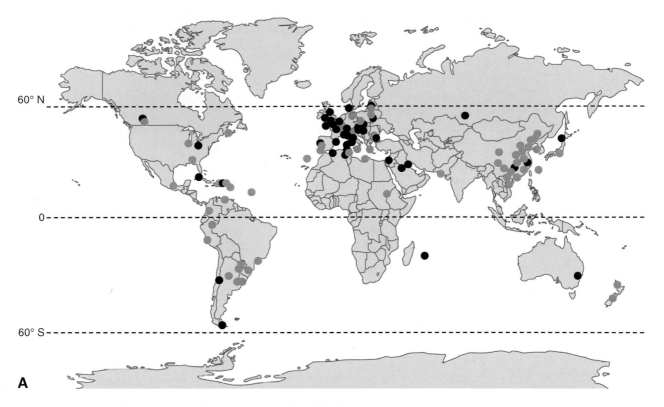

A

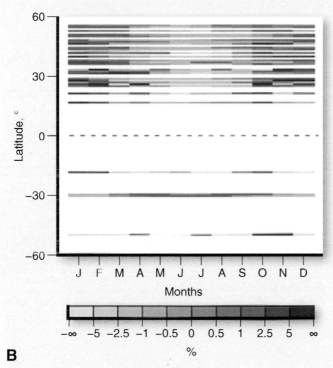

B

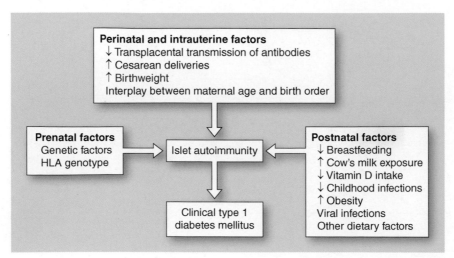

Figure 4-5. Prenatal, perinatal, and postnatal factors implicated in the development of type 1 diabetes. Apart from genetic factors, environmental factors, such as delivery by Cesarean section, high birth weight, vitamin D deficiency, viral infections, and obesity, may interact in a complex manner to cause autoimmunity and clinical type 1 diabetes (adapted from Ma and Chan [5]).

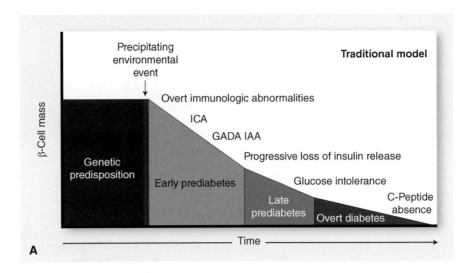

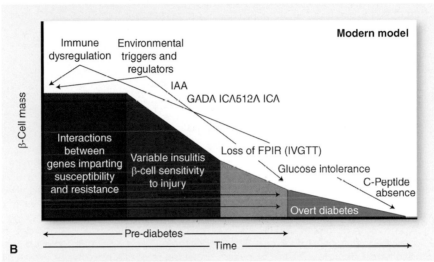

Figure 4-6. Traditional and modern models of the pathogenesis and natural history of type 1 diabetes. The traditional model (**A**) represents common features cited in numerous publications and presentations from 1986 to the present. The modern model (**B**) expands and updates the traditional model by including information gained through an improved understanding of the roles of genetics, immunology, and the environment in the natural history of type 1 diabetes. In the modern model, the natural history of type 1 diabetes that has been modeled into a disease comprises four stages. Stage 1 includes genetic susceptibility and resistance [major histocompatibility complex (MHC) and non-MHC] with intact β-cell mass. The interaction between the genetics surrounding this disorder, immune dysregulation, and environmental encounters results in stage 2, a process that in some cases can begin in the first few months or years of life. At that time, insulitis is initiated and, again, owing to a genetic predisposition that does not properly regulate immune responses, the process of β-cell destruction begins. Autoantibodies to islet cell antigens develop, marking the autoimmune disease process; however, no measurable β-cell dysfunction occurs at this stage. In stage 3, a gradual decline in β-cell mass occurs, with the slope being highly variable between persons (i.e., months to years). Incipient β-cell damage is first detectable as an abnormal intravenous glucose tolerance test (IVGTT) with a deficient first-phase insulin response (FPIR). In stage 4, an advanced degree of β-cell damage, hyperglycemia symptomatic of type 1 diabetes onset (with minimal C peptide), and exogenous insulin dependence occur. With complete β-cell destruction, the C peptide becomes undetectable and autoantibody markers of disease disappear. *IAA* insulin autoantibodies, *ICAs* islet cell cytoplasmic autoantibodies, *GADAs* glutamic acid decarboxylase autoantibodies (adapted from Atkinson and Eisenbarth [1], Eisenbarth [6], and Devendra [7]).

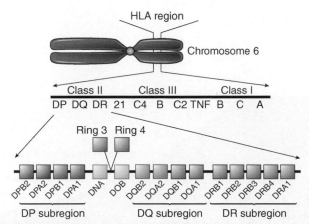

Figure 4-7. Genetics of type 1 diabetes. The HLA region is located on the short arm of chromosome 6. This region is approximately 3.5 centimorgans long and includes classes I, II, and III loci. Class I gene products (i.e., HLA-A, HLA-B, and HLA-C) are expressed on all nucleated cells and serve as the classic transplantation antigens. These proteins present antigenic peptides to CD8+ T lymphocytes. Class II gene products are restricted in expression to antigen-presenting cells (e.g., macrophages, dendritic cells, and B lymphocytes) and function to present peptides to CD4+ T lymphocytes. Class III gene products include complement proteins (e.g., B, C2, and C4) and tumor necrosis factor (TNF).

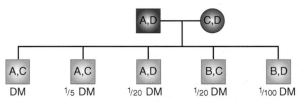

Figure 4-8. Familial risk of developing type 1 diabetes as a function of the relationship to the disease proband. The prevalence of disease (DM) is 30–50% in twins (not shown), 20% in HLA–identical siblings (patient A,C), 5% in haploidentical siblings (A,D; B,C), and 1% in nonidentical siblings (B,D).The mode of inheritance remains an enigma. Both dominant and recessive patterns of inheritance have been proposed; however, neither model adequately addresses type 1 diabetes. This line of investigation is further complicated by the potential interactions between genes and environmental factors, as well as evidence of the polygenic nature (i.e., currently over 40 additional loci) of the disorder. Furthermore, the risk of developing diabetes is higher in offspring of a father with type 1 diabetes than in offspring of a mother with the disorder. The lifetime risk for first-degree relatives is 5–8%. The probability is shown relative to the inheritance of HLA haplotypes, which is indicated as A–D.

HLA-DR and HLA-DQ Types and the Risk for Type 1 Diabetes			
Risk	**Genotype**	**Risk**	**Genotype**
Susceptible	DR3	Resistant	DR2
	DR4		DR5 (< DR2)
	DR1 (< DR3 or DR4)		DQB1*0602
	DQA1*0301		DQB1*0301
	DQA1*0501		
	DQB1*0201		
	DQB1*0302		

Figure 4-9. HLA-DR and HLA-DQ types and the risk for type 1 diabetes. Note that these associations are representative of those most often observed in whites with a strong northern Europe genetic influence. Interestingly, a variance in susceptibility and resistance of HLA types have been noted with type 1 diabetes in patients of different ethnic admixtures, especially those of Asian descent. Approximately 95% of whites with type 1 diabetes have either HLA-DR3 or HLA-DR4. However, susceptibility appears to reside predominantly in the HLA-DQ alleles under the influence of HLA-DR. Furthermore, depending on the specific haplotype inherited, risk can be modified by the presence of a strong susceptibility or resistance allele (e.g., DQB1*0602).

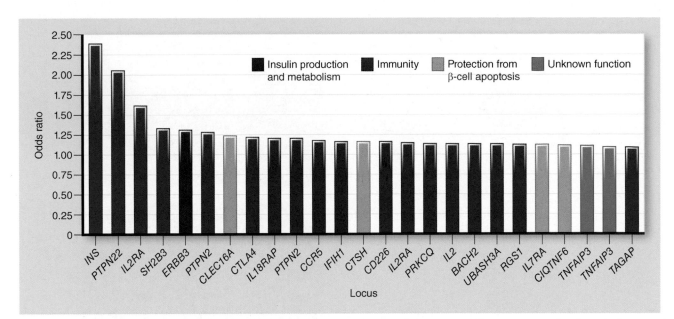

Figure 4-10. Putative functions of non-HLA-associated loci in type 1 diabetes. The y-axis indicates the best estimate of the odds ratio for risk alleles at each of the indicated loci on the basis of currently published data. Although not shown, the HLA region has a predicted odds ratio of approximately 6.8. On the x-axis, there are indicated possible candidate genes within genomic regions in which convincing associations with type 1 diabetes have been reported. On the basis of the known functions of these candidate genes, the corresponding bars in the graph depicting odds ratios have been color coded to suggest possible roles of these loci in susceptibility to type 1 diabetes. At IL2RA and TNFAIP3, there is evidence of two independent effects on risk with different odds ratios, so these loci both appear twice in the figure. An excellent resource for current information on all aspects of genes implicated in type 1 diabetes is T1DBase (see http://www.t1dbase.org) (adapted from Concannon et al. [8]).

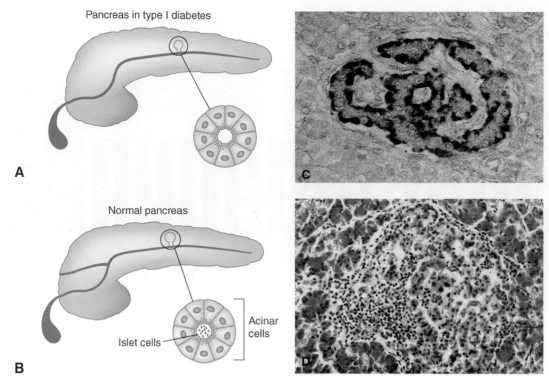

Figure 4-11. Effect of type 1 diabetes on the pancreas and islet cells. The pancreas of a person with type 1 diabetes (**A**) is often smaller and weighs less (i.e., approximately 50% of total organ weight and 30% of endocrine weight) than its healthy counterpart (**B**). This difference is a consequence of the progressive atrophy of exocrine tissue that comprises about 98% of the total pancreatic volume. (**C, D**) demonstrate the pathology of pancreatic specimens from a patient with recent-onset type 1 diabetes. (**C**) shows insulin-deficient islet stained for glucagon, somatostatin, and pancreatic polypeptide. All endocrine cells appear to have been stained, confirming the lack of β cells. (**D**) Shows insulitis, an elusive lesion to detect in the human pancreas, with only rare detection after 1 year of overt type 1 diabetes. A chronic inflammatory cell infiltrate is centered on the islet. With prolonged duration of disease, a progressive distortion of islet architecture develops, with a tendency for α and β cells to leave the islet and spread as single cells into the exocrine parenchyma. [(**C**) Immuno-alkaline phosphatase stain, ×1,150 and (**D**), hematoxylin and eosin, ×300]. [(**C, D**) from Foulis [9] with permission].

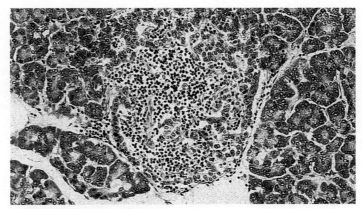

FIGURE 4-12. Islet of a patient with type 1 diabetes. An islet of a patient recently diagnosed with type 1 diabetes is shown, demonstrating a diffuse lymphocytic infiltration (insulitis) with the onset of atrophy of the islet cords (hematoxylin and eosin, ×300) (from Foulis [9] with permission).

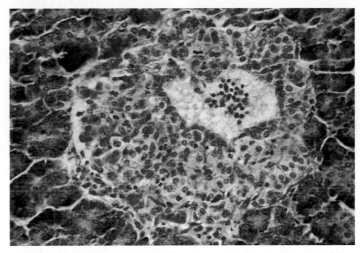

FIGURE 4-13. Pathology of a regenerating islet in the pancreas of a patient recently diagnosed with type 1 diabetes. Newly formed islet cells are derived from the epithelium of a duct. Lymphocytes are present in the lumen of the duct and, in some places, at the periphery. Evidence of such regeneration is rare in the pancreatic organs of patients with type 1 diabetes and is usually limited to those who die shortly after the disease's onset (hematoxylin and eosin, ×400) (from Foulis [9] with permission).

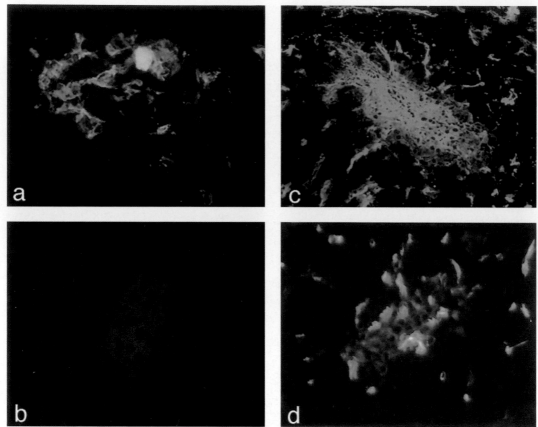

FIGURE 4-14. Cellular composition of the insulitis lesion in human type 1 diabetes before the symptomatic onset of disease. One of the earliest indicators suggestive of an autoimmune pathogenesis for type 1 diabetes was the finding of lymphocytic infiltration of the pancreatic islet cells, findings that were derived predominantly from studies of autopsy specimens from subjects after the disease's onset. Strength of animal models of the disease (e.g., BioBreeding rats, NOD mice) has been that the natural history and composition of the insulitis lesion can be analyzed at any time, including that before disease onset. Only recently have there been attempts to obtain biopsies of the pancreas in humans, of patients with recent onset diabetes and people who are at increased risk for the disease. Shown in this figure are photomicrographs of pancreatic biopsy specimens from such a study involving analysis of subjects with type 1 diabetes of recent onset. T-cell-predominant infiltration to islets and the hyperexpression of major histocompatibility complex class I antigens on islet cells were the two major findings observed in 17 of 29 recent-onset type 1 diabetic patients. CD3+ T lymphocytes (*green*) are infiltrating into the islet and insulin-containing pancreatic β cells (*red*) in one patient (*top left*), but are not observed in another patient (*bottom left*). The expression of major histocompatibility complex class I antigens were increased in one patient (*top right*), but did not increase in another patient (*bottom right*). Original magnification ×3,280 (*top left, bottom left*, and *bottom right*) and ×3,200 (*top right*) (from Imagawa et al. [10]; with permission).

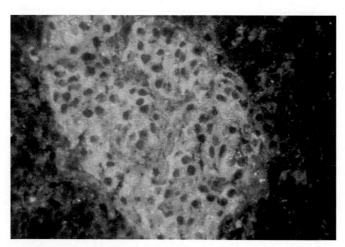

FIGURE 4-15. ICAs. Autoantibodies are present in the serum of approximately 75% of people at the onset of type 1 diabetes versus 0.4% of healthy people. The first autoantibody ascribed to type 1 diabetes, the presence of islet cell autoantibodies (ICA) is identified by indirect immunofluorescent assay using human blood group O pancreas. ICAs specific for β cells have been identified. However, the autoantibodies react with all cells within the islet, including those that secrete insulin (β cells), glucagon (α cells), somatostatin cells (δ cells), and pancreatic polypeptide (PP) cells. Autoantigens thus far ascribed to be responsible for the ICA reaction include sialoglycolipids, glutamic acid decarboxylase, and ICA512/IA-2.

Autoantibody Markers of Islet Immunity in Human Type 1 Diabetes		
Described in the 1970s	Described in the 1990s	Described in the 2000s
Islet cell cytoplasmic autoantibodies	37kd/40kD tryptic fragment autoantibodies	Carbonic anhydrase I autoantibodies
Islet cell surface autoantibodies	52kD rat insulinoma autoantibodies	Carbonic anhydrase II autoantibodies
Described in the 1980s	51kD aromatic-L-amino-acid decarboxylase autoantibodies	SOX-13 autoantibodies
64kD autoantibodies	128kD autoantibodies 152kD autoantibodies	ZnT8 autoantibodies
Carboxypeptidase-H autoantibodies	Chymotrypsinogen-related 30 kD pancreatic autoantibodies	
Heat shock protein autoantibodies	DNA topoisomerase II autoantibodies	
Insulin autoantibodies	Glucose transporter 2 autoantibodies	
Insulin receptor autoantibodies	Glutamic acid decarboxylase 65 autoantibodies	
Proinsulin autoantibodies	Glutamic acid decarboxylase 67 autoantibodies	
	Glima 38 autoantibodies	
	Glycolipid autoantibodies	
	GM2-1 islet ganglioside autoantibodies ICA512/IA-2 autoantibodies	
	IA-2 autoantibodies	
	Phogrin autoantibodies	

ZnTA—zinc transporter8 antibody.

Figure 4-16. Autoantibody markers of islet immunity in human type 1 diabetes. Since the first description of ICAs in 1974 (see Fig. 4.15), many new autoantibody markers of anti-islet immunity have been identified in patients with type 1 diabetes. In addition to their presence at disease onset, many of these markers have proved useful in identifying patients in the presymptomatic period, months to years before the clinical onset of type 1 diabetes. Of these, five markers have gained the most acceptance owing to scientific confirmation, high frequency of expression, and superior disease sensitivity and specificity, including ICA, insulin autoantibodies, glutamic acid decarboxylase, IA-2, and ZnT8 autoantibodies.

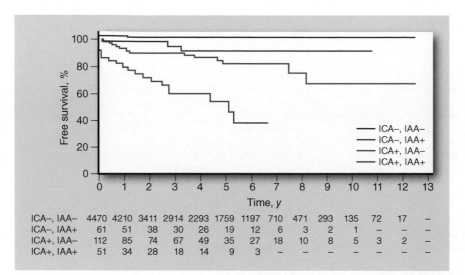

ICA–, IAA–	4470	4210	3411	2914	2293	1759	1197	710	471	293	135	72	17	–
ICA–, IAA+	61	51	38	30	26	19	12	6	3	2	1	–	–	–
ICA+, IAA–	112	85	74	67	49	35	27	18	10	8	5	3	2	–
ICA+, IAA+	51	34	28	18	14	9	3	–	–	–	–	–	–	–

FIGURE 4-17. Using autoantibodies to islet cell autoantigens to predict future cases of type 1 diabetes. This life-table analysis indicates the probability of remaining disease-free, stratified by the appearance of ICAs and IAAs in relatives of probands who have the disease. The number of relatives followed since iden-tification of the autoantibody is displayed at the bottom for each group. As can be observed, the probability of develop-ing type 1 diabetes is highest in people who have two autoan-tibodies, with approximately half of these persons developing the disease within 4 years (adapted from Krischer et al. [11]).

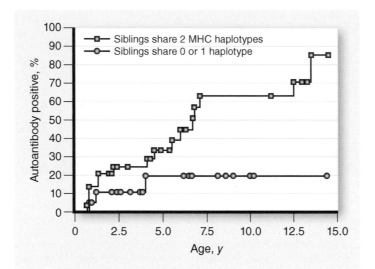

FIGURE 4-18. Extreme risk for type 1 diabetes autoimmunity. Shown are the results of life-table analysis of DR3/4-DQ2/8 siblings of patients with type 1 diabetes in the Diabetes Autoimmunity Study in the Young study followed from birth for the develop-ment of anti-islet autoantibodies. Relatives with the highest risk DR3/4-DQ2/8 HLA genotype were subdivided by the number of HLA haplotypes inherited identical by descent to their proband diabetic sibling. High-risk cohorts are DR3/4-DQ8 siblings that share both MHC haplotypes identical by descent with their proband, n=29. Low-risk cohorts are DR3/4-DQ8 siblings that do not share both MHC haplotypes identical by descent with their proband, n=19 (adapted from Aly et al. [12]).

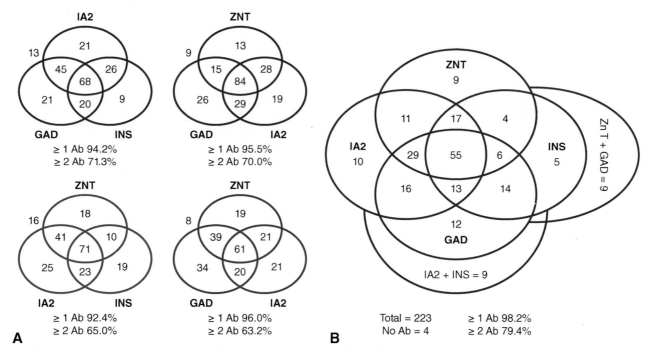

Figure 4-19. Overlapping prevalence of ZnT8A, GADA, protein tyrosine phosphatase (IA2A), and IAAs at the onset. (**A**) Seropositive individuals evaluated with the three-autoantibody standard or with ZnT8A substituted for GADA, IA2A, or IAA are shown. The ZnT8A assay incorporates both C-terminal and N/C assays in the one measurement. (**B**) Seropositive individuals evaluated with the four-autoantibody standard are shown. ZnT8As were found in 26% of T1D subjects classified as autoantibody-negative on the basis of existing markers (GADA, IA2A, IAA, and ICA). The combined measurement of ZnT8A, GADA, IA2A, and IAA raised autoimmunity detection rates to 98% at disease onset, a level that approaches what is needed to detect prediabetes in a general pediatric population (adapted from Wezlau et al. [13]) *GAD* glutamic acid decarboxylase; *INS* insulin autoantibodies.

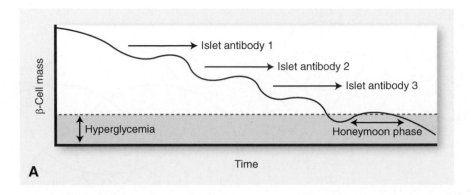

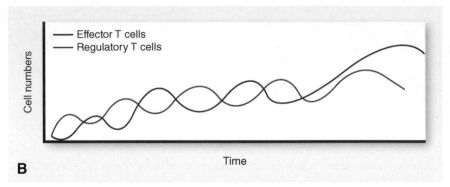

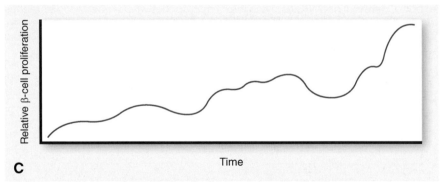

Figure 4-20. Type 1 diabetes: a relapsing remitting disease? (**A**) The nonlinear decline of β-cell mass over time is shown, as well as the development of autoantibodies that are associated with hyperglycemia; that is, the onset of type 1 diabetes. (**B**) The immunological response to type 1 diabetes is cyclic. An increase in the number of autoreactive effector T lymphocytes is controlled by an increase in the number of regulatory T lymphocytes. However, over time, a gradual disequilibrium of the cyclical behavior could occur, leading to the number of autoreactive effector T lymphocytes surpassing the number of regulatory T lymphocytes, which would no longer be capable of containing autoreactive effector T lymphocyte responses and thereby lead to a decline in pancreatic islet function. (**C**) β-cell proliferation increases in a cyclical fashion over time. This figure indirectly depicts the biological trends of

the development of type 1 diabetes, which may be attributed to the cyclical nature of the immunological events that lead to the attack or protection of β cells. Such a phenomenon is usually the result of feedback-loop mechanisms that, in the case of type 1 diabetes, could be due to misdirected effector T lymphocytes that are not easily controlled by regulatory T lymphocytes. The inflammatory process of the pancreatic islets themselves may enhance β-cell proliferation and antigenic presentation, ultimately leading to the generation of more effector and regulatory T lymphocytes. In addition, as β-cell mass declines, the pressure on each β cell to produce insulin increases, which may be sufficient to alter the recognition of β cells by the immune system and to alter their ability to regenerate and increase insulin production (adapted from Von Herrath et al. [14]).

NOD Mouse Model of Type 1 Diabetes	
Characteristic	NOD Mice
Disease onset	Spontaneous, age 13–30+ wk
Gender bias	Female predominance
Disease frequency	Strong intercolony variation. Typical rates at age 26 weeks: 50%–80% female and 20%–50% male
Clinical presentation	Hyperglycemia, mild ketosis, polydipsia, polyuria, weight loss, insulin dependency
Additional disease model	Thyroiditis, sialadenitis (Sjögren syndrome), deafness
Insulitis	Appears in nondestructive (5–12 wk) and destructive (13+ wk) phases; macrophages, dendritic cells, T and B lymphocytes, NK cells
Genetic susceptibility	MHC and > 15 non-MHC loci
Immune markers	Autoantibodies, autoreactive T cells

FIGURE 4-21. NOD model for type 1 diabetes. The NOD mouse model of type 1 diabetes is described here.

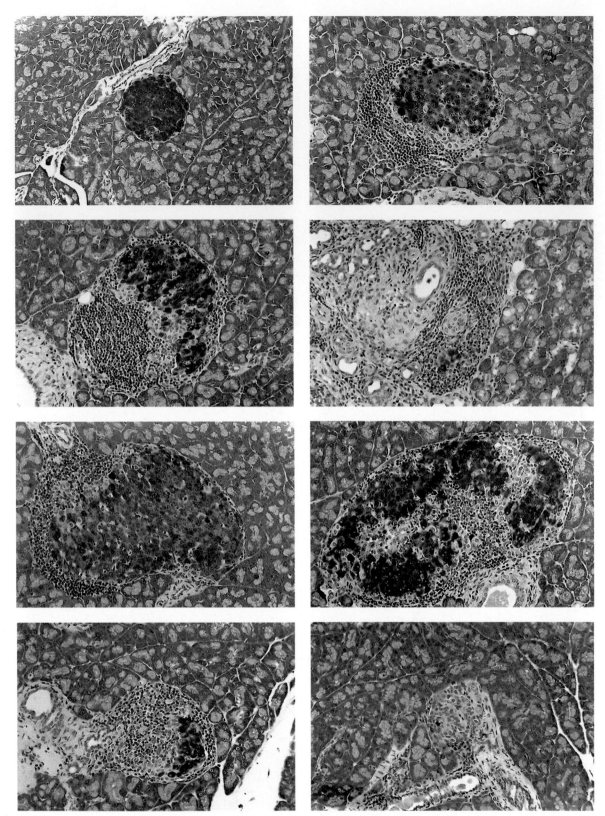

Figure 4-22. Developmental stages of the insulitis lesion in NOD mice. The pathology of pancreatic specimens from a normal islet cell devoid of leukocytic infiltrate (**A**) and at various stages of infiltration (**B–H**) are shown. Beginning at 5–7 weeks of age, leukocytes surround and eventually infiltrate the islets in increasing numbers. Beginning at 12–14 weeks of age, this early insulitis (often termed *nondestructive*) is replaced with an insulitis that destroys the insulin-producing β cells. When the islet is devoid of β cells the leukocytic infiltrate disappears, leaving only α, δ, and PP cells (**H**). (Hematoxylin eosin stain followed by counterstaining with an anti-insulin antibody and avidin-biotin, ×300) (courtesy of A. Peck, University of Florida).

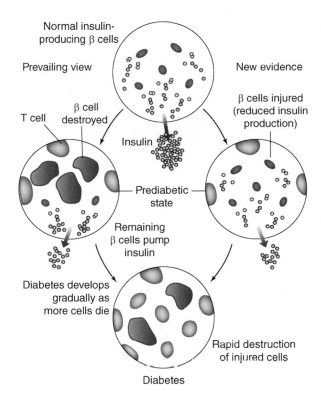

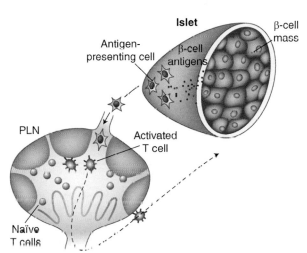

Figure 4-23. New model showing rapid destruction of β cells in the pathogenesis of type 1 diabetes. Until recently, most models assessing the rate of β-cell destruction have presumed a gradual (i.e., modified linear; see Fig. 4.6) endocrine cell loss characterized by small periods of "waxing and waning" in the immune response. However, recent investigations of NOD mice have suggested that actual β-cell destruction occurs in a very limited time period immediately before symptomatic onset. The composition of the insulitic lesion, destructive activity, or both before this event would be of nondestructive or limited destructive capacity. Although limited evidence exists for this model in terms of human type 1 diabetes, it is the subject of ongoing investigation.

Figure 4-24. Hypothetical model for the initiation of type 1 diabetes. Native T lymphocytes circulate through the blood and lymphoid organs, including pancreatic lymph nodes (PLNs). In the nodes, they encounter antigen-presenting cells (most likely mature dendritic cells) displaying on their surface MHC molecules carrying antigens in the form of peptide fragments. In this case, the antigens derive from proteins synthesized by pancreatic islet β cells, picked up (in soluble form, as cell bits or as apoptotic cells) when the antigen-presenting cells resided in the islets. A minute fraction of the naïve T lymphocytes recognize MHC molecule/β-cell antigen complexes, become activated, and then access tissues, including the pancreas, where they re-encounter cognate antigen, are reactivated, and are retained (adapted from Mathis et al. [15]).

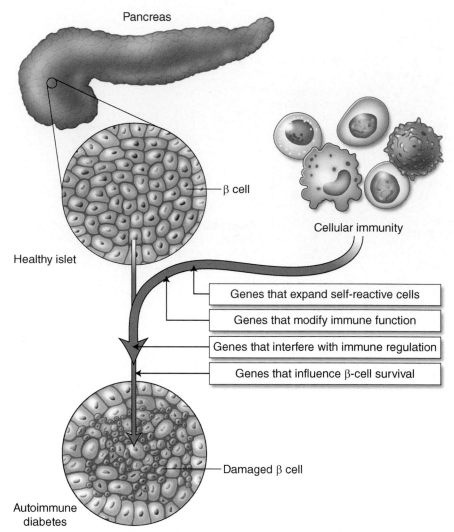

Pancreas

β cell

Cellular immunity

Healthy islet

Genes that expand self-reactive cells

Genes that modify immune function

Genes that interfere with immune regulation

Genes that influence β-cell survival

Damaged β cell

Autoimmune diabetes

FIGURE 4-25. Current data suggest that many risk loci for type 1 diabetes may exert their effects through the immune system. Within the immune response, these genes can act at multiple levels, affecting the establishment of the immune repertoire, the function of cell types in the immune system, or the regulation of cellular responses that can lead to autoimmunity (adapted from Concannon et al. [8]).

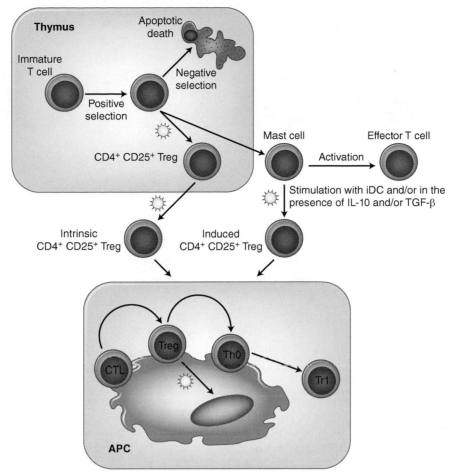

FIGURE 4-26. Two modes for the development of regulatory T lymphocytes and their modes of action in modulating the immune response. Regulatory T lymphocytes are thought to develop in two locations: from cells emanating directly from the thymus and those directed into this phenotype from the periphery. For years, immunologists have worked with a model in which positive selection ensures that only T lymphocytes bearing a relevant T-lymphocyte receptor (capable of interacting with self-MHC molecules) develop and migrate into the periphery. In contrast, negative selection eliminates T lymphocytes bearing high-affinity T-lymphocyte receptors for peptide–MHC complexes, thereby preventing these cells from entering the periphery and causing autoimmune diseases, including type 1 diabetes. More recently, studies of thymectomized mice have indicated that the thymus also generates cells that have a regulatory capacity, the so-called *T-reg cells*. T-reg cells generated in the thymus recognize self-peptide–MHC complexes with high-affinity T-lymphocyte receptors and escape the fate of apoptotic death that occurs during negative selection. These T lymphocytes differentiate into the naturally occurring (intrinsic) T-reg cells, a population phenotypically characterized by their co-expression of CD4 and CD25. Naïve cells can also differentiate into T-reg cells by a process that requires immature dendritic cells (as a source of antigen-presenting cells [APC]) during the priming of an immune response. Additionally, this process can be promoted by the cytokines interleukin-10 (IL-10) and transforming growth factor-β (TGF-β). Without such activation, these cells have the potential to generate into effector T lymphocytes. In terms of their immune-modulating capabilities, T reg cells that recognize antigen presented by APC suppress other lymphocytes; for example, cytotoxic T lymphocytes (CTLs) and helper T lymphocytes (Th cells) through a mechanism that requires direct T-lymphocyte–cell contact. In terms of their importance to type 1 diabetes formation, studies from NOD mice have supported the notion that such cells do have the capacity to prevent diabetes and, additionally, many forms of therapy capable of interrupting disease in this animal model are associated with the production of CD4+ CD25+ T lymphocytes. In humans, we and others have associated type 1 diabetes with abnormal function of these regulatory T lymphocytes. Although it is premature to speculate how these cells may in actuality influence the development of type 1 diabetes, a picture is rapidly emerging in the field that understanding T-reg function may provide important clues to aspects ranging from pathogenesis to therapy (adapted from Sutmuller et al. [16]).

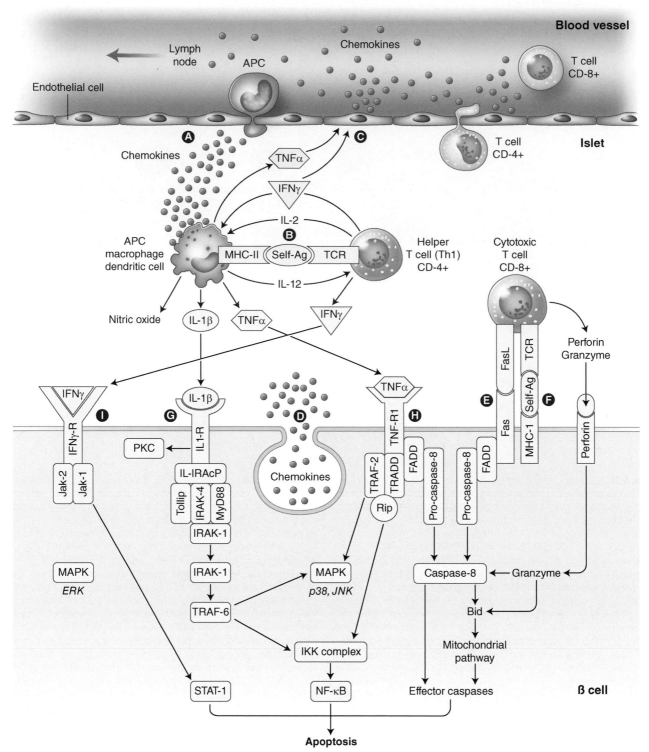

FIGURE 4-27. Schematic representation of the auto-immune attack to the β cells in type 1 diabetes. At the early stages of insulitis, activated local APCs recruit and activate CD4+ helper T lymphocytes via migration to the pancreatic lymph nodes, presentation of β-cell antigens, and release of chemokines/cytokines (*A*). CD4+ helper T lymphocytes, in turn, stimulate APC secretion of cytokines and nitric oxide (*B*). Cytokines induce the secretion of chemokines by endothelial cells, which enhance the recruitment of immune cells into the islets and, together with cytokines, activate CD8+ cytotoxic T lympho-cytes (*C*). The β cells themselves also secrete chemokines in response to viral infection or cytokines, further enhancing the recruitment and activation of immune cells (*D*). Activated CD8+ cytotoxic T lymphocytes, in turn, induce β-cell apoptosis via (*E*), the Fas pathway, and (*F*), the granzyme/perforin system. Cytokines also bind to receptors at the surface of β cells. (*G*) IL-1β activates nuclear factor (NF)-κB and the kinases PKC, p38, and JNK. (*H*) TNF-α (TNFα) activates caspase-8, NF-κB, and the MAPK p38 and JNK. (*I*) Interferon-γ (IFNγ) activates Stat-1 and the kinase ERK (adapted from Pirot et al. [17]).

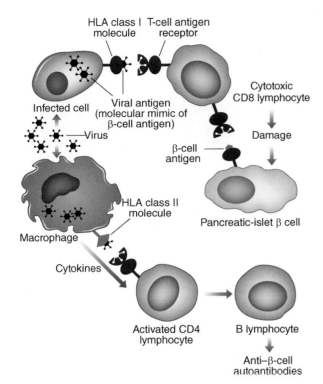

FIGURE 4-28. Potential role for viruses in the pathogenesis of type 1 diabetes: the molecular mimicry model. In this model, the autoimmune process begins after a "normal" immune response to a cell infected with a virus whose proteins share a similar sequence to that of a β-cell protein. The infected cells display processed viral antigens (by way of class I molecules) to CD8+ T lymphocytes. Macrophages having phagocytosed and processed virus present the viral peptides to CD4+ T lymphocytes through class II molecules. The CD4+ T lymphocytes amplify the actions of the CD8+ T lymphocytes to become cytotoxic effector cells that can kill β cells that express a peptide common to the viral protein. Despite exhaustive research efforts to demonstrate molecular mimicry as an underlying cause of type 1 diabetes, it remains an unproved model. Contemporary support predominantly derives from studies demonstrating an amino acid sequence similarity between β-cell proteins (e.g., glutamic acid decarboxylase and IA-2) with those of viruses (e.g., coxsackie and rotavirus) and the ability of HLA molecules with susceptibility and resistance to type I disease to bind these regions of mimicry. Studies, particularly those of cellular immunity, of the natural history of diabetes in humans and NOD mice have failed to elevate this model beyond the hypothetical stage (adapted from Atkinson and Eisenbarth [1]).

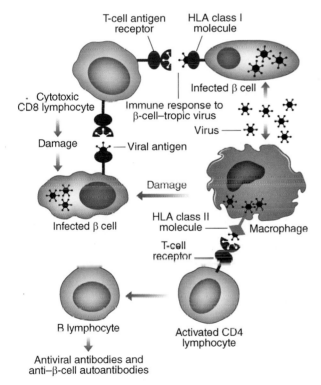

FIGURE 4-29. Potential role for viruses in the pathogenesis of type 1 diabetes: β-tropic virus–viral superantigen models. In these models, initiation of the autoimmune process follows direct viral infection of β cells or the expression in β cells of a virus acting as a superantigen. In both situations, leukocytes are recruited to pancreatic islets. Recruitment increases the release of cytokines (e.g., interferon-α) and the adhesion of leukocytes within the pancreatic islets. In the β-cell tropic model, the infected β cell is susceptible to a direct attack by antiviral cytotoxic lymphocytes. In both models, cytokines and free radicals produced by macrophages activated within the islet cells may augment the cytotoxic response to the β cells; the cytokines also recruit CD4+ T lymphocytes to the lesion. Macrophages present autoantigens derived from virus-damaged β cells, thus leading to the development of lymphocytes and autoantibodies that react with β-cell proteins. Support for both of these models exists, yet they remain hypothetical. Whereas viruses capable of β-cell destruction have been isolated from an extremely limited number of human pancreatic organs, an examination of a large number of these tissues from patients with type 1 diabetes has failed to reveal the presence of such viruses. Support for the superantigen model exists through the identification of T lymphocytes characteristic of superantigen activation in the pancreatic organs of a limited number of patients with new-onset type 1 diabetes. To date, however, no such viral superantigen has been unequivocally identified (adapted from Atkinson and Eisenbarth [1]).

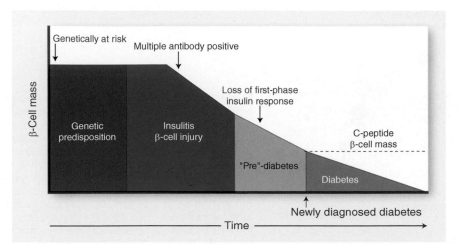

FIGURE 4-30. Potential timing of interventions to interdict the type 1 diabetes disease process. Through a combination of analyzing previous studies involving humans and animal models of type 1 diabetes (i.e., NOD mice), a model has recently emerged supporting specific "windows of opportunity" for interventions aimed at type 1 diabetes prevention. These would include studies at the time of diagnosis, aimed at preserving β-cell function as measured by C-peptide; studies in "prediabetes" in multiple autoantibody-positive individuals or in those who have lost the first-phase insulin response or have some glucose abnormality already, to prevent diabetes; and studies in those genetically at risk, to prevent autoimmunity. Key principles to this model include that of matching risk versus reward (i.e., more benign therapies in newborns in which the progression to type 1 diabetes is less certain) and the utilization of agents when they may provide the most therapeutic effectiveness (adapted from Skyler [18]).

Results of Studies to Prevent Type 1 Diabetes in People at Increased Risk for the Disease				
	DPT-1 parenteral insulin	DPT-1 oral insulin	ENDIT nicotinamide	DIPP nasal insulin
	At 5years	At 5 years	At 4 years	At 4 years
Control	61%	35%	24%	~50%
Treated	58%	33%	27%	~50%

FIGURE 4-31. Results of three large clinical trials designed to prevent the development of type 1 diabetes in humans. The Diabetes Prevention Trial (DPT-1) addressed this goal through the administration of parenteral and oral insulin, whereas the European Nicotinamide Diabetes Intervention Trial (ENDIT) utilized nicotinamide. Both of these studies analyzed relatives of patients with type 1 diabetes and, through a combination of genetic, immunologic, and metabolic markers, identified subjects who were at increased risk of developing the disease. The Type 1 Diabetes Prediction and Prevention (DIPP) study investigated whether nasal insulin reduced the incidence of type 1 diabetes in children from the general population, with genotypes and autoantibodies increasing the risk of developing the disease. Each trial posed the question of whether the given therapy could delay the onset of type 1 diabetes. In the case of DPT-1, based on the degree of risk, high or intermediate, study subjects were placed onto parenteral or oral insulin, respectively. More detailed results of the DPT-1 parenteral insulin trial are shown in Fig. 4.32 (adapted from Skyler and Marks [19]).

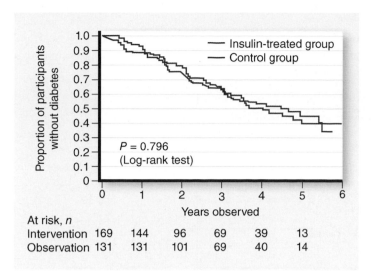

At risk, n
Intervention 169 144 96 69 39 13
Observation 131 131 101 69 40 14

Figure 4-32. Kaplan–Meier curves showing the proportion of subjects without type 1 diabetes during the Diabetes Prevention Trial-1 parenteral insulin trial, by treatment assignment. The insulin-treated group is depicted by the *pink line*, whereas the control group is indicated by the *purple line*. There is no difference between the two curves in terms of the rate of progression to overt type 1 diabetes. The proportion of subjects without type 1 diabetes is indicated on the y-axis, whereas the x-axis depicts the number of at risk subjects (intervention, *top*; observation, *bottom*) observed for a given duration in years (adapted from Diabetes Prevention Trial Type 1 Diabetes Study Group [20]).

Interventions Studied in Human Type 1 Diabetes
New-onset diabetes to preserve β-cell function
Completed studies with a suggestion of metabolic benefit
Cyclosporin
Azathioprine with glucocorticoids
Anti-CD5 monoclonal antibody with ricin-A chain (immunotoxin)
Insulin-intensive therapy
Nicotinamide
Plasmapheresis
Anti-CD3 monoclonal antibody
GAD vaccine
Anti-CD20 monoclonal antibody (rituxamab)
Completed studies without benefit
Bacille Calmette-Guérin
Intravenous immune globulin
Oral insulin
Oral interferon
Mycophenolate mofetil alone and with anti-CD25 antibody (daclizumab)
Insulin B9-23 altered peptide ligand
Heat-shock protein-60 p277 peptide (+/–)
Vitamin D in adults
Diazoxide
Studies in progress
Anti-CD3 (repeated doses)
Thymoglobulin
IL-2 plus rapamycin (sirolimus)
Abatacept (CTLA4-Ig)
Anakinra
Canakinumab (Anti-IL1β)
Intensive metabolic control
Antibody-positive relatives at risk
Completed studies without benefit
Parenteral insulin
Nicotinamide
Oral Insulin (except suggested benefit in a subgroup)
Nasal insulin
Studies in progress
Oral insulin
Anti-CD3
Newborns or neonates to prevent autoimmunity and diabetes
Studies in progress
Omission of cow milk protein
Omega-3 fatty acids

Figure 4-33. Studied interventions. Interventions that have been studied, or are being studied, in human type 1 diabetes, at the various stages discussed in Fig. 4.30, are presented here.

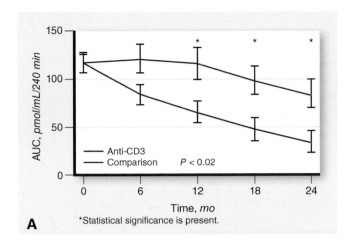

A

*Statistical significance is present.

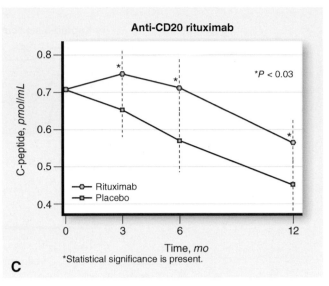

C

*Statistical significance is present.

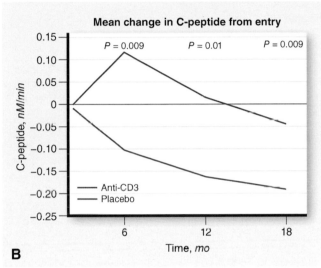

B

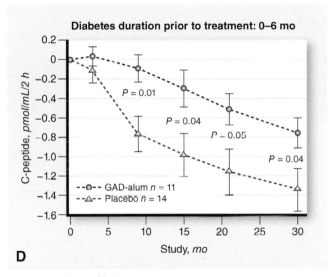

D

FIGURE 4-34. Results of recent intervention studies. The results of recent intervention studies in new-onset type 1 diabetes show beneficial effects, but nonetheless a progressive decline of β-cell function (measured by C-peptide). These results include an intervention with the anti-CD3 monoclonal antibodies teplizumab (**A**) [21] and otelixizumab (**B**) [22], the anti-CD20 monoclonal antibody rituximab (**C**) [23], and a GAD vaccine (**D**) [24]. *AUC* area under the curve.

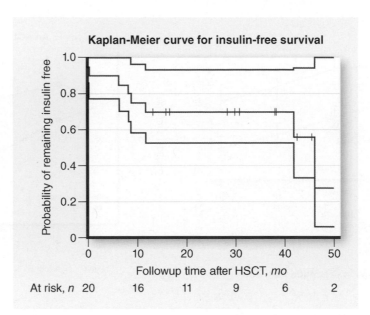

Figure 4-35. Results: insulin-free survival of patients with type 1 diabetes. One study, which unfortunately did not include a control group, showed prolonged insulin-free survival of subjects with type 1 diabetes and was conducted in Brazil. In this study, patients were treated with high-dose immunosuppression – with cyclophosphamide and antithymocyte globulin – followed by rescue with autologous nonmyeloablative hematopoietic stem cell transplantation (data from Couri et al. [25] and Voltarelli et al. [26]).

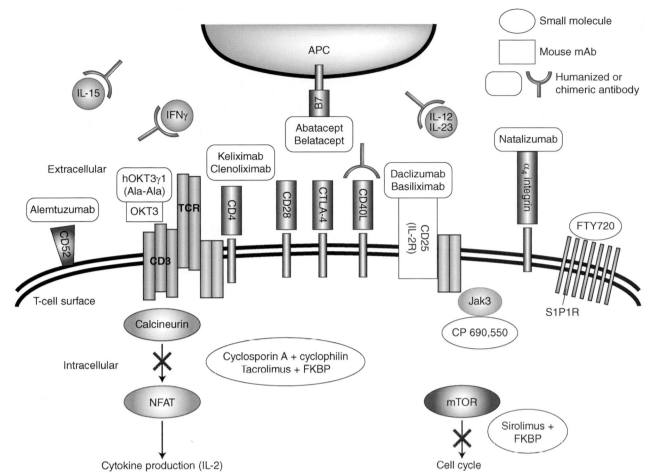

FIGURE 4-36. Molecular targets that modulate T-lymphocyte function. Conceptually, T-lymphocyte-directed therapy can be thought of in several ways. First, polyclonal antibodies, such as antithymocyte globulin or OKT3 simply delete T lymphocytes. TCR-mediated signals are inhibited by classical drugs, such as cyclosporin A and tacrolimus (FK506), which inhibit the phosphatase calcineurin. That in turn blocks the activation of NFAT. However, NFAT and calcineurin are not T-lymphocyte-specific factors and those drugs are toxic beyond immunosuppression. Cytokines regulate all aspects of T-lymphocyte development and differentiation, and so are also important targets. At present, mAbs to IL-15, IL-12, IL-23, and IFNγ are being studied, and mAbs to IL-2 receptor α (CD25) are approved for use in transplant rejection. The small molecule CP 690,550 inhibits Jak3 and blocks signaling via IL-2 and related cytokines. Sirolimus also blocks cytokine signaling, but its target, mammalian target of rapamycin (mTOR), is a ubiquitous molecule. Newer mAbs have been devised, which target costimulatory molecules and adhesion molecules, such as CD28 and α4 integrin. Chemokines are critical in lymphocyte trafficking and, thus, represent logical targets. FTY720 is an agonist of the sphingosine 1-phosphate type 1 receptor (S1P1R), which, like chemokine receptors, is a seven-transmembrane, G protein-coupled receptor. FTY720 interferes with egress of lymphocytes from lymphoid tissues. *APC* antigen-presenting cell, *IL-2R* IL-2 receptor, *FKBP* FK506-binding protein, *CD40L* CD40 ligand (adapted from Liu et al. [27]).

References

1. Atkinson M, Eisenbarth G: Type 1 diabetes: new perspectives on disease pathogenesis and treatment. *Lancet* 2001, 358:221–229.

2. Karvonen M, Viik M, Moltchanova E *et al.*: *Diabetes Care* 2000, 23:1516–1526.

3. Harjutsalo V, Sjoberg L, Tuomilehto J: Time trends in the incidence of type 1 diabetes in Finnish children: a cohort study. *Lancet* 2008, 371:1777–1782.

4. Moltchanova EV, Schreier N, Lammi N, Karvonen M: Seasonal variation of diagnosis of type 1 diabetes mellitus in children worldwide. *Diabetic Med* 2009, 26:673–678.

5. Ma RCW, Chan JCN: Incidence of childhood type 1 diabetes: a worrying trend. *Nat Rev Endocrin* 2009, 5:529–530.

6. Eisenbarth GS: Type 1 diabetes mellitus. A chronic autoimmune disease. *N Engl J Med* 1986, 314:1360–1368.

7. Devendra D, Liu E, Eisenbarth GS: Type 1 diabetes: recent developments. *BMJ* 2004, 328:750–754.

8. Concannon P, Rich SS, Nepom GT: Genetics of type 1A diabetes. *N Engl J Med* 2009, 360:1646–1654.

9. Foulis AK: In *Textbook of Diabetes*, vol 1. Edited by Pickup J, Williams G. Oxford, UK: Blackwell Scientific; 1991.

10. Imagawa A, Hanafusa T, Tamura S, *et al.*: Pancreatic biopsy as a procedure for detecting in situ autoimmune phenomena in type 1 diabetes: close correlation between serological markers and histological evidence of cellular autoimmunity. *Diabetes* 2001, 50:1269–1273.

11. Krischer JP, Schatz D, Riley WJ, *et al.*: Insulin and islet cell autoantibodies as time-dependent covariates in the development of insulin-dependent diabetes. *J Clin Endocrinol Metab* 1993, 77:743–749.

12. Aly TA, Ide A, Jahromi MM, *et al.*: Extreme genetic risk for type 1A diabetes. *Proc Natl Acad Sci U S A* 2006, 38:14074–14079.

13. Wezlau JM, Frisch LM, Gardner TJ, *et al.*: Novel antigens in type 1 diabetes: the importance of ZnT8. *Curr Diab Rep* 2009, 9:105–112.

14. Von Herrath M, Sanda S, Herold K: Type 1 diabetes as a relapsing-remitting disease? *Nat Reviews Immunol* 2007, 7:998–994.

15. Mathis D, Vence L, Benoist C: Beta-cell death during progression to diabetes. *Nature* 2001, 414:729–798.

16. Sutmuller RPM, Offringa R, Melief CJM: Revival of the regulatory T-lymphocyte: new targets for drug development. *Drug Discov Today* 2004, 9:310–317.

17. Pirot P, Cardozo AK, Eizirik DL: Mediators and mechanisms of pancreatic beta cell death in type 1 diabetes. *Arq Bras Endrocrinol Metab* 2008, 52:156–165.

18. Skyler JS: Immunotherapy for interdicting the type 1 diabetes disease process. In *Textbook of Diabetes*, edn 3. Edited by Pickup J, Williams G. Oxford, UK: Blackwell; 2003:74-1–74-12.

19. Skyler JS, Marks JB: Immune intervention. In *Diabetes Mellitus: A Fundamental and Clinical Text*, edn 3. Edited by LeRoith D, Taylor SI, Olefsky JM. Philadelphia: Lippincott Williams & Wilkins; 2004:701–709.

20. Diabetes Prevention Trial Type 1 Diabetes Study Group: Effects of insulin in relatives of patients with type 1 diabetes mellitus. *N Engl J Med* 2002, 346:1685–1691.

21. Herold KC, Hagopian W, Auger J, *et al.*: Anti-CD3 monoclonal antibody in new onset type 1 diabetes mellitus. *N Engl J Med* 2002, 346:1692–1698.

22. Keymeulen B, Vandemeulebroucke E, Ziegler AG, *et al.*: Insulin needs after CD3-antibody therapy in new-onset type 1 diabetes. *N Engl J Med* 2005, 352:2598–2608.

23. Pescovitz MD, Greenbaum CJ, Krause-Steinrauf H, *et al.*: Rituximab, B-lymphocyte depletion and preservation of beta-cell function. *N Engl J Med* 2009, 361:2143–2152.

24. Ludvigsson J, Faresjö M, Hjorth M, *et al.*: GAD treatment and insulin secretion in recent-onset type 1 diabetes. *N Engl J Med* 2008, 359:1909–1920.

25. Couri CE, Oliveira MC, Stracieri AB, *et al.*: C-peptide levels and insulin independence following autologous nonmyeloablative hematopoietic stem cell transplantation in newly diagnosed type 1 diabetes mellitus. *JAMA* 2009, 301:1573–1579.

26. Voltarelli JC, Martinez ED, Burt RK: Autologous nonmyeloablative hematopoietic stem cell transplantation in newly diagnosed type 1 diabetes mellitus. Author's reply. *JAMA* 2009, 302:624–625.

27. Liu EH, Siegal RM, Harlan DH, O'Shea JJ: T-lymphocyte-directed therapies: lessons learned and future prospects. *Nat Immunol* 2007, 8:25–30.

5 Management of Type 1 Diabetes

Irl B. Hirsch and Jay S. Skyler

The treatment of type 1 diabetes has a relatively short history; the disease was uniformly fatal before the discovery of insulin in 1922. It is interesting to note that by the late 1920s, it was observed that insulin tended to make "fat people fatter"; however, it was not until the mid-1930s that some basic differences were noted between the two major types of diabetes. Although insulin therapy has prevented certain death in patients with type 1 diabetes, it brought on a new era of problems not formally appreciated. This "era of complications" was notable for the grim realization that about half the patients developed proliferative diabetic retinopathy and between 30 and 40% developed diabetic nephropathy. One of the most important scientific debates of the twentieth century was the relationship between diabetic complications and glycemic control. By the 1980s, new tools, such as home self-monitoring of blood glucose (SMBG), assessment of integrated glycemic control by glycated hemoglobin HbA$_{1c}$ (A$_{1c}$), continuous subcutaneous insulin infusion (CSII), and human insulins, made it possible to attempt near-normal glycemic control. The announcement of the results of the Diabetes Control and Complications Trial (DCCT) in 1993 ended the debate by demonstrating a strong relationship between blood glucose control and the microvascular and neuropathic complications of type 1 diabetes. Since then, the goals have been to further improve our tools for managing type 1 diabetes and to develop new strategies for treating diabetes-related complications once they develop.

Rationale for Improved Glycemic Control

Several small studies in the 1980s suggested that "intensive therapy" with improved glycemic control could reduce the risk of developing the microvascular complications of diabetes. Despite this long-standing debate dating back decades, it was not until the 1980s that this question could be adequately addressed. During the early part of that decade, there was a dramatic change in the management tools for type 1 diabetes. SMBG, A$_{1c}$, purified insulins, and CSII therapy all were being routinely (although not necessarily widely) used in the management of this patient population.

The landmark study that ended all the debate was the DCCT [1]. Starting in 1982 and ending in 1993, this study of 1,441 subjects addressed the fundamental question regarding the relationship between glycemic control and microvascular and neuropathic complications. Follow-up examinations occurred after a mean of 6.5 years. The DCCT actually asked two questions: Does an intensive therapy program prevent the appearance of microvascular disease (primary prevention), and does this therapy retard the progression of early preexisting disease (secondary intervention)? *Intensive therapy* was defined as either a multiple daily injection regimen (at least three injections per day) or CSII, in combination with a minimum of premeal and bedtime SMBG measurements, monthly clinic visits, and psychological and nutritional support.

This intensive therapy resulted in a mean A$_{1c}$ difference of about 2% over the course of the study. Compared with conventional therapy for both primary prevention and

J.S. Skyler (ed.), *Atlas of Diabetes: Fourth Edition*,
DOI 10.1007/978-1-4614-1028-7_5, © Springer Science+Business Media, LLC 2012

secondary intervention, intensive therapy reduced the development of both early and later manifestations of diabetic retinopathy, microalbuminuria, clinical grade proteinuria, and peripheral and autonomic neuropathy. However, in this young population of subjects with type 1 diabetes, the reduction in cardiovascular events – which were few – did not reach statistical significance. Intensive therapy did result in a threefold increased risk of severe hypoglycemia (requiring the assistance of another person) and weight gain. No cognitive impairment was found in those with severe hypoglycemia. It is important to note that the DCCT ended before the introduction of insulin analogues.

Subjects from the DCCT have had continued follow-up in a study known as the Epidemiology of Diabetes Interventions and Complications (EDIC). After the formal DCCT was completed, the two treatment groups had a merging of A_{1c} levels to about 8%. Despite that, there appeared to be a "metabolic memory" in that over the next 12 years, the progression of retinopathy, nephropathy, and even carotid artery intimal thickness was reduced in the group previously randomly assigned to receive intensive therapy [2, 3]. Then, in 2005, the EDIC investigators reported a 57% reduction in cardiovascular events in the group originally assigned to intensive therapy [4]. Although the mechanism of "metabolic memory" is unknown because the DCCT population initiated the study with disease durations of about 2.5 years (primary prevention) and 8.7 years (secondary intervention), it is clear that early and aggressive glycemic management is critical. As a consequence, after three decades of type 1 diabetes, there was a dramatic reduction in complications [5].

Available Forms of Insulin

When insulin therapy became available in the 1920s, preparations were somewhat crude, required reasonably large volumes, and were relatively short acting. Therefore, most patients receiving insulin were treated with three or more daily injections. In the 1930s and 1940s, protein chemists modified the existing soluble (regular) insulin with the goal of prolonging its duration of action, thus making insulin therapy less cumbersome. The result was the development of protamine zinc insulin, neutral protamine Hagedorn (NPH) or isophane insulin, globin insulin, and the Lente series of insulins (Semilente, Lente, and Ultralente) [6]. By the 1960s, several clinicians realized that convenience resulted in a deterioration of glycemic control, and the classical "split mix" program of twice-daily NPH and regular insulin was popularized [7]. Although this insulin regimen was an improvement in physiologic insulin replacement, it still was far from perfect.

The quantity of insulin impurities declined, and human insulin was introduced in 1984 [8]. Although the introduction of purified human insulin did not alter the treatment of diabetes as much as some had predicted, it provided the first example of recombinant DNA technology having a major impact on the pharmacologic treatment of a disease.

Traditionally, insulin has been classified based on its pharmacokinetic characteristics as short, intermediate, or long acting. By understanding pharmacokinetics (the appearance of insulin in the blood) and pharmacodynamics (the time of insulin action on blood glucose levels), it is quite clear that the traditional classification strategy based on time actions is problematic. A better way to conceptualize insulin is by considering its physiologic role. *Basal insulin* is the insulin injected to suppress hepatic glucose production overnight and between meals. *Prandial insulin* (also known as "bolus" or mealtime insulin) is insulin injected to minimize glucose excursions after food ingestion. Classifying insulin in this way, it is clear why the older nomenclature is problematic. The only two standard insulins available today – regular and NPH – because of their peaks and long durations of action have both prandial and basal components [9]. The implications of the pharmacodynamics of these insulins are important to appreciate. Regular insulin, for example, has a pharmacodynamic peak long after carbohydrate is consumed, but more importantly the long "tail" of action of regular insulin necessitates that either a snack or meal be consumed after the previous meal is digested. NPH insulin, on the other hand, has a peak that traditionally has been used for lunchtime insulin coverage; however, its insulin action profile, especially when combined with regular insulin, causes the two preparations to overlap (also termed *insulin stacking*), aggravating the need for frequent snacks to avoid hypoglycemia.

Although the evolution of multiple daily injections and even CSII improved some of the problems with insulin stacking, the real seminal change in the treatment of type 1 diabetes occurred with the introduction of insulin analogues. The three prandial insulin analogues—insulin lispro, insulin aspart, and insulin glulisine—more selectively match prandial insulin requirements. The two basal insulins—insulin glargine and insulin detemir—are true basal insulin preparations in that if they are dosed correctly, there is no requirement for additional snacking. On the other hand, for someone using both prandial and basal analogues, snacking usually requires an additional injection of prandial insulin.

The major advantage of the analogues compared with standard insulins is that less hypoglycemia has been consistently seen with all the analogues. Although some of this observation is related to the fact that each analogue has a single function, in general these insulins also vary less in their absorption compared with their standard insulin comparators [10].

There is one other insulin category: "correction dose" or supplemental insulin [9]. This type of insulin is used to correct hyperglycemia regardless of the time in relation to the meal, although it is usually provided with the prandial insulin. There have been no studies comparing rapid-acting insulin analogues (lispro, aspart, glulisine) with regular insulin for correction dose insulin, although the analogues would be expected to correct the hyperglycemia more quickly and provide less risk of insulin stacking than regular insulin.

The goal of modern insulin replacement in type 1 diabetes is to replace physiologic insulin to maintain near-normal glycemia. Current goals for this approach include maintaining A_{1c} below 7% with preprandial and postprandial glucose targets of 90–130 mg/dL and less than 180 mg/dL, respectively [11].

One strategy for achieving these goals is to provide insulin injections in a physiologic replacement manner.

There are two components to doing this: (1) replacing basal insulin, usually with insulin glargine or insulin detemir and (2) providing prandial insulin, usually with insulin lispro, insulin aspart, or insulin glulisine. Occasionally, one may opt to use a standard insulin instead of an analogue. This approach might include using regular insulin at lunchtime for school-aged children to provide greater insulinemia for a late afternoon snack; using regular insulin for meals low in carbohydrate and high in protein and fat, for which prolonged action is desired; or adding a dose of bedtime NPH when significant early-morning insulin resistance is present (the "dawn phenomenon"). Others prefer to use regular insulin as the prandial insulin in situations where gastric emptying is prolonged, such as in patients using pramlintide (see later) or those with gastroparesis.

Another strategy for physiologic insulin replacement to achieve the glycemic goals is CSII. Insulin pump therapy has been an option since 1980, and it has slowly gained in popularity. Basal insulin and prandial insulin both are provided by a subcutaneous pump connected to a catheter, which is changed every 2 or 3 days. Not surprisingly, the rapid-acting insulin analogues have resulted in better glycemic control than regular insulin when used in pumps [12]. A meta-analysis comparing CSII with multiple injections in 12 randomized, controlled trials showed an improvement in A_{1c} with CSII [13]. The authors concluded that even this relatively small improvement (equivalent to an A_{1c} of 0.51%) significantly reduces the risk of microvascular complications. The major risks of CSII include unexplained hyperglycemia/ketoacidosis and skin infection; both can be minimized with strict attention to detail.

It must be emphasized that for any insulin regimen to be successful, sufficient SMBG is required. Specific recommendations are difficult because the ideal frequency of blood glucose testing has never been studied. At the least, before-meal and bedtime SMBG is recommended for type 1 diabetes, but between-meal tests also are suggested, particularly if it is unknown how much insulin should be injected for a food not usually consumed or to confirm that adequate insulin was given for the treatment of premeal hyperglycemia. Surveys of both pediatric and nonpediatric diabetes centers show that SMBG typically is performed an average of six times daily.

The other critical factor required to ensure success is a basic understanding of prandial insulin dosing for meals. Trial and error based on SMBG is attempted by some, but a more quantitative strategy often proves more successful. This approach is best accomplished with the assistance of a nutritionist, and several methods have been tested. One popular method is "carbohydrate counting." In this approach, carbohydrate is quantified, either by estimating the number of grams of carbohydrates in a portion of food (e.g., one piece of bread has 15 g of carbohydrate) or noting how much carbohydrate is present in a serving based on package information. Many patients learn this by actually weighing their food during their initial education. The *carbohydrate ratio*, then, refers to the number of grams of carbohydrate required for 1 U of insulin. For example, a carbohydrate ratio of 1/15 refers to one unit of insulin injected for every 15 g of carbohydrate. The ratio can then be altered based on frequent SMBG results.

New Tools for Managing Type 1 Diabetes

Although there have been tremendous advances with the development of insulin analogues, several new developments are further improving the management of type 1 diabetes.

The first new tool is the development of the analogue of the naturally occurring hormone amylin, called pramlintide [14]. Native amylin is cosecreted with insulin and appears to improve glycemia by inhibiting the paradoxic increase in postprandial glucagon concentrations that occurs in type 1 diabetes. It also appears to have a direct effect on modulating gastric emptying. Thus, the net effect is a reduction of postprandial hyperglycemia. Small but consistent weight loss has been observed with pramlintide.

There also is continued interest in the development of pulmonary inhaled insulin. This mode of delivery eliminates the need for prandial injections and may be used to replace these injections in patients with type 1 diabetes, without deterioration in glycemic control [15]. Although the first pulmonary insulin product was not commercially successful and was removed from the market, a newer product still in development has two potential beneficial features compared with the discontinued product: (1) a simpler, smaller delivery system and (2) more rapid onset of action with the potential to better control postprandial glycemia [16].

Another goal of new technology in type 1 diabetes is the development of a real-time continuous glucose monitor (CGM). Continuous glucose monitoring devices, the first of which was introduced in 2000 [17], measure interstitial fluid glucose from a subcutaneous glucose sensor. Initially, glucose readings could be reviewed only retrospectively after downloading them to a computer. In the mid 2000s, real time CGM was introduced [18]. This approach uses the same principle of interstitial fluid glucose transmitting a signal based on the degree of glycemia, only now the results are almost real time.

The introduction of CGM is quickly changing the standard of type 1 diabetes therapies. The Juvenile Diabetes Research Foundation (JDRF) Continuous Glucose Monitoring Study Group has shown the benefit of CGM in improving glycemic control (A_{1c} levels) [19] and reducing hypoglycemic exposure in patients already well-controlled [20]. CGM may be used with a multiple daily injection regimen or integrated with an insulin pump [21]. However, the technology is not a panacea because patient success is still based on behavioral changes; the JDRF study demonstrated that improvement was seen only when patients wore their CGM devices consistently [22]. The accuracy and size of the devices likely will further improve acceptability and usage. Presumably, CGM will continue to grow in popularity as more patients and providers appreciate the benefits.

Conclusions

The changes in the management of type 1 diabetes in a relatively short period have been dramatic. Less than 100 years ago, children diagnosed with diabetes rarely lived more than a few months, and those who lived longer had a poor quality of life. The current tools allow most patients to live relatively normal lives, although teaching both patients and providers how to use these tools has proven to be a challenge. The translation of the DCCT has not been as smooth as was originally predicted for several reasons; most importantly, the tools of that era were still relatively crude by today's standards. On the other hand, with the introduction of insulin analogues, improved insulin pumps, and CGM devices, the future for type 1 diabetes treatment appears even brighter, and the practical goal for both patients and providers is to extrapolate the research and use the new tools as efficiently as possible so that the morbidity and early mortality of this once fatal disease can be eliminated.

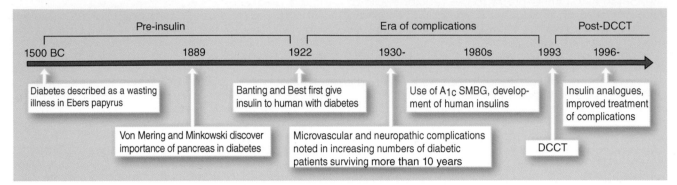

Figure 5-1. The three eras in the history of type 1 diabetes. The history of type 1 diabetes can be divided into three distinct eras. In the preinsulin era, diabetes was usually fatal within 1–2 years of its development. In the era of complications, acute mortality was almost eliminated but chronic complications were first noted. The DCCT [1] proved that intensive diabetes therapy with a multidisciplinary team, frequent SMBG, and an insulin regimen consisting of either multiple injections or CSII could dramatically reduce the appearance and progression of microvascular and neuropathic complications. In the post-DCCT era, newer tools have been developed to manage hyperglycemia as well as its complications.

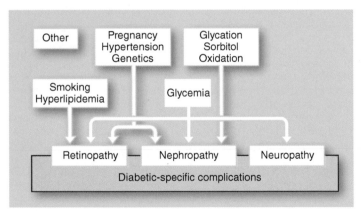

Figure 5-2. Pathogenesis of complications. The specific mechanism or mechanisms that cause the microvascular and neurologic complications of diabetes remain unidentified. Several obvious contributing factors, however, have been noted in epidemiologic studies, animal models, and interventional studies. Although no single mechanism likely explains the myriad complications, glycemia appears to be an underlying cause for all of them, as demonstrated in interventional studies, such as the DCCT [1]. It is probable that different clinical stages of specific complications – for example, nonproliferative and proliferative retinopathy – have different causes. Genetic factors likely contribute to the risk of both retinopathy [23] and nephropathy [24]. Hypertension and pregnancy are well-known to accelerate the development of retinopathy and nephropathy. In addition, interventional studies using antihypertensive agents, especially renin-angiotensin-aldosterone system blockers, have demonstrated attenuation of the otherwise inexorable progression of nephropathy [25, 26].

LONG-TERM COMPLICATIONS OF TYPE 1 DIABETES AND THE RISK OF DEVELOPING CLINICAL MANIFESTATIONS OF SPECIFIED COMPLICATIONS
Cataract: 25%–30% lifetime risk with 3%–5% requiring cataract extraction
Glaucoma (open angle): 10% risk after 30 years
Retinopathy: 90% develop some degree over lifetime; 40%–50% require laser and 3%–5% are blind after 30 years' duration
Adhesive capsulitis: frozen shoulder, prevalence 10%
Coronary artery disease: major cause of mortality
Gastroparesis: 1%–5% develop symptoms—lifetime risk
Carpal tunnel syndrome: 30% with electrophysiologic evidence; 9% with symptoms (prevalence)
Nephropathy: 35% develop end-stage renal disease over lifetime
Trigger finger, Dupuytren's contractures: 10% prevalence
Autonomic neuropathy (prevalence): bladder, 1%–5% with dysfunction; impotence, 10%–40%; diarrhea, 1%
Peripheral vascular disease
Peripheral neuropathy: 54% lifetime risk; 2%–3% foot ulcers/year

FIGURE 5-3. Long-term complications of type 1 diabetes and the risks of developing clinical manifestations of specified complications. Data for some complications are sparse. The estimates provided reflect the era before the DCCT. Intensive therapy of type 1 diabetes is anticipated to reduce the lifelong risk of development of retinopathy, nephropathy, and neuropathy by 50–80%. The overall effect of diabetic complications results in a substantial 15-year reduction in the life span, predominantly owing to the development of nephropathy and cardiovascular disease.

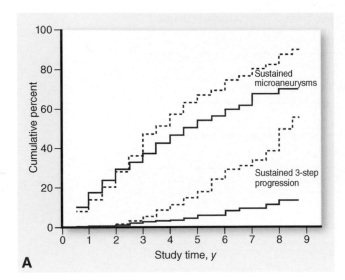

A

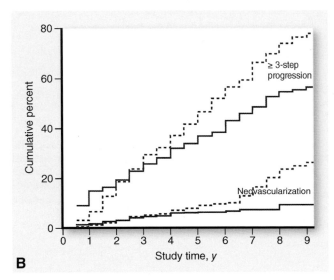

B

Figure 5-4. Retinopathy. In the DCCT, retinopathy was measured in 18,000 sets of photographs with seven-field stereoscopic fundus photography performed every 6 months. The development and progression of retinopathy at virtually every stage were decreased by intensive therapy. (**A**) The primary prevention cohort had 1–5 years' duration of diabetes and no retinopathy at baseline. In the primary cohort, the development of sustained microaneurysms, defined as one or more microaneurysms detected at two consecutive 6-month examinations, and of sustained three-step or greater progression according to the Early Treatment of Diabetic Retinopathy Study (ETDRS) scale was decreased by 27 and 76% ($P<0.002$), respectively. (**B**) The secondary intervention cohort was defined as having 1–15 years' duration of diabetes and at least one microaneurysm in either eye at baseline. In the secondary intervention cohort, intensive therapy was highly effective at reducing the progression to more severe levels of retinopathy, including a 34% reduction in three-step or greater progression ($P<0.02$). The development of even more severe retinopathy, defined as neovascularization on the disc or elsewhere, was reduced by 48% ($P<0.02$) (adapted from DCCT Research Group [27]).

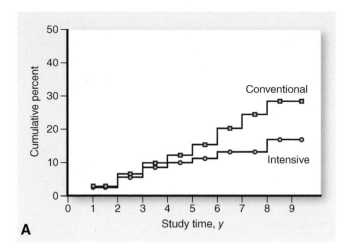

A

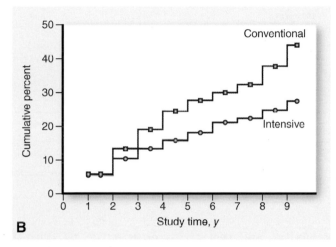

B

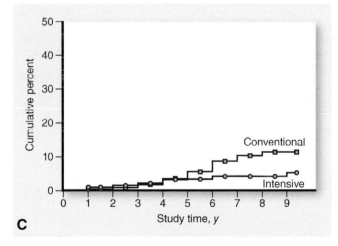

C

Figure 5-5. Nephropathy. Nephropathy in patients with type 1 diabetes progresses through several stages, usually over 15–25 years. The development of microalbuminuria, defined as between 20 and 40 mg of albumin excretion per 24 h, is the first detectable stage, progressing to clinical albuminuria (>300 mg albumin excretion/24 h), usually over more than a decade. Albumin excretion progresses to the level consistent with nephrotic syndrome followed by decreasing glomerular filtration rate and culminating in end-stage renal disease. Hypertension uniformly accompanies the development of nephropathy. Treatment of hypertension, especially with angiotensin-converting enzyme (ACE) inhibitors, and use of ACE inhibitors during the microalbuminuric stage, even in the absence of hypertension, retard the progression of microalbuminuria. The DCCT demonstrated a uniformly beneficial effect of intensive therapy on the development of microalbuminuria (40 mg/24 h). (**A**) In patients with primary prevention, a 34% risk reduction (P=0.04). (**B**) In patients with secondary prevention, a 43% reduction (P<0.001). (**C**) A 56% reduction in the development of more advanced stages of nephropathy, such as clinical albuminuria (P<0.01) (adapted from DCCT Research Group [28]).

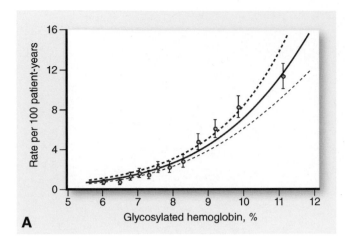

A

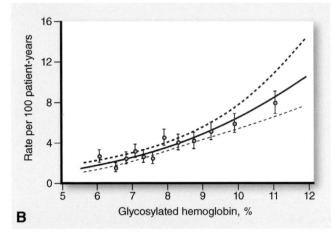

B

C. CALCULATED RELATIVE RISK REDUCTIONS ASSOCIATED WITH 10% LOWER MEAN HEMOGLOBIN A_{1c}	
Complication	Risk Reduction, %*
Retinopathy	
Onset	35
Sustained progression	39
Severe nonproliferative	37
Nephropathy	
Microalbuminuria	
≥ 40 mg/24 h	25
≥ 100 mg/24 h	39
Albuminuria, ≥ 300 mg/24 h	34
Neuropathy	30
*Calculated reduction in risk for every 10% decrease in HbA_{1c}.	

C

FIGURE 5-6. Glycemia and complications. The DCCT performed primary analyses comparing the effects of intensive and conventional therapy on long-term complications. In addition, the DCCT performed secondary analyses examining the relationship of glycemia (mean of all HbA_{1c} values for each subject during the trial) and the development or progression of complications, independent of treatment assignment. These analyses provide an assessment of the expected risk for different complications based on HbA_{1c} achieved. (**A**) Rate of retinopathy progression in combined treatment groups. (**B**) Rate of development of microalbuminuria (>40 mg/24 h) in combined treatment groups. (**C**) In addition, the risk reduction for a specified decrease in HbA_{1c} can be calculated (adapted from DCCT Research Group [29]).

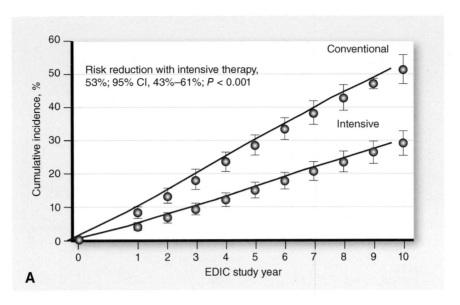

A

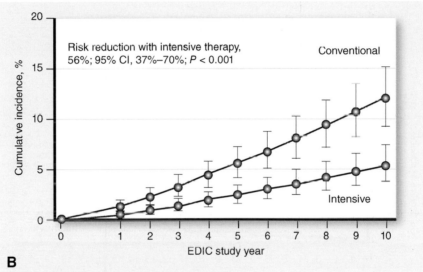

B

Figure 5-7. Retinopathy in DCCT/EDIC long-term follow-up. Cumulative incidence of further progression of retinopathy in the former conventional therapy and intensive therapy groups over the 10 years after DCCT closeout. (**A**) Three-step progression of retinopathy. (**B**) Progression to proliferative retinopathy (adapted from DCCT/EDIC Research Group [2]).

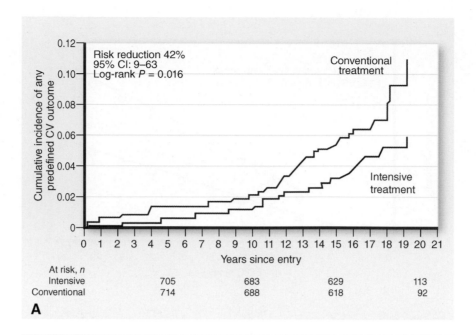

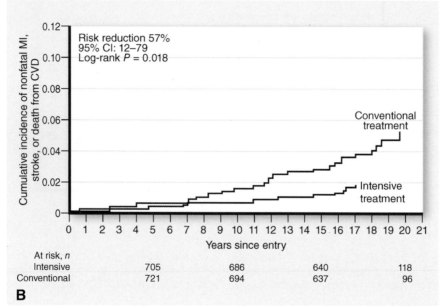

Figure 5-8. Cardiovascular complications in DCCT/EDIC long-term follow-up. (**A**) Cumulative incidence of the first of any of the predefined cardiovascular disease outcomes (nonfatal myocardial infarction or stroke, death judged to be secondary to cardiovascular disease, subclinical myocardial infarction, angina confirmed by ischemic changes with exercise tolerance testing or by clinically significant obstruction on coronary angiography, or revascularization with angioplasty or coronary artery bypass). (**B**) Cumulative incidence of the first occurrence of nonfatal myocardial infarction, stroke, or death from cardiovascular disease (adapted from DCCT/EDIC Research Group [4]).

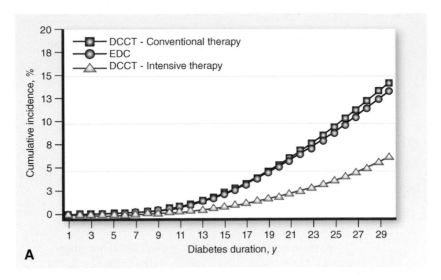

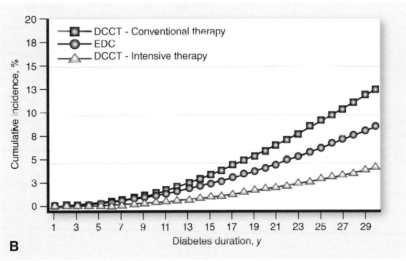

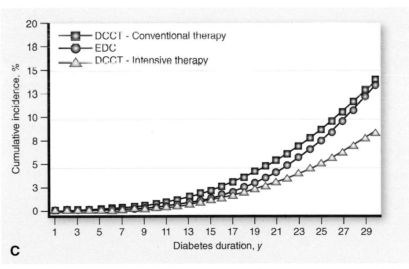

Figure 5-9. Estimated cumulative incidences over time up to 30 years' duration of diabetes in DCCT/EDIC and the Pittsburgh Epidemiology of Diabetes Complications (EDC) study [5]. (**A**) Proliferative retinopathy or worse. (**B**) Nephropathy, defined as an albumin excretion rate ≥300 mg/24 h, a serum creatinine level ≥2 mg/dL, or dialysis or renal transplant. (**C**) Cardiovascular disease, defined as in Fig. 5.8a.

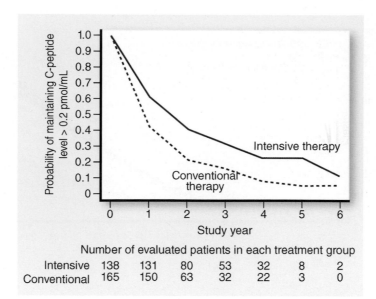

Figure 5-10. Preservation of endogenous insulin secretion with intensive therapy. In the DCCT, patients with less than 5 years' duration of diabetes could have a modest degree of residual insulin secretion (C-peptide level 0.2–0.5 pmol/mL 90 min after a standardized meal). Of the patients, 303 fulfilled this criterion; 138 were randomly assigned to intensive therapy and 165 to conventional therapy. During the DCCT, repeated tests of endogenous insulin secretion were performed. As shown, intensive therapy was more likely than conventional therapy to preserve endogenous secretion of insulin, extending the residual secretion by at least 2 years. Compared with patients having intensive treatments without residual insulin secretion, those having intensive treatment with residual insulin secretion maintained lower hemoglobin A$_{1c}$ levels with less exogenous insulin and had less-frequent severe hypoglycemia and a lower risk of retinopathy progression. Thus, preservation of endogenous insulin secretion is clinically important, facilitating the safe implementation of intensive therapy. Intensive therapy should be initiated as early as possible in the course of type 1 diabetes (adapted from DCCT Research Group [30]).

CLASSIFICATION OF INSULIN PREPARATIONS AND INSULIN ANALOGUES			
Insulin	Onset	Peak	Effective Duration, *h*
Rapid acting (insulin lispro, insulin aspart, insulin glulisine	5–15 min	30–90 min	5
Short acting (regular)	30–60 min	2–3 h	5–8
Intermediate acting (NPH)	2–4 h	4–10 h	10–16
Long acting			
Glargine	2–4 h	None	20–24
Detemir	2–4 h	4–12 h	14–20

Figure 5-11. Classification of insulin preparations and insulin analogues.

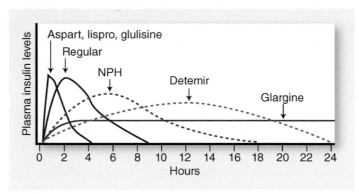

Figure 5-12. Idealized insulin appearance curves after subcutaneous injection.

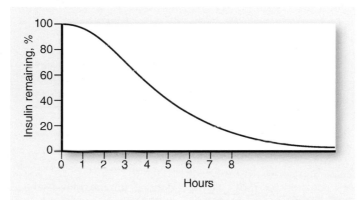

Figure 5-13. The appearance of insulin in the bloodstream (pharmacokinetics) is different from the measurement of insulin action (pharmacodynamics). The figure represents timing of insulin action for insulin aspart from euglycemic clamp (0.2 U/kg injected into the abdomen). This graph may be used to help patients avoid "insulin stacking." For example, 3 h after administration of 10 U of insulin aspart, one can estimate that 40% of the 10 U – or 4 U of insulin – remains. By way of comparison, the pharmacodynamics of regular insulin are approximately twice that of insulin aspart or insulin lispro. Currently used insulin pumps keep track of this "insulin on board" to avoid insulin stacking (adapted from Mudaliar et al. [31]).

FACTORS THAT AFFECT INSULIN ABSORPTION
Insulin dose
Site of injection
Depth of injection (intramuscular vs subcutaneous)
Exercise
Local heat/massage
Mixing insulins
Poor resuspension of nonsoluble insulin preparations
Smoking

Figure 5-14. Factors that affect insulin absorption.

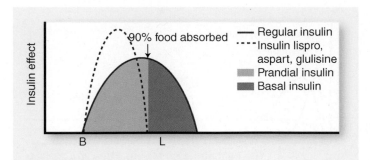

FIGURE 5-15. Idealized insulin action curves for morning regular insulin and rapid-acting insulin analogues (lispro, aspart, glulisine). The rapid-acting analogues contribute only to prandial insulin, whereas the regular insulin contributes to both prandial and basal insulin. *B* breakfast, *L* lunch.

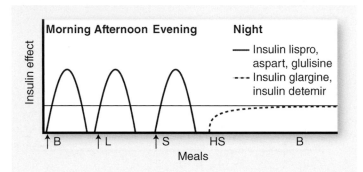

FIGURE 5-16. Idealized insulin curves for prandial insulin with a rapid-acting insulin analogue (lispro, aspart, glulisine) together with basal insulin as insulin glargine or insulin detemir. Each insulin is responsible for either the prandial or basal component. Some patients find that the insulin glargine or insulin detemir does not last the entire 24 h, so they give the insulin twice daily. In addition, giving half on arising and half on retiring adds flexibility in times of arising and retiring. To date, there have been no clinical trials testing these points. *B* breakfast, *HS* bedtime, *L* lunch, *S* supper.

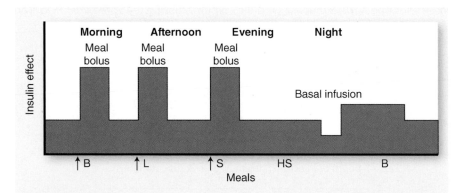

FIGURE 5-17. Idealized insulin curves for CSII with a rapid-acting insulin analogue (lispro, aspart, glulisine). Note that the basal insulin component may be altered based on changing basal insulin requirements. Typically, insulin rates may be lowered between midnight and 4 a.m. (predawn sleep hypoglycemia phenomenon) and raised between 4 and 8 a.m. (dawn phenomenon). The basal rate of the rest of the day is usually intermediate to the other two. Modern pumps can calculate prandial insulin dose by the patient's entering into the pump the blood glucose concentration and the anticipated amount of carbohydrate to be consumed. The pump calculates how much previous prandial insulin is still available and provides the patient with a final suggested dose, which the patient may activate or override.

UNEXPLAINED HYPERGLYCEMIA WITH CSII: FACTORS TO CONSIDER
Pump
1. Basal rate programmed incorrectly
2. Battery discharged
3. Pump malfunction
4. Cartridge does not advance properly
Cartridge
1. Improper placement
2. Insulin depleted
3. Insulin leakage
Infusion set
1. Insulin leakage
2. Dislodged catheter
3. Air in tubing
4. Insulin occlusion
5. Tear in tubing
Infusion site
1. Redness, irritation, inflammation
2. Placement in area of lipohypertrophy
Insulin
1. Expired or exposed to extreme temperature (hot or cold) and not at normal potency

Figure 5-18. Possible etiologies for unexplained hyperglycemia with CSII.

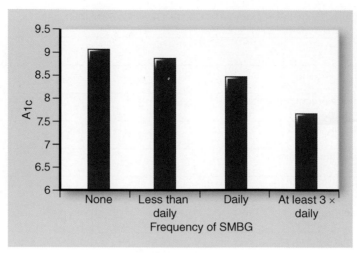

Figure 5-19. Estimated A$_{1c}$ for a population (N=1,159) of patients with type 1 diabetes in a large health maintenance organization. As SMBG frequency increased, A$_{1c}$ improved (adapted from Karter et al. [32]).

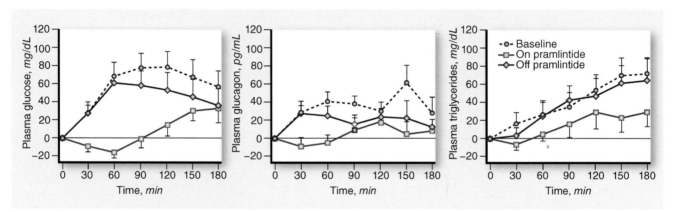

Figure 5-20. Effect of pramlintide on postprandial glucose, glucagon, and triglycerides in type 1 diabetes. This study had 18 evaluable patients, with pramlintide provided at 30 µg three times daily for 4 weeks. Data are presented as change from baseline (adapted from Levetan et al. [14]).

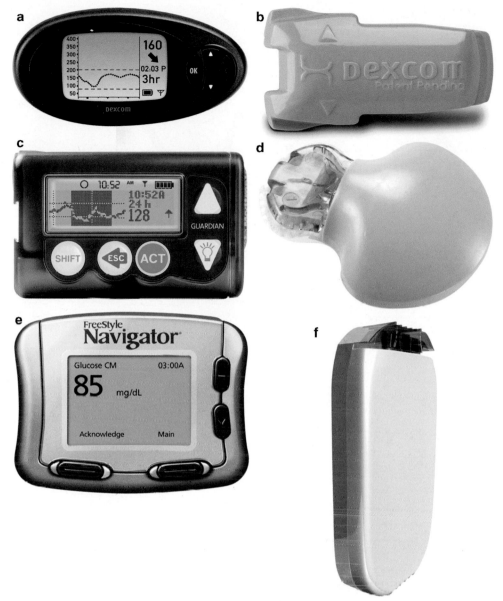

Figure 5-21. Continuous glucose monitors. (**A**, **B**) Seven Plus (DexCom, San Diego, CA). (**C**, **D**) Guardian Real-Time (Medtronic Diabetes, Northridge, CA). (**E**, **F**) FreeStyle Navigator (Abbott Laboratories, Abbott Park, IL). Each device is depicted with its receiver on the left and transmitter on the right. The transmitter is placed subcutaneously and remains in place for 7, 3, or 5 days, respectively, for the CGMs shown.

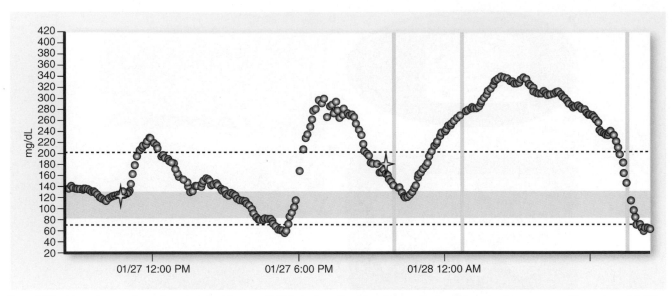

FIGURE 5-22. Glucose readings downloaded from a CGM device. These data are from a 31-year-old woman with an A₁c of 6.8%.

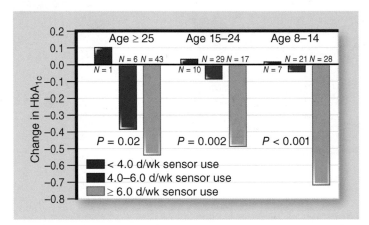

FIGURE 5-23. Change in A₁c from baseline to 6 months in subjects with baseline A₁c≥7.0% according to average amount of CGM use over the 6-month period in the JDRF CGM study. The *N*s refer to the number of subjects in each CGM use category. The *P* values are for the association between sensor use over the 6 months and the change in A₁c from baseline to 26 weeks, evaluated in a general linear model, with sensor use as a continuous variable adjusted for baseline A₁c (adapted from Juvenile Diabetes Research Foundation Continuous Glucose Monitoring Study Group [22]).

References

1. Diabetes Control and Complications Trial Research Group: The effect of intensive treatment of diabetes on the development and progression of long-term complications in insulin-dependent diabetes mellitus. *N Engl J Med* 1993, 329:977–986.

2. White NH, Sun W, Cleary PA, *et al.*: Prolonged effect of intensive therapy on the risk of retinopathy complications in patients with type 1 diabetes mellitus: 10 years after the Diabetes Control and Complications Trial. *Arch Ophthalmol* 2008, 126:1707–1715.

3. The Diabetes Control and Complications Trial/Epidemiology of Diabetes Interventions and Complications Research Group: Retinopathy and nephropathy in patients with type 1 diabetes four years after a trial of intensive therapy. *N Engl J Med* 2000, 342:381–389.

4. Nathan DM, Cleary PA, Backlund JY, *et al.*; Diabetes Control and Complications Trial/Epidemiology of Diabetes Interventions and Complications (DCCT/EDIC) Study Research Group: Intensive diabetes treatment and cardiovascular disease in patients with type 1 diabetes. *N Engl J Med* 2005, 353:2643–2653.

5. Diabetes Control and Complications Trial/Epidemiology of Diabetes Interventions and Complications (DCCT/EDIC) Research Group; Nathan DM, Zinman B, Cleary PA, *et al.*: Modern-day clinical course of type 1 diabetes mellitus after 30 years' duration: the diabetes control and complications trial/epidemiology of diabetes interventions and complications and Pittsburgh epidemiology of diabetes complications experience (1983–2005). *Arch Intern Med* 2009, 169:1307–1316.

6. Skyler JS: Insulin pharmacology. *Med Clin North Am* 1988, 72:1337–1354.

7. Jackson RL: Historical background. In *The Physiologic Management of Diabetes in Children*. Edited by Jackson RL, Guthrie RA. New York: Medical Examination Publishing Company; 1986:6–16.

8. Skyler JS: Human insulin of recombinant DNA origin: clinical potential. *Diabetes Care* 1982, 5(suppl 2):181–186.

9. Dewitt DE, Hirsch IB: Outpatient insulin therapy in type 1 and type 2 diabetes mellitus: scientific review. *JAMA* 2003, 289:2254–2264.

10. Rossetti P, Porcellati F, Fanelli CG, *et al.*: Superiority of insulin analogues versus human insulin in the treatment of diabetes mellitus. *Arch Physiol Biochem* 2008, 114:3–10.

11. American Diabetes Association: Standards of medical care in diabetes – 2010. *Diabetes Care* 2010, 33:(suppl 1):S11–S61.

12. Colquitt J, Royle P, Waugh N: Are analogue insulins better than soluble in continuous subcutaneous insulin infusion? Results of a meta-analysis. *Diabet Med* 2003, 20:863–866.

13. Pickup J, Mattock M, Kerry S: Glycaemic control with continuous subcutaneous insulin infusion compared with intensive insulin injections in patients with type 1 diabetes; meta-analysis of randomized controlled trials. *BMJ* 2002, 324:1–6.

14. Levetan C, Want LL, Weyer C, *et al.*: Impact of pramlintide on glucose fluctuations and postprandial glucose, glucagon, and triglyceride excursions among patients with type 1 diabetes intensively treated with insulin pumps. *Diabetes Care* 2003, 26:1–8.

15. Skyler JS, Cefalu WT, Kourides IA, *et al.*: Efficacy of inhaled human insulin in type 1 diabetes mellitus: a randomized proof-of-concept study. *Lancet* 2001, 3:331–335.

16. Neumiller JJ, Campbell RK, Wood LD: A review of inhaled technosphere insulin. *Ann Pharmacother* 2010, 44:1231–1239.

17. Skyler JS (ed): Advances in continuous glucose monitoring in diabetes mellitus. *Diabetes Technol Ther* 2000, 2(suppl 1):S1–S97.

18. Skyler JS: Continuous glucose monitoring: an overview of its development. *Diabetes Technol Ther* 2009, 11(suppl 1):S5–S10.

19. Juvenile Diabetes Research Foundation Continuous Glucose Monitoring Study Group; Tamborlane WV, Beck RW, Bode BW, *et al.*: Continuous glucose monitoring and intensive treatment of type 1 diabetes. *N Engl J Med* 2008, 359:1464–1476.

20. Juvenile Diabetes Research Foundation Continuous Glucose Monitoring Study Group: The effect of continuous glucose monitoring in well-controlled type 1 diabetes. *Diabetes Care* 2009, 32:1378–1383.

21. Bergenstal RM, Tamborlane WV, Ahmann AB, *et al.*; for the STAR 3 Study Group: Effectiveness of sensor-augmented insulin-pump therapy in type 1 diabetes. *N Engl J Med* 2010, 363:311–320.

22. Juvenile Diabetes Research Foundation Continuous Glucose Monitoring Study Group; Beck RW, Buckingham B, Miller K, *et al.*: Factors predictive of use and of benefit from continuous glucose monitoring in type 1 diabetes. *Diabetes Care* 2009, 32:1947–1953.

23. Abhary S, Hewitt AW, Burdon KP, Craig JE: A systematic meta-analysis of genetic association studies for diabetic retinopathy. *Diabetes* 2009, 58:2137–2147.

24. Pezzolesi MG, Poznik GD, Mychaleckyj JC, *et al.*; DCCT/EDIC Research Group: Genome-wide association scan for diabetic nephropathy susceptibility genes in type 1 diabetes. *Diabetes* 2009, 58:1403–1410.

25. Lewis EJ, Hunsicker LG, Bain RP, Rohde RD for the Collaborative Study Group: The effect of angiotensin-converting-enzyme inhibition on diabetic nephropathy. *N Engl J Med* 1993, 329:1456–1462.

26. Mauer M, Zinman B, Gardiner R, *et al.*: Renal and retinal effects of enalapril and losartan in type 1 diabetes. *N Engl J Med* 2009, 361:40–51.

27. Diabetes Control and Complications Trial Research Group: Progression of retinopathy with intensive versus conventional treatment in the Diabetes Control and Complications Trial. *Ophthalmology* 1995, 102:647–661.

28. Effect of intensive therapy on the development and progression of diabetic nephropathy in the Diabetes Control and Complications Trial (DCCT) Research Group. *Kidney Int* 1995, 47:1703–1720.

29. Diabetes Control and Complications Trial Research Group: The absence of a glycemic threshold for the development of long-term complications. *Diabetes* 1996, 45:1289–1298.

30. Diabetes Control and Complications Trial Research Group: Effect of intensive therapy on residual b cell function in patients with type 1 diabetes in the Diabetes Control and Complications Trial. *Ann Int Med* 1998, 128:517–523.

31. Mudaliar S, Lindberg FA, Joyce M, *et al.*: Insulin aspart (B28 Asp-insulin): a fast-acting analog of human insulin. *Diabetes Care* 1999, 22:1501–1506.

32. Karter AJ, Ackerson LM, Darbinian JA, *et al.*: Self-monitoring of blood glucose levels and glycemic control: the Northern California Kaiser Permanente Diabetes registry. *Am J Med* 2001, 111:1–9.

6

Childhood Diabetes

Jamie R. Wood and Francine R. Kaufman

Diabetes, one of the most common chronic diseases of childhood, has a unique impact on children and their families. The daily life of children and youth is affected by the rigors of the diabetes regimen and the need to frequently monitor blood glucose levels, provide glucose-lowering agents, and balance the effect of activity and food. Despite this, pediatric patients must still strive to reach the normal developmental milestones of childhood and adolescence, succeed in school, and develop eventual autonomy. To accomplish these tasks, an organized system of diabetes care utilizing a multidisciplinary team versed in pediatric issues must be in place to assure optimal physical and emotional health for the affected child, and support and education for the family, caregivers, and school personnel. In this way, children with type 1 or type 2 diabetes can succeed in reaching adulthood with as little adverse impact on their physical and emotional well-being as possible.

Upon diagnosis, the type of diabetes should be determined. In the neonatal period and up to 6 months of age, diabetes may be transient or due to one of a number of molecular defects. For children 6 months to 10 years old, diabetes is most likely immune-mediated type 1; after age 10, type 2 diabetes is increasingly diagnosed, particularly in children from ethnic minorities.

One of the major risks of type 1 diabetes for children is the development of diabetic ketoacidosis (DKA). DKA remains a major source of morbidity and mortality in pediatric patients as a consequence of cerebral edema. The treatment of DKA in patients younger than age 20 years involves meticulous rehydration with electrolyte-containing solutions, intravenous insulin administration via a low-dose continuous infusion, avoidance of bolus bicarbonate therapy, and extremely close monitoring of neurologic status. There is increasing evidence that risk factors for cerebral edema include severe dehydration as evidenced by a high initial blood urea nitrogen concentration and failure of the serum sodium level to rise with therapy. It remains controversial as to the etiology of brain swelling, which may be due to fluid shifts, hypoperfusion followed by vasogenic edema, or disruption of the blood–brain barrier triggering inflammatory mediators. In addition to brain swelling, brain infarction can be a consequence of DKA and its treatment and can lead to persistent neurologic deficit. Because it remains unclear how to avoid the neurologic sequelae of DKA-associated cerebral edema, it becomes imperative to avoid DKA altogether. Efforts aimed at increasing public and professional awareness have occurred and have been effective in reducing DKA at diagnosis in certain geographies. For established patients, detailed sick day guidelines provided to families can help avoid dehydration, acidosis, and severe hyperglycemia during intercurrent illness.

Since the completion of the Diabetes Control and Complications Trial, the benefits for infants, children, and youth with type 1 diabetes of following a diabetes management system allowing for optimal glycemia has become increasingly apparent. The benefit not only appears to be immediate but also long-term, up to 30 years, and should be instituted in pre- and postpubertal children. Systems of diabetes management that improve glycemic

J.S. Skyler (ed.), *Atlas of Diabetes: Fourth Edition*,
DOI 10.1007/978-1-4614-1028-7_6, © Springer Science+Business Media, LLC 2012

control must be well-defined, have age-specific targets, be carefully taught to patients and families, and allow for flexibility of lifestyle. The use of technology, insulin pumps, continuous glucose sensors, and sensor augmented pumps are viable treatment options in children and teens. Close multidisciplinary follow-up care with screening for diabetes complications and comorbidities is imperative. Finally, certain aspects of diabetes care must also be conveyed to school personnel and other caregivers if pediatric subjects are to maximally benefit from an intensive management approach.

The psychological stress of diabetes, with the fear of immediate and long-term complications, must be addressed by providers of pediatric diabetes care. The child or teen with diabetes, as well as other family members including parents and siblings, should be evaluated to assure that there is not a negative effect on family functioning. Quality of life must be an outcome measure. As such, there is evidence that improved diabetes control, with all of its demands, actually improves quality of life.

As found in the adult population, type 2 diabetes in children and youth is due to the combination of insulin resistance coupled with relative β-cell failure. Although there appears to be a host of potential genetic and environmental risk factors for insulin resistance and limited β-cell reserve, perhaps the most significant risk factor is obesity. The intrauterine environment does appear to have a significant effect with a U-shaped curve for birth weight and risk of type 2 diabetes. Youth with phenotypic type 2 diabetes should still be assessed for the presence of islet autoimmunity because this affects insulin sensitivity and secretion. Because fewer than 10% of youth with type 2 diabetes can be treated with diet and exercise alone, pharmacologic intervention is required for these patients to achieve glycemic targets. In most surveys, practitioners use metformin or insulin or both and less commonly one or another oral agents. Treatment guidelines have been developed to enable target hemoglobin A_{1c} levels to be met and maintained.

Although diabetes management remains demanding, children and families can succeed in achieving glycemic targets and in having physical and psychological well-being. The multidisciplinary team, able to appropriately assess and follow up the patient, can play a major role in preparing children and youth for the most complication-free possible future.

Continued high rates of diabetic ketoacidosis (DKA) and the risk of mortality. The overall frequency of DKA at the onset of diabetes ranges from 15% to 70% in Europe and North America and results in death in 0.15–0.3%. In an ongoing evaluation of DKA performed in 106 pediatric diabetes centers in Germany and Austria, 14,664 type 1 patients were assessed between 1995 and 2007. The DKA rate was 21.1% and the frequency of DKA, including the severe form, remained unchanged throughout the 13-year period. The frequency of DKA was particularly striking among children younger than 5 years of age at 16.5% [5].

Types of Diabetes in the Pediatric Population

Classification of Disorders of Glycemia

Type 1	
Immune mediated	
Idiopathic	
Type 2	
Other specific types	
Genetic defects if β-cell function	
Chromosome 12, HNF-1α (MODY3)	
Chromosome 7, glucokinase (MODY2)	
Chromosome 20, HNF-4α (MODY1)	
Chromosome 13, insulin promoter factor (IPF-1; MODY4)	
Chromosome 17, HNF-1β (MODY5)	
Chromosome 2, NeuroD1 (MODY6)	
Mitochondrial DNA mutation	
Chromosome 7, KCNJ11 (Kir6.2)	
Others	
Genetic defects in insulin action	
Type A insulin resistance	
Leprechaunism	
Rabson-Mendenhall syndrome	
Lipoatrophic diabetes	
Others	
Diseases of the exocrine pancreas	
Pancreatitis	
Cystic fibrosis	
Others	

Endocrinopathies
Cushing's syndrome
Pheochromocytoma
Hyperthyroidism
Others
Drug- or chemical-induced
Infections
Congenital rubella
Cytomegalovirus
Others
Uncommon forms of immune-mediated diabetes
Other genetic syndromes sometimes associated with diabetes
Down syndrome
Klinefelter syndrome
Turner syndrome
Wolfram syndrome
Friedreich's ataxia
Huntington's chorea
Laurence-Moon-Biedl syndrome
Myotonic dystrophy
Porphyria
Prader-Willi syndrome
Others

FIGURE 6-1. Diabetes mellitus is a group of metabolic diseases that either cause defects in insulin action, insulin secretion, or a combination of both, resulting in hyperglycemia. Diabetes mellitus can be diagnosed in children and youth with the same criteria that are used in adults: (1) symptoms of diabetes plus casual glucose concentration ≥200 mg/dL; (2) fasting plasma glucose ≥126 mg/dL; or (3) 2-h postload glucose ≥200 mg/dL during an oral glucose tolerance test. Hyperglycemia must be confirmed on a subsequent day in the absence of unequivocal hyperglycemia. Although A_{1c} may also be used for diabetes diagnosis, exact criteria for children have not been established. The American Diabetes Association and World Health Organization expert committee on the classification and diagnosis of diabetes have recommended the following classification of types of diabetes [1]. The distinction between type 1 diabetes, type 2 diabetes, and monogenic diabetes in children and adolescents is made by considering together the presentation (degree of hyperglycemia and metabolic derangement, presence of ketones), physical examination (body mass index, presence of acanthosis nigricans), family history, and laboratory evaluation (genetic markers, c-peptide and insulin levels, presence of diabetes associated autoantibody markers). *HNF* hepatocyte nuclear factor (adapted from Craig et al. [1]; with permission).

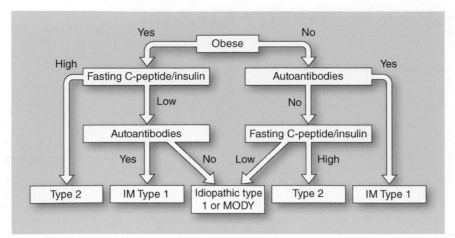

FIGURE 6-2. Research schema for classification of diabetes in children and youth to determine the presence of type 2 diabetes. The vast majority, in some reports up to 90%, of youth with type 2 diabetes, have a body mass index more than 27 kg/m² or are in higher than the 85th percentile for their age. Those children who are obese and have a high fasting C-peptide or insulin level are presumed to have type 2 disease. Obese children with low fasting C-peptide or insulin levels should have autoantibodies measured. If they are present, the patient likely has type 1 diabetes. If autoantibodies are absent, the subject could have idiopathic diabetes or maturity onset diabetes of the young (MODY). In nonobese children and youth, the presence of autoantibodies indicates type 1. Nonobese children with absent antibodies should have C-peptide and insulin assessed. If high, the patient likely has type 2 diabetes; if low, the patient may have idiopathic diabetes or MODY. The final diagnostic classification may require following up the patient's clinical course for a few years after diagnosis [2]. *IM* immune mediated.

Gene clinical syndrome inheritance	PNDM or TNDM	Consanguineous or isolated populations, %	Median birth weight, g (SDS)	Median age of diagnosis, wk (range)	Pancreatic appearance	Other features
ZAC/HYAMI imprinting defect on 6q24	TNDM	Rare	2100 (2.94)	0.5 (0–4)	Normal	Macroglossia (23%)
Kir6.2 (KCNJ11)	PNDM TNDM (10%)	Rare	2580 (1.73)	6 (0–260)	Normal	Developmental delay (20%), epilepsy (6%), DKA (30%)
SUR1 (ABCO8)	PNDM TNDM (78%)	Rare	2600 (1.7)	6 (0–17)	Normal	Developmental delay
EIF2AK3 Wolcott-Rallison syndrome recessive	PNDM	90%	3000 (1.0)	13 (6–65)	Atrophy of pancreas (?), exocrine dysfunction (25%)	Epiphyseal dysplasia (90%) , osteopenia (50%), acute liver failure (75%), developmental delay (80%), hypothyroidism (25%)
INS	PNDM	Rare	2600 (1.7)	9 (0–26)	Normal	None
FOXP3 IPEX syndrome X linked	PNDM	Rare	2860 (1.2)	6 (0–30)	?	Only boys affected Chronic diarrhea with villous atrophy (95%); pancreatic and thyroid autoantibodies (75%); thyroiditis (20%); eczema (50%), anemia (30%); often die young (first year)
GCK (glucokinase) recessive	PNDM	85%	1720 (2.75)		Normal	Parents have fasting hyperglycemia as heterozygotes
IPF1 recessive	PNDM	50%	2140 (2.97)		Absent	Parents may have early-onset diabetes as heterozygotes
HNF-1β dominant (60%) spontaneous	TNDM	2 rare	1900 (3.21)		Atrophy	Renal developmental disorders
PTF1A recessive	PNDM	100%	1390 (3.8)		Atrophy	Severe neurological dysfunction and cerebellar hypoplasia

Figure 6-3. Types and characteristics of diabetes presenting in the first 6 months of life. Diabetes diagnosed in the first 6 months of life is very rarely type 1 diabetes and can be classified into transient neonatal diabetes mellitus (TNDM) or permanent neonatal diabetes mellitus (PNDM). In the past decade, there have been significant advances in the understanding of the molecular genetic etiology of neonatal diabetes that have also resulted in successful treatment with oral sulfonylureas in some cases (Kir6.2 mutations). *DKA* diabetic ketoacidosis, *SDS* standard deviation score (adapted from Hattersley et al. [3]; with permission).

Diabetic Ketoacidosis in the Pediatric Population with Type 1 Diabetes

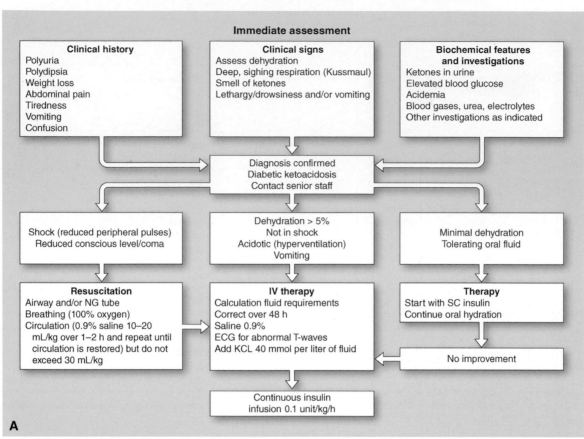

Immediate assessment

Clinical history
Polyuria
Polydipsia
Weight loss
Abdominal pain
Tiredness
Vomiting
Confusion

Clinical signs
Assess dehydration
Deep, sighing respiration (Kussmaul)
Smell of ketones
Lethargy/drowsiness and/or vomiting

Biochemical features and investigations
Ketones in urine
Elevated blood glucose
Acidemia
Blood gases, urea, electrolytes
Other investigations as indicated

Diagnosis confirmed
Diabetic ketoacidosis
Contact senior staff

Shock (reduced peripheral pulses)
Reduced conscious level/coma

Dehydration > 5%
Not in shock
Acidotic (hyperventilation)
Vomiting

Minimal dehydration
Tolerating oral fluid

Resuscitation
Airway and/or NG tube
Breathing (100% oxygen)
Circulation (0.9% saline 10–20 mL/kg over 1–2 h and repeat until circulation is restored) but do not exceed 30 mL/kg

IV therapy
Calculation fluid requirements
Correct over 48 h
Saline 0.9%
ECG for abnormal T-waves
Add KCL 40 mmol per liter of fluid

Therapy
Start with SC insulin
Continue oral hydration

No improvement

Continuous insulin
infusion 0.1 unit/kg/h

A

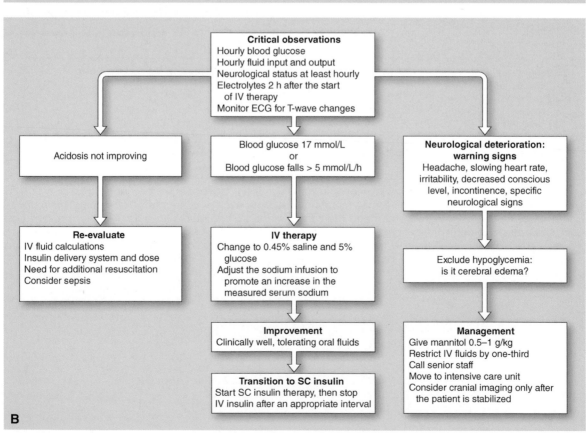

Critical observations
Hourly blood glucose
Hourly fluid input and output
Neurological status at least hourly
Electrolytes 2 h after the start of IV therapy
Monitor ECG for T-wave changes

Acidosis not improving

Blood glucose 17 mmol/L
or
Blood glucose falls > 5 mmol/L/h

Neurological deterioration: warning signs
Headache, slowing heart rate, irritability, decreased conscious level, incontinence, specific neurological signs

Re-evaluate
IV fluid calculations
Insulin delivery system and dose
Need for additional resuscitation
Consider sepsis

IV therapy
Change to 0.45% saline and 5% glucose
Adjust the sodium infusion to promote an increase in the measured serum sodium

Exclude hypoglycemia:
is it cerebral edema?

Improvement
Clinically well, tolerating oral fluids

Management
Give mannitol 0.5–1 g/kg
Restrict IV fluids by one-third
Call senior staff
Move to intensive care unit
Consider cranial imaging only after the patient is stabilized

Transition to SC insulin
Start SC insulin therapy, then stop IV insulin after an appropriate interval

B

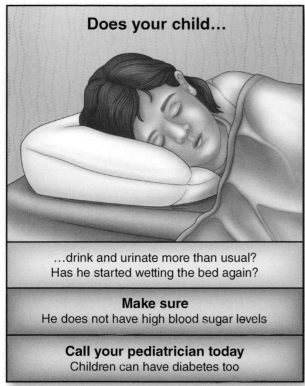

A

B

FIGURE 6-5. A large, ethnically diverse cohort of youth with diabetes in Chicago was studied to determine the risk factors for mortality. Using the Chicago Diabetes Registry, 1,238 cases were assessed during a 15-year period ending in 2000. The crude mortality rate was 2.4% with six subjects dying in DKA at presentation, as well as seven subjects dying with DKA after onset. In total, DKA accounted for 13 of the 30 deaths. The high proportion of deaths from DKA, including at onset, suggests that there is still a lack of understanding regarding warning signs and severity [6]. Given the high rate of DKA at onset of diabetes and significant morbidity and mortality, prevention of DKA at onset of diabetes should be a top priority. Vanelli et al. [7] from Parma, Italy began a campaign in schools and pediatrician's offices in the province of Parma to educate about the early signs of diabetes in children. The campaign involved the use of posters similar to the one shown in (**A**). They were able to demonstrate a dramatic reduction in the frequency of DKA at onset of diabetes up to 8 years after the initial campaign. During the 8 years of the campaign, the cumulative frequency of DKA dropped from 78 to 12.5%. The International Diabetes Federation in 2006 to 2008 launched an international effort using similar posters, as shown in (**B**), to increase awareness about the early signs and symptoms of diabetes in children as part of its World Diabetes Day campaign [8]. ((**A**) adapted from Vanelli et al. [7]; (**B**) adapted from the International Diabetes Federation [0]).

FIGURE 6-4. Management of pediatric patients (<20 years old) with diabetic ketoacidosis (DKA). (**A, B**) The protocol for the management of pediatric patients (<20 years old) with DKA [4] begins with intravenous (IV) fluid therapy to restore circulation. The rate of fluid administration is dependent on the presence or absence of hypovolemic shock and typically ranges from 10 to 20 mL/kg of 0.9% normal saline (NS). Repeat IV fluid boluses should only be given in the presence of continued hypovolemia and the total should rarely exceed 30 mL/kg. After fluid resuscitation, IV fluid administration is given at a rate that will complete rehydration in 48 h. The sodium concentration of the fluid replacement solution is typically 0.9% for at least 4 h and then is adjusted to 0.45–0.75% normal saline depending on sodium, corrected sodium, and mental status. Insulin infusion is begun after fluid resuscitation; the rate of administration of regular insulin is 0.1 U/kg/h. Insulin can be administered intramuscularly if IV access cannot be secured. Potassium is added to the replacement fluids at a variable infusion rate depending on the serum potassium level. Bicarbonate is given only for severe acidosis and pH less than 7.0, administered for more than 1 h but not as IV bolus therapy. Addition of glucose to the IV solution occurs as the serum glucose level drops. The key to successful management is close monitoring of glucose and electrolytes, and appropriate level of care to detect and treat early neurologic compromise. *NG* nasogastric, *KCl* potassium chloride, *SC* subcutaneous (adapted from Wolfsdorf et al. [4]; with permission).

Multivariate Analysis of Risk Factors for Cerebral Edema in Children with Cerebral Edema Compared With a Matched Control Group [*]		
Variable [†]	Relative risk (95% CI)	P value
Male sex	0.6 (0.3–1.4)	0.27
Age (per 1-y increase)	0.9 (0.6–1.3)	0.53
Initial serum sodium concentration (per increase of 5.8 mmol/L)	0.7 (0.5–1.02)	0.06
Initial serum glucose concentration (per increase of 244 mg/dL)	1.4 (0.5–3.9)	0.58
Initial serum urea nitrogen concentration (per increase of 9 mg/dL)	1.8 (1.2–2.7)	0.008
Initial serum bicarbonate concentration (per increase of 3.6 mmol/L)	1.2 (0.5–2.6)	0.73
Initial partial pressure of arterial carbon dioxide (per decrease of 7.8 mm Hg)	2.7 (1.4–5.1)	0.002
Rate of increase in serum sodium concentration during therapy (per increase of 5.8 mmol/L/h)	0.6 (0.4–0.9)	0.01
Rate of increase in serum glucose concentration during therapy (per decrease of 190 mg/dL/h)	0.8 (0.5–1.4)	0.41
Rare of increase in serum bicarbonate concentration during therapy (per increase of 3 mmol/L/h)	0.8 (0.5–1.1)	0.15
Administration of insulin bolus	0.8 (0.3–2.2)	0.62
Treatment of bicarbonate	4.2 (1.5–12.1)	0.008
Rate of infusion of intravenous fluid (per increase of 5 mL/kg of body weight/h)	1.1 (0.4–3.0)	0.91
Rate of infusion of sodium (per increase of 0.6 mmol/kg/hr)	1.2 (0.6–2.7)	0.59
Rate of infusion of insulin (per increase of 0.04 unit/kg/hr)	1.2 (0.8–1.8)	0.30

[*]*This analysis compared the cerebral edema group with the matched control group by means of conditional logistic regression. To convert values for serum glucose to mmol/L, multiply by 0.056; to convert values for serum urea nitrogen to mmol/L, multiply by 0.36.*

[†]*The increase or decrease used in the analysis of each continuous variable (except age) represents a change of 1 standard deviation in the variable in the randomly selected control children with diabetic ketoacidosis.*

FIGURE 6-6. Risk factors for cerebral edema in children with diabetic ketoacidosis (DKA). In a multicenter study, 61 children who developed symptomatic cerebral edema associated with DKA were compared with 181 randomly selected children with DKA and 174 children with DKA matched based on age, new onset versus known case, initial pH, and initial serum glucose concentration [9]. Multivariate statistical methods showed that children with DKA-related cerebral edema had lower initial PCO_2 values and higher serum urea nitrogen concentrations than the control groups. A lesser rise in serum sodium concentration during treatment was seen in those with cerebral edema, although it is unclear whether this was due to therapy itself or a physiologic response to cerebral injury. The administration of bicarbonate bolus was also associated with the development of cerebral edema, suggesting that bicarbonate therapy, for the most part, is contraindicated in children with DKA (adapted from Glaser et al. [9]; with permission).

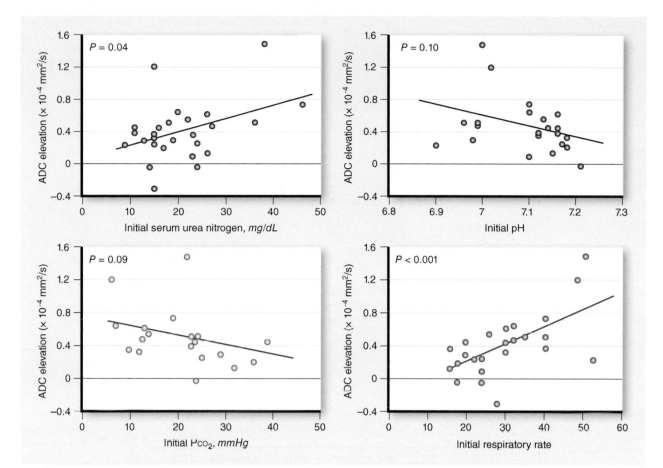

FIGURE 6-7. Pathogenesis of cerebral edema in children with diabetic ketoacidosis (DKA). The pathogenesis of cerebral edema is not well understood. Glaser et al. [9] identified some factors associated with the development of cerebral edema in the setting of DKA (see Fig. 6.6). In a follow up study, Glaser et al. [10] used magnetic resonance diffusion-weighted imaging to quantify edema formation and measured the apparent diffusion coefficient (ADC) of brain water during and after DKA treatment in 26 children. They hypothesized that DKA-related cerebral edema might be caused by cerebral hypoperfusion before treatment, with vasogenic edema occurring as a result of reperfusion injury. They observed more elevated ADC values during DKA treatment compared with baseline and children with altered mental status had greater elevation in ADC. ADC elevation during DKA was associated with degree of initial dehydration and hyperventilation at presentation, but was not correlated with initial glucose, change in glucose with treatment, initial osmolality, or with change in osmolality. The authors concluded that formation of cerebral edema during DKA is related to cerebral hypoperfusion during DKA and that osmotic fluctuations during DKA treatment are not the causal factors.

Hoffman et al. [11] studied the brains from two cases of fatal brain edema associated with DKA and evaluated the blood–brain barrier integrity and the potential involvement of inflammatory mediators in the breakdown of the blood–brain barrier. In both cases, the blood–brain barrier was disrupted and the inflammation was localized to the perivascular areas of the disrupted blood–brain barrier (adapted from Glaser et al. [10]; with permission).

Sick day management guidelines

1. Warning signs
   Call the health team if there is:
   - Vomiting (> two times or > 4 h)
   - Elevated blood glucose level (two or more readings outside the target range or > 250 mg/dL)
   - Presence of blood or large urinary ketones
   - Weakness, dry mouth, or signs of dehydration, excessive thirst
   - Heavy breathing, shortness of breath
   - Abdominal pain, diarrheal stools
   - Evidence of bacterial infection
   - Altered state of consciousness or a change in mental status
2. Never stop insulin
3. Phone numbers
   - Pediatrician_____
   - Diabetes team_____
   - Emergency_____
4. Log

	1st h	2nd h	3rd h	4th h	5th h	6th h	7th h
Blood sugar							
Ketone level							
Temperature							
Fluid input							
Urine output							
Insulin dose							

5. Principles for low blood sugar
   - Glucose-containing fluids should be given in small quantities
   - Insulin should be decreased by 20%–50%
   - If persistent hypoglycemia occurs and patients are not able to retain glucose-containing solutions, consider a mini-dose of glucagon (for children ≤ 2 y, 20 µg or two "units" on the insulin syringe; for children > 2 y, 150 µg, or 15 "units")
6. Management of hyperglycemia—how to calculate the amount of extra insulin on sick days (*see* Fig. 6-9.)

Figure 6-8. Sick day guidelines for the prevention of diabetic ketoacidosis (DKA). Early signs of DKA need to be treated aggressively and the results of treatment carefully monitored to avoid the development of moderate-to-severe dehydration, hyperglycemia, and acidosis. Antecedents of DKA in children and youth with established diabetes include intercurrent illness, infection, incorrect insulin dosage for the glycemic level, inappropriate insulin administration, omission of insulin, psychological trauma, or surgery. Patients, parents, baby sitters, school personnel, and day care workers need to understand the early signs of DKA and how to access the health-care team so that DKA can be reversed at home. The use of a sick day management guideline [12, 13] can be of benefit in promoting the early institution of monitoring and treatment to avoid the need for hospitalization and emergency room visits. Blood ketone monitoring during sick days may be more effective at reducing the need for hospitalization and emergency room visit compared with urine ketone testing [14].

Calculation of Amount of Extra Insulin on Sick Days

Ketones		Blood glucose				
Blood ketones, *mmol/L*	Urine ketones	< 5.5 mmol/L; < 100 mg/dL	5.5–10 mmol/L; 100–180 mg/dL	10–14 mmol/L; 180–250 mg/dL	14–22 mmol/L; 250–400 mg/dL	> 22 mmol/L; > 400 mg/dL
< 0.6	Negative or trace	Do not give extra insulin. May need to consider minidoses of glucagon (*see* Fig. 6-9) if < 4 mmol (70 mg/dL). Check BG and ketones again in 2 h.	No need to worry .	Increase dose of insulin for next meal if BG is still elevated	Give extra 5% of TDD or 0.05 U/kg.	Give extra 10% of TDD or 0.1 U/kg. Repeat if needed.
0.6–0.9	Trace or small	Check BG and ketones. Extra carbohydrates and fluid are needed.	Starvation ketones. Extra carbohydrates and fluid are needed.	Give extra 5% of TDD or 0.05 U/kg	Give extra 5%–10% of TDD or 0.05–0.1 U/kg.	Give extra 10% of TDD or 0.1 U/kg. Repeat if needed.
1.0–1.4	Small or moderate	Starvation ketones. Extra carbohydrates and fluid are n eeded.	Starvation ketones. Extra carbohydrates and fluid are needed. Give ordinary bolus dose.	Extra carbohydrates and fluid are needed. Give 5%–10% of TDD or 0.05–0.1 U/kg.	Give extra 10% of TDD or 0.1 U/kg.	Give extra 10% of TDD or 0.1 U/kg. Repeat if needed.
1.5–2.9	Moderate or large	High levels of starvation ketones. Check BG meter. Recheck BG and ketones. Extra carbohydrates and fluid are needed. May need IV glucose if child cannot eat or drink. Risk of developing ketoacidosis. Check BG and ketones every hour.	High levels of starvation ketones. Extra carbohydrates and fluid are needed. Give 5% of TDD or 0.05 U/kg. Repeat when blood glucose has risen. *Risk of developing ketoacidosis.*	Extra carbohydrates and fluid are needed. Give 10% of TDD or 0.1 U/kg.	Give extra 10%–20% of TDD or 0.1–0.2 U/kg. Repeat dose after 2 h if ketones do not decrease.	
≥ 3	Large	Very high levels of starvation ketones. Check BG meter. Recheck BG and ketones. Extra carbohydrates and fluid are needed.	Very high levels of starvation ketones. Extra carbohydrates and fluid are needed. Give 5% of TDD or 0.05 U/kg. Repeat when blood glucose has risen.	Extra carbohydrates and fluid are needed. Give 10% of TDD or 0.1 U/kg.	Give extra 10%–20% of TDD or 0.1–0.2 U/kg. Repeat dose after 2 h if ketones do not decrease.	
		There is an immediate risk of ketoacidosis if the blood ketone level is ≥ 3 mmol/L. Insulin treatment is needed urgently. Consider evaluation of patient at emergency department.				

Figure 6-9. Management of hyperglycemia: how to calculate the amount of extra insulin on sick days. To calculate the total daily dose (TDD), add up all the insulin given on a usual day (i.e., rapid-/short-acting+intermediate/long-acting) or sum of basal rate and boluses in a pump. Do not include additional boluses given for unexpected hyperglycemia. High-blood glucose (BG) and elevated ketones indicate a lack of insulin. "Starvation blood ketones" are usually less than 3 mmol/L. When children are feeling sick or vomit, and the BG is below 10–14 mmol/L (180–250 mg/dL), they must try to drink sugar-containing fluids in small portions to keep BG level up. When ketone levels are raised, priority is to give extra insulin; this is difficult if BG is low. Extra insulin may be given as rapid-acting analogs or short-acting regular insulin, but rapid-acting if available is preferred. Short-acting insulin can be given intramuscularly to accelerate absorption. The ketones level may increase slightly (10–20%) within the first hour after administration of extra insulin, but after that it should decrease (adapted from Brink et al. [15]; with permission).

Type 1 Diabetes in Children and Youth: Population Distribution and Importance of Intensive Management

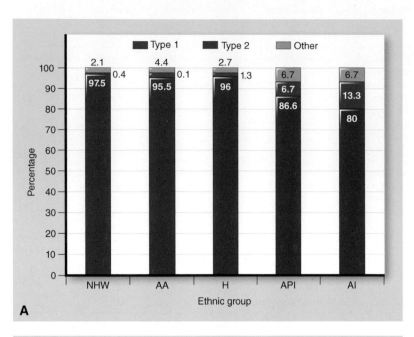

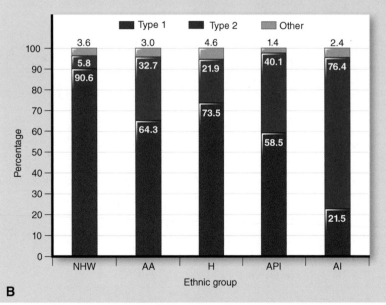

Figure 6-10. Prevalence and incidence of childhood diabetes in the USA: The SEARCH Study. The SEARCH for Diabetes in Youth Study [16] began in 2000 with the objective to estimate the prevalence and incidence of physician-diagnosed diabetes in youth younger than 20 years old by age, sex, race/ethnicity, and diabetes type and to characterize key risk factors for diabetes complications, according to race/ethnicity and diabetes type. The six centers in the SEARCH Study conducted a population-based ascertainment of physician-diagnosed diabetes. In 2001, they identified 6,379 US youth with diabetes in a population of approximately 3.5 million. The crude estimated prevalence was 1.82 cases per 1,000 youth, with lower prevalence in youth 0–9 years old (0.79 cases per 1,000 youth) and higher prevalence in youth 10–19 years old (2.80 cases per 1,000 youth). Among children 0–9 years old (**A**), the highest prevalence was in non-Hispanic white (NHW) youth (1.06 cases per 1,000 youth); among 10–19 year olds (**B**), African American (AA) youth (3.22 cases per 1,000 youth) and NHW youth (3.18 cases per 1,000 youth) had the highest rates, followed by American Indian (AI) youth (2.28 cases per 1,000 youth), Hispanic (H) youth (2.18 cases per 1,000 youth), and Asian/Pacific Islander (API) youth (1.34 cases per 1,000 youth). In the 0–9 year age group, type 1 diabetes accounted for more than 80% of cases, but in the older group, the proportion of type 2 diabetes increased and ranged from 6% in NHW youth to 76% in AI youth. Overall, the prevalence of diabetes was estimated to be 0.18% for all children and youth in the USA, with approximately 154,369 pediatric diabetes patients in 2001 (adapted from The Writing Group for the SEARCH for Diabetes in Youth Study Group [17]; with permission).

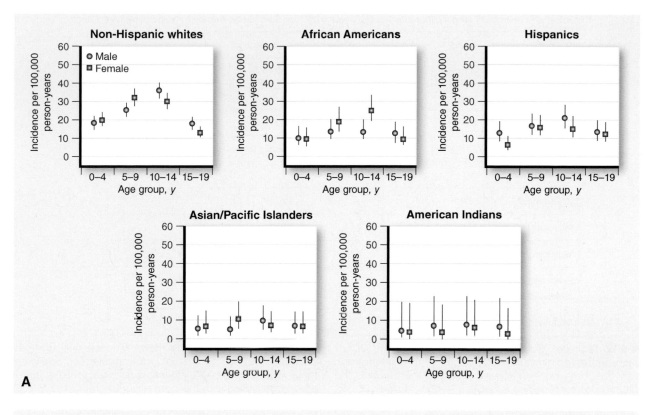

A

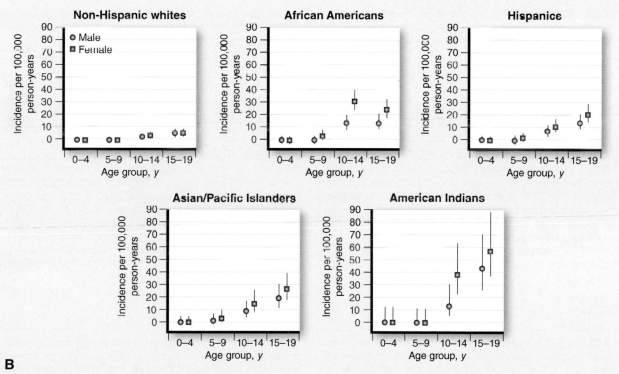

B

FIGURE 6-11. In 2002 to 2003, 2,435 youth with newly diagnosed diabetes were identified by the SEARCH Study [17] at 10 locations in the USA, in a population covering 10 million person-years. Diabetes type was differentiated by GAD65 autoantibodies and C-peptide measurements. The overall incidence of diabetes (per 100,000 person-years) was 24.3. In children younger than 10 years old, type 1 diabetes was most frequent; the rate in non-Hispanic white youth was 18.6, 28.1, and 32.9 for age groups 0–4, 5–9, and 10–14 years, respectively. (**A**) In children older than 10 years of age, type 1 diabetes was frequent among non-Hispanic white, Hispanic, and African American groups. (**B**) Type 2 was relatively infrequent, with the highest rates of 17–49.4 per 100,000 person-years in groups other than non-white 15–19 year olds. The overall estimates were that 15,000 youth were diagnosed with type 1 diabetes in 2002 to 2003 and 3,700 youth were diagnosed with type 2 diabetes.

Diabetes Control and Complications Trial Results: Comparison of Adults Versus Adolescents and Long-Term Effect

	Adults		Adolescents	
	Intensive	Conventional	Intensive	Conventional
Glycemia				
Mean BG, mg/dL	155 $\pm$ 30	231 $\pm$ 55	171 $\pm$ 31	260 $\pm$ 52
HbA$_{1c}$ (90)	7.12 $\pm$ 0.03	9.02 $\pm$ 0.05	8.06 $\pm$ 0.03	9.76 $\pm$ 0.12
Risk reduction				
Retinopathy	63%		61%	
Microalbuminuria	54%		35%	
Hypoglycemia				
Episodes/100 patient-years	61.2	18.7	85.7	29.6
Relative risk	3.3		2.8	

FIGURE 6-12. Diabetes Control and Complications Trial (DCCT) results: comparison of adults versus adolescents and long-term effect. The main impetus for improving diabetes care, the DCCT, did not enroll subjects under 13 years of age [18, 19]. The DCCT did enroll adolescent patients; 14% were between 13 and 17 years old at the time of entry into the study. Compared with adult subjects, the teens had higher blood glucose (BG) and hemoglobin A$_{1c}$ (HbA$_{1c}$) levels in both the intensive and the conventional groups. Nevertheless, there was still a difference in the mean glucose and HbA$_{1c}$ level between the two groups of adolescents. For adolescents, there was a 1.7%±0.2% decrease in HbA$_{1c}$ in the intensive group compared with the conventional group. The reduction in the development of complications seen in youth as a result of achieving improved glycemia was similar to the reduction appreciated in adults. This reduction was coupled with a greater absolute rate of severe hypoglycemia in adolescents compared with adults.

In the follow-up of the DCCT, the Epidemiology of Diabetes Interventions and Complications (EDIC) study [20], 175 of the 195 adolescent subjects were reevaluated with fundus photography and measurement of albumin excretion rate. During 4 years of assessment with the EDIC study, the mean HbA$_{1c}$ levels were similar between the former intensive and the former conventional groups (8.38% vs. 8.45%). The prevalence of retinopathy remained reduced in the former intensive therapy group compared with the conventional group (74%; $P<0.007$) for three steps or more worsening of retinopathy (78%; $P<0.007$) to proliferative or severe nonproliferative retinopathy. The EDIC findings indicate that the benefit of optimal glycemic control for adolescents with type 1 diabetes is not only immediate but also enduring. The durable effect of intensive management was further enhanced by the 30-year follow-up report from the DCCT/EDIC cohort from 2009. Although this report did not differentiate the cohort by age, it did show that after 30 years of diabetes, the cumulative incidences of proliferative retinopathy, nephropathy, and cardiovascular disease were 50%, 25%, and 14%, respectively, in the DCCT conventional treatment group and 21%, 9%, and 9%, respectively, in the DCCT intensive therapy group. The frequencies of serious diabetes complications can be substantially reduced by intensive management [21].

FIGURE 6-13. Targets for glycemia in the pediatric age range: American Diabetes Association and International Society for Pediatric and Adolescent Diabetes Targets (ISPAD). (**A**) The management goal for infants, children, and teens with type 1 diabetes is to have blood glucose (BG) and hemoglobin A$_{1c}$ (HbA$_{1c}$) levels fall within an age-specific target range that takes into account the developmental, cognitive and communicative abilities, and resources of the patient and family. Because it appears that young children are more susceptible to severe hypoglycemia, the target ranges for BG and HbA$_{1c}$ levels are generally higher. However, as children age, the primary concern shifts from avoidance of excessive hypoglycemia to avoidance of hyperglycemia as a means to decrease long-term diabetes complications. (**B**) The ISPAD targets include a stratification of glucose and HbA$_{1c}$ values that should be used to determine the level of action required. *DCCT* Diabetes Control and Complications Trial, *PG* plasma glucose, *SBGM* self blood glucose monitoring (adapted from American Diabetes Association Clinical Practice Recommendations 2009 [22] and International Society for Pediatric and Adolescent Diabetes Targets Clinical Practice Consensus Guidelines 2006–2007 [23]; with permission).

A   Plasma Blood Glucose and HbA$_{1c}$ Goals for Type 1 Diabetes by Age Group

Values by age, y	Plasma blood glucose goal range (mg/dL)		HbA$_{1c}$	Rationale
	Before meals	Bedtime/overnight		
Toddlers and preschoolers (0–6 y)	100–180	110–200	< 8.5% (but > 7.5%)	High risk and vulnerability to hypoglycemia
School age (6–12)	90–180	100–180	< 8%	Risks of hypoglycemia and relatively low risk of complications before puberty
Adolescents and young adults (13–19)	90–130	90–150	< 7.5%	Risk of severe hypoglycemia; developmental and psychological issues; a lower goal (< 7%) if it can be achieved without excessive hypoglycemia

B   Target Indicators of Glycemic Control

Level of control	Ideal (nondiabetic)	Optimal	Suboptimal (action suggested)	High-risk (action required)
Clinical assessment				
Raised BG	Not raised	No symptoms	Polyuria, polydipsia, and enuresis	Blurred vision, poor weight gain, poor growth, delayed puberty, poor school attendance, skin or genital infections, and signs of vascular complications
Low BG	Not low	Few mild and no severe hypoglycemias	Episodes of severe hypoglycemia (unconscious and/or convulsions)	–
Biochemical assessment[*]				
SBGM values				
AM fasting or preprandial	3.6–5.6 (65–100)	5–8 (90–145)	> 8 (> 145)	> 9 (> 162)
PG in mmol/L (mg/dl)				
Postprandial PG[†]	4.5–7 (80–126)	5–10 (90–180)	10–14 (180–250)	> 14 (> 250)
Bedtime PG[†]	4–5.6 (80–100)	6.7–10 (120–180)	< 6.7 or 10–11 (< 120 or 180–200)	< 4.4 or > 11 (< 80 or > 200)
Nocturnal PG[†]	3.6–5.6 (65–100)	4.5–9 (80–162)	< 4.2 or > 9 (< 75 or > 162)	< 4 or > 11 (< 70 or > 200)
HbA$_{1c}$ (%) (DCCT standardized)	< 6.05	< 7.5[†]	7.5–9[†]	> 9[‡]

*These population-based target indicators must be adjusted according to individual circumstances. Different targets will be appropriate for various individuals such as those who have experienced severe hypoglycemia or those with hypoglycemic unawareness.

†These figures are based on clinical studies and expert opinion, but no strict evidence-based recommendations are available. PG levels are given because BG meters are internally calibrated to reflect the plasma glucose level.

‡DCCT conventional adult cohort had a mean HbA$_{1c}$ value of 8.9% and both DCCT and Epidemiology of Diabetes Interventions and Complications Study have shown poor outcomes with this level; therefore, it seems prudent to recommend levels below this value.

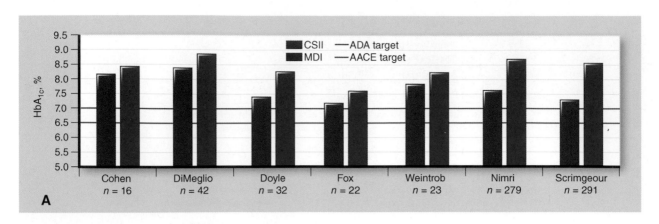

B   CSII Supportive Care

The child and caregivers should be aware of the following:
Nutrition therapy including carbohydrate counting/estimation
Principles of basal-bolus therapy
Insulin kinetics and pump failure
Recognition and management of hypoglycemia and hyperglycemia
The effects of activity and exercise on blood glucose
Sick day management

Figure 6-14. Use of pump therapy in children and youth. Numerous observational studies [24–31] involving more than 760 pediatric patients with type 1 diabetes have shown decreases in hemoglobin A_{1c} (HbA$_{1c}$) with pump therapy. The mean HbA$_{1c}$ level in these studies was comparable to or lower than that reported in the adolescent cohort of the Diabetes Control and Complications Trial. However, most of the studies were 6–12 months in duration, and only four had a follow-up period of 2–5 years. (**A**) Data are shown from seven studies done between 2004 and 2007 in children as young as 1.6 years. As illustrated, the continuous subcutaneous insulin infusion (CSII) groups all had lower HbA$_{1c}$ levels than the multiple daily injection (MDI) groups. In addition, several observational pediatric trials have shown a decrease in the rate of severe hypoglycemia with CSII, whereas simultaneously lowering HbA$_{1c}$. Quality of life measures, patient satisfaction, and disease-related satisfaction are generally improved or unchanged with CSII therapy. In some studies, parents of infants and toddlers have reported more freedom, flexibility, and spontaneity, as well as reduced parental stress and worry. CSII should be considered for children and youth with recurrent severe hypoglycemia, wide fluctuations in blood glucose levels regardless of HbA$_{1c}$, suboptimal diabetes control, microvascular complications, and/or risk factors for macrovascular complications and good metabolic control. In addition, young children and especially infants and neonates, adolescents with eating disorders, youth with pronounced dawn phenomenon, pregnant adolescents, ketosis-prone individuals, and competitive athletes are candidates for pump therapy. (**B**) With a specific education program, appropriate programming of the insulin pump, glucose monitoring, data management, and team care, the consensus statement indicates that children and youth, with their families, can succeed with CSII.

Due to the increasing numbers of children with diabetes who use insulin pump technology and the disparity in access to pediatric endocrine care, which is mainly centered in academic medical centers, the use of the Internet-based insulin pump monitoring system, CareLink (Medtronic; Minneapolis, MN), was evaluated to determine if it could improve glycemic control in children and youth living in a rural setting. The records of children treated with insulin pump therapy in New Mexico from 2004 to 2007 revealed that use of the Internet-based diabetes management system improved glycemic control in the 41 children who used CareLink; they had a reduction in HbA_{1c} from 8.0±0.1 to 7.7±0.1 (P=0.002), a subset of 18 youth living in rural areas had a reduction in HbA_{1c} from 7.9±0.2 to 7.4±0.2 (P=0.001), even though they had fewer clinic visits per year compared with urban patients (2.8±0.2 vs. 3.5±0.1; P=0.001) [32].

Continuous Glucose Monitoring of Children with Type 1 Diabetes

	Adults (≥ 25 y; n = 98)		Adolescents (15–24 y; n = 110)		Children (8–14 y; n = 114)	
HbA_{1c}	CGM (n = 52)	Control (n = 46)	CGM (n = 57)	Control (n = 53)	CGM (n = 56)	Control (n = 58)
HbA_{1c} change from baseline to 26 wk (%)	−0.50 ± 0.56	0.02 ± 0.45	−0.18 ± 0.65	−0.21 ± 0.61	−0.37 ± 0.90	−0.22 ± 0.54
HbA_{1c} < 7% at week 26 (no severe hypoglycemic events) (number %)	15 (30%)	3 (7%)	7 (13%)	7 (14%)	14 (25%)	6 (10%)
Sensor usage for at least 6 d	83%	–	30%	–	50%	–

FIGURE 6-15. Continuous glucose monitoring (CGM) of children with type 1 diabetes. Real-time CGM provides patients, family members, and health-care providers with detailed information regarding glucose trends, including postprandial and overnight glucose profiles, which are rarely obtained with conventional self-monitoring of blood glucose with home glucose monitoring systems. CGM provides the current glucose value, the direction and rate of change of glucose concentrations and alarms for actual (and in some devices impending) hypoglycemia and hyperglycemia. Patients, parents, and health-care providers can also retrospectively review days to months of data to look for trends and patterns that would allow for adjustments in diabetes management. For real-time CGM to be accepted, the sensors must be comfortable and the system must be easy to use, not be burdensome or annoying to the wearer. A number of studies have evaluated the efficacy of CGM in children and youth, either with sensor augmented pump therapy or with those who take multiple daily injections. The Juvenile Diabetes Research Foundation (JDRF) sponsored study [33] of 322 subjects 8–72 years of age, divided the cohort by age 8–14 years (children), 15–24 years (adolescents), and older than 25 years old (adults). The results at 26 weeks showed all age groups experienced similar hemoglobin A_{1c} (HbA_{1c}) reduction with near-daily use of CGM. Adults experienced a statistically significant HbA_{1c} absolute reduction of 0.53% and spent more time in the target glucose range. The children did not achieve a statistically significant change in HbA_{1c}, but a greater percentage of CGM users achieved a 0.5% or greater absolute reduction in HbA_{1c}, a 10% or greater relative reduction in HbA_{1c}, and an HbA_{1c} level less than 7.0% compared with the control group. The adolescents showed no statistically significant change in HbA_{1c} and this age group had the lowest CGM utilization. However, when CGM was used at least six times per week, all age groups achieved at least a 0.5% absolute reduction in HbA_{1c} without an increase in hypoglycemia. In a follow-up analysis of the JDRF study, the study group evaluated those who entered the study with HbA_{1c} less than 7.0%. Approximately half of the cohort was children or adolescents. At 26 weeks, there was a significant treatment group difference in the CGM group in mean HbA_{1c} adjusted for baseline (P<0.001). The challenge for those caring for children and youth who would benefit from CGM is to determine how to increase motivation to use CGM, and it also underscores the need to develop new strategies to increase acceptance, effectiveness, and long-term use (adapted from The Juvenile Diabetes Research Foundation Continuous Glucose Monitoring Study Group [34]; with permission).

Components of the Outpatient Visit

Medical History	Physical Examination
Symptoms and results of laboratory tests related to the diagnosis of diabetes	Height, weight, and BMI calculation (and comparison to age - and sex-specific norms)
Recent or current infections or illnesses	Blood pressure determination and comparison to age-, sex-, and height-specific norms
Previous growth record, including growth chart, and pubertal development	Funduscopic examination
Family history of diabetes, diabetes complications, and other endocrine disorders	Oral examination
Current or recent use of medications that may affect blood glucose levels (eg, glucocorticoids, chemotherapeutic agents, atypical antipsychotics)	Thyroid palpation
History and treatment of other conditions, including endocrine and eating disorders, and diseases known to cause secondary diabetes (eg, cystic fibrosis)	Cardiac examination
Lifestyle, cultural, psychosocial, educational, and economic factors that might influence the management of diabetes	Abdominal examination (eg, for hepatomegaly)
Use of tobacco, alcohol, and/or recreational drugs	Staging of sexual maturation
Physical activity and exercise	Evaluation of pulses
Contraception and sexual activity (if applicable)	Hand/finger examination
Risk factors for atherosclerosis: smoking, hypertension, obesity, dyslipidemia, and family history	Foot examination
ROS should include gastrointestinal function (including symptoms of celiac disease) and symptoms of other endocrine disorders (especially hypothyroidism and Addison's disease)	Skin examination (for acanthosis nigricans SMBG testing sites and insulin-injection sites*)
Prior HbA$_{1c}$ records*	Neurologic examination
Details of previous treatment programs, including nutrition and diabetes self-management education, attitudes, and health beliefs*	Laboratory evaluation
Results of past testing for chronic diabetes complications, including ophthalmologic examination and microalbumin screening*	If clinical evidence of DKA: serum glucose, electrolytes, arterial, or venous pH, serum or urine ketones
Frequency, severity, and cause of acute complications such as ketoacidosis and hypoglycemia*	If signs and symptoms are suggestive of type 2 diabetes: evidence of islet autoimmunity (eg, islet cell [ICA] 512 or 1A -2, GAD, and insulin autoantibodies); evidence of β -cell secretory capacity (eg, C-peptide levels) after 1 -year, if diagnosis is in doubt
Current treatment of diabetes, including medications, meal plan, and results of glucose monitoring and patients' use of data *	HbA$_{1c}$
Referrals and screening	Lipid profile
Yearly ophthalmologic evaluation	Annual screening for microalbuminuria
Medical nutrition therapy (by a registered dietician). As part of initial team education, or referral as needed; generally requires a series of sessions during the initial 3 months of diagnosis, then at least annual reeducation	Thyroid-secreting hormone levels
Behavioral specialist. As part of initial team education or referral as needed optimally for evaluation and counseling of patient and family at diagnosis, then as indicated to enhance support and empowerment to maintain family involvement in diabetes care tasks to identify and discuss ways to overcome barriers in successful diabetes management	Celiac antibodies at diagnosis or initial visit if not done previously
Depression screening annual for children ≥ 10 y of age, with referral as indicated	
*Pertain only to previously diagnosed patients at time of initial referral, assuming prior medical management.	

Figure 6-16. At the time of diagnosis, the patient should be assessed with a medical history, physical examination, laboratory evaluation, and series of referrals and screening as shown in the American Diabetes Association Initial Assessment form [35]. After that, pediatric patients with diabetes should have comprehensive, multidisciplinary outpatient visits at regular intervals [36]. The purpose of these visits is to assess health status, adjust the diabetes regimen as indicated, promote diabetes knowledge and competency, and motivate patients and families to improve short and long-term outcomes. Diabetes health-care providers should ensure that the patient has routine pediatric care for well-child visits to diagnose and treat other medical/psychological problems and to administer immunizations and anticipatory guidance. At quarterly visits, hemoglobin A$_{1c}$ (HbA$_{1c}$) levels should be obtained. Preferably, the results are available at the time of the clinic visit to allow for a face-to-face discussion if glycemic targets are not met. Thyroid function tests should be done yearly. Thyroid autoantibodies are present in 20–30% of pediatric type 1 subjects; however, overt hypothyroidism occurs in 1–5% and compensated hypothyroidism in 5–10%. A fasting lipid profile that includes total cholesterol, high-density lipoprotein cholesterol, low-density lipoprotein cholesterol, and triglycerides should be obtained in children and adolescents after glucose control has been established. Microalbumin levels can be measured using a random microalbumin-to-creatinine ratio, timed overnight microalbumin assay-to-albumin excretion rate assessment, or 24-h timed urinary microalbumin-to-albumin excretion rate measurement. Celiac disease has been reported to occur 10–50 times more often in children with diabetes compared with the general population. Depending on the study, celiac disease may be present in 1–10% of children and adolescents with type 1 diabetes. Celiac disease should be considered in children and youth with gastrointestinal symptoms such as diarrhea, pain, flatulence, dyspepsia, or aphthous ulcers. Unexplained hypoglycemia, dermatitis herpetiformis, and delayed growth or pubertal development can also be associated with celiac disease. A celiac screen, including antiendomysial IgA antibody quantitation, should be obtained. At the time of diagnosis, patients should have liver function tests and a creatinine and urinalysis. Assessment of islet autoimmunity should be made by obtaining specific antibodies to islet antigens. *BMI* body mass index, *ROS* review of systems, *SMBG* self blood glucose monitoring (adapted from American Diabetes Association Care for Children [35]; with permission).

A ISPAD Clinical Practice Consensus Guidelines 2009 Compendium : Screening, Risk Factors, and Interventions for Vascular Complications

	When to commence screening?	Screening methods	Risk factors	Potential intervention
Retinopathy	Annually from age 11 y with 2 y duration and from 9 y with 5 y duration (E)	Fundal photography or mydriatic ophthalmoscopy (less sensitive) (E)	Hyperglycemia (A); high blood pressure (B); lipid abnormalities (B); higher BMI (C)	Improved glycemic control (A); laser therapy (A)
Nephropathy	Annually from age 11 y with 2 y duration and from 9 y with 5 y duration (E)	Urinary albumin/creatinine ratio or first morning albumin concentration (E)	High blood pressure (B); lipid abnormalities (B); smoking (B)	Improved glycemic control (A); ACEI and AIIRA (A); blood pressure lowering (B)
Neuropathy	Unclear	History and physical examination	Hyperglycemia (A); higher BMI (C)	Improved glycemic control (A)
Macrovascular disease	After age 12 y (E)	Lipid profile every 5 y, blood pressure annually (E)	Hyperglycemia (A); high blood pressure (A); lipid abnormalit ies (B); higher BMI (B); smoking (B)	Improved glycemic control (A); blood pressure control (B); statins (A)

Levels of evidence (A, B, C, E) for risk factors and interventions pertain to adult studies, except for improved glycemic control.

FIGURE 6-17. Complication screening. Although clinically significant diabetes-related micro- and macrovascular complications are rare in childhood and adolescence, the prevention of such complications through optimization of glycemic control, blood pressure, body mass index (BMI), and lipids is paramount during this time. Thus, International Society for Pediatric and Adolescent Diabetes (ISPAD) recommends routine annual screening for the presence of diabetes-related complications beginning at 11 years of age and slightly earlier (9 years old) if diabetes duration is longer than 5 years [37] (**A**). The guidelines from the American Diabetes Association (ADA) are similar with the recommendation to begin annual screening for retinopathy and nephropathy when the child has more than 5 years of diabetes duration and is older than 10 years old [35] (**B**). Autoimmune thyroid disease and celiac disease are fairly common comorbid conditions of type 1 diabetes, and therefore, regular screening is important so treatment can be started. Both the ISPAD and ADA recommend that children and adolescents are screened for autoimmune thyroid disease at the onset of diabetes with a measurement of both thyroid-stimulating hormone and thyroid antibodies [35, 37]. This should be repeated every 1–2 years or sooner if symptoms or a goiter develop. Although ISPAD and ADA differ slightly on the frequency of screening for celiac disease, both groups recommend screening at onset of diabetes. *AIIRA* angiotensin II receptor antagonist, *ACEI* angiotensin converting enzyme inhibitor, *CVD* cardiovascular disease, *DCCT* Diabetes Control and Complications Trial, *HbA$_{1c}$* hemoglobin A$_{1c}$, *HDL* high-density lipoprotein, *LDL* low-density lipoprotein (adapted from ISPAD Clinical Practice Consensus Guidelines 2009 Compendium [37]; with permission).

B   Target Levels for Different Parameters to Reduce the Risk of Microvascular and CVD in Children and Adolescents with Type 1 Diabetes

Parameter	Target level	Level of evidence
HbA$_{1c}$ (DCCT standard)	≤ 7.5% without severe hypoglycemia	A
LDL cholesterol	< 2.6 mmol/L	A
HDL cholesterol	≥ 1.1 mmol/L	C
Triglycerides	< 1.7 mmol/L	C
Blood pressure	< 90th percentile by age, sex, and height; < 130/80 mm Hg	C/B
Body mass index	< 95th percentile (nonobese)	E
Smoking	None	A
Physical activity	> 1 h if moderate physical activity daily	B
Sedentary activities	< 2 h daily	B
Healthy diet	Caloric intake appropriate for age and normal growth. Fat < 30% of caloric intake, saturated fat < 10% of caloric intake. Fiber intake 25 −35 g daily. Increased intake of fresh fruit and vegetables .	E
Levels of evidence pertain to adult studies.		

FIGURE 6-17. (continued)

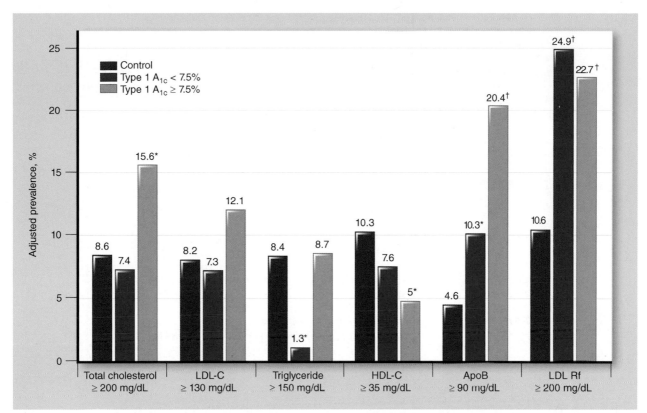

FIGURE 6-18. Dyslipidemia. Dyslipidemia is a very important and modifiable risk factor for cardiovascular disease (CVD) and CVD is the leading cause of death in people with type 1 and type 2 diabetes. The SEARCH for Diabetes in Youth (SEARCH) study demonstrated that 3% of youth with type 1 diabetes mellitus (T1DM) had low density lipoprotein cholesterol (LDL-C) levels higher than 160 mg/dL, 14% had LDL-C levels higher than 130 mg/dL, and 48% had LDL-C levels higher than 100 mg/dL [38]. The SEARCH study group also completed a cross-sectional study of 512 youth with T1DM (age, 10–22 y; mean duration, 4.22 y) and 188 healthy controls [39]. They compared fasting lipid profiles of youth with well-controlled diabetes (hemoglobin A$_{1c}$ [A$_{1c}$] < 7.5%) and less well-controlled diabetes (A$_{1c}$ ≥ 7.5%) with the healthy controls. They found that youth with optimal glycemic control had similar mean levels of total cholesterol, LDL-C, non-high-density lipoprotein (HDL) cholesterol, and LDL particle size. They had lower mean levels of triglyceride and higher HDL cholesterol compared with healthy controls. However, they had higher mean apolipoprotein B (apoB) levels. By contrast, the youth with suboptimal glycemic control had more atherogenic lipid profiles. *Asterisk* indicates P < 0.05, type 1 diabetes with optimal or suboptimal A$_{1c}$ versus healthy youth. *Dagger* indicates P < 0.01, type 1 diabetes with optimal or suboptimal A$_{1c}$ versus healthy youth. *Rf* relative flotation (adapted from Guy et al. [39]; with permission).

A   ADA Recommendations on Lipid Screening and Management in Youth with Diabetes

Diabetes Care 2003, 26:2194; *Diabetes Care* 2005, 28:186	Type 1 diabetes	Type 2 diabetes
Initial screening age (once glycemic control obtained)	>2 y at diagnosis if unknown or positive family history; otherwise at 12 y (puberty)	At diagnosis
Rescreening if lipids normal	5 y	2 y
Optimal concentration	LDL-C < 100 mg/dL HDL-C > 35 mg/dL Triglyceride < 150 mg/dL	
Management of elevated LDL-C	Goal LDL-C < 100 mg/dL	
Initial therapy	Glycemic control, MNT, physical activity, weight control, tobacco cessation	
After 3–6 mo	LDL-C > 160 mg/dL: begin medication LDL-C 130–159 mg/dL: "recommended" after MNT failure based on other CVD risk factors Counsel on pregnancy if statin started	

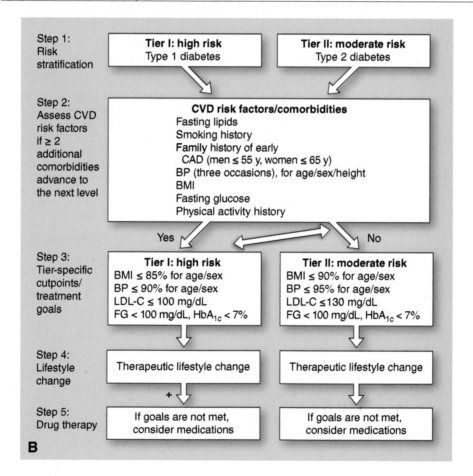

School Health Care Plans
Diabetes Medical Management Plan: Prepared by the student's personal diabetes health care team
Individualized Health Care Plan: Prepared by the school nurse
Emergency Care Plans: Prepared by the school nurse
Diabetes Medical Management Plan: Prepared by the student's personal diabetes health care team

FIGURE 6-20. Diabetes in the school and day care center. Approximately 125,000 children of school age have diabetes in the USA. The health, safety, and educational progress of a student with diabetes depend on cooperation and collaboration among the student, the parents/guardian, the school nurse, and other school staff members. Working together, they form the school health team that implements the provisions of the student's health-care and education plans and provides the necessary assistance in the school setting. There are three federal laws that protect children with diabetes including the Rehabilitation Act of 1973, the Individuals with Disabilities Education Act of 1991, and the Americans with Disabilities Act of 1992. These laws make it illegal for schools to discriminate and any school that receives federal funding or is considered open to the public must reasonably accommodate the special needs of children with diabetes. Accommodations must be made within the child's usual school setting with as little disruption to the routine of the school and child as is possible and allowing for full participation in all school activities. To ensure this, the American Diabetes Association has issued a position statement including general guidelines for the care of the child in the school and day-care setting [41]. These guidelines include explaining the responsibilities of the various stakeholders, the parent/guardian, the school/day-care provider, the health-care team, and the student/child. Key to the successful implementation of these guidelines is the development of the individualized diabetes care plan that provides specific instructions about blood-glucose monitoring, insulin administration, recognition and treatment of hypoglycemia and hyperglycemia, the meal plan, and testing for ketones (adapted from American Diabetes Association [41], with permission; and National Institutes of Health and Centers for Disease Control and Prevention [42], with permission).

FIGURE 6-19. The International Society for Pediatric and Adolescent Diabetes (ISPAD), American Diabetes Association (ADA), and the American Heart Association (AHA) have all developed recommendations for the screening and treatment of dyslipidemia in youth with diabetes. ISPAD recommends screening lipids every 5 years starting at 12 years old, dietary intervention if low-density lipoprotein cholesterol (LDL-C) levels are higher than 2.6 mmol/L, and initiation of lipid-lowering agents if LDL levels are higher than 3.4 mmol/L in the presence of one or more cardiovascular disease (CVD) risk factors [37]. (**A**) The ADA has an added recommendation of screening at more than 2 yrs of age at diagnosis if family history is unknown or positive for dyslipidemia. In addition, they recommend initiation of screening at diagnosis of type 2 diabetes regardless of age and more frequent screening of patients (every 2 y). Threshold for initiating therapy and treatment goals are outlined. (**B**) The AHA includes individuals with type 1 diabetes in tier 1 (high risk) and individuals with type 2 diabetes in tier II (moderate risk). Treatment goals and threshold for treatment is then determined by tier level and presence of additional CVD risk factors, such that an individual with type 1 diabetes and ≥ two CVD risk factors would have an LDL-C cutpoint of ≤100 mg/dL. *BMI* body mass index, *BP* blood pressure, *CAD* coronary artery disease, *FG* fasting glucose, *HbA$_{1c}$* hemoglobin A$_{1c}$, *HDL-C* high-density lipoprotein cholesterol, *MNT* medical nutrition therapy (adapted from Maahs et al. [40]; with permission).

Adjustment to Childhood Diabetes

Psychosocial Issues in Pediatric Diabetes

Psychosocial factors affecting initial diabetes management
Patient's and family's adjustment to losses and uncertainties inherent in diagnosis
Cultural and health beliefs competing with treatment requirements
Emotional reactions to diabetes-specific tasks and complications (fear of injections, blood-glucose monitoring, responses to hypo- and hyperglycemia, long-term complications)
Psychiatric and social problems preceding diagnosis
Community and social support surrounding the family
Relationship and communication with health care team
Financial resources for treatment and access to good caretakers
Important factors in psychosocial management
Self-care tasks appropriate to maturity rather than age
Complete supervision in children, discrete supervision in adolescents
Avoidance of extremes of overprotection or total independence
Clear attribution and sharing of responsibilities among family members and patients
Realistic treatment goals according to the patient's acceptance
Empathic understanding of the stresses of living with diabetes
Encouragement of open communication and venting of negative feelings toward diabetes
Recognition of diabetes burnout
Problem-solving skills practiced regularly
Help form mental health professionals if necessary
Focus on overall success: age-appropriate developmental skills, adequate social and family relationships, good glycemic control

FIGURE 6-21. Psychosocial issues in pediatric diabetes. The majority of patients diagnosed with diabetes exhibit mild depression, anxiety, and somatic complaints at the time of diagnosis [43]. In most cases, these symptoms are usually self-limited and resolve within 6–9 months. However, in a subset of patients, depressive symptoms increase over time and anxiety worsens, more often in girls than boys. Patient adjustment to diabetes at the time of diagnosis predicts later adjustment. The psychosocial factors affecting initial diabetes management are given below. Family characteristics have a major influence on adjustment to diabetes, self-management, and quality of life. Children and adolescents living in families with a high degree of conflict or with parents who are less caring have less optimal metabolic control. To improve psychological stability and glycemic control, early assessment of family dynamics and, when appropriate, psychological intervention, as listed below, should be done by a multidisciplinary diabetes team equipped to provide social and psychological support.

Type 2 Diabetes in Children and Youth

A   Testing for Type 2 Diabetes in Children

Criteria
Overweight (BMI > 85th% for age and sex, weight for height > 85th percentile or weight > 120% ideal for height)   *Plus any two of the following risk factors:*   Family history of type 2 diabetes in first - or second-degree relative   Race/ethnicity (American Indian, African American, Hispanic, Asian/Pacific Islander)   Signs of insulin resistance or condition associated with insulin resistance (Acanthosis nigricans, hypertension, dyslipidemia, PCOS)
Age of initiation : Age 10 years or at onset of puberty if puberty occurs at a younger age
Frequency : Every 2 years
Test: Fasting plasma glucose preferred

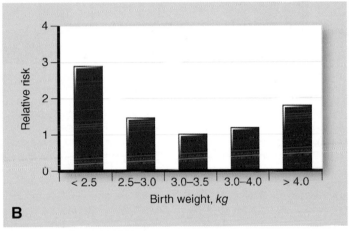

B

Figure 6-22. Risk factors and screening for type 2 diabetes. (**A**) Type 2 diabetes in children and youth is due to insulin resistance and relative insulin deficiency. Risk factors for type 2 diabetes in youth include overweight/obesity associated with poor diet and decreased physical inactivity, race/ethnicity, family history, diabetic gestation, underweight or overweight for gestational age, and signs of insulin resistance including hyperandrogenism (polycystic ovary syndrome), hypertension, dyslipidemia, and other atherosclerosis risk factors [2, 45]. Studies have shown that youth with type 2 diabetes have a strong family history with 45–80% having at least one parent with diabetes and 74–100% having a first- or second-degree relative with type 2 diabetes. Children with type 2 diabetes are also more likely to have a family history of cardiovascular disease and in Pima youth, the cumulative incidence of type 2 diabetes was highest in offspring if both parents had diabetes. The intrauterine environment has also been recognized as an increasingly important contributor to diabetes. (**B**) Both low birth weight (<2,500 g) and high birth weight are associated with type 2 diabetes even in children as young as 10 years of age. This relationship is likely mediated by both genetic and environmental factors. A survey from Taiwan showed a U-shaped curve for birth weight and risk of type 2 diabetes [46]. The risk increased in those with high birth weight (≥4,000 g; OR, 1.78; 95% CI, 1.04–3.06) and low birth weight (<2,500 g; OR, 2.91; 95% CI, 1.25–6.76). These results were still valid after accounting for age, sex, and family history of type 2 diabetes. These two extremes of birth weight likely represent two separate types of risk for diabetes, the thrifty phenotype for low birth weight, and the genetic, and possibly, environmental risk associated with high birth weight and maternal diabetes during pregnancy. *BMI* body mass index, *PCOS* polycystic ovarian syndrome. [(**A**) adapted from The American Diabetes Association [2], with permission; and (**B**) adapted from Shaw [44], with permission].

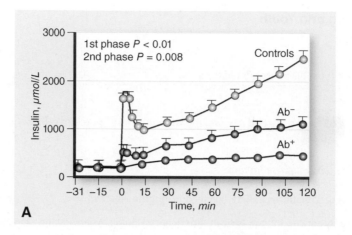

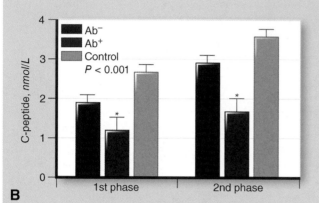

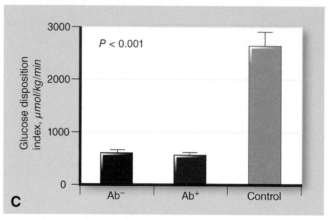

FIGURE 6-23. Phenotypic type 2 diabetes in obese youth. It is important to determine if youth diagnosed with type 2 diabetes have the presence of islet autoantibodies (Ab). These phenotypic type 2 diabetes subjects with positive autoantibodies have distinct patterns of insulin secretion, insulin sensitivity, and body composition/adiposity compared with phenotypic type 2 diabetes subjects who are autoantibody negative. In a small sample, including 16 antibody-negative, 26 antibody-positive, and 39 obese controls, severe insulin resistance was noted in those subjects who were antibody-negative with type 2 diabetes [47]. They had significantly lower insulin-stimulated total, oxidative, and nonoxidative glucose disposal and suppression of fat oxidation during hyperinsulinemia compared with those who were antibody-positive or who were obese controls. The responses of antibody-positive type 2 subjects were equivalent to those of the obese controls. Antibody-positive subjects had significantly lower first- and second-phase insulin secretion (**A**) and C-peptide values (**B**) compared with those who were anti-

body-negative. Glucose disposition index (**C**) was equivalent between the type 2 diabetes antibody-positive and antibody-negative groups, and lower than the controls. Ketonuria at the onset of diabetes was higher in the antibody-positive subjects than the antibody-negative subjects, as would have been expected. Autoantibody-positive youth diagnosed with type 2 diabetes had severe insulin deficiency due to β-cell failure, similar to youth with type 1 diabetes. By contrast, autoantibody-negative youth were characterized by severe insulin resistance and relative insulin deficiency, as expected with type 2. These differences in metabolic findings should influence the course of this diverse disease in youth, particularly with regard to clinical outcomes and the potential for insulin treatment. As a result, assessing autoantibody status in phenotypic type 2 diabetes in obese youth is clinically relevant. *Asterisk* in panel B indicates post-hoc Bonferroni correction; $P < 0.05$ Ab+ vs. AB−, Ab+ vs. control subjects (adapted from Tfayli et al. [47]; with permission).

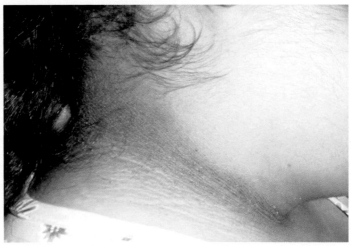

FIGURE 6-24. Acanthosis nigricans. Acanthosis nigricans is a marker of insulin resistance. It is frequently associated with type 2 diabetes; 60–90% of youth with type 2 diabetes have acanthosis nigricans. The skin is hyperpigmented in intertriginous areas. In a survey from 1,412 students in Galveston, TX, 7.1% had acanthosis nigricans [48]. The prevalence was highest in African American children (13.3%), followed by Hispanics (5.5%) and Caucasians (0.5%) [48]. Acanthosis nigricans is highly associated with obesity. The prevalence of diabetes is six times higher in African American subjects with acanthosis nigricans than it is in African Americans without this skin lesion. Because acanthosis nigricans is so highly associated with diabetes, it can potentially be used as a screening tool to help identify those at high risk for type 2 diabetes [49].

Prevalence of High BMI for Age Among US Children, 2003 –2006[*]

	All[*]		Non-Hispanic White		Non-Hispanic Black		Mexican Americans	
	Patients, n	% (SE)	Patients, n	% (SE)	Patients, n	% (SE)	Patients, n	% (SE)
BMI ≥ 97th percentile of the CDC Growth Charts								
Age of both sexes, y								
2–19	8165	11.3 (0.8)	2194	9.6 (1.1)	2695	15.9 (0.8)	2582	15.5 (1.2)
2–5	1770	8.5 (0.8)	497	6.7 (1.3)	517	10.8 (1.3)	558	13.4 (1.9)
6–11	2095	11.4 (0.9)	558	8.9 (1.4)	673	17.0 (1.6)	670	17.6 (1.9)
12–19	4300	12.6 (1.0)	1139	11.2 (1.4)	1505	17.4 (1.0)	1354	15.0 (1.2)
Boys' age, y								
2–19	4117	12.2 (0.9)	1113	10.6 (1.3)	1396	13.0 (0.9)	1279	17.7 (1.5)
2–5	875	9.0 (1.3)	260	7.6 (2.1)	254	10.1 (2.5)	269	16.0 (2.7)
6–11	1013	11.7 (1.2)	265	8.7 (2.0)	335	14.4 (2.1)	321	21.0 (2.6)
12–19	2229	13.9 (1.3)	588	13.1 (1.7)	807	15.3 (1.5)	689	15.9 (1.6)
Girls' age, y								
2–19	4048	10.5 (0.9)	1081	8.5 (1.2)	1299	19.0 (1.0)	1303	13.2 (1.4)
2–5	895	7.9 (1.1)	237	5.8 (1.8)	263	11.6 (1.3)	289	10.8 (2.1)
6–11	1082	11.1 (1.1)	293	9.1 (1.7)	338	19.7 (1.9)	349	14.0 (2.1)
12–19	2071	11.1 (1.2)	551	9.1 (1.6)	698	19.6 (1.5)	1354	14.1 (1.3)
BMI ≥ 95th percentile of the CDC Growth Charts								
Age of both sexes, y								
2–19	8165	16.3 (0.9)	2194	14.6 (1.3)	2695	20.7 (1.0)	2582	20.9 (1.3)
2–5	1770	12.4 (1.0)	497	10.7 (1.5)	517	14.9 (1.3)	558	16.7 (2.3)
6–11	2095	17.0 (1.3)	558	15.0 (1.9)	673	21.3 (1.8)	60	23.8 (2.0)
12–19	4300	17.6 (1.2)	1139	16.0 (1.7)	1505	22.9 (1.1)	1354	21.1 (1.4)
Boys' age, y								
2–19	4117	17.1 (1.1)	1113	15.6 (1.5)	1396	17.4 (1.0)	1279	23.2 (1.6)
2–5	876	12.3 (1.2)	260	11.1 (2.2)	254	13.3 (2.5)	269	18.8 (2.8)
6–11	1013	18.0 (1.7)	265	15.5 (2.8)	335	18.6 (2.6)	321	27.5 (2.1)
12–19	2229	18.2 (1.5)	588	17.3 (2.0)	807	18.5 (1.3)	689	22.1 (2.2)
Girls' age, y								
2–19	4048	15.5 (1.1)	1081	13.6 (1.4)	1299	24.1 (1.3)	1303	18.5 (1.5)
2–5	895	12.8 (1.3)	237	10.2 (1.9)	263	16.6 (2.3)	289	14.5 (2.7)
6–11	1082	15.8 (1.4)	293	14.4 (2.1)	338	24.0 (2.0)	349	19.7 (2.6)
12–19	2071	16.8 (1.5)	551	14.5 (2.0)	698	27.7 (1.9)	665	19.9 (1.4)
BMI ≥ 85th percentile of the CDC Growth Charts								
Age of both sexes, y								
2–10	8165	31.9 (1.2)	2194	30.7 (1.7)	2695	34.9 (1.3)	2582	38.0 (1.4)
2–5	1770	24.4 (1.6)	497	23.2 (2.2)	517	24.8 (2.1)	558	29.9 (2.5)
6–11	2095	33.3 (2.0)	558	31.6 (3.0)	673	36.9 (2.5)	670	42.8 (2.3)
12–19	4300	34.1 (1.5)	1139	33.1 (2.1)	1505	38.1 (1.4)	1354	38.9 (1.6)
Boys' age, y								
2–19	4117	32.7 (1.4)	1113	31.9 (2.0)	1396	30.8 (1.6)	1279	40.8 (1.6)
2–5	875	25.5 (2.0)	260	25.4 (2.9)	254	23.2 (3.3)	269	32.4 (3.2)
6–11	1013	33.9 (2.2)	265	31.7 (3.6)	335	33.8 (3.6)	321	47.1 (2.5)
12–19	2229	34.9 (1.9)	588	34.5 (2.6)	807	32.1 (1.8)	689	40.5 (2.6)
Girls' age, y								
2–19	4048	31.0 (1.3)	1081	29.5 (1.8)	1299	39.2 (1.1)	1303	35.0 (1.7)
2–5	895	23.3 (1.8)	237	20.9 (2.6)	263	26.4 (2.8)	289	27.3 (2.8)
6–11	1092	32.6 (2.4)	293	31.5 (3.6)	338	40.1 (2.3)	349	38.1 (3.3)
12–19	2071	33.3 (1.8)	551	31.7 (2.4)	698	44.5 (1.5)	665	37.1 (1.9)

Figure 6-25. Prevalence of overweight, obesity, and severe obesity in boys and girls 12–19 years of age. Although there had been a marked increase in the prevalence of obesity in girls and boys across all ethnic groups, except Caucasian girls, during the past two to three decades, no further increase in overweight/obesity rates was seen from 2003 to 2006. Overall, 11.3% of children and youth 2–19 years of age had a body mass index (BMI) higher than the 97th percentile of the 2000 BMI-for-age growth charts, 16.3% were higher than the 95th percentile, and 31.9% were higher than the 85th percentile. Although prevalence varied by age and race/ethnicity, the overall analysis of trends showed no statistically significant trend over the periods from 1999 to 2006 [50]. *CDC* Centers for Disease Control and Prevention, *SE* standard error (adapted from Ogden et al. [50]; with permission).

Sixth-Grade Student Characteristics[*]

Age, *y*	11.8 ± 0.6 (9–15)
Sex (male)	47.6
Race/ethnicity	
Hispanic	53.1
Black	19.7
White	18.8
Other	8.4
Positive self-report first-degree family history of diabetes	16.4
Tanner stage (self-report Pubertal Development Scale)	
Male	
1	15.5
2	38.6
3	38.1
4	6.5
5	0.3
Female	
1	5.8
2	13.0
3	42.7
4	34.9
5	3.6
BMI, *kg/m²*	22.3 ± 5.5
Male	22.4 ± 5.5
Female	22.2 ± 5.5
BMI percentile (categorical, adjusted for age and sex)	
< 85%	50.7
85%–94%	19.7
≥ 95%	29.6
Fasting glucose, *mg/dL*	93.4 ± 6.7
Fasting glucose (categorical)	
< 100 mg/dL	84.0
100–109 mg/dL	14.7
110–125 mg/dL	1.2
≥ 126 mg/dL	0.1[†]
Fasting insulin (µU/mL)	13.3 ± 11.6
Fasting insulin ≥ 30 µU/mL (categorical)	6.8

[*]Data are means ± SD (minimum –maximum) or percent unless otherwise indicated , based on 6358 patients.

[†]Six subjects had fasting glucose > 126 mg/dL at screening; only one of these values was confirmed on follow-up clinical testing.

Figure 6-26. Diabetes risk factors in multiracial youth. The HEALTHY study [51] was designed to determine the prevalence of risk factors for type 2 diabetes in a multiracial cohort of sixth grade students followed through to eighth grade in seven cities across the USA. The intervention was comprehensive and aimed at improving the overall school environment (involving food services, physical education, a health curriculum, social marketing, outreach to families). Assessment from the students at baseline during sixth grade showed a high rate of overweight and obesity (49.3% had a body mass index ≥85th percentile) and 15.9% had a fasting glucose value ≥100 mg/dL, the impaired fasting glucose value range. However, the rate of undiagnosed diabetes found during the assessment period was extremely low at 0.1% (six subjects were initially found on screening but only one confirmed to have diabetes) (adapted from The HEALTHY Study Group [51]; with permission).

Characteristic	Metformin	Placebo
Sex	42	40
Male	12 (28.6)	13 (32.5)
Female	30 (71.4)	27 (67.5)
Age, y		
Mean	13.9 ± 1.8	13.6 ± 1.8
Median	14	14
Range	10–16	10–17[*]
Age, y		
8 to < 10	0	0
10 to < 12	5 (11.9)	7 (17.5)
12 to < 14	9 (21.4)	12 (30)
14 to < 16	18 (42.9)	14 (35)
≥ 16	10 (23.8)	7 (17.5)
Race		
White	17 (40.5)	13 (32.5)
Black	11 (26.2)	13 (32.5)
Asian/Pacific Islander	3 (7.1)	1 (2.5)
Hispanic/Latino	9 (21.4)	9 (22.5)
Other	2 (4.8)	4 (10)
Weight, kg		
Mean	92.8 ± 31.8	90.3 ± 38.1
Median	91	87.9
Range	43–160.5	32–196.4

BMI (kg/m^2)		
Mean	34.2 ± 10.6	33.9 ± 12.7
Median	33.2	32
Range	19.2–58.4	18.1–82.8
BMI (kg/m^2)		
< 75th percentile for age	6 (14.3)	8 (20)
≥ 75th percentile for age	36 (85.7)	32 (80)
FPG (mmol/L) [†]		
Mean	9.2 ± 2.8	11 ± 3.3
< 7	10 (23.8)[§]	4 (10)[§]
7 to < 8.9	12 (28.6)	7 (17.5)
8.9 to < 11.1	11 (26.2)	9 (22.5)
11.1 to < 13.3	2 (4.8)	11 (27.5)
≥ 13.3	7 (16.7)	9 (22.5)
HbA$_{1c}$ (%) [†]		
Mean	8.3 ± 1.3	9 ± 1.4
< 7	5 (11.9)[§]	1 (2.5)[‡]
7 to < 8	14 (33.3)	7 (17.5)
8 to < 9	12 (28.6)	17 (42.5)
9 to < 10	5 (11.9)	7 (17.5)
≥ 10	6 (14.3)	8 (20)
Stimulated C-peptide (nmol/L)	2.4 (1.1)	2.2 (1.1)
Total cholesterol (mmol/L) [§]	4.5 (1.0)	4.9 (1.0)
HDL cholesterol (mmol/L) [§]	1.1 (0.3)	1.1 (0.3)
LDL cholesterol (mmol/L) [§]	2.6 (0.8)	2.9 (0.7)
Triglycerides (mmol/L) [¶]	1.7 (1.3)	2.3 (2.2)[¶]

[*]*One subject was 10 years old when the informed consent was signed but had a birthday between the signing date and the screening visit.*

[†]*The PPG and HbA$_{1c}$ values provided were the values at the randomization visit (visit 2). The inclusion criteria had to be met only at screening (visit 1), consequently, at randomization some subjects had levels outside the range given in the inclusion criteria.*

[‡]*To convert cholesterol levels from mmol/L to mg/dL, divide by 0.259. Data are rounded.*

[§]*To convert triglyceride levels from mmol/L to mg/dL, divide by 0.0113.*
[¶]*One subject had a triglyceride level of 12 mmol/L, which contributed to the higher mean for the placebo group.*

FIGURE 6-27. Use of metformin in pediatric type 2 subjects and obese youth. Metformin has been shown to be effective in children and youth with type 2 diabetes. It is the first oral hypoglycemic agent to gain US Food and Drug Administration approval for type treatment of type 2 diabetes in children. A multicenter study evaluated 82 subjects with doses of metformin up to 1,000 mg twice daily [52]. Subjects were 10–16 years of age and treated for up to 16 weeks in a randomized, double-blind, placebo-controlled trial. Entry criteria were a fasting plasma glucose (FPG) of ≥126 and ≤240 mg/dL and hemoglobin A$_{1c}$ (HbA$_{1c}$) ≥7.0% and C-peptide ≥0.5 nmol/L. Subjects had a body mass index (BMI) higher than the 50th percentile for age. The table shows the beneficial effect of metformin compared with placebo. Improvement in FPG occurred in both sexes and all race groups. Metformin did not have a negative impact on body weight or lipid profile, and the adverse events were similar to those seen in adults. Metformin is the first oral agent to be proven safe and effective for the treatment of type 2 diabetes in pediatric subjects.

A systematic review and meta-analysis of randomized controlled trials evaluated the effect of metformin on BMI and measures of insulin sensitivity [53] in obese youth. Five trials showed that, compared with placebo, metformin reduced BMI by 1.42 kg/m² and homeostatic model assessment insulin resistance score of 2.01.

Therefore, metformin appears to be moderately affective in reducing BMI and insulin resistance in hyperinsulinemic obese youth in the short term. However, insufficient long-term data exist to determine if metformin has a role in the treatment of adolescent obesity.

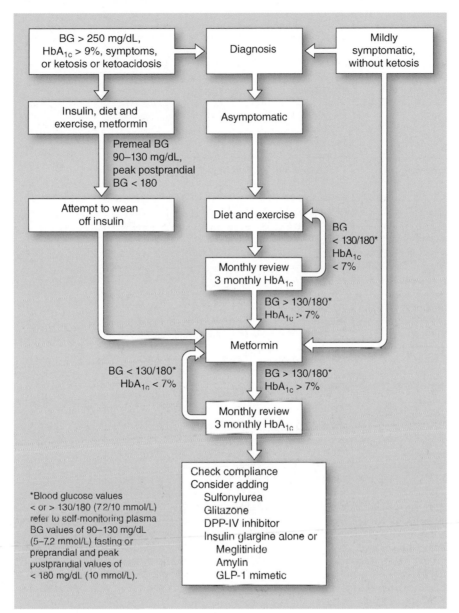

FIGURE 6-28. Algorithm of treatment of type 2 diabetes. The treatment of type 2 diabetes in pediatric patients must include diabetes education to both the family and patient, with emphasis on the importance of regular exercise and appropriate nutrition. Glycemic targets should be established. Goals of maintaining hemoglobin A₁c (HbA₁c) less than 7.0% and fasting plasma glucose levels as near to 126 mg/dL as possible are difficult to achieve in adolescents [54]. *BG* blood glucose, *DPP-IV* dipeptidyl peptidase-4, *GLP-1* glucagon-like peptide-1 (adapted from Rosenbloom et al. [55], with permission).

Comparison of Clinical Characteristics and Complication Rates in Youth with Type 1 and Type 2 Diabetes in New South Wales from 1996 to 2005

Variable	Type 1 diabetes	Type 2 diabetes	P value
Patients, n	1433	68	–
Age at last assessment, y	15.7 (13.9–17.0)	15.3 (13.6–16.4)	0.23
Age at diagnosis, y	8.1 (4.8–10.8)	13.2 (11.6–15.0)	< 0.0001
Sex (male/female)	674/759	34/34	0.63
Duration, y	6.8 (4.7–9.6)	1.3 (0.6–3.1)	< 0.0001
HbA_{1c}, %	8.5 (7.8–9.5)	7.3 (6.0–8.3)	< 0.0001
HbA_{1c} < 7.5%	230/1393 (17%)	42/66 (64%)	< 0.0001
Insulin/weight	1.15 (0.96–1.39)	0.89 (0.51–1.31) (n = 9)	0.063
BMI SD score	0.80 (0.25–1.27)	1.86 (1.28–2.40)	< 0.0001
Social disadvantage risk score	0.23 (–0.17 to –0.80)	0.14 (–0.47 to –0.56)	0.058
From urban area	957/1419 (67%)	46/63 (73%)	0.56
Microalbuminuria	81/1325 (6%)	10/36 (28%)	< 0.0001
Hypertension	223/1393 (16%)	21/58 (36%)	< 0.0001
Retinopathy	254/1264 (20%)	1/25 (4%)	0.043
Peripheral nerve abnormality	375/1376 (27%)	5/24 (21%)	0.48
Pupillary abnormality	568/928 (61%)	13/23 (57%)	0.65
Overweight	452/1411 (32%)	16/64 (25%)	0.24
Obese	100/1411 (7%)	36/64 (56%)	< 0.0001

FIGURE 6-29. Comparing the complication rate between type 1 and type 2 diabetes. In a study of 1,433 type 1 and 68 type 2 youth from 1996 to 2005 in Australia, youth with type 2 diabetes were found to have significantly higher rates of microalbuminuria and hypertension than those with type 1 diabetes, at a shorter duration of diabetes. Patients with type 1 diabetes had significantly more retinopathy, whereas rates of peripheral and autonomic neuropathy were equal in both types of diabetes. Microalbuminuria was significantly associated with older age and systolic hypertension in type 1 diabetes and with only higher hemoglobin A_{1c} (HbA_{1c}) in type 2 diabetes. Screening for the complications of diabetes in youth remains imperative, as does improving HbA_{1c}. [56]. *BMI* body mass index (adapted from Eppin et al. [56]; with permission).

References

1. Craig ME, Hattersley A, Donaghue KC: Definition, epidemiology and classification of diabetes in children and adolescents. *Pediatric Diabetes* 2009, 10(Suppl 12):3–12.

2. American Diabetes Association: Type 2 diabetes in children and adolescents. *Diabetes Care* 2000, 23:381–389.

3. Hattersley A, Bruining J, Shield J, *et al.*: The diagnosis and management of monogenic diabetes in children and adolescents. *Pediatric Diabetes* 2009, 10(Suppl 12):33–42.

4. Wolfsdorf J, Craig ME, Daneman D, *et al.*: Diabetic ketoacidosis in children and adolescents with diabetes. *Pediatric Diabetes* 2009, 10(Suppl 12):118–133.

5. Neu A, Hofer SE, Karges B, et al.: Ketoacidosis at diabetes onset is still frequent in children and adolescents: a multicenter analysis of 14,664 patients from 106 institutions. *Diabetes Care* 2009, 32:1647–1648.

6. Burnet DL, Cooper AJ, Drum ML, Lipton RB: Risk factors for mortality in a diverse cohort of patients with childhood-onset diabetes in Chicago. *Diabetes Care* 2007, 30:2559–2563 .

7. Vanelli M, Scarabello C, Fainardi V: Available tools for primary ketoacidosis prevention at diabetes diagnosis in children and adolescents—"The Parma campaign." *Acta Biomed* 2008, 79:73–78.

8. International Diabetes Federation: World Diabetes Day posters. Accessible at http://www.worlddiabetesday.org/en/materials/campaign-posters-0. Accessed March 2010.

9. Glaser N, Barnett P, McCaslin I, et al.: Risk factors for cerebral edema in children with diabetic ketoacidosis. *N Engl J Med* 2001, 344:264–269.

10. Glaser NS, Marcin JP, Wootton-Gorges SL, et al.: Correlation of clinical and biochemical findings with diabetic ketoacidosis–related cerebral edema in children using magnetic resonance diffusion–weighted imaging. *J Pediatrics* 2008, 153:541–546.

11. Hoffman WH, Stamatovic SM, Andjelkovic AV: Inflammatory mediators and blood brain barrier disruption in fatal brain edema of diabetic ketoacidosis. *Brain Res* 2009, 1254:138–148.

12. Kaufman FR, Halvorson M: The treatment and prevention of diabetic ketoacidosis in children and adolescents with type 1 diabetes mellitus. *Pediatr Ann* 1999, 28:576–582.

13. Karvonen M, Viik-Kajander M, Moltchanova E, et al.: Incidence of childhood type 1 diabetes worldwide. *Diabetes Care* 2000, 23:1516–1526.

14. Laffel LM, Wentzell K, Loughlin C, et al.: Sick day management using blood 3-hydroxybutyrate (3-OHB) compared with urine ketone monitoring reduces hospital visits in young people with T1DM: a randomized clinical trial. *Diabetic Medicine* 2006, 23:278–284.

15. Brink S, Laffel L, Likitmaskul S, et al.: Sick day management in children and adolescents with diabetes. *Pediatric Diabetes* 2009, 10(Supp 12):146–153.

16. The SEARCH for Diabetes in Youth Study Group: The burden of diabetes mellitus among US youth: prevalence estimated from the SEARCH for diabetes in youth study. *Pediatrics* 2006,118:1510–1518.

17. The Writing Group for the SEARCH for Diabetes in Youth Study Group: Incidence of diabetes in youth in the united states. *JAMA* 2007, 297:2716–2724.

18. The Diabetes Control and Complications Trial Research Group: The effect of intensive treatment of diabetes on the development and progression of long-term complications in insulin dependent diabetes mellitus. *N Engl J Med* 1993, 329:977–986.

19. Diabetes Control and Complications Trial Research Group: Effect of intensive diabetes treatment on the development and progression of long-term complications in adolescents with insulin-dependent diabetes. *J Pediatr* 1994, 125:177–188.

20. Diabetes Control and Complications Group (DCCT)/Epidemiology of Diabetes Interventions and Complications (EDIC) Research Group: Beneficial effects of intensive therapy of diabetes during adolescence: outcomes after the conclusion of the diabetes control and complications trial (DCCT). *J Pediatr* 2001, 139:804–812.

21. The Diabetes Control and Complications Group (DCCT)/Epidemiology of Diabetes Interventions and Complications (EDIC) Research Group: Modern day clinical course of type 1 diabetes mellitus after 30 years' duration. *Arch Intern Med* 2009, 169:1307–1316.

22. American Diabetes Association: Standards of medical care in diabetes. *Diabetes Care* 2009, 32(Supp 1):S13–S61.

23. Rewers M, Pihoker C, Donaghue K, et al.: ISPAD Clinical Practice Consensus Guidelines 2006–2007: assessment and monitoring of glycemic control in children and adolescents with diabetes. *Pediatric Diabetes* 2007, 8:408–418.

24. Phillip M, Battelino T, Rodriguez H, et al.: Use of insulin pump therapy in the pediatric age-group: Consensus Statement from the European Society for Pediatric Endocrinology, the Lawson Wilkins Pediatric Endocrine Society, the International Society for Pediatric and Adolescent Diabetes, endorsed by the American Diabetes Association and the European Association for the Study of Diabetes. *Diabetes Care* 2007, 30:1653–1662.

25. Cohen D, Weintrob N, Benzaquen H, et al.: Continuous subcutaneous insulin infusion versus multiple daily injections in adolescents with type 1 diabetes mellitus: a randomized open crossover trial. *J Pediatr Endocrin Metab* 2003, 16:1047–1050.

26. DiMeglio LA, Pottorff TM, Boyd SR, et al.: A randomized, controlled study of insulin pump therapy in diabetic preschoolers. *J Pediatr* 2004, 145:380–384.

27. Doyle EA, Weinzimer SA, Steffen AT, et al.: A randomized, prospective trial comparing the efficacy of continuous subcutaneous insulin infusion with multiple daily injections using insulin glargine. *Diabetes Care* 2004, 27:1554–1558.

28. Fox LA, Buckloh LM, Smith SD, et al.: A randomized controlled trial of insulin pump therapy in young children with type 1 diabetes. *Diabetes Care* 2005, 28:1277–1281.

29. Weintrob N, Benzaquen H, Galatzer A, et al.: Comparison of continuous subcutaneous insulin infusion and multiple daily injection regimens in children with type 1 diabetes. a randomized open crossover trial. *Pediatrics* 2003, 112:559–564.

30. Nimri R, Weintrob N, Benzaquen H, et al.: Insulin pump therapy in youth with type 1 diabetes: a retrospective paired study. *Pediatrics* 2006, 117:2126–2131.

31. Scrimgeour L, Cobry E, McFann K, et al.: Improved glycemic control after long-term insulin pump use in pediatric patients with type 1 diabetes. *Diabetes Technol Ther* 2007, 9:421–428.

32. Corriveau EA, Durso PJ, Kaufman LD, et al.: Effect of CareLink, an internet-based insulin pump monitoring system, on glycemic control in rural and urban children with type 1 diabetes mellitus. *Pediatric Diabetes* 2008, 9(Part II):360–366.

33. The Juvenile Diabetes Research Foundation Continuous Glucose Monitoring Study Group: Continuous glucose monitoring and intensive treatment of type 1 diabetes. *N Engl J Med* 2008, 359:1464–1476.

34. The Juvenile Diabetes Research Foundation Continuous Glucose Monitoring Study Group: The effect of continuous glucose monitoring in well-controlled type 1 diabetes. *Diabetes Care* 2009, 32:1378–1383.

35. Silverstein J, Klingensmith G, Copeland K, et al.: Care of children and adolescents with type 1 diabetes. A statement of the American Diabetes Association. *Diabetes Care* 2005, 28:186–212.

36. Kaufman FR, Halvorson M: New trends in managing type 1 diabetes. *Contemp Pediatr* 1999,16:112–123.

37. Donaghue KC, Chiarelli F, Trotta D, et al.: Microvascular and macrovascular complications associated with diabetes in children and adolescents. *Pediatric Diabetes* 2009, 10(Supp 12):195–203.

38. Kershnar AK, Daniels SR, Imperatore G, et al.: Lipid abnormalities are prevalent in youth with type 1 and type 2 diabetes: The search for diabetes in youth study. *J Pediatrics* 2006, 149:314–319.

39. Guy J, Ogden L, Wadwa RP, *et al.*: Lipid and lipoprotein profiles in youth with and without type 1 diabetes: the SEARCH for diabetes in youth case-control study. *Diabetes Care* 2009, 32:416–420.

40. Maahs DM, Wadwa RP, Bishop F, et al.: Dyslipidemia in youth with diabetes: to treat or not to treat? *J Pediatr* 2008, 153:458–465.

41. American Diabetes Association: Care of children with diabetes in the school and day care setting, position Statement. *Diabetes Care* 1999, 22:163–166.

42. National Institutes of Health and the Centers for Disease Control and Prevention: National Diabetes Education Program School Guide: Helping the Student with Diabetes Succeed: A Guide for School Personnel, Updated 2009 Edition. Available at http://www.ndep.nih.gov/media/Youth_NDEPSchoolGuide.pdf. Accessed March 2010.

43. Schiffrin A: Psychosocial issues in pediatric diabetes. *Curr Diabetes Rep* 2001, 1:33–40.

44. Shaw J: Epidemiology of childhood type 2 diabetes and obesity. *Pediatric Diabetes* 2007, 8(Suppl. 9):7–15.

45. Silverstein JH, Rosenbloom AL: Type 2 diabetes in children. *Curr Diabetes Rep* 2001, 1:19–27.

46. Wei JN, Sung FC, Li CY, *et al.*: Low birth weight and high birth weight infants are both at an increased risk to have type 2 diabetes among school children in Taiwan. *Diabetes Care* 2003, 26:343–348.

47. Tfayli H, Bacha F, Arslanian S: Phenotypic type 2 diabetes in obese youth: insulin sensitivity and secretion in islet cell antibody-negative versus -positive patients. *Diabetes* 2009, 58:738–744.

48. Stuart CA, Pate CJ, Peters EJ: Prevalence of acanthosis nigricans in an unselected population. *Am J Med* 1989, 87:269–272.

49. Arslanian SA: Type 2 diabetes mellitus in children: pathophysiology and risk factors. *J Pediatr Endocrinol Metab* 2000, 13(Suppl 6):1385–1394.

50. Ogden CL, Carroll MD, Flegel KM: High body mass index for age among US children and adolescents, 2003–2006. *JAMA* 2008, 299:2401–2405.

51. HEALTHY Study Group: Risk factors for type 2 diabetes in a sixth grade multiracial cohort. *Diabetes Care* 2009, 32:953–955.

52. Jones KL, Arslanian S, Peterokova VA, *et al.*: Effect of metformin in pediatric patients with type 2 diabetes. *Diabetes Care* 2002, 25:89–94.

53. Park MH, Kinra S, Ward KJ, *et al.*: Metformin for obesity in children and adolescents: a systemic review. *Diabetes Care* 2009, 32:1743–1745.

54. Silverstein JH, Rosenbloom AL: Treatment of type 2 diabetes mellitus in children and adolescents. *J Pediatr Endocrinol Metab* 2000, 13(Suppl 6):1403–1409.

55. Rosenbloom AL, Silverstein JH, Amemiya S, *et al.*: Type 2 diabetes in children and adolescents. *Pediatric Diabetes* 2009, 10(Suppl 12):17–32.

56. Eppens MC, Craig ME, Cusumano J, *et al.*: Prevalence of diabetes complications in adolescents with type 2 compared with type 1 diabetes. *Diabetes Care* 2006, 29:1300–1306.

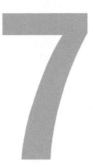

7 Pathogenesis of Type 2 Diabetes

Mazen Alsahli and John E. Gerich

Type 2 diabetes is one of the most common chronic diseases. In the USA, it affects about 8% of the population. In addition to 18 million people with diagnosed diabetes, 6 million have undiagnosed diabetes and 57 million have prediabetes [i.e., impaired fasting glucose (IFG) or impaired glucose tolerance (IGT)] [1]. Phenotypically, more than 90% of people with diabetes mellitus have type 2 diabetes. This disorder, however, is extremely heterogeneous (see Fig. 7.1). Approximately 10% of patients have late-onset type 1 diabetes; about another 5% develop diabetes as a result of rare monogenic defects in either insulin secretion or insulin action. The remaining patients have "garden variety" type 2 diabetes. The number of people with type 2 diabetes worldwide is expected to increase from 135 million to more than 300 million by 2025, with most of this increase occurring in developing countries. In addition to the increase in the prevalence of obesity, better awareness of the disease among the population and health care providers may be responsible for the increase in diagnosed cases. The prevalence of type 2 diabetes in the USA has increased rapidly over the past 50 years (see Fig. 7.2) and is highest in minority populations, including blacks, Hispanics, and especially Native Americans. In the Pima Indians of Arizona, 50% of adults older than 35 years have the disease [2]. In all populations, the prevalence increases with age; in whites, the prevalence reaches 20% by age 80 years (see Fig. 7.3) [3].

The pathogenesis of type 2 diabetes involves the interaction of genetic and environmental (acquired) factors that adversely affect insulin secretion (pancreatic β-cell function) and tissue responses to insulin (insulin sensitivity; see Fig. 7.4). Impaired β-cell function and insulin resistance are present before the onset of type 2 diabetes and are predictive of its subsequent development [4–7]. Type 2 diabetes is a polygenic disorder [8]; the additive effects of an as yet unknown number of genetic polymorphisms (risk factors) are required for development of the disorder, although they may not be sufficient necessarily in the absence of environmental (acquired) risk factors (see Fig. 7.5). Searches for candidate genes based on various proteins involved in mediating insulin action have generally failed to find diabetic genes in this category [8]. To date, only a few polymorphisms have been identified as risk factors with confidence: one involves an amino acid polymorphism Pro 12 Ala in the peroxisome proliferator-activated receptor γ (PPARγ), which is expressed in insulin target tissues and β cells [9]; this apparently conveys susceptibility to adverse effects of free fatty acids (FFAs) on insulin release. A second involves the gene encoding calpain-10, a cysteine protease that modulates insulin release as well as insulin effects on muscle and adipose tissue [10]. A third is the E23K variant of the KIR6.2 gene (potassium inwardly rectifying channel J11 gene), which has been shown in a large association study to increase the risk of type 2 diabetes presumably through its effect on β cells' potassium channel and, in turn, on insulin secretion [11, 12]. More recently, variants of the transcription factor 7-like 2 gene (TCF7L2) were found to be associated with increased risk of type 2 diabetes [13–15]. Insulin secretion is decreased in carriers of the at-risk alleles [13]. It is of note that the expression of glucagon-like peptide 1 (GLP-1), a peptide encoded by the human glucagon gene in gut endocrine cells, is regulated by TCF7L2 [16]. Use of knockout techniques in mice have identified several elements of the insulin-signaling cascade that might be potential sites where genetic polymorphisms might affect β-cell function, but to date none of these have been found to occur in people with type 2 diabetes [17].

J.S. Skyler (ed.), *Atlas of Diabetes: Fourth Edition*,
DOI 10.1007/978-1-4614-1028-7_7, © Springer Science+Business Media, LLC 2012

The importance of inheritable factors is underscored by the fact that a person with both parents or a monozygotic twin with type 2 diabetes has up to an 80% lifetime risk of developing this disorder [18]. Having a single parent or sibling with type 2 diabetes carries a risk of about 30%, which represents a two- to fourfold increase above that of the general population [19, 20]. Impaired β-cell function is the earliest detectable defect in people with normal glucose tolerance who are genetically predisposed to developing type 2 diabetes [6, 7, 21] (e.g., first-degree relatives of individuals with type 2 diabetes; see Fig. 7.9) [22]. The strongest evidence for this finding comes from studies of monozygotic twins in which one twin has type 2 diabetes but the other has normal glucose tolerance [23]. The twin with normal glucose tolerance has about an 80% chance of developing type 2 diabetes and, thus, can be considered to be a true genetically prediabetic individual. All four studies of such twin pairs have found that the twin with normal glucose tolerance had impaired β-cell function [23–26]; the only study that simultaneously assessed insulin sensitivity found it to be normal [23].

Environmental (acquired) factors, however, are also critical for developing diabetes because without these, genetic factors may be insufficient to cause type 2 diabetes. The most important factors are those that influence insulin sensitivity: obesity (especially visceral obesity), physical inactivity, high-fat/low-fiber diets, smoking, and low birth weight (see Fig. 7.6) [20, 27–32]. Intervention trials have consistently demonstrated that the risk for developing type 2 diabetes can be reduced by up to 60% by caloric restriction, diet modification, and increased physical activity (see Fig. 7.7) [33–41]. Bariatric surgery is associated with a 60–80% remission rate of type 2 diabetes (remission is generally defined as normoglycemia with no diabetes medications) [42, 43]. Diabetes improves rapidly after surgery, before any significant weight loss [43, 44]. This is especially true for malabsorptive procedures such as biliopancreatic diversion (BPD) and combined malabsorptive and restrictive procedures such as Roux-en-y gastric bypass (RYGB) [42]. The mechanism is poorly understood but probably involves gastrointestinal hormonal and neural changes. Incretins are hormones released by the gut in response to food ingestion, which augment insulin release by what is known as the incretin effect (i.e., more insulin responses after oral than intravenous glucose despite comparable glycemia). Two major incretins are GLP-1 and glucose-dependent insulinotropic polypeptide (GIP). Other gut hormones that influence glucose homeostasis include ghrelin and peptide YY (PYY). Ghrelin acts on the hypothalamus to stimulate appetite. It also inhibits insulin secretion [45, 46]. PYY, on the contrary, increases satiety and decreases food intake [47]. Bariatric surgeries that expedite nutrient delivery to the distal ileum, such as BPD and RYGB, increase GLP-1 and PYY levels [48–52]. The effects of gastric bypass on ghrelin and GIP are inconsistent [42, 50, 53–55]. The combination of changes in gut hormones' secretion pattern and caloric restriction following gastric bypass improve insulin secretion and sensitivity and, ultimately, especially with the ensuing weight loss, lead to remission of type 2 diabetes [42]. An alternative explanation is the foregut exclusion hypothesis, which suggests that bypassing the proximal gut prevents the secretion of an as-yet unidentified diabetogenic factor [42, 56, 57]. Although most (>90%) patients with classic type 2 diabetes are obese (and, therefore, insulin resistant), most insulin-resistant obese individuals are not diabetic. What distinguishes obese individuals with and without diabetes is the ability to compensate for insulin resistance with increased insulin secretion (see Fig. 7.8) [58].

There are numerous examples in the literature in which type 2 diabetes can occur solely as a result of impaired insulin secretion in the absence of insulin resistance [59–67]. Virtually, all the insulin resistance found in people with type 2 diabetes can be ascribed to environmental (acquired) factors such as obesity, physical inactivity, high-fat diets, and glucose and lipid toxicity [68]. After binding to its receptor, insulin triggers a complex series of events (see Fig. 7.11). The insulin resistance of obesity is associated with reduced numbers of insulin receptors, reduced insulin receptor kinase activity, and reduced activation of insulin-signaling proteins and glucose transport [69]. Quantitatively similar defects have been found in obese individuals with type 2 diabetes compared with obese individuals without type 2 diabetes [69]. Several factors may be involved in the insulin resistance associated with obesity: altered release from adipose tissue of FFAs [70], tumor necrosis factor-α [71], resistin [72], leptin [73], adepsine [74], and adiponectin [17], as well as accumulation of lipid in insulin target organs [75, 76] (see Fig. 7.12).

People destined to develop type 2 diabetes initially have IGT, a state characterized by isolated postprandial hyperglycemia in which impaired early insulin release and, to some extent, excessive glucagon release and insulin resistance result in increased postprandial glucose production – the key factor responsible for postprandial hyperglycemia (see Figs. 7.13, 7.15 and 7.16). In type 2 diabetes, the basic metabolic derangements are the same as in IGT except that progressive deterioration in β-cell function and a modest decrease in insulin sensitivity now result in overproduction of glucose by the liver and kidney in the postabsorptive state (i.e., fasting hyperglycemia) and impaired splanchnic glucose sequestration (i.e., glycogen formation) in the postprandial state [77, 78]. Fasting hyperglycemia is directly related to rates of glucose production (see Fig. 7.17). Because of the mass action effect of hyperglycemia and prevailing insulin levels, glucose utilization rates are still, in an absolute sense, normal in type 2 diabetes, although the distribution of tissue uptake and metabolic fates may be altered (see Fig. 7.18) [78]. For example, in type 2 diabetes [79], overall postprandial tissue glucose uptake, glycolysis, and storage are normal, but glucose oxidation is reduced; nonoxidative glycolysis is increased; glucose storage via the direct pathway is increased, but glucose storage via the indirect pathway is reduced because gluconeogenic carbons are released into plasma as glucose rather than being stored as glycogen. As a result of increased glycogenolysis, net hepatic glucose storage is reduced (e.g., increased glycogen cycling). Thus, it appears that the mass action effects of hyperglycemia can overcome the major defect in peripheral glucose metabolism [80] but cannot overcome defects in intracellular pathways that appear to be related to oxidative processes [81]. Poorly controlled diabetes leads to microvascular complications (retinopathy, nephropathy, neuropathy) and macrovascular complications (premature atherosclerosis). Interventional clinical trials [e.g., the Diabetes Control and Complications Trial (DCCT), UK Prospective Diabetes Study (UKPDS), Kumamoto Study, Stockholm Diabetes Intervention Study, and Action in Diabetes and Vascular Disease: Preterax and Diamicron MR Controlled Evaluation (ADVANCE) trial] [82–85] have shown that microvascular complications can be prevented if HbA_{1c} levels are maintained below 7% (upper limit of normal, 6%) (see Fig. 7.19). The beneficial effect of intensive therapy on macrovascular outcomes has been difficult to demonstrate consistently. Some trials lacked sufficient statistical power [i.e., the Action to Control Cardiovascular Risk in Diabetes (ACCORD) and ADVANCE trials] [82, 86] or were of a relatively short duration (<7 years) and included patients with advanced disease (≥8 years) who would be unlikely to benefit (i.e., the Veterans Affairs Diabetes Trial, ACCORD, and ADVANCE trials) [82, 86, 87]. However, a beneficial effect was seen in the UKPDS and the DCCT trials, both of which were primary prevention trials [88–90]. The DCCT randomized 1,441 patients with type 1 diabetes to receive either conventional or intensive insulin therapy. At the end of the average follow-up length of 6.5 years, a nonsignificant trend toward fewer cardiovascular events with intensive therapy (3.2 vs. 5.4%; P=0.08) was noted [90]. A total of 93% of patients from the DCCT were subsequently followed up for 11 years in the observational Epidemiology of Diabetes Interventions and Complications (EDIC) study [91]. A 42% reduction in the risk of any cardiovascular disease event was noted in patients who were in the intensive treatment group during DCCT (95% CI, 9–63%; P=0.02). The UKPDS compared the efficacy of conventional therapy (dietary restriction) or intensive therapy (either sulfonylurea or insulin or, in overweight patients, metformin) on glycemic control and on complications of type 2 diabetes in about 4,000 newly diagnosed patients. Intervention lasted 10 years and surviving patients were observed for an additional 10 years in a post-trial follow-up period. Substantial risk reduction for myocardial infarction (39%; P=0.01) was observed in the intensive metformin therapy group during the original trial. In the post-trial period, a 15–33% risk reduction for myocardial infarction was noted in patients who received intensive therapy during the original trial [88, 89].

Because IGT is associated with an approximately twofold increase in cardiovascular mortality [92] and because a clinical trial [93] has shown that reduction in postprandial hyperglycemia reduces cardiovascular events, in the future considerable attention will be paid to reducing hyperglycemia. Currently, the American Association of Clinical Endocrinologists recommends a target of less than 6.5% [94]; the American Diabetes Association and the European Association for the Study of Diabetes recommend a target HbA_{1c} of less than 7 [95]. These associations recognize that this goal is not appropriate or practical for some patients, and clinical judgment, based on the potential benefits and risks of a more intensified regimen, needs to be applied for every patient. Less strict goals need to be considered; for example, for patients with limited life expectancies, patients with a history of severe hypoglycemia, or in very young children. The main difference between people with HbA_{1c} values of 7 and 6.5 is their postprandial glucose levels [96]. Improved insulin preparations and new oral agents that specifically target impaired insulin secretion and insulin resistance are now available, which can achieve this degree of glycemic control (see Fig. 7.20). Furthermore, lifestyle changes (e.g., weight loss, exercise) and drugs that reduce insulin resistance can reverse IGT and prevent its progression to type 2 diabetes. Because of the progressive deterioration in insulin secretion, most patients initially successfully managed on one oral agent will need additional drugs and up to 50% may ultimately need some form of insulin therapy to maintain adequate glycemic control [97–108].

Heterogeneity of phenotypic type 2 diabetes	
Subtype	Patients (%)
LADA [109]	~10%
MODY [110]	~3%
MODY 1: HNF-4α	
MODY 2: Glucokinase	
MODY 3: HNF-1α	
MODY 4: PDX-1 (IPF-1)	
MODY 5: HFN-1β	
MODY 6: Neuro D1-β2	
Maternally inherited diabetes and deafness (mutations in mitochondrial DNA, RNA) [175]	<1%
Insulin receptor defects [176]	<1%
Leprechaunism	
Type A insulin resistance and acanthosis nigricans	
Rabson–Mendenhall syndrome	
Type 2 diabetes mellitus	~85%

Figure 7-1. Heterogeneity of phenotypic type 2 diabetes. Patients with late-onset autoimmune diabetes (LADA) [109] experience the onset of disease after age 30 years, are generally lean, have islet cell or glutamic acid decarboxylase antibodies, and usually progress to insulin dependence in less than 5 years. Patients with maturity-onset diabetes of youth (MODY) [110] generally experience the onset of disease between ages 15 and 30 years, can be either obese or lean, and have a strong family history of diabetes consistent with an autosomal dominant inheritance that results in impaired insulin release but little or no insulin resistance. Five monogenetic mutations have been identified and more are expected. *HNF* hepatic nuclear factor, *IPF* insulin-promoting factor, neuro D1/β2 – D1/β-cell box transactivator 2, *PDX* pancreatic development factor.

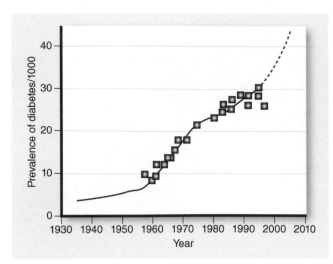

Figure 7-2. Increasing prevalence of diabetes in the USA. The prevalence of diagnosed diabetes in the USA has risen steadily since 1930 and is expected to continue to increase rapidly in the early part of the twenty-first century. About 90% of cases of diagnosed diabetes are of type 2 diabetes. It is estimated that at any given time, at least one-third of persons with type 2 diabetes are undiagnosed (adapted from Diabetes in America [111]).

Prevalence of diabetes			
Population group	**1999–2002 (*n*=8,526)**	**2003–2006 (*n*=8,780)**	***P* value**
Overall	6.6	7.7	0.03
Age			
20–39 years	1.7	1.8	0.47
40–59 years	6.5	8.2	0.05
≥60 years	15.2	16.9	0.08
Sex			
Male	7	7.5	0.58
Female	6.2	7.9	0.003
Race/ethnicity			
Non-Hispanic white	5.3	6.3	0.04
Non-Hispanic black	10.9	12.6	0.12
Mexican American	10.4	12.4	0.16
Other	11.2	11.5	0.81
BMI			
<25.0 kg/m^2	3.7	4	0.77
25.0–29.9 kg/m^2	5.5	6.1	0.3
≥30.0 kg/m^2	10	12.7	0.03

Figure 7-3. Prevalence of diagnosed diabetes in the USA from 1999 to 2002 and 2003 to 2006. The prevalence increased from 6.6% during the period from 1999 to 2002 to 7.8% from 2003 to 2006. The increase was significant among women, non-Hispanic whites, and obese people. *BMI* body mass index (data from Cheung et al. [3]).

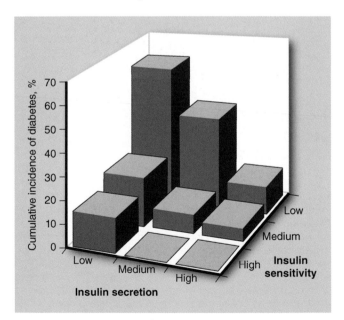

Figure 7-4. Incidence of diabetes among Pima Indians. The relative impact of variations in β-cell function and insulin sensitivity on the subsequent development of diabetes among 262 Pima Indians is shown. The acute insulin secretory response to intravenous glucose and insulin action at baseline was measured in patients who initially had normal glucose tolerance. The patients were divided into tertiles of insulin secretion and insulin sensitivity and were followed for an average of 7 years. The observations, however, do not take into consideration whether the β-cell function was appropriate for the degree of insulin resistance; they merely illustrate the fact that both factors influence the risk for developing type 2 diabetes (adapted from Pratley and Weyer [7]).

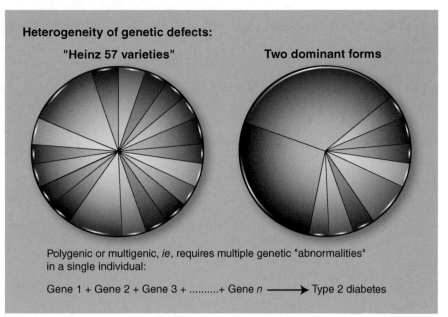

Heterogeneity of genetic defects:

"Heinz 57 varieties"   Two dominant forms

Polygenic or multigenic, *ie*, requires multiple genetic "abnormalities" in a single individual:

Gene 1 + Gene 2 + Gene 3 + ...+ Gene *n* ⟶ Type 2 diabetes

FIGURE 7-5. Two major features of the genetics of type 2 diabetes in the general population. First, this disease is a genetically heterogeneous disorder. At present, however, it is not clear how many forms of diabetes exist, whether there are one or two predominant forms, or whether each form represents only a small percentage of the total population. For most patients, the disease is polygenic: some abnormality or sequence polymorphism is present in several genes, each contributing a small amount to the overall pathogenesis. Although there is no definitive information on the number of genes involved in each form, most investigators believe that at least three genes – and perhaps as many as 10 or 20 – may contribute to the final phenotype. Most likely, these are "normal" genetic variants or sequence polymorphisms, which slightly alter insulin action or insulin secretion [112].

RR for type 2 diabetes of three common factors

Factor	Relative risk
Obesity (BMI, kg/m^2)	
<23	1
23–25	3
25–30	8
30–35	20
>35	40
Physical activity (exercise, h/week)	
>7	1
4–7	1.1
2–4	1.2
0.5–2	1.5
<0.5	1.8
Healthy diet (quintiles based on fat/fiber content)	
5	1
4	1.15
3	1.30
2	1.50
1	2

FIGURE 7-6. Relative risks for developing type 2 diabetes. A physically inactive individual (<30 min/week of exercise) who consumes an unhealthy diet (level 1) and is modestly overweight (BMI of 25–30) would approximately have a 30-fold increased risk of developing type 2 diabetes compared with the general population, which would translate to a lifetime risk of nearly 100% (adapted from Choi and Shi [28]).

Interventions to reduce the development of type 2 diabetes

Study	Patients, n	Interventions	Reduction
Eriksson and Lindgarde [37]	181	Diet and exercise in nonobese IGT	37% (11 vs. 29%/6 years)
Pan et al. [36]	577	Diet and exercise in nonobese IGT	~40% (9 vs. 16%/6 years)
Tuomilehto et al. [35]	522	Diet and exercise in obese IGT	~58% (11 vs. 23%/6 years)
Knowler et al. [34]	3,234	Diet and exercise in obese high-risk IGT	58% (14 vs. 29%/4 years)
		Metformin (500 mg BID) in obese high-risk IGT	31% (22 vs. 29%/4 years)
Wenying et al. [38]	321	Diet and exercise	30% (11 vs. 8%/year)
		Acarbose	80%
		Metformin	64%
Chiasson et al. [39]	1,348	Acarbose (100 mg three times daily) in obese IGT	25% (32 vs. 42%/4 years)
Buchanan et al. [40]	266	Troglitazone (400 mg/dL) in postgestational diabetic obese Hispanic women (72% IGT)	50% (6 vs. 12%/2.5 years)
Torgerson et al. [41]	794	Lifestyle vs. lifestyle and orlistat in obese IGT	35% (19 vs. 29%/4 years)
Beals [113]	602	Pioglitazone (45 mg/dL)	81% (1.5 vs. 7%/year)
Gerstein et al. [114]	5,269	Rosiglitazone (8 mg/dL)	60% (12 vs. 26%/3 years)

Figure 7-7. Use of lifestyle modifications and drugs to reduce the development of type 2 diabetes in people with IGT. People with IGT have a 20–40% risk of developing type 2 diabetes over a 5-year period. Numerous clinical trials [34–41, 113, 114] have demonstrated that lifestyle modifications (e.g., diet and exercise) or drugs that reduce insulin resistance (metformin, pioglitazone) or obesity (orlistat) can decrease the development of type 2 diabetes in individuals with IGT.

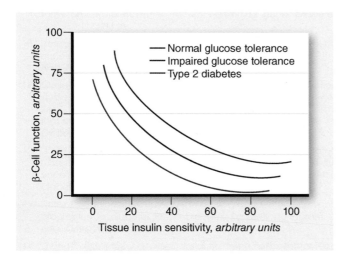

Figure 7-8. Reciprocal relationship between β-cell function and tissue insulin sensitivity. A hyperbolic function relates β-cell function to tissue insulin sensitivity such that when insulin decreases, β-cell function increases to maintain normal glucose homeostasis. Patients who develop impaired glucose tolerance or type 2 diabetes have an inadequate β-cell compensation for insulin resistance in that for any degree of reduced tissue insulin sensitivity, the β-cell response is below normal [5–7, 115].

Figure 7-10. Nutrient sensing and insulin secretion by the pancreatic β cell. The β cell takes up glucose and amino acids via specific transporters on the cell membrane, such as the GLUT2 glucose transporter. This isoform of transporter is expressed only by the β cell and the liver, and has a Km in the physiologic range. After it is inside the cell, glucose is phosphorylated by a specialized form of hexokinase called glucokinase. The subsequent metabolism of glucose results in a change in the ratio of adenosine triphosphate (ATP) to adenosine diphosphate (ADP) in the cell, which in turn causes activation of the ATP-sensitive potassium channel. This results in depolarization of the cell, an influx of calcium, and the subsequent release of insulin from secretory granules. The sulfonylurea receptor can also activate the ATP-sensitive potassium channel, mimicking the effect of glucose. Other secretagogues, such as GLP-1, bypass this system by changing cellular cyclic adenosine monophosphate (cAMP) levels. The level of expression of the several molecules involved in glucose sensing, including the GLUT2 glucose transporter and the development of the β cell, are controlled by several nuclear transcription factors. The best studied of these are HNF-1α, HNF-1β, HNF-4α, and pancreatic duodenal homeobox-1 (PDX-1; IPF-1). Maturity-onset diabetes of youth can result from genetic defects in any of these transcription factors or a genetic defect in glucokinase. In type 2 diabetes, the exact site of the defect in glucose sensing is unknown, but studies in animal models of disease have suggested that this may be the result of a downregulation of the GLUT2 glucose transporter [116].

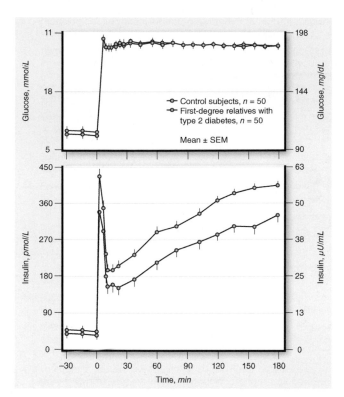

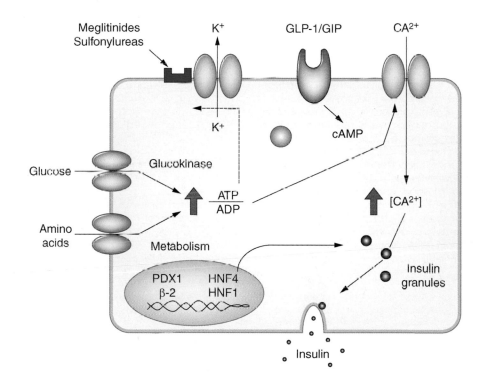

FIGURE 7-9. Plasma glucose (*top*) and insulin (*bottom*) concentrations in hyperglycemic clamp experiments. In response to an acute elevation of blood glucose concentrations, insulin is secreted in a biphasic manner; a first phase lasts approximately 10 min followed by a gradually increasing second phase. The first phase of insulin release has been linked to insulin granules located near the β-cell membrane (rapidly releasable pool). Second-phase insulin release depends partly on mobilizing insulin granules from a storage pool to the rapidly releasable pool, as well as increased synthesis of insulin. In this study, subjects with normal glucose tolerance but a first-degree relative with type 2 diabetes were studied using a hyperglycemic clamp to assess their β-cell function and insulin sensitivity relative to a group of subjects with normal glucose tolerance but no family history of diabetes [22]. Subjects were matched for age, gender, and obesity to exclude environmental (acquired) risk factors. It was demonstrated that individuals with a first-degree relative with type 2 diabetes had reduced early (first-phase) and late (second-phase) insulin release and were not insulin resistant (adapted from Pimenta et al. [22]).

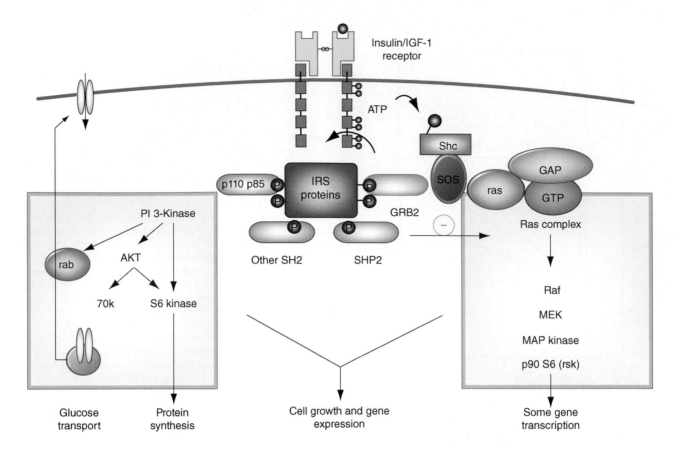

Insulin/IGF-1
receptor

ATP

Shc

SOS

GAP

ras

GTP

Ras complex

p110 p85

IRS
proteins

GRB2

Other SH2

SHP2

PI 3-Kinase

rab

AKT

70k

S6 kinase

Raf

MEK

MAP kinase

p90 S6 (rsk)

Glucose
transport

Protein
synthesis

Cell growth and gene
expression

Some gene
transcription

Lipid and glycogen synthesis

FIGURE 7-11. Insulin signaling network. The full network is complex and can be divided into five levels (1) activation of the insulin receptor tyrosine kinase and closely linked events; (2) phosphorylation of a family of substrate proteins; (3) interaction of the receptor and its substrates with several intermediate signaling molecules via SH2 (src homology 2) and other recognition domains; (4) activation of serine and lipid kinases, resulting in a broad range of phosphorylation–dephosphorylation events; and (5) regulation of the final biological effectors of insulin action, such as glucose transport, lipid synthesis, gene expression, and mitogenesis. The SH2 proteins link the insulin receptor substrate (IRS) proteins to a series of cascading reactions involving serine/threonine kinases and phosphatases such as the mitogen-activated protein (MAP) kinases, S6 kinases, and protein phosphatase-1A. These serine kinases act on enzymes such as glycogen synthase, transcription factors, and other proteins to produce many of the final biological effects of the hormone. In adipose tissue and muscle, insulin stimulation also increases glucose uptake by promoting translocation of an intracellular pool of glucose transporters to the plasma membrane. Exactly how this action is linked to the phosphorylation cascade is unknown, but several studies suggest that this important action of insulin, as well as most metabolic effects, is downstream of the enzyme phosphatidylinositol 3-kinase (PI 3-kinase). Other effects of insulin, such as stimulation of glycogen and lipid synthesis, occur through additional intracellular effects to stimulate the enzymes involved in these reactions. *GAP* GTPase-activating protein, *GRB2* growth-factor receptor binding protein 2, *GTP* guanosine triphosphate, *IGF* insulin-like growth factor, *MEK* MAP-Erk kinase, *SOS* son-of-sevenless.

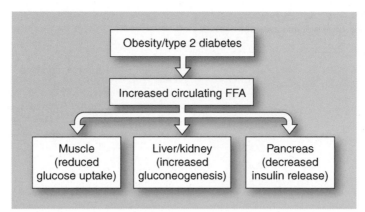

Figure 7-12. Insulin resistance and obesity. The insulin resistance associated with type 2 diabetes can be largely explained by obesity because comparably obese individuals with and without type 2 diabetes have quantitatively similar reductions in insulin-receptor binding, insulin-receptor tyrosine kinase activity, and muscle glucose transport [69, 117]. Most of these abnormalities in patients with type 2 diabetes can be normalized by weight loss [118]. Current evidence indicates that the most important factor involved in the insulin resistance of obesity in humans is the increased circulating levels of plasma FFAs [70]. The experimental elevation of FFAs in normal humans decreases muscle glucose uptake and increases endogenous glucose production; in animal models, this elevation impairs insulin secretion [119, 120]. All of these actions would promote hyperglycemia by altering rates of the balance between entry and the removal of glucose from the circulation. The mechanisms for the effects of FFAs are twofold: substrate competition [121] and impaired insulin signaling [122]. Acetylated products of FFA metabolism decrease glucose oxidation via the inhibition of pyruvate dehydrogenase and activate serine/threonine kinases, possibly through increases in protein kinase C (theta), leading to reduced activity of IRS proteins. The main effect of the latter appears to be a reduction in glucose transport [123–125].

Stages of type 2 diabetes mellitus	Impaired β-cell function	Insulin resistance	Glucose tolerance
Stage 1	Demonstrable on testing (+)	Absent	Normal
Stage 2	Demonstrable on testing (++)	Present (variable)	Normal
Stage 3	Clearly abnormal (+++)	Worse than above	IGT[a]
Stage 4	More abnormal (++++)	Worse than above	IGT+IFG[b]
Stage 5	Markedly abnormal (+++++)	Worse than above	Type 2 diabetes mellitus[c]

[a]Fasting plasma glucose is generally normal, <110 mg/dL (6.1 mM), but 2-h postprandial is >140 mg/dL (7.8 mM) < 200 mg/dL (11.1 mM)

[b]Fasting plasma glucose >110 mg/dL (6.1 mM) but less than 126 mg/dL (7.0 mM), and 2-h postprandial

[c]Fasting plasma glucose >126 mg/dL (7.0 mM) or 2-h postprandial >200 mg/dL (11.1 mM)

Figure 7-13. Stages in the development of type 2 diabetes. Longitudinal and cross-sectional studies indicate that individuals who are destined to develop type 2 diabetes pass through five stages. The first stage begins at birth, when glucose homeostasis is normal but individuals are at risk for type 2 diabetes because of genetic polymorphisms that predispose them to become obese and limit the ability of their pancreatic β cells to compensate for insulin resistance. During stage 2, decreases in insulin sensitivity emerge as a result of a genetic predisposition and unhealthy lifestyle, which is initially compensated for by an increase in β-cell function so that glucose tolerance remains normal. During stage 3, β-cell function and insulin sensitivity both deteriorate so that when challenged, as during a glucose tolerance test or a standardized meal, postprandial glucose tolerance becomes abnormal. At this point, β-cell function is clearly abnormal but sufficient to maintain normal fasting plasma glucose concentrations. In stage 4, as a result of further deterioration in β-cell functioning and worsening of insulin sensitivity (probably a result of postprandial hyperglycemia), fasting plasma glucose concentrations increase due to an increase in basal endogenous glucose production. Finally, in stage 5, as a result of further deterioration in β-cell function (due to genetic and environmental factors such as glucose and lipotoxicity), both fasting and postprandial glucose levels reach diabetic levels.

β-Cell mass in type 2 diabetes mellitus

Study	β-cell mass
Butler et al. [126]	Reduced
Yoon et al. [127]	Reduced
Guiot et al. [128]	Reduced
Stefan et al. [129]	Reduced
Sakuraba et al. [130]	Reduced
Clark et al. [131]	Reduced
Kloppel et al. [132]	Reduced
Gepts et al. [133]	Reduced
Saito et al. [134]	Reduced
MacLean et al. [135]	Reduced
Westermark and Wilander [136]	Reduced
Rahier et al. [137]	Reduced
Deng et al. [138]	Reduced

FIGURE 7-14. Study results: β-cell mass and diabetes. Thirteen of 13 studies have reported β-cell mass to be reduced in patients with type 2 diabetes [126–138], and one has found β-cell mass to be reduced in people with IGT [126]. Islet cells from patients with type 2 diabetes have increased rates of apoptosis, but normal rates of replication and regeneration [126]. To what extent this decrease in β-cell mass is acquired or genetically programmed is unclear. Various factors have been implicated: intrauterine malnutrition [139, 140], glucose toxicity [141–146], lipotoxicity [119, 147–149], cytokines [150–152], and an accumulation of amyloid within islet cells [153, 154]. In addition to a reduced β-cell mass, isolated islet cells from patients with type 2 diabetes secrete less insulin than islet cells from nondiabetic individuals [138], indicating that functional as well as structural abnormalities exist.

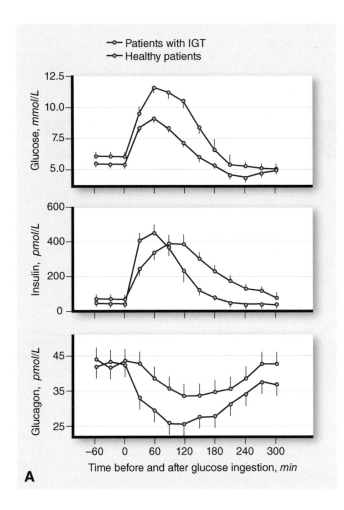

A

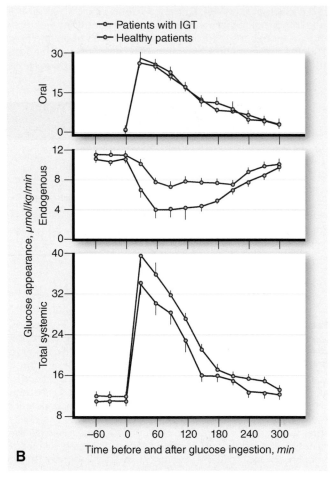

B

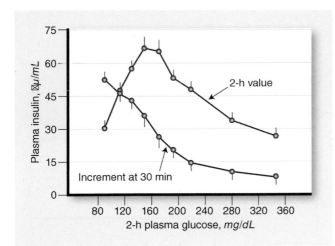

FIGURE 7-16. Comparison of early and late plasma insulin responses during oral glucose tolerance tests. The decrease in early (30 min) postprandial insulin secretion has been correlated with the reduced suppression of endogenous glucose production [155] and decreases progressively as glucose tolerance deteriorates [157]. By contrast, 2-h insulin levels increase initially and only decrease after 2-h plasma glucose levels reach diabetic values [21]. The latter phenomenon had been erroneously interpreted to imply that insulin resistance occurs earlier than impaired insulin secretion in the evolution of type 2 diabetes [158], but it is now evident that this results from the hyperglycemia caused by delayed early insulin release [6, 7, 21, 159].

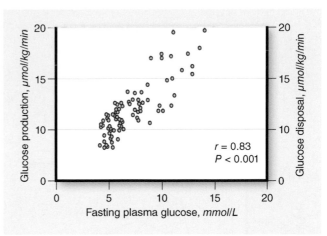

FIGURE 7-17. Glucose production and disposal in the postabsorptive state. With further deterioration in β-cell function, plasma glucose levels in the fasting state increase as a result of impaired suppression of hepatic and renal glucose release by insulin [78]. This is largely due to increased gluconeogenesis [160–163]. As shown in this figure, glucose removal from the circulation also increases as fasting blood glucose levels increase, illustrating that the primary cause of fasting hyperglycemia is an overproduction of glucose, not reduced glucose utilization. The increased glucose production results from impaired β-cell function as well as insulin resistance, indirectly mediated in part by increased plasma FFAs, an increased availability of gluconeogenic substrates, and a lack of appropriate suppression of glucagon secretion (adapted from Dinneen et al. [78])

FIGURE 7-15. Comparison of changes in hormones (insulin and glucagon) and rates of glucose production and utilization after glucose ingestion in patients with IGT (*closed circles*) and in healthy patients (*open circles*). Patients with IGT have normal fasting plasma glucose, insulin, and glucagon levels as well as normal fasting rates of glucose production and utilization. However, after an oral glucose challenge or a meal, they have a reduced early release of insulin during the initial 30–60 min accompanied by a reduced decrease in plasma glucagon levels (**A**). These hormonal abnormalities lead to a reduced suppression of endogenous glucose production with the preservation of normal splanchnic sequestration of the ingested glucose. Consequently, more than a normal amount of glucose enters the systemic circulation (**B**). This exceeds the rates of glucose removal from the circulation during the first 1–2 h so that plasma glucose levels increase more than normal. The hyperglycemia eventually leads to delayed and greater-than-normal plasma insulin levels that, along with the hyperglycemia, cause glucose utilization to exceed glucose production so that plasma glucose eventually returns to normal fasting levels [155, 156]. During the 4- to 6-h postprandial period, a greater-than-normal amount of glucose enters the circulation, and plasma glucose levels start at a normal level and return to a normal level; therefore, it is obvious that a greater-than-normal amount of glucose has been removed from circulation. Although tissue glucose utilization is not reduced in patients with IGT, it is less than would have been found in patients with normal glucose tolerance whose plasma glucose and insulin levels match those of patients with IGT, indicating that patients with IGT are insulin resistant [157] (adapted from Mitrakou et al. [155]).

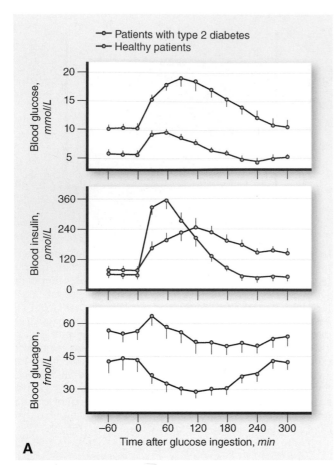

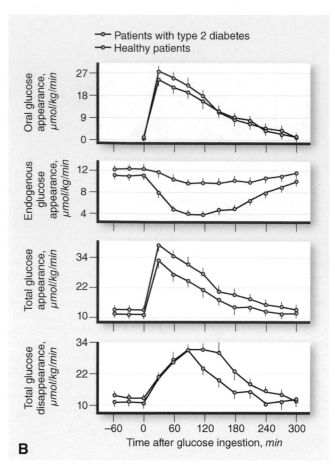

Figure 7-18. Comparison of postprandial changes in plasma insulin and glucagon levels (**A**) and rates of glucose appearance and removal from plasma (**B**) in patients with type 2 diabetes and healthy patients. The postprandial abnormalities in patients with type 2 diabetes (*closed circles*) are quite similar to those of people with impaired glucose tolerance (*open circles*), except that they are more exaggerated. The only major difference is that with excessive glycosuria, the uptake of glucose in liver is diminished [77, 78, 164, 165] (adapted from Mitrakou et al. [77]).

UKPDS: Effect of intensive treatment of type 2 diabetes

Reduced HbA$_{1c}$ by 11% with intensive therapy (7.9 vs. 7%)

This leads to:

   12% decrease in any diabetes-related endpoint

   25% decrease in microvascular endpoints

   21% decrease in retinopathy at 12 years

   33% decrease in microalbuminuria at 12 years

   25% decrease in cataract

   16% decrease in myocardial infarction (ns)

   5% decrease in stroke (ns)

Figure 7-19. Effects of intensive treatment of type 2 diabetes. Results of the UKPDS showed an unequivocal effect of intensive insulin therapy on long-term complications of diabetes and mortality [88, 166]. *HbA$_{1c}$* glycated hemoglobin.

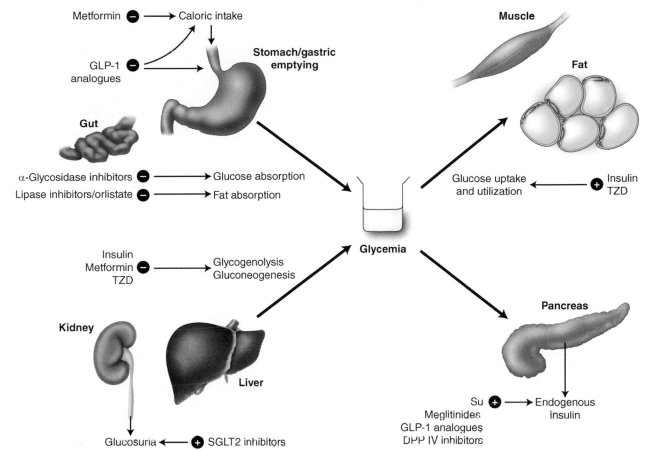

Figure 7-20. Sites of action of drugs used to treat type 2 diabetes. In addition to insulin, various agents are available for the treatment of type 2 diabetes. These agents differ in their modes of action, efficacy, pharmacokinetics, and side effects. Sulfonylureas and meglitinides are insulin secretagogues that act directly on the pancreatic β cells via inhibiting ATP-sensitive potassium channels [97]. Metformin, a biguanide, and the thiazolidinediones (TZDs) are classified as insulin sensitizers. Both agents improve insulin sensitivity in liver and peripheral tissues [101, 167]. Metformin may act on gluconeogenic and mitochondrial enzymes, and appears to work preferentially in the liver to inhibit glucose production. It also reduces appetite [168]. The exact mechanism of action of TZDs on a molecular level still is poorly understood. They are selective ligands of the nuclear transcription factor PPARγ and are thought to work primarily on adipose tissue and muscle, where they reduce FFA release and increase the efficiency of glucose uptake, respectively [102, 169]. By contrast, the mechanism of action of the alphaglucosidase inhibitors (acarbose) is well established [170]. By inhibiting the digestion of dietary starches, they slow the postprandial absorption of glucose. Lipase inhibitors (orlistat), on the contrary, inhibit pancreatic and gastric lipases and thus reduce the absorption of ingested fat and cause clinically meaningful weight loss. In diabetic patients, the weight loss induced by orlistat is associated with an improvement in glycemic control, making orlistat a useful adjunct therapy for patients with type 2 diabetes [171, 172]. Antidiabetic drugs that enhance incretins' activity or level (GLP-1 analogues and dipeptidyl peptidase [DPP]-IV inhibitors) are currently available and have proven to be effective in lowering glucose in type 2 diabetes. GLP-1 analogues also have other noninsulinotropic effects that are beneficial for treating diabetes, such as slowing gastric emptying and gut motility [173]. The sodium–glucose cotransporter-2 (SGLT2) inhibitors are the newest class of glucose-lowering agents and are currently undergoing clinical trials. SGLT2 is the major transporter responsible for the renal reabsorption of glucose. Inhibition of this reabsorption process reduces the renal threshold for glucose, thus promoting the excretion of excess glucose in the urine, which lowers plasma glucose levels and ameliorates glucose toxicity [174]. *Su* sulfonylureas.

References

1. American Diabetes Association: Total prevalence of diabetes and pre-diabetes, 2007. Available at http://diabetes.org. Accessed September 2009.

2. Bogardus C, Lillioja S, Bennett P: Pathogenesis of NIDDM in Pima Indians. *Diabetes Care* 1991, 14:685–690.

3. Cheung BM, Ong KL, Cherny SS, *et al.*: Diabetes prevalence and therapeutic target achievement in the United States, 1999 to 2006. *Am J Med* 2009, 122:443–453.

4. Weyer C, Tataranni PA, Bogardus C, Pratley R: Insulin resistance and insulin secretory dysfunction are independent predictors of worsening of glucose tolerance during each stage of type 2 diabetes development. *Diabetes Care* 2000, 24:89–94.

5. Weyer C, Bogardus C, Mott D, Pratley R: The natural history of insulin secretory dysfunction and insulin resistance in the pathogenesis of type 2 diabetes mellitus. *J Clin Invest* 1999, 104:787–794.

6. Kahn S: The importance of ß-cell failure in the development and progression of type 2 diabetes. *J Clin Endocrinol Metab* 2001, 86:4047–4058.

7. Pratley R, Weyer C: The role of impaired early insulin secretion in the pathogenesis of type II diabetes mellitus. *Diabetologia* 2001, 44:929–945.

8. Hamman R: Genetic and environmental determinants of noninsulin dependent diabetes mellitus (NIDDM). *Diabetes Metab Rev* 1992, 8:287–338.

9. Stefan N, Fritsche A, Haring H, Stumvoll M: Effect of experimental elevation of free fatty acids on insulin secretion and insulin sensitivity in healthy carriers of the Pro12Ala polymorphism of the peroxisome proliferator-activated receptor-gamma2 gene. *Diabetes* 2001, 50:1143–1148.

10. Horikawa Y, Oda N, Cox N, *et al.*: Genetic variation in the gene encoding calpain-10 is associated with type 2 diabetes mellitus. *Nat Genet* 2000, 26:163–175.

11. Gloyn AL, Weedon MN, Owen KR, *et al.*: Large-scale association studies of variants in genes encoding the pancreatic beta-cell KATP channel subunits Kir6.2 (KCNJ11) and SUR1 (ABCC8) confirm that the KCNJ11 E23K variant is associated with type 2 diabetes. *Diabetes* 2003, 52:568–572.

12. Florez JC, Jablonski KA, Kahn SE, *et al.*: Type 2 diabetes-associated missense polymorphisms KCNJ11 E23K and ABCC8 A1369S influence progression to diabetes and response to interventions in the Diabetes Prevention Program. *Diabetes* 2007, 56:531–536.

13. Florez JC, Jablonski KA, Bayley N, *et al.*: TCF7L2 polymorphisms and progression to diabetes in the Diabetes Prevention Program. *N Engl J Med* 2006, 355:241–250.

14. Zhang C, Qi L, Hunter DJ, *et al.*: Variant of transcription factor 7-like 2 (TCF7L2) gene and the risk of type 2 diabetes in large cohorts of U.S. women and men. *Diabetes* 2006, 55:2645–2648.

15. Grant SF, Thorleifsson G, Reynisdottir I, *et al.*: Variant of transcription factor 7-like 2 (TCF7L2) gene confers risk of type 2 diabetes. *Nat Genet* 2006, 38:320–323.

16. Yi F, Brubaker PL, Jin T: TCF-4 mediates cell type-specific regulation of proglucagon gene expression by beta-catenin and glycogen synthase kinase-3beta. *J Biol Chem* 2005, 280:1457–1464.

17. Saltiel A, Kahn C: Insulin signalling and the regulation of glucose and lipid metabolism. *Nature* 2001, 414:799–806.

18. Gloyn A: The genetics of diabetes: a progress report. *Practical Diabetes Int* 2001, 18:246–250.

19. Shaw J, Purdie D, Neil H, *et al.*: The relative risks of hyperglycemia, obesity and dyslipidemia in relatives of patients with type II diabetes mellitus. *Diabetologia* 1999, 42:24–27.

20. Shatten B, Smith G, Kuller L, Neation J: Risk factors for the development of type 2 diabetes among men enrolled in the usual care group of the multiple risk factor intervention trial. *Diabetes* 1993, 16:1331–1338.

21. Gerich J, Van Haeften T: Insulin resistance versus impaired insulin secretion as the genetic basis for type 2 diabetes. *Curr Opin Endocrinol Diabetes* 1998, 5:144–148.

22. Pimenta W, Kortytkowski M, Mitrakou A, *et al.*: Pancreatic beta-cell dysfunction as the primary genetic lesion in NIDDM. Evidence from studies in normal glucose-tolerant individuals with a first-degree NIDDM relative. *JAMA* 1995, 273:1855–1861.

23. Vaag A, Alford F, Beck-Nielsen H: Intracellular glucose and fat metabolism in identical twins discordant for non-insulin-dependent diabetes mellitus (NIDDM): acquired versus genetic metabolic defects. *Diabetic Med* 1996, 13:806–815.

24. Cerasi E, Luft R: Insulin response to glucose infusion in diabetic and nondiabetic monozygotic twin pairs: genetic control of insulin response. *Acta Endocrinol* 1967, 55:330–345.

25. Barnett A, Spiliopoulos A, Pyke D, *et al.*: Metabolic studies in unaffected co-twins of noninsulin dependent diabetics. *Br Med J* 1981, 282:1656–1658.

26. Pyke D, Taylor K: Glucose tolerance and serum insulin in unaffected identical twins of diabetics. *Br Med J* 1967, 4:21–22.

27. Hu F, Manson J, Stampfer M, *et al.*: Diet, lifestyle, and the risk of type 2 diabetes mellitus in women. *N Engl J Med* 2001, 345:790–797.

28. Choi B, Shi F: Risk factors for diabetes mellitus by age and sex: results of the national population health survey. *Diabetologia* 2001, 44:1221–1231.

29. Marshall J, Hoag S, Shetterly S, Hammon R: Dietary fat predicts conversion of impaired glucose tolerance to NIDDM. *Diabetes Care* 1994, 17:50–56.

30. Wei M, Schweitner H, Blair S: The association between physical activity, physical fitness and type 2 diabetes mellitus. *Compr Ther* 2000, 26:176–182.

31. Wannamethee S, Shaper A, Perry I: Smoking as a modifiable risk factor for type 2 diabetes in middle aged men. *Diabetes Care* 2001, 24:1590–1595.

32. Rich-Edwards J, Colditz G, Stampfer M, *et al.*: Birthweight and the risk for type 2 diabetes mellitus in adult women. *Ann Intern Med* 1999, 130:278–284.

33. Eriksson J, Lindstrom J, Tuomilehto J: Potential for prevention of type 2 diabetes. *Br Med Bull* 2001, 60:183–199.

34. Knowler W, Barrett-Connor E, Fowler S, *et al.*: Reduction in the incidence of type 2 diabetes with lifestyle intervention or metformin. *N Engl J Med* 2002, 346:393–403.

35. Tuomilehto J, Lindström J, Eriksson J, *et al.*: Prevention of type 2 diabetes mellitus by changes in lifestyle among subjects with impaired glucose tolerance. *N Engl J Med* 2001, 344:1343–1350.

36. Pan X-R, Li G-W, Hu Y-H, *et al.*: Effects of diet and exercise in preventing NIDDM in people with impaired glucose tolerance: the Da Qing IGT and Diabetes Study. *Diabetes Care* 1997, 20:537–544.

37. Eriksson K, Lindgarde F: Prevention of type 2 (noninsulin dependent) diabetes mellitus by diet and exercise. *Diabetologia* 1991, 34:891–898.

38. Wenying Y, Lixiang L, Jinwu Q, *et al.*: The preventive effect of acarbose and metformin on the progression to diabetes mellitus in the IGT population: a 3-year multicenter prospective study. *Chin J Endocrinol Metab* 2001, 17:131–136.

39. Chiasson J, Josse R, Gomis R, *et al.*: Acarbose for prevention of type 2 diabetes mellitus: the STOP-NIDDM randomised trial. *Lancet* 2002, 359:2072–2077.

40. Buchanan TA, Xiang AH, Peters RK, *et al.*: Preservation of pancreatic beta-cell function and prevention of type 2 diabetes by phar-

macological treatment of insulin resistance in high-risk hispanic women. *Diabetes* 2002, 51:2796–2803.

41. Torgerson JS, Hauptman J, Boldrin MN, Sjostrom L: XENical in the prevention of diabetes in obese subjects (XENDOS) study: a randomized study of orlistat as an adjunct to lifestyle changes for the prevention of type 2 diabetes in obese patients. *Diabetes Care* 2004, 27:155–161.

42. Vetter ML, Cardillo S, Rickels MR, Iqbal N: Narrative review: effect of bariatric surgery on type 2 diabetes mellitus. *Ann Intern Med* 2009, 150:94–103.

43. Buchwald H, Avidor Y, Braunwald E, et al.: Bariatric surgery: a systematic review and meta-analysis. *JAMA* 2004, 292:1724–1737.

44. Pories WJ, Swanson MS, MacDonald KG, et al.: Who would have thought it? An operation proves to be the most effective therapy for adult-onset diabetes mellitus. *Ann Surg* 1995, 222:339–350.

45. Cummings DE, Overduin J: Gastrointestinal regulation of food intake. *J Clin Invest* 2007, 117:13–23.

46. Kageyama H, Funahashi H, Hirayama M, et al.: Morphological analysis of ghrelin and its receptor distribution in the rat pancreas. *Regul Pept* 2005, 126:67–71.

47. Ballantyne GH: Peptide YY(1–36) and peptide YY(3–36): Part I. Distribution, release and actions. *Obes Surg* 2006, 16:651–658.

48. Clements RH, Gonzalez QH, Long CI, et al.: Hormonal changes after Roux-en Y gastric bypass for morbid obesity and the control of type-II diabetes mellitus. *Am Surg* 2004, 70:1–4.

49. Laferrere B, Teixeira J, McGinty J, et al.: Effect of weight loss by gastric bypass surgery versus hypocaloric diet on glucose and incretin levels in patients with type 2 diabetes. *J Clin Endocrinol Metab* 2008, 93:2479–2485.

50. Korner J, Bessler M, Inabnet W, et al.: Exaggerated glucagon-like peptide-1 and blunted glucose-dependent insulinotropic peptide secretion are associated with Roux-en-Y gastric bypass but not adjustable gastric banding. *Surg Obes Relat Dis* 2007, 3:597–601.

51. le Roux CW, Welbourn R, Werling M, et al.: Gut hormones as mediators of appetite and weight loss after Roux-en-Y gastric bypass. *Ann Surg* 2007, 246:780–785.

52. Morinigo R, Moize V, Musri M, et al.: Glucagon-like peptide-1, peptide YY, hunger, and satiety after gastric bypass surgery in morbidly obese subjects. *J Clin Endocrinol Metab* 2006, 91:1735–1740.

53. Cummings DE, Weigle DS, Frayo RS, et al.: Plasma ghrelin levels after diet-induced weight loss or gastric bypass surgery. *N Engl J Med* 2002, 346:1623–1630.

54. Faraj M, Havel PJ, Phelis S, et al.: Plasma acylation-stimulating protein, adiponectin, leptin, and ghrelin before and after weight loss induced by gastric bypass surgery in morbidly obese subjects. *J Clin Endocrinol Metab* 2003, 88:1594–1602.

55. Holdstock C, Engstrom BE, Ohrvall M, et al.: Ghrelin and adipose tissue regulatory peptides: effect of gastric bypass surgery in obese humans. *J Clin Endocrinol Metab* 2003, 88:3177–3183.

56. Cummings DE, Overduin J, Foster Schubert KE, Carlson MJ: Role of the bypassed proximal intestine in the anti-diabetic effects of bariatric surgery. *Surg Obes Relat Dis* 2007, 3:109–115.

57. Rubino F: Is type 2 diabetes an operable intestinal disease? A provocative yet reasonable hypothesis. *Diabetes Care* 2008, 31(Suppl 2):S290–S296.

58. Porte D Jr, Kahn S: Beta-cell dysfunction and failure in type 2 diabetes: potential mechanisms. *Diabetes* 2001, 50(Suppl 1):S160–S163.

59. Carey D, Jenkins A, Campbell L, et al.: Abdominal fat and insulin resistance in normal and overweight women: direct measurements reveal a strong relationship in subjects at both low and high risk of NIDDM. *Diabetes* 1996, 45:633–638.

60. Banerji M, Chaiken R, Gordon D, et al.: Does intra-abdominal adipose tissue in black men determine whether NIDDM is insulin-resistant or insulin-sensitive? *Diabetes* 1995, 44:141–146.

61. Byrne M, Sturgis J, Sobel R, Polonsky K: Elevated plasma glucose 2h postchallenge predicts defects in B-cell function. *Am J Physiol* 1996, 270:E572–E579.

62. Nesher R, Casa Della L, Litvin Y, et al.: Insulin deficiency and insulin resistance in type II (noninsulin dependent) diabetes: quantitative contributions of pancreatic and peripheral responses to glucose homeostasis. *Eur J Clin Invest* 1987, 17:266–274.

63. Campbell P, Mandarino L, Gerich J: Quantification of the relative impairment in actions of insulin on hepatic glucose production and peripheral glucose uptake in non-insulin-dependent diabetes mellitus. *Metabolism* 1988, 37:15–21.

64. Kalant N, Leibovici D, Fukushima N, et al.: Insulin responsiveness of superficial forearm tissues in type 2 (noninsulin-dependent) diabetes. *Diabetologia* 1982, 22:239–244.

65. Bonora E, Bonadonna R, DelPrato S, et al.: In vivo glucose metabolism in obese and type II diabetic subjects with or without hypertension. *Diabetes* 1993, 42:764–772.

66. Nosadini R, Solini A, Velussi M, et al.: Impaired insulin-induced glucose uptake by extrahepatic tissue is hallmark of NIDDM patients who have or will develop hypertension and microalbuminuria. *Diabetes* 1994, 43:491–499.

67. Groop L, Ekstrand A, Forsblom C, et al.: Insulin resistance, hypertension and microalbuminuria in patients with type 2 (non-insulin-dependent) diabetes mellitus. *Diabetologia* 1993, 36:642–647.

68. Gerich J: The genetic basis of type 2 diabetes mellitus: Impaired insulin secretion versus impaired insulin sensitivity. *Endocr Rev* 1998, 19:491–503.

69. Dohm GL, Tapscott E, Pories W, et al.: An in vitro human muscle preparation suitable for metabolic studies. Decreased insulin stimulation of glucose transport in muscle from morbidly obese and diabetic subjects. *J Clin Invest* 1988, 82:486–494.

70. Boden G: Role of fatty acids in the pathogenesis of insulin resistance and NIDDM. *Diabetes* 1997, 46:3–10.

71. Hotamisligil G, Spiegelman B: Tumor necrosis factor alpha: a key component of the obesity diabetes link. *Diabetes* 1994, 43:1271–1278.

72. Steppan C, Bailey S, Bhat S, et al.: The hormone resistin links obesity to diabetes. *Nature* 2001, 409:307–312.

73. Ahima R, Flier J: Leptin. *Annu Rev Physiol* 2000, 62:413–437.

74. Ahima R, Flier J: Adipose tissue as an endocrine organ. *Trends Endocrinol Metab* 2000, 11:327–332.

75. Kelley D, Goodpaster B: Skeletal muscle triglyceride: an aspect of regional adiposity and insulin resistance. *Diabetes Care* 2001, 24:933–941.

76. Virkamaki A, Korsheninnikova E, Seppala-Lindroos A, et al.: Intramyocellular lipid is associated with resistance to in vivo insulin actions on glucose uptake, antilipolysis, and early insulin signaling pathways in human skeletal muscle. *Diabetes* 2001, 50:2337–2343.

77. Mitrakou A, Kelley D, Veneman T, et al.: Contribution of abnormal muscle and liver glucose metabolism in postprandial hyperglycemia in noninsulin-dependent diabetes mellitus. *Diabetes* 1990, 39:1381–1390.

78. Dinneen S, Gerich J, Rizza R: Carbohydrate metabolism in noninsulin-dependent diabetes mellitus. *N Engl J Med* 1992, 327:707–713.

79. Woerle HJ, Szoke E, Meyer C, et al.: Mechanisms for abnormal postprandial glucose metabolism in type 2 diabetes. *Am J Physiol Endocrinol Metab* 2006, 290:E67–E77.

80. Perseghin G, Petersen K, Shulman GI: Cellular mechanism of insulin resistance: potential links with inflammation. *Int J Obes Relat Metab Disord* 2003, 27 Suppl 3:S6–11.

81. Petersen KF, Dufour S, Befroy D, et al.: Impaired mitochondrial activity in the insulin-resistant offspring of patients with type 2 diabetes. *N Engl J Med* 2004, 350:664–671.

82. Patel A, MacMahon S, Chalmers J, et al.: Intensive blood glucose control and vascular outcomes in patients with type 2 diabetes. *N Engl J Med* 2008, 358:2560–2572.

83. DCCT Research Group: The effect of intensive treatment of diabetes on the development and progression of long-term complications in insulin dependent diabetes mellitus. *N Engl J Med* 1993, 329:977–986.

84. UK Prospective Diabetes Study (UKPDS) Group: Effect of intensive blood-glucose control with metformin on complications in overweight patients with type 2 diabetes (UKPDS 34). *Lancet* 1998, 352:854–865.

85. Reichard P, Pihl M, Rosenqvist U, Sule J: Complications in IDDM are caused by elevated blood glucose level: The Stockholm Diabetes Intervention Study (SDIS) at 10-year follow up. *Diabetologia* 1996, 39:1483–1488.

86. Gerstein HC, Miller ME, Byington RP, et al.: Effects of intensive glucose lowering in type 2 diabetes. *N Engl J Med* 2008, 358:2545–2559.

87. Abraira C, Duckworth WC, Moritz T: Glycaemic separation and risk factor control in the Veterans Affairs Diabetes Trial: an interim report. *Diabetes Obes Metab* 2009, 11:150–156.

88. UK Prospective Diabetes Study (UKPDS) Group: Intensive blood-glucose control with sulphonylureas or insulin compared with conventional treatment and risk of complications in patients with type 2 diabetes (UKPDS 33). *Lancet* 1998, 352:837–853.

89. Holman RR, Paul SK, Bethel MA, et al.: 10-year follow-up of intensive glucose control in type 2 diabetes. *N Engl J Med* 2008, 359:1577–1589.

90. DCCT Research Group: Effect of intensive diabetes management on macrovascular events and risk factors in the Diabetes Control and Complications Trial. *Am J Cardiol* 1995, 75:894–903.

91. Nathan DM, Cleary PA, Backlund JY, et al.: Intensive diabetes treatment and cardiovascular disease in patients with type 1 diabetes. *N Engl J Med* 2005, 353:2643–2653.

92. Gerich JE: Clinical significance, pathogenesis, and management of postprandial hyperglycemia. *Arch Intern Med* 2003, 163:1306–1316.

93. Chiasson JL, Josse RG, Gomis R, et al.: Acarbose treatment and the risk of cardiovascular disease and hypertension in patients with impaired glucose tolerance: the STOP-NIDDM trial. *JAMA* 2003, 290:486–494.

94. Rodbard HW, Blonde L, Braithwaite SS, et al.: American Association of Clinical Endocrinologists medical guidelines for clinical practice for the management of diabetes mellitus. *Endocr Pract* 2007, 13(Suppl 1):1–68.

95. Nathan DM, Buse JB, Davidson MB, et al.: Management of hyperglycemia in type 2 diabetes: a consensus algorithm for the initiation and adjustment of therapy: a consensus statement from the American Diabetes Association and the European Association for the Study of Diabetes. *Diabetes Care* 2006, 29:1963–1972.

96. Woerle HJ, Pimenta W, Meyer C, et al.: Diagnostic and therapeutic implications of relationships between fasting, 2 hour postchallenge plasma glucose and HbA$_{1c}$ values. *Arch Intern Med* 2004, 164:1627–1632.

97. Lebovitz H: Insulin secretogogues: old and new. *Diab Rev* 1999, 7:139–153.

98. Langtry H, Balfour J: Glimepiride. A review of its use in the management of type 2 diabetes mellitus. *Drugs* 1998, 55:563–584.

99. Dunn C, Faulds D: Nateglinide. *Drugs* 2000, 60:607–615.

100. Lee Y, Hirose H, Ohneda M, et al.: Beta-cell lipotoxicity in the pathogenesis of non-insulin-dependent diabetes mellitus of obese rats: impairment in adipocyte-beta-cell relationships. *Proc Natl Acad Sci U S A* 1994, 91:10878–10882.

101. Mudaliar S, Henry R: New oral therapies for type 2 diabetes mellitus: the glitazones or insulin sensitizers. *Annu Rev Med* 2001, 52:239–257.

102. Inzucchi S, Maggs D, Spollett G, et al.: Efficacy and metabolic effects of metformin and troglitazone in type II diabetes mellitus. *N Engl J Med* 1998, 338:867–872.

103. Campbell L, Baker D, Campbell RK: Miglitol: assessment of its role in the treatment of patients with diabetes mellitus. *Ann Pharmacother* 2000, 34:1291–1301.

104. Bolli G, Di Marchi R, Park G, et al.: Insulin analogues and their potential in the management of diabetes mellitus. *Diabetologia* 1999, 42:1151–1167.

105. Lepore M, Pampanelli S, Fanelli C, et al.: Pharmacokinetics and pharmacodynamics of subcutaneous injection of long-acting human insulin analog glargine, NPH insulin, and ultralente human insulin and continuous subcutaneous infusion of insulin lispro. *Diabetes* 2000, 49:2142–2148.

106. Abraira C, Henderson W, Colwell J, et al.: Response to intensive therapy steps and glipizide dose in combination with insulin in type 2 diabetes. *Diabetes Care* 1998, 21:574–579.

107. Turner R, Cull C, Frighi V, Holman R: Glycemic control with diet, sulfonylurea, metformin, or insulin in patients with type 2 diabetes mellitus. Progressive requirement for multiple therapies (UKPDS 49). *JAMA* 1999, 281:2005–2012.

108. Siegel E, Mayer G, Nauck M, Creutzfeldt W: [Factitious hypoglycemia caused by taking a sulfonylurea drug] [German]. *Dtsch Med Wochenschr* 1987, 112:1575–1579.

109. Wroblewski M, Gottsater A, Lindgarde F, et al.: Gender, autoantibodies, and obesity in newly diagnosed diabetic patients aged 40–75 years. *Diabetes Care* 1998, 21:250–255.

110. Bell G, Polonsky K: Diabetes mellitus and genetically programmed defects in beta-cell function. *Nature* 2001, 414:788–791.

111. *Diabetes in America*, edn 2. Bethesda, MD: National Institutes of Health; 1995.

112. Kahn C: Insulin action, diabetogenes, and the cause of type II diabetes. *Diabetes* 1994, 43:1066–1084.

113. Beals JK: Pioglitazone reduces conversion from impaired glucose tolerance to type 2 diabetes. Presented at the American Diabetes Association 68th Scientific Sessions: Late Breaking Clinical Studies. San Francisco, CA; June 9, 2008. Medscape Medical News 2008. Accessible at http://www.medscape.com/viewarticle/575860. Accessed September 3, 2009.

114. Gerstein HC, Yusuf S, Bosch J, et al.: Effect of rosiglitazone on the frequency of diabetes in patients with impaired glucose tolerance or impaired fasting glucose: a randomised controlled trial. *Lancet* 2006, 368:1096–1105.

115. Kahn S: The importance of the ß-cell in the pathogenesis of type 2 diabetes mellitus. *Am J Med* 2000, 108(Suppl 6A):2S–8S.

116. Thorens B, Wu Y, Leahy J, Weir G: The loss of GLUT2 expression by glucose-unresponsive beta cells of db/db mice is reversible and is induced by the diabetic environment. *J Clin Invest* 1992, 90:77–85.

117. Caro J, Sinha M, Raju SM, et al.: Insulin receptor kinase in human skeletal muscle from obese subjects with and without noninsulin dependent diabetes. *J Clin Invest* 1987, 79:1330–1337.

118. Bak J, Moller N, Schmitz O, et al.: In vivo action and muscle glycogen synthase activity in type II (noninsulin dependent) diabetes mellitus: effects of diet treatment. *Diabetologia* 1992, 35:777–784.

119. McGarry J, Dobbins R: Fatty acids, lipotoxity and insulin secretion. *Diabetologia* 1999, 42:128–138.

120. Unger R, Zhou Y: Lipotoxity of beta-cells in obesity and in other causes of fatty acid spillover. *Diabetes* 2001, 50(Suppl 1):S118–S121.

121. Randle P, Priestman D, Mistry S, Halsall A: Glucose fatty acid interactions and the regulation of glucose disposal. *J Cell Biochem* 1994, 55S:1–11.

122. Shulman G: Cellular mechanisms of insulin resistance. *J Clin Invest* 2000, 106:171–176.

123. Garvey W, Huecksteadt T, Matthaei S, Olefsky J: Role of glucose transporters in the cellular insulin resistance of type II noninsulin-dependent diabetes mellitus. *J Clin Invest* 1988, 81:1528–1536.

124. Kelley D, Mintun M, Watkins S, *et al.*: The effect of non-insulin-dependent diabetes mellitus and obesity on glucose transport and phosphorylation in skeletal muscle. *J Clin Invest* 1996, 97:2705–2713.

125. Cline G, Petersen K, Krssak M, *et al.*: Impaired glucose transport as a cause of decreased insulin-stimulated muscle glycogen synthesis in type 2 diabetes. *N Engl J Med* 1999, 341:240–246.

126. Butler AE, Janson J, Bonner-Weir S, *et al.*: Beta-cell deficit and increased beta-cell apoptosis in humans with type 2 diabetes. *Diabetes* 2003, 52:102–110.

127. Yoon KH, Ko SH, Cho JH, *et al.*: Selective beta-cell loss and alpha-cell expansion in patients with type 2 diabetes mellitus in Korea. *J Clin Endocrinol Metab* 2003, 88:2300–2308.

128. Guiot Y, Sempoux C, Moulin P, Rahier J: No decrease of the beta-cell mass in type 2 diabetic patients. *Diabetes* 2001, 50(Suppl 1):S188.

129. Stefan Y, Orci L, Malaisse-Lagae F, *et al.*: Quantitation of endocrine cell content in the pancreas of nondiabetic and diabetic humans. *Diabetes* 1982, 31:694–700.

130. Sakuraba H, Mizukami H, Yagihashi N, *et al.*: Reduced beta-cell mass and expression of oxidative stress-related DNA damage in the islet of Japanese Type II diabetic patients. *Diabetologia* 2002, 45:85–96.

131. Clark A, Wells C, Buley I, *et al.*: Islet amyloid, increased alpha cells, reduced beta-cells and exocrine fibrosis: quantitative changes in the pancreas in type 2 diabetes. *Diabetes Res* 1988, 9:151–159.

132. Kloppel G, Lohr M, Habich K, *et al.*: Islet pathology and the pathogenesis of type 1 and type 2 diabetes mellitus revisited. *Surv Synth Pathol Res* 1985, 4:110–125.

133. Gepts W: Contribution to the morphological study of the islands of Langerhans in diabetes; study of the quantitative variations of the different insular constituents. *Ann Soc R Sci Med Nat Brux* 1957, 10:5–108.

134. Saito K, Yaginuma N, Takahashi T: Differential volumetry of A, B, and D cells in the pancreatic islets of diabetic and nondiabetic subjects. *Tohoku J Exp Med* 1979, 129.273–283.

135. MacLean N, Ogilvie RF: Quantitative estimation of the pancreatic islet tissue in diabetic subjects. *Diabetes* 1955, 4:367–376.

136. Westermark P, Wilander E: The influence of amyloid deposits on the islet volume in maturity onset diabetes mellitus. *Diabetologia* 1978, 15:417–421.

137. Rahier J, Guiot Y, Goebbels RM, *et al.*: Pancreatic beta-cell mass in European subjects with type 2 diabetes. *Diabetes Obes Metab* 2008, 10(Suppl 4):32–42.

138. Deng S, Vatamaniuk M, Huang X, *et al.*: Structural and functional abnormalities in the islets isolated from type 2 diabetic subjects. *Diabetes* 2004, 53:624–632.

139. Hales C, Barker D, Clark P, *et al.*: Fetal and infant growth and impaired glucose tolerance at age 64. *BMJ* 1991, 303:1019–1022.

140. Dahri S, Snoeck A, Reusens-Billen B, *et al.*: Islet function in offspring of mothers on low-protein diet during gestation. *Diabetes* 1991, 40(Suppl 2):115–120.

141. Moran A, Zhang HJ, Olson LK, *et al.*: Differentiation of glucose toxicity from beta cell exhaustion during the evolution of defective insulin gene expression in the pancreatic islet cell line, HIT-T15. *J Clin Invest* 1997, 99:534–539.

142. Olson LK, Redmon JB, Towle HC, Robertson RP: Chronic exposure of HIT cells to high glucose concentrations paradoxically decreases insulin gene transcription and alters binding of insulin gene regulatory protein. *J Clin Invest* 1993, 92:514–519.

143. Lu M, Seufert J, Habener JF: Pancreatic beta-cell-specific repression of insulin gene transcription by CCAAT/enhancer-binding protein beta. Inhibitory interactions with basic helix-loop-helix transcription factor E47. *J Biol Chem* 1997, 272:28349–28359.

144. Jonas JC, Sharma A, Hasenkamp W, *et al.*: Chronic hyperglycemia triggers loss of pancreatic beta cell differentiation in an animal model of diabetes. *J Biol Chem* 1999, 274:14112–14121.

145. Tanaka Y, Gleason CE, Tran PO, *et al.*: Prevention of glucose toxicity in HIT-T15 cells and Zucker diabetic fatty rats by antioxidants. *Proc Natl Acad Sci U S A* 1999, 96:10857–10862.

146. Tajiri Y, Moller C, Grill V: Long-term effects of aminoguanidine on insulin release and biosynthesis: evidence that the formation of advanced glycosylation end products inhibits B cell function. *Endocrinology* 1997, 138:273–280.

147. Cnop M, Hannaert JC, Hoorens A, *et al.*: Inverse relationship between cytotoxicity of free fatty acids in pancreatic islet cells and cellular triglyceride accumulation. *Diabetes* 2001, 50:1771–1777.

148. Maedler K, Spinas GA, Dyntar D, *et al.*: Distinct effects of saturated and monounsaturated fatty acids on beta-cell turnover and function. *Diabetes* 2001, 50:69–76.

149. Gremlich S, Bonny C, Waeber G, Thorens B: Fatty acids decrease IDX-1 expression in rat pancreatic islets and reduce GLUT2, glucokinase, insulin, and somatostatin levels. *J Biol Chem* 1997, 272:30261–30269.

150. Farney AC, Xenos E, Sutherland DE, *et al.*: Inhibition of pancreatic islet beta cell function by tumor necrosis factor is blocked by a soluble tumor necrosis factor receptor. *Transplant Proc* 1993, 25:865–866.

151. Bolaffi JL, Rodd GG, Wang J, Grodsky GM: Interrelationship of changes in islet nicotine adenine nucleotide, insulin secretion, and cell viability induced by interleukin-1 beta. *Endocrinology* 1994, 134:537–542.

152. Campbell IL, Oxbrow L, Harrison LC: Interferon-gamma: pleiotropic effects on a rat pancreatic beta cell line. *Mol Cell Endocrinol* 1987, 52:161–167.

153. Janson J, Ashley R, Harrison D, *et al.*: The mechanism of islet amyloid polypeptide toxicity is membrane disruption by intermediate-sized toxic amyloid particles. *Diabetes* 1999, 48:491–498.

154. Clark A, Nilsson MR: Islet amyloid: a complication of islet dysfunction or an aetiological factor in Type 2 diabetes? *Diabetologia* 2004, 47:157–169.

155. Mitrakou A, Kelley D, Mokan M, *et al.*: Role of reduced suppression of glucose production and diminished early insulin release in impaired glucose tolerance. *N Engl J Med* 1992, 326:22–29.

156. Gerich J: Metabolic abnormalities in impaired glucose tolerance. *Metabolism* 1997, 46(Suppl 1):40–43.

157. Van Haeften T, Pimenta W, Mitrakou A, *et al.*: Relative contributions of β-cell function and tissue insulin sensitivity to fasting and postglucose-load glycemia. *Metabolism* 2000, 49:1318–1325.

158. DeFronzo R: The triumvirate: B-cell, muscle, and liver: a collusion responsible for NIDDM. *Diabetes* 1988, 37:667–687.

159. Calles-Escandon J, Robbins D: Loss of early phase of insulin release in humans impairs glucose tolerance and blunts thermic effect of glucose. *Diabetes* 1987, 36:1167–1172.

160. Meyer C, Stumvoll M, Nadkarni V, *et al.*: Abnormal renal and hepatic glucose metabolism in type 2 diabetes mellitus. *J Clin Invest* 1998, 102:619–624.

161. Consoli A, Nurjhan N, Capani F, Gerich J: Predominant role of gluconeogenesis in increased hepatic glucose production in NIDDM. *Diabetes* 1989, 38:550–561.

162. Magnusson I, Rothman D, Katz L, *et al.*: Increased rate of gluconeogenesis in type II diabetes. A 13C nuclear magnetic resonance study. *J Clin Invest* 1992, 90:1323–1327.

163. Nurjhan N, Consoli A, Gerich J: Increased lipolysis and its consequences on gluconeogenesis in noninsulin-dependent diabetes mellitus. *J Clin Invest* 1992, 89:169–175.

164. Kelley D, Mokan M, Veneman T: Impaired postprandial glucose utilization in non-insulin-dependent diabetes mellitus. *Metabolism* 1994, 43:1549–1557.

165. Roden M, Petersen K, Shulman G: Nuclear magnetic resonance studies of hepatic glucose metabolism in humans. *Recent Prog Horm Res* 2001, 56:219–237.

166. Turner R: The U.K. Prospective Diabetes Study. A review. *Diabetes Care* 1998, 21(Suppl 3):C35–C38.

167. Cusi K, DeFronzo R: Metformin: a review of its metabolic effects. *Diab Rev* 1998, 6:89–131.

168. Stumvoll M, Nurjhan N, Perriello G, *et al.*: Metabolic effects of metformin in non-insulin-dependent diabetes mellitus. *N Engl J Med* 1995, 333:550–554.

169. Yki-Jarvinen H: Thiazolidinediones. *N Engl J Med* 2004, 351:1106–1118.

170. Göke B, Herrmann-Rinke C: The evolving role of alpha-glucosidase inhibitors. *Diabetes Metab Rev* 1998, 14:S31–S38.

171. Hollander PA, Elbein SC, Hirsch IB, *et al.*: Role of orlistat in the treatment of obese patients with type 2 diabetes. A 1-year randomized double-blind study. *Diabetes Care* 1998, 21:1288–1294.

172. Miles JM, Leiter L, Hollander P, *et al.*: Effect of orlistat in overweight and obese patients with type 2 diabetes treated with metformin. *Diabetes Care* 2002, 25:1123–1128.

173. Amori RE, Lau J, Pittas AG: Efficacy and safety of incretin therapy in type 2 diabetes: systematic review and meta-analysis. *JAMA* 2007, 298:194–206.

174. Idris I, Donnelly R: Sodium-glucose co-transporter-2 inhibitors: an emerging new class of oral antidiabetic drug. *Diabetes Obes Metab* 2009, 11:79–88.

175. Maassen J, Kadowaki T: Maternally inherited diabetes and deafness: a new diabetes subtype. *Diabetologia* 1996, 39:375–382.

176. Taylor S, Cama S, Accili D, *et al.*: Mutations in the insulin receptor gene. *Endocr Rev* 1992, 13:566–595.

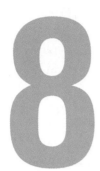

Management of Type 2 Diabetes Mellitus

Jennifer B. Marks

Diabetes and its complications are a significant cause of morbidity and mortality in the USA. The prevalence of diabetes has been steadily increasing in the adult population, based on national household surveys that were conducted (see Fig. 8.1) [1, 2]. Undiagnosed diabetes and abnormal glucose tolerance are considered to have substantial clinical importance (see Fig. 8.2) [1, 3–6].

Approximately 90–95% of people with diabetes have type 2 diabetes [7]. The pathogenesis of type 2 diabetes involves inadequate insulin secretion from pancreatic β-cells and inadequate insulin action in target tissues, or insulin resistance (see Fig. 8.3). When these tissues become insulin resistant, hepatic glucose production (HGP) increases, glucose uptake is decreased, and lipolysis is enhanced. Increased free fatty acids (FFAs) from lipolysis stimulate the cellular uptake of FFAs and lipid oxidation. In muscle, the increased FFA availability accelerates fat oxidation, resulting in decreased insulin-mediated glucose uptake and disposal. In the liver, elevated FFAs stimulate gluconeogenesis and increase hepatic glucose output. The coupling of insulin resistance in the target tissues and β-cell dysfunction leads to hyperglycemia, elevated plasma FFA levels, and the development of type 2 diabetes [4, 8]. DeFronzo has expanded the pathogenetic scheme to include the so-called "ominous octet," depicted in Fig. 8.4, in which it is noted that many other organs also contribute to the metabolic defects in type 2 diabetes [8].

Insulin resistance is present prior to the onset of clinical disease and is a predictor of its development [8–11]. In the natural history of the development of type 2 diabetes, insulin resistance is present prior to the onset of clinical disease. β-cells increase insulin secretion in response to insulin resistance and, for a period of time, are able to effectively overcome insulin resistance and maintain glucose levels below the diabetic range. However, when β-cell function begins to decline, insulin production is insufficient to overcome the insulin resistance and blood glucose levels rise. As illustrated, the rise in glycemia is paralleled by a decline in β-cell function. Note that once established, insulin resistance remains relatively stable over time. Therefore, the progression of diabetes is a result of worsening β-cell function with preexisting established insulin resistance (see Fig 8.5).

J.S. Skyler (ed.), *Atlas of Diabetes: Fourth Edition*,
DOI 10.1007/978-1-4614-1028-7_8, © Springer Science+Business Media, LLC 2012

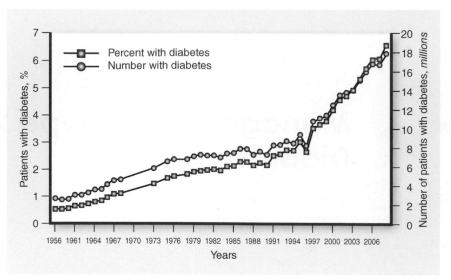

Figure 8-1. Number and percent of the US population with diagnosed diabetes, from 1958 to 2008 (adapted from the National Health Interview Survey).

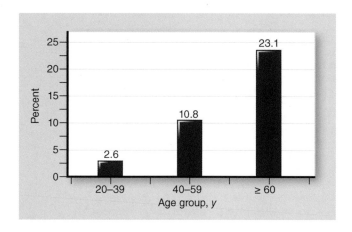

Figure 8-2. Estimated prevalence of diagnosed and undiagnosed diabetes. Shown are estimated rates of diagnosed and undiagnosed diabetes in people 20 years of age or older in the USA, by age group, in 2007. Data are from the 2003 to 2006 National Health and Nutrition Examination Survey estimates of total prevalence (both diagnosed and undiagnosed), projected to year 2007.

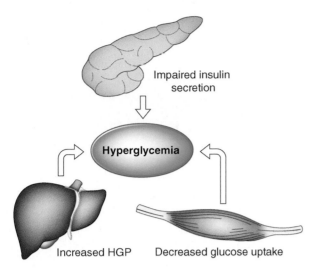

Figure 8-3. Mechanism of the pathogenesis of type 2 diabetes. Insulin resistance is manifested in the liver by increased HGP due to failure to suppress HGP and is manifested in muscle by decreased glucose uptake.

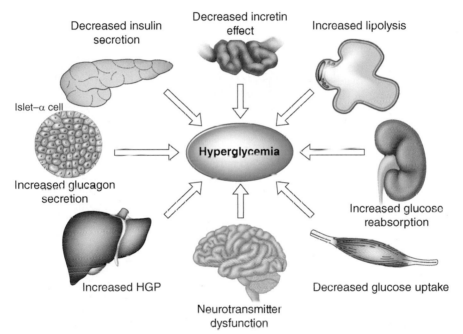

Figure 8-4. DeFronzo's "ominous octet," showing how many organs contribute to the metabolic defects in type 2 diabetes. In addition to the three defects noted in Fig. 8.3, also included is adipose tissue with increased lipolysis, the gut with diminished incretin secretion and consequent decreased incretin effect, the pancreatic α cell with increased glucagon secretion, the kidney with increased glucose reabsorption, and the brain with neurotransmitter dysfunction.

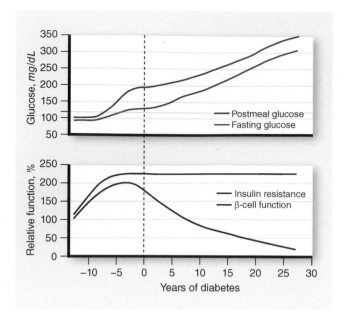

Figure 8-5. Natural history of type 2 diabetes. The dynamics between glucose levels, insulin resistance, and β-cell function that lead to the onset of type 2 diabetes is illustrated. Note also that the rise in postmeal glucose in this graph occurs before the rise in fasting glucose, a commonly seen occurrence in the prediabetic phase (adapted from International Diabetes Center, Minneapolis, MN).

Environmental factors, particularly abdominal obesity and a sedentary lifestyle, are important contributors to the development of type 2 diabetes, due at least in part to their effects on insulin sensitivity [1, 3, 4, 12–18]. Specific population subgroups have a higher prevalence of diabetes than the population as a whole (see Fig. 8.6) [19]. The greater the number of risk factors present in an individual, the greater the chance of that individual developing diabetes. The risk of developing diabetes increases with increasing age (≥45 years), obesity [body mass index (BMI) ≥25 kg/m²], and lack of physical activity. Diabetes is more common in individuals with a family history of the disease and in members of certain racial or ethnic groups (e.g., African Americans, Hispanic Americans, Native Americans, Asian Americans, and Pacific Islanders). Diabetes occurs frequently in women with a history of prior gestational diabetes or polycystic ovarian syndrome, and in individuals with hypertension, dyslipidemia [high-density lipoprotein (HDL) cholesterol ≤35 mg/dL or triglyceride level ≥250 mg/dL], vascular disease, impaired glucose tolerance (IGT), or impaired fasting glucose (IFG). Routine screening for diabetes is recommended for people 45 years of age or older. However, individuals who fall into any of these higher risk categories should be screened earlier [19].

Risk for Type 2 Diabetes
Age ≥ 45 y
Overweight or obesity (BMI ≥ 25 kg/m²)
Family history of type 2 diabetes
Habitual physical inactivity
Race/ethnicity
IGT or IFG
History of gestational diabetes or delivery of baby > 9 lb
Hypertension
HDL cholesterol ≤ 35 mg/dL or triglyceride level ≥ 250 mg/d
Polycystic ovarian syndrome
History of vascular disease

Figure 8-6. Populations at increased risk for type 2 diabetes are listed.

A recent International Expert Committee report has dramatically changed the recommended diagnostic criteria for diabetes [20]. The new recommendation is that diabetes should be diagnosed when A_{1C} is greater than or equal to 6.5%. This is a major change over previous criteria, which were based on plasma glucose (PG) measurements. The reason for the recommendation is because the A_{1C} assay is an accurate, precise measure of chronic glycemic levels and correlates with the risk of diabetes complications. The new recommendation suggests that the diagnosis should be confirmed with a repeat A_{1C} test, except in symptomatic subjects with PG levels greater than or equal to 200 mg/dL (11.1 mmol/L). This threshold for diabetes may not be appropriate for all racial and ethnic groups and leaves an "A_{1C} diagnostic hiatus" between the upper limit of normal A_{1C} and the new diagnostic threshold. Therefore, the Committee recommended that "those with A_{1C} levels below the threshold for diabetes but greater than or equal to 6.0% should receive demonstrably effective preventive interventions" and that "those with A_{1C} below this range may still be at risk and, depending on the presence of other diabetes risk factors, may also benefit from prevention efforts" [20, p. 1332]. Previously, the diagnostic criteria for diabetes was based on PG, with diabetes defined as a fasting PG (FPG) of 126 mg/dL or more, or either a postchallenge or casual PG of 200 mg/dL or more. In addition, two high-risk states of abnormal glucose metabolism, IFG and IGT, were defined (see Fig. 8.7) [7, 19]. It may be desirable to use a combination of A_{1C} and PG criteria to establish the diagnosis in any given individual.

Diagnostic Criteria for Diabetes		
Normal	Prediabetes IFG or IGT	Diabetes
FPG < 100	FPG ≥ 100–125 (IFG)	FPG ≥ 126
2-h PG < 140	2-h PG 140–199 (IGT)	2-h PG ≥ 200
A_{1C} < 5.7%	A_{1C} 5.7%–6.4%	A_{1C} ≥ 6.5%

A_{1C} ≥ 6.5% (test performed NGSP certified and standardized to DCCT)*

FPG ≥ 126 mg/dL (no caloric intake for at least 8 h)

2-h glucose ≥ 200 mg/dL during an OGTT (test performed as per WHO; 75-g glucose)

Classic symptoms of hyperglycemia equal random glucose ≥ 200 mg/dL

FIGURE 8-7. Diagnostic criteria for diabetes. It is possible to diagnose diabetes based on either A_{1C} criteria or PG criteria. The PG-based diagnostic criteria distinguish diabetes and abnormal states of glucose metabolism, i.e., IFG and IGT. In the absence of unequivocal hyperglycemia, the diagnosis of diabetes is confirmed on a subsequent day by measurement of FPG, or 2-h PG (2-h post 75-g glucose load). A casual PG greater than 200 mg/dL is diagnostic if symptoms are present.

Chronic poor glucose control is associated with the development of diabetic vascular complications, which include microvascular (retinopathy, neuropathy, and nephropathy) and macrovascular (premature cardiovascular disease [CVD]). CVD (coronary and cerebrovascular disease) accounts for 65–70% of deaths in patients with type 2 diabetes (see Fig. 8.8) [21, 22]. Epidemiologic studies have shown that the risk of a myocardial infarction (MI) or CVD death in a diabetic individual who has no prior history of CVD is similar to that of an individual who has had a previous CVD event (see Fig. 8.9) [23, 24].

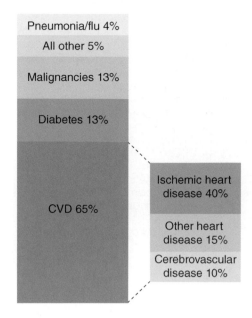

Pneumonia/flu 4%

All other 5%

Malignancies 13%

Diabetes 13%

CVD 65%

Ischemic heart disease 40%

Other heart disease 15%

Cerebrovascular disease 10%

Figure 8-8. Causes of death in diabetic individuals. CVDs (coronary and cerebrovascular) account for 65% of deaths in patients with diabetes (adapted from Geiss et al. [22]).

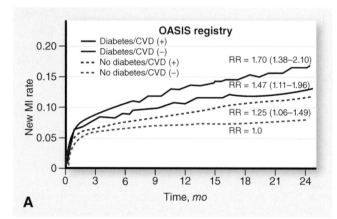

A

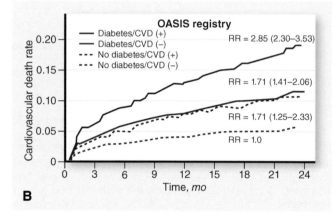

B

Figure 8-9. Organization to Assess Strategies for Ischemic Syndromes (OASIS) registry: rate of new MIs in patients with and without diabetes, and with and without CVD. The OASIS registry was a multicenter European registry of individuals with and without diabetes and risk for new coronary events. (**A**) The data demonstrated that, across this population, patients with diabetes and a history of previous CVD had the highest risk for a subsequent event over the follow-up period of 2 years. Those without diabetes or CVD had the lowest risk. Most significantly, the data demonstrated that the risk of a MI in a diabetic individual with no prior history of CVD was very similar to that of an individual who had already had a previous CVD event. (**B**) The OASIS study also demonstrated that the risk of cardiac death in a patient with diabetes with no prior history of CVD was exactly the same as that of an individual who had previous CVD (adapted from Malmberg et al. [23]).

In addition to hyperglycemia, individuals with type 2 diabetes often have a myriad of other metabolic abnormalities that increase their cardiovascular risk, including dyslipidemia, hypertension, and abnormalities of fibrinolysis and coagulation [25–30]. The Multiple Risk Factor Intervention Trial (MRFIT), which studied 347,978 men 35–57 years of age, demonstrated the absolute risk of CVD death to be approximately three times higher for men with diabetes than for those without diabetes, regardless of age, ethnic background, or risk factor level (see Fig. 8.10). With progressively less favorable baseline risk factor status, the CVD mortality rate rose much more steeply for men with diabetes than for their nondiabetic counterparts [31]. In the UK Prospective Diabetes Study (UKPDS), coronary heart disease (CHD) risk factors were evaluated by inclusion in a Cox proportional hazards model [32]. In order, and all statistically significant, the variables were low-density lipoprotein (LDL) cholesterol, high-density lipoprotein (HDL) cholesterol, A_{1c}, and systolic blood pressure (SBP) [10] (see Fig. 8.11).

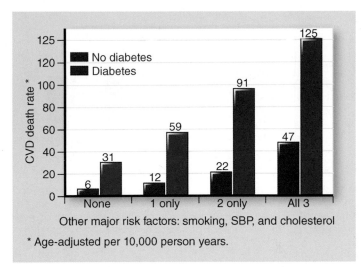

* Age-adjusted per 10,000 person years.

Figure 8-10. Interaction of diabetes with other risk factors in the risk of CVD death: the MRFIT. In the MRFIT, 347,978 men 35–57 years of age were followed up for 12 years and demonstrated that the absolute risk of CVD death was approximately three times higher for men with diabetes than for those without diabetes, regardless of their age, ethnic background, and risk factor level. The significant predictors in both groups of men were serum cholesterol level, SBP, and cigarette smoking. With progressively less favorable baseline risk factor status, the CVD mortality rate rose much more steeply for men with diabetes than for their nondiabetic counterparts. Therefore, the absolute excess risk of CVD death became progressively greater for diabetic than for nondiabetic men, and those men with diabetes and poorer baseline risk factors had a worse prognosis. This graph shows that the men with diabetes in this trial had a five-fold increased risk of CVD mortality during an average 12-year interval, even in the absence of the three other major CVD risk factors (cholesterol level >200 mg/dL, SBP >120 mmHg, and cigarette smoking). In addition, diabetes was associated with a much higher risk of CVD death in the presence of any one, two, or three of these other factors (with relative risks 4.82, 4.05, and 2.64, respectively) (adapted from Stamler et al. [31]).

Risk Factors in the UKPDS Evaluated by the Cox Proportional Hazards Model		
Position in model	**Variable**	**P value**
First	LDL cholesterol	< 0.0001
Second	HDL cholesterol	0.0001
Third	HbA$_{1C}$	0.0022
Fourth	SBP	0.0065
Fifth	Smoking	0.056

Coronary artery disease: n = 280. Adjusted for age and gender.

Figure 8-11. Stepwise selection of risk factors in 2,693 white patients with type 2 diabetes with a dependent variable as time to first event: UKPDS. In the UKPDS, CHD risk factors were evaluated by their inclusion in a Cox proportional hazards model. In order, the variables included in the model were LDL cholesterol, HDL cholesterol, hemoglobin A$_{1c}$ (HbA$_{1c}$), SBP, and smoking. While HbA$_{1c}$ was highly statistically significant, so were conventional cardiovascular risk factors, the most important of which seem to be LDL and HDL. Triglycerides did not enter the multivariate analysis and were not a powerful predictor even when HDL was not in the model (adapted from Turner et al. [32]).

A number of interventional trials, such as The Diabetes Control and Complications Trial (DCCT), the UKPDS, The Kumamoto Study, and the Stockholm Diabetes Intervention Study, demonstrated that microvascular complications can be delayed or prevented by maintaining excellent glycemic control [33–38]. Data from the UKPDS are shown in Fig. 8.12.

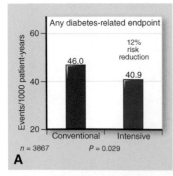
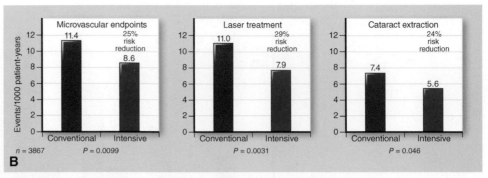

Figure 8-12. Impact of improved glycemic control. **(A)** The impact of improved glycemic control on "any diabetes related end point" in the UKPDS is illustrated, showing both absolute risk reduction and relative risk reduction [36]. **(B)** The impact of improved glycemic control on microvascular end points, laser photocoagulation for retinopathy, and cataract extraction in the UKPDS is illustrated, showing both absolute risk reduction and relative risk reduction [36].

In the intervention trial phase of the UKPDS, a 16% reduction in the risk of MI, including nonfatal and fatal MI and sudden death, was observed in the cohort of recently diagnosed type 2 diabetic individuals randomized to tight blood glucose control, just missing the level for statistical significance [36], although an epidemiologic analysis of UKPDS suggested a relationship between A_{1C} and MI (see Fig. 8.13) [39]. More importantly, longer term follow-up of the UKPDS cohort demonstrated a beneficial impact of earlier glycemic control; in the observational phase of the UKPDS, a glycemic difference between the two groups was lost in the first year, but a continued reduction in microvascular risk and risk reductions for MI and death from any cause were observed over the next 10 years (see Fig. 8.14) [40]. These findings are consistent with those of the Epidemiology of Diabetes Interventions and Complications (EDIC) study [41, 42], the follow-up study of the type 1 diabetes participants in the DCCT, which reported similar long-term benefits over several more years of follow-up from prior improved glycemic control. In both these trials, risk reductions were seen despite the loss of glycemic difference after the intervention phases. These studies support the hypothesis that glycemic control early in the course of disease management may impart CVD and microvascular benefit later on, the so-called "legacy" or "metabolic memory" effect.

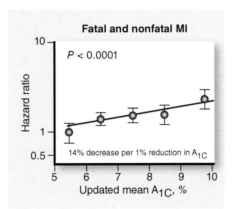

Figure 8-13. Glycemia-associated risk reduction for MI in the UKPDS. In the UKPDS, a 16% reduction ($P=0.052$) in the risk of MI, including nonfatal and fatal MI and sudden death, was observed in the cohort of type 2 diabetic patients randomized to tight blood glucose control, just missing the level for statistical significance. Yet, a secondary multivariate observational analysis of the UKPDS cohort was performed to evaluate the relationship between exposure to hyperglycemia over time (measured as the updated mean of annual measurements of A_{1C}) and the development of vascular complications. Shown are the hazard ratios for fatal and nonfatal MI as a log-linear plot of the estimated association with the updated mean A_{1C}. The reference category (hazard ratio = 1.0) was A_{1C} less than 6.0%. A reduction in the risk of fatal and nonfatal MI for each 1.0% reduction in updated A_{1C} was 14% (8–21%, $P<0.0001$) (adapted from Stratton et al. [39]).

UKPDS Legacy of Earlier Glucose Control, Median 8.5 Years Post-trial Followup				
Aggregate endpoint	RRR, *1997*	RRR, *2007*	P, *1997*	P, *2007*
Any diabetes-related endpoint	12%	9%	0.029	0.40
Microvascular disease	25%	24%	0.0099	0.001
MI	16%	15%	0.052	0.014
All-cause mortality	6%	13%	0.44	0.007

FIGURE 8-14. UKPDS legacy effect of earlier glucose control. At the end of the original UKPDS observation period (1997), there were significant reductions in "any diabetes related end point" and in microvascular disease, but not in MI or all-cause mortality [36]. With an additional decade of follow-up, despite similar glycemic control during that follow-up, the impact of previous glycemic control became evident for both MI and all-cause mortality and was sustained for any diabetes-related end point and microvascular disease. *P* log-rank; *RRR* relative risk reduction (adapted from Holman et al. [40]).

Direct evidence of the benefit of improved glycemic control on macrovascular complications is less clear. Three trials recently failed to show the benefit of intensive versus standard glycemic control. The Action in Diabetes and Vascular Disease: Preterax and Diamicron Modified Release Controlled Evaluation (ADVANCE) trial [43] followed 11,140 subjects with type 2 diabetes with a risk for, or a history of, vascular disease, who received either intensive or standard glucose control, with a difference in mean A_{1C} level of 0.8%. While a significant reduction in microvascular events was observed, there was no significant reduction in major macrovascular events after 5 years of follow-up. In the Action to Control Cardiovascular Risk in Diabetes (ACCORD) trial [44], 10,251 subjects with type 2 diabetes and either a history of CVD or increased risk for CVD were randomized to intensive versus standard glycemic control and were followed up for 3.5 years. At that point, the trial was stopped early due to an unexplained excess rate of death from any cause (22%; $P=0.04$) in the intensive group, whose mean A_{1C} was 6.4%, versus the mean in the standard group of 7.5%. The Veterans Affairs Diabetes Trial (VADT) [45] randomized 1,791 subjects with uncontrolled diabetes (mean A_{1C} at entry 9.4%) to either intensive glycemic control, with a goal A_{1C} of less than 6%, or to standard glycemic control, with a goal A_{1C} of 8% to 9%, and achieved a glycemic separation between the two groups of 1.6%. After a mean follow-up of 5.6 years, there were less overall CVD events, but more CVD deaths, in the intensive arm than the standard arm; however, the differences were not statistically significant. In all three of these trials, other CVD risk factors were treated moderately to highly aggressively and, probably due to this treatment, the three standard arms all had lower rates of CVD than were predicted. All trials were carried out in subjects with well-established diabetes and either known CVD or multiple risk factors for CVD, suggesting that macrovascular disease was likely present at the start of the trials and, thus, perhaps not reversible by glycemic improvement. A summary of the outcomes of these studies, as well as DCCT-EDIC and UKPDS, is shown in Fig. 8.15. Multiple meta-analyses have also been performed to evaluate the impact of glycemic control on both CVD events and death, and all have shown that there is likely a reduction in CVD events and no increase in mortality with improved glycemic control. One of these analyses was conducted by the combined authors of UKPDS, ADVANCE, ACCORD, and VADT [46]; Fig. 8.16 depicts the principal results from that meta-analysis.

Intensive Therapy in Diabetes: Summary of Results from Major Trials						
Study	Microvascular	Microvascular, *long term followup*	CVD	CVD, *long-term followup*	Mortality	Mortality, *long-term followup*
DCCT/EDIC	↓	↓	↔	↓	↔	↔
UKPDS	↓	↓	↔	↓	↔	↓
ACCORD	↓		↔		↑	
ADVANCE	↓		↔		↔	
VADT	↓		↔		↔	

FIGURE 8-15. Impact of intensive therapy in diabetes: summary of major clinical trials. All five of the trials listed here demonstrated a statistically significant reduction of microvascular disease, including a sustained "legacy" benefit in both DCCT-EDIC and UKPDS. Yet, during the initial phase of the studies, none demonstrated a change in macrovascular disease (CVD), while on longer follow-up a benefit was seen in both DCCT-EDIC and UKPDS. Mortality was increased only in ACCORD and there was a mortality benefit to long-term follow-up in UKPDS.

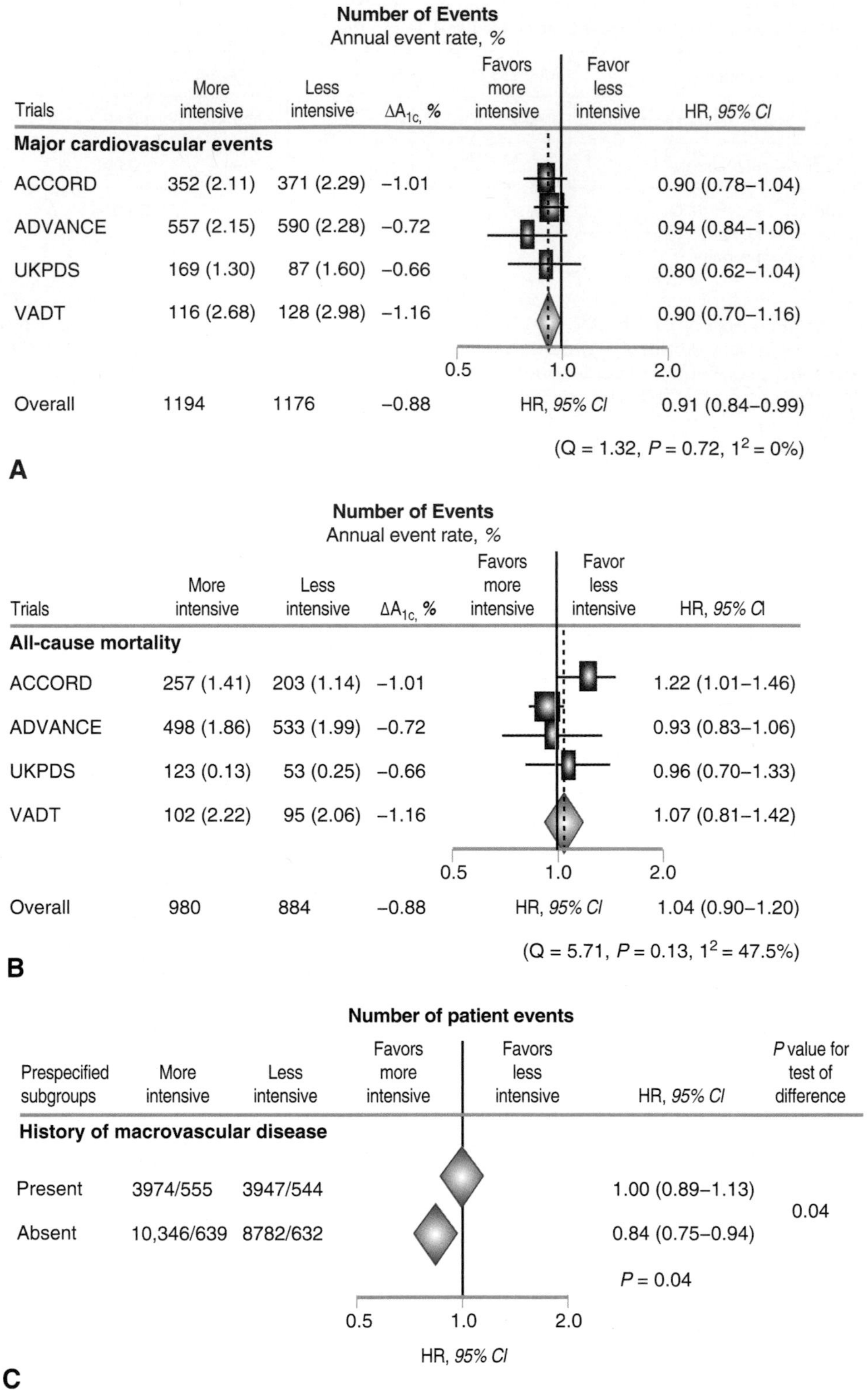

Number of Events
Annual event rate, %

Trials	More intensive	Less intensive	ΔA$_{1c,}$ %	Favors more intensive / Favor less intensive	HR, 95% CI
Major cardiovascular events					
ACCORD	352 (2.11)	371 (2.29)	−1.01		0.90 (0.78–1.04)
ADVANCE	557 (2.15)	590 (2.28)	−0.72		0.94 (0.84–1.06)
UKPDS	169 (1.30)	87 (1.60)	−0.66		0.80 (0.62–1.04)
VADT	116 (2.68)	128 (2.98)	−1.16		0.90 (0.70–1.16)
Overall	1194	1176	−0.88	HR, 95% CI	0.91 (0.84–0.99)

(Q = 1.32, P = 0.72, I^2 = 0%)

A

Number of Events
Annual event rate, %

Trials	More intensive	Less intensive	ΔA$_{1c,}$ %	Favors more intensive / Favor less intensive	HR, 95% CI
All-cause mortality					
ACCORD	257 (1.41)	203 (1.14)	−1.01		1.22 (1.01–1.46)
ADVANCE	498 (1.86)	533 (1.99)	−0.72		0.93 (0.83–1.06)
UKPDS	123 (0.13)	53 (0.25)	−0.66		0.96 (0.70–1.33)
VADT	102 (2.22)	95 (2.06)	−1.16		1.07 (0.81–1.42)
Overall	980	884	−0.88	HR, 95% CI	1.04 (0.90–1.20)

(Q = 5.71, P = 0.13, I^2 = 47.5%)

B

Number of patient events

Prespecified subgroups	More intensive	Less intensive	Favors more intensive / Favors less intensive	HR, 95% CI	P value for test of difference
History of macrovascular disease					
Present	3974/555	3947/544		1.00 (0.89–1.13)	0.04
Absent	10,346/639	8782/632		0.84 (0.75–0.94)	

P = 0.04

HR, 95% CI

C

FIGURE 8-16. Meta-analysis of CVD. (**A**) Results of a meta-analysis of major CVD events, conducted by the investigators from ACCORD, ADVANCE, UKPDS, and VADT, are shown. Overall, there is a hazard ratio of 0.91, indicating a 9% risk reduction of CVD, which is significant. (**B**) Results of a meta-analysis of mortality, conducted by the investigators from ACCORD, ADVANCE, UKPDS, and VADT, are shown. Overall, there is a hazard ratio of 1.04, which is not significant, imply-ing no increased mortality risk. (**C**) Results of subgroup analysis within a meta-analysis of major CVD events, conducted by the investigators from ACCORD, ADVANCE, UKPDS, and VADT, are shown. Overall, there is a reduction of risk for those subjects with no previous history of CVD (hazard ratio of 0.84 or 16% risk reduction) and no effect for those with a previous history of CVD (hazard ratio of 1.00) (adapted from Turnbull et al. [46]).

Based on the results of clinical trials such as those reviewed above, recommendations for targets of glycemic control have been put forth (see Fig. 8.17) [47, 48]. Other nonglycemic interventions have demonstrated effectiveness in reducing CVD in type 2 diabetes. The Microalbuminuria, Cardiovascular, and Renal Outcomes in the Heart Outcomes Prevention Evaluation (MICRO-HOPE) Study included 3,577 patients with types 1 and 2 diabetes, with and without hypertension, and compared the cardiovascular event rates with the angiotensin-converting enzyme (ACE) inhibitor, ramipril,

versus placebo [50]. The results demonstrated that treatment with ramipril lowered the risk of the combined primary outcome of combined MI, stroke, or CVD mortality by 25%, MI by 22%, stroke by 33%, and cardiovascular death by 37% (see Fig. 8.18). The Hypertension Optimum Treatment (HOT) study randomized subjects to diastolic blood pressure targets of 90, 85, or 80 mmHg [51]. Among people with diabetes, there was benefit in achieving a diastolic blood pressure of 80 mmHg both for CVD events and CVD mortality (see Fig. 8.19).

Recommended Glycemic Goals		
	ADA	AACE
HbA$_{1c}$	< 7%	< 6.5%
FPG, *mg/dL*	80–120	< 110
2-h BG, *mg/dL*	< 180	< 140
HS BG, *mg/dL*	100–140	100–140

Figure 8-17. Recommended glycemic goals. Glycemic goals (whole blood values) as recommended by the American Diabetes Association (ADA) and the American Association of Clinical Endocrinologists (AACE), are shown. *BG* blood glucose, *HS* hours of sleep (adapted from ADA [48] and AACE Diabetes Mellitus Clinical Practice Guidelines Task Force [49]).

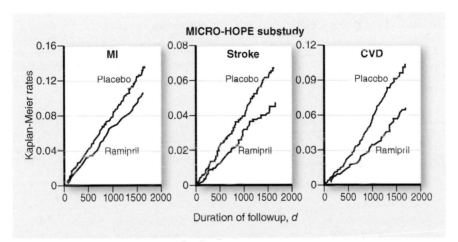

Figure 8-18. ACE inhibitor effects on CVD. The MICRO-HOPE Study included 9,297 high-risk patients, 3,577 with types 1 and 2 diabetes, with and without hypertension, and compared the cardiovascular event rates with the ACE inhibitor, ramipril, versus placebo. The primary end point was combined MI, stroke, or CVD mortality. The results demonstrated that treatment with ramipril lowered the risk of the combined primary outcome by 25% (95% CI 12–36, *P*=0.0004), MI by 22% (6–36), stroke by 33% (10–50), CVD by 37% (21–51), total mortality by 24% (8–37), revascularization by 17% (2–30), and overt nephropathy by 24% (3–40, *P*=0.027). After adjusting for the changes in systolic (2.4 mm Hg) and diastolic (1.0 mm Hg) blood pressures, ramipril still lowered the risk of the combined primary outcome by 25% (12–36, *P*=0.0004) (adapted from Heart Outcomes Prevention Evaluation Study Investigators [50]).

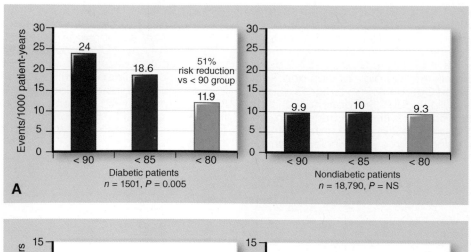

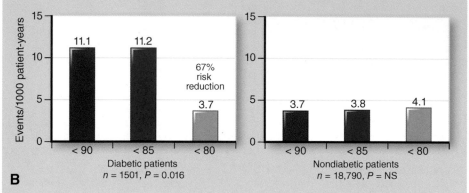

FIGURE 8-19. HOT Trial results. (**A**) In the HOT Trial, subjects with diabetes who were randomized to a diastolic blood pressure of less than 80 had a 51% reduction in major cardiovascular events at 4 years, whereas no difference was seen in those without diabetes. (**B**) Also in the HOT Trial, subjects with diabetes who were randomized to a diastolic blood pressure of less than 80 had a 67% reduction in cardiovascular mortality at 4 years, whereas no difference was seen in those without diabetes (adapted from Hansson et al. [51]).

Lowering serum cholesterol has been demonstrated in many studies to be effective at reducing CDV risks, both as primary and secondary prevention, in patients with diabetes (see Figs. 8.20 and 8.21) [52, 53]. Further studies, although not specifically in people with diabetes, have suggested that more aggressive LDL cholesterol-lowering in high-risk individuals should be the appropriate target of such treatment (see Fig. 8.22) [54].

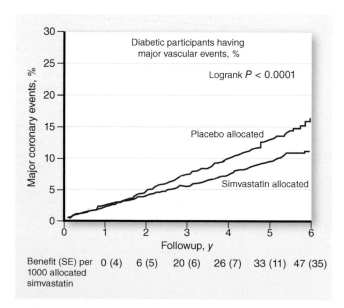

FIGURE 8-20. Heart protection study: effect of cholesterol lowering on vascular events in diabetic subjects. A total of 5,963 adults with diabetes and 14,573 patients with occlusive arterial disease, 40–80 years of age, were randomized to simvastatin 40 mg daily or placebo and were followed up for 5 years. The average difference in total cholesterol between the two groups was 39 mg/dL.

The results of the study for individuals with diabetes were as follows: lowering LDL cholesterol by 1 mmol/L (40 mg/dL) reduces the risk of major vascular events by about one-quarter during 5 years of treatment. Continued statin treatment prevents not only first but also subsequent major vascular events (adapted from Collins et al. [52])

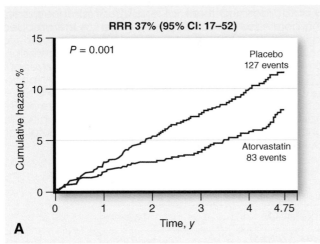

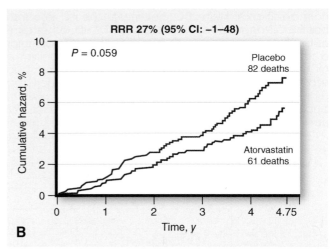

Figure 8-21. Collaborative Atorvastatin Diabetes Study (CARDS) results. (**A**) Over 4.75 years, there was a RRR for major cardio-vascular events of 37% in CARDS, a primary prevention study in 2,838 patients in type 2 diabetes, which used atorvastatin or placebo. (**B**) In CARDS, there also was a 27% reduction in all-cause mortality with atorvastatin versus placebo, as shown (adapted from Colhoun et al. [53]).

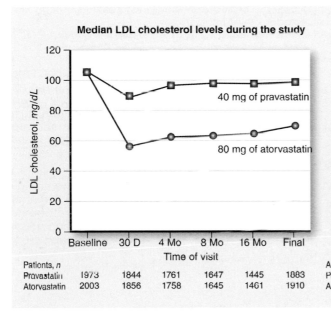

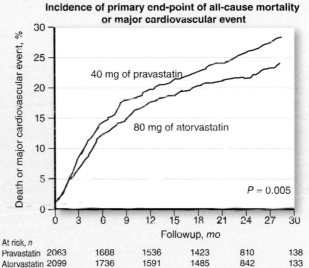

Figure 8-22. Pravastatin or Atorvastatin Evaluation and Infection Therapy–Thrombolysis in Myocardial Infarction 22 (PROVE IT–TIMI 22): effect of cholesterol lowering in patients with acute coronary events. A total of 4,162 patients who had been hospitalized for an acute coronary syndrome within the preceding 10 days, 40–80 years of age, were randomized to pravastatin 40 mg daily or atorvastatin 80 mg daily and were followed up for 18–36 months. Approximately 17.5% of each group had diabetes. The primary end point was a composite of death, MI, unstable angina, revascularization, or stroke. Median levels of LDL cholesterol in the two groups were 95 and 62 mg/dL, respectively.

Kaplan–Meier estimates of the rates of the primary end point at 2 years were 26.3% in the pravastatin group and 22.4% in the atorvastatin group, reflecting a 16% reduction in the hazard ratio in favor of the group with the lower LDL levels ($P=0.005$; 95% CI, 5%–26%) (adapted from Cannon et al. [54])

In addition to high LDL cholesterol, the risk determinants of CVD include the presence of CHD, other clinical forms of atherosclerotic disease, and several major non-LDL cholesterol risk factors such as cigarette smoking, hypertension, low HDL, family history of premature CHD, and age (men ≥ 45 years, women ≥ 55 years). Based on these other risk determinants, the Expert Panel on Detection, Evaluation, and Treatment of High Blood Cholesterol in Adults [Adult Treatment Panel III (ATP III)] identifies three categories of risk that modify the goals and modalities of LDL-lowering therapy (see Fig. 8.23) [55].

NCEP ATP III: LDL Goals and Therapy	
CHD or CHD equivalent (10-y risk > 20%)	Goal: < 100 mg/dL
LDL ≥ 100 mg/dL	Drug prescription ≥ 130 mg/dL
2 or more risk factors (10-y risk ≤ 20%)	Goal: < 130 mg/dL
LDL ≥ 130 mg/dL	Drug prescription at 10-y risk ≤ 20% 130–160 mg/dL
0–1 risk factors	Goal: < 160 mg/dL
LDL > 160 mg/dL	Drug prescription at > 190 mg/dL

Figure 8-23. National Cholesterol Education Program (NCEP) ATP III LDL goals and therapy according to risk category. Risk determinants in addition to LDL cholesterol include the presence or absence of CHD, other clinical forms of atherosclerotic disease, and the major risk factors other than LDL (i.e., cigarette smoking, hypertension, low HDL, family history of premature CHD, and age [men ≥ 45 years, women ≥ 55 years]). Based on these other risk determinants, ATP III identifies three categories of risk that modify the goals and modalities of LDL-lowering therapy (adapted from Expert Panel on Detection, Evaluation, and Treatment of High Blood Cholesterol in Adults [55]).

In the Steno-2 Study, an intensive, multifactor risk-reduction strategy targeting blood pressure, lipids, and smoking cessation was tested, and benefits were observed in patients with type 2 diabetes after 7.8 years of follow-up [56]. Further, in the observational Steno-2, postinterventional benefits were seen after a total follow-up period of 13.3 years, demonstrating that there may be a legacy effect for other, nonglycemic, metabolic interventions as well (see Fig. 8.24) [57]. The multifactor risk-reduction strategy emphasized in Steno-2 study has been adopted by the ADA [7]. The current ADA recommendations for diabetes treatment targets are summarized in Fig. 8.25. The components of therapy, inherent from these targets, are listed in Fig. 8.26.

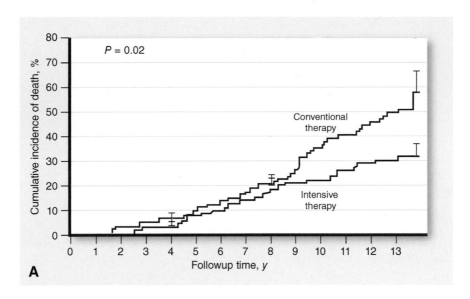

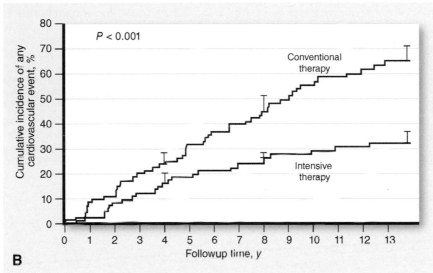

FIGURE 8-24. Steno-2 Study results. (**A**) The cumulative incidence of the risk of death from any cause (the study's primary end point) during the 13.3-year study period is shown. (**B**) The cumulative incidence of a secondary composite end point of cardiovascular events are shown, including death from cardiovascular causes, nonfatal stroke, nonfatal MI, coronary-artery bypass grafting (CABG), percutaneous coronary intervention (PCI), revascularization for peripheral atherosclerotic artery disease, and amputation (adapted from Gaede et al. [57]).

ADA Treatment Goals in Diabetes	
A_{1c}	< 7%
Blood pressure	< 130/80 mm Hg
LDL cholesterol	< 100 mg/dL (2.6 mmol/L) or < 70 mg/dL (1.8 mmol/L) or ~30–40% reduction from baseline
Serum triglycerides	< 150 mg/dL (1.7 mmol/L)
HDL cholesterol	Men: > 40 mg/dL (1.04 mmol/L) Women: > 50 mg/dL (1.3 mmol/L)
Smoking cessation	Yes
Aspirin therapy	If history (or increased risk) of CVD

FIGURE 8-25. ADA treatment goals. The ADA treatment goals for patients with diabetes are listed, emphasizing a multifactor risk approach (adapted from ADA Position Statement [7]).

Diabetes Treatment Components
Aspirin/anti-platelet therapy
Blood pressure control
Cholesterol control/statin therapy
Diet
Exercise
Fat (decrease body weight)
Glucose control

FIGURE 8-26. Diabetes treatment components. The components of diabetes treatment are listed following an ABC approach.

The management of glycemia in type 2 diabetes involves both lifestyle and medications. Lifestyle is a fundamental component of treatment and should entail attention to both medical nutrition therapy ("diet") and physical activity ("exercise"). In addition, education about all of the elements of diabetes management is essential to treatment success. Optimally, this involves a diabetes team that includes, as a minimum, a physician, a nurse educator, and a dietitian.

There are many classes of medications to control glycemia in type 2 diabetes available today. Of course, insulin treatment can be given, but there are a number of noninsulin antidiabetic agents available. There currently are a variety of insulin preparations and insulin analogs available (see Fig. 8.27), which serve to increase circulating insulin levels. In type 2 diabetes, it is common to commence insulin therapy with a basal insulin preparation to control basal (fasting) hyperglycemia (see Fig. 8.28), with the addition of prandial insulin as necessary to control incremental hyperglycemia after meals. An example of the effectiveness of basal insulin therapy, from the Treating to Target in Type 2 (4-T) study, is shown in Fig. 8.29 [59]. A recent study, the 4-T study, compared insulin initiation with basal insulin alone, versus prandial insulin alone, versus premixed insulin [60, 61]. Ultimately, it was found that the majority of patients required both basal and prandial insulin (see Fig. 8.30).

Diabetes Treatment Components
Aspirin/anti-platelet therapy
Blood pressure control
Cholesterol control/statin therapy
Diet
Exercise
Fat (decrease body weight)
Glucose control

FIGURE 8-27. Comparison of human insulins and analogs. Human insulins [regular and neutral protamine Hagedorn (NPH)] are made by recombinant DNA technology. Regular insulin is similar to that produced in the human pancreas, but NPH insulin has been modified to slow subcutaneous absorption. Genetically engineered insulin preparations have been modified either to show a rapid onset of action (insulin lispro, insulin aspart, and insulin glulisine) or to have prolonged action and a relatively flat action profile (insulin glargine and insulin detemir).

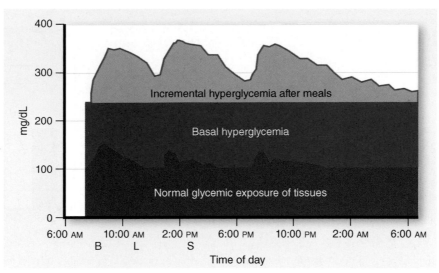

FIGURE 8-28. Basal versus mealtime hyperglycemia in type 2 diabetes mellitus. This schematic distinguishes basal (fasting) hypergly-cemia and prandial (incremental) meal-related hyperglycemia.

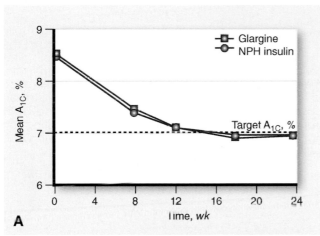

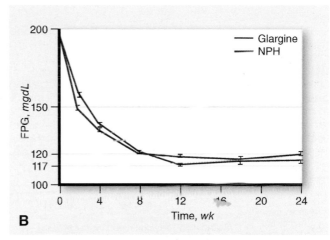

FIGURE 8-29. Treat to Target Study results: mean A_{1C} levels. (**A**) Mean A_{1C} levels during the Treat to Target are shown. The forced-titra-tion schedule of insulin glargine and NPH insulin also produced a decline in mean A_{1C} levels. The mean A_{1C} value of 8.6% was decreased to 6.94% in both insulin glargine and NPH insulin groups. The A_{1C} target of less than or equal to 7% was achieved by 58% of patients receiving insulin glargine and 57% of patients receiving NPH insulin. The average amount of insulin at the study's end was approximately 44 units or 0.46 μm/kg/day. (**B**) Mean fasting glucose levels in the Treat to Target Study are shown (adapted from Riddle et al. [58]).

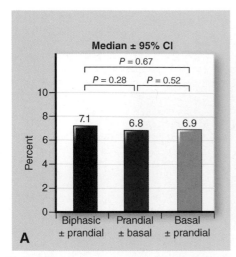
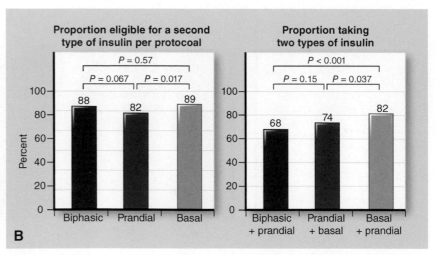

Figure 8-30. 4-T Study results: primary outcomes. (**A**) Primary outcome: HbA$_{1c}$ at 3 years. In the 4-T Study, insulin initiation with basal insulin alone was compared with prandial insulin alone and with premixed (biphasic) insulin. If there was inadequate control, prandial insulin was added to basal and biphasic insulin, and basal insulin was added to prandial insulin. In the end, excellent glycemic control was achieved in all three groups, as noted above. (**B**) In the 4-T Study, although insulin was initiated with a single insulin, most subjects required an additional type of insulin to attain the target glycemic control (adapted from Holman [59]).

The many available types of noninsulin antidiabetic agents target different mechanisms of the underlying pathogenesis of the disease (see Fig. 8.31). Figure 8.32 lists current glucose-lowering agents. The use of agents with complementary mechanisms of action greatly enhances the ability to optimally manage hyperglycemia. Sulfonylureas and the glinides (i.e., repaglinide, nateglinide) are two classes of insulin secretagogues that work by stimulating the release of insulin from the pancreas. Metformin, a biguanide, improves insulin sensitivity primarily by reducing insulin resistance in the liver, thereby decreasing HGP. The thiazolidinediones (TZDs, i.e., rosiglitazone, pioglitazone) improve insulin sensitivity primarily in the muscle, thereby increasing peripheral uptake and utilization of glucose. The α-glucosidase inhibitors (i.e., acarbose, miglitol, voglibose) prevent the breakdown of carbohydrates to glucose in the gut by inhibiting the enzymes that catalyze this process, thus delaying carbohydrate absorption.

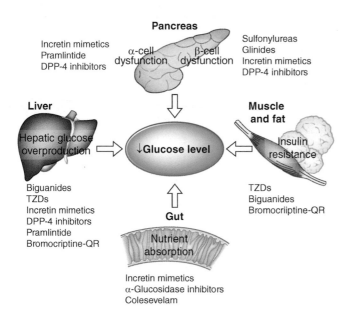

Figure 8-31. Major targeted sites of various drug classes to control hyperglycemia in type 2 diabetes. Different drug classes with different but complementary mechanisms may be suitable for combination therapy to address multiple pathophysiologic defects and improve A$_{1c}$ control.

Sulfonylureas act in the pancreas, stimulating insulin release by binding to the sulfonylurea receptor of β-cell membranes. Glinides (i.e., repaglinide and nateglinide), another class of short-acting insulin secretagogues, also act in the pancreas, stimulating insulin release by binding to several sites on the β-cells. The glinides are used to control postprandial hyperglycemia. TZDs are selective peroxisome proliferator-activated receptor γ (PPAR-γ) agonists and act primarily in the muscle, and also exert effects in the liver and adipose tissue. These agents reduce insulin resistance and decrease hepatic glucose output. The α-glucosidase inhibitors lower postprandial blood glucose concentrations by inhibiting disaccharidase enzymes in the gut, thereby delaying carbohydrate absorption. This action retards glucose entry into the systemic circulation.

Biguanides (metformin) act primarily in the liver by decreasing hepatic glucose output through a mechanism that has not been fully elucidated; metformin also enhances insulin sensitivity in muscle and decreases intestinal absorption of glucose. The incretin mimetics (GLP-1 receptor agonists) and incretin enhancers [dipeptidyl peptidase-4 (DPP-4) inhibitors] have multiple actions, including glucose-dependent secretion, inhibition of glucagon secretion, and slowing of glucose absorption from the gut. Colesevelam is a bile acid sequestrant, administered orally, that binds bile acids in the intestine and causes more of the bile acids to be excreted in the stool; it is unclear how this lowers blood glucose. Pramlintide is a synthetic analog of the hormone amylin, which is secreted together with insulin from the β-cell; it inhibits glucagon secretion, slows glucose absorption from the gut, and works in the brain to stimulate satiety and decrease appetite. Bromocriptine quick release (QR) is a formulation of bromocriptine that works in the brain to impact body rhythms and has consequent effects on decreasing insulin resistance.

Over the last few years, a number of new classes of therapeutic agents have been introduced. A newer class of oral agents is the DPP-IV inhibitors (i.e., sitagliptin, vildagliptin, saxagliptin) [61–65]. The DPP-IV inhibitors work via enhancement of the activity of the glucoregulatory incretin hormone GLP-1 by inhibiting its rapid degradation by the enzyme DPP-IV. Thus, these drugs have also been called "incretin enhancers." The net results are an improvement in insulin secretion and a suppression of glucagon secretion, both in a glucose-dependent manner.

There are two other oral drugs whose mechanisms of glucose-lowering action are not completely understood: colesevelam and bromocriptine. As a bile acid sequestrant, colesevelam lowers cholesterol but has also been found to lower glucose as well, perhaps by a similar mechanism [66]. Bromocriptine is a dopamine receptor agonist used primarily to treat hyperprolactinemia, a QR version of which appears to reset rhythms in the hypothalamus and, consequently, reduce insulin resistance [67]. Intriguingly, in a safety study, bromocriptine-QR was associated with reduced cardiovascular risk [68].

Two new injectable classes are on the market: GLP-1 receptor agonists, also known as "incretin mimetics" [61, 63–65], and the amylin mimetic pramlintide [69, 70]. The first GLP-1 receptor agonist is exenatide, a synthetic version of the peptide exendin-4 that is formed in the salivary gland of the Gila monster. By virtue of its amino acid sequence, it escapes degradation by DPP-IV. It comes in two versions, an unmodified form requiring injection at least twice daily and a newer once-weekly preparation. Liraglutide is another GLP-1 receptor agonist, which is administered once daily independent of meals. Other GLP-1 receptor agonists are in development. Their antiglycemic effects are via enhancement of glucose-dependent insulin secretion, suppression of glucagon secretion, and delay of gastric emptying [61, 63–65]. Pramlintide is an analog of the human hormone amylin, which is normally cosecreted with insulin and becomes deficient as insulin levels decline. It is injected two or three times a day before meals. Its antiglycemic effects are via suppression of glucagon secretion, delay of gastric emptying, and increased satiety.

The newer antidiabetic drugs are discussed in more detail in Chap. 18. The oral agents and the GLP-1 receptor agonists are generally utilized in, and effective in, patients with some preserved β-cell secretory capacity or in combination with exogenous insulin. Since type 2 diabetes is a progressive disease, driven by diminishing endogenous insulin secretion, most patients will reach a point in their disease at which time they will require insulin replacement. The sequence of use of agents, and their combinations, has attracted much attention in the literature. The ADA and the European Association for the Study of Diabetes (EASD) have published a consensus algorithm suggesting a strategy for the approach to the initiation and intensification of management of type 2 diabetes (see Fig. 8.32) [71]. Likewise, the American Association of Clinical Endocrinologists (AACE) and the American College of Endocrinology (ACE) also have published a somewhat different consensus algorithm (see Fig. 8.33) [72]. Another algorithm has been developed by the International Diabetes Federation (IDF) (see Fig. 8.34) [73]. Also, DeFronzo, in his Banting Lecture to the ADA, championed yet another algorithm, claiming it to be based more on the pathophysiology of the type 2 diabetes (see Fig. 8.35) [8].

Insulins and Insulin Analogs		Biguanides
Rapid-acting preparations		Metformin: Glucophage, now generic
Insulin lispro: Humalog		Phenformin: DBI, removed from the market in the United States
Insulin aspart: Novolog		Buformin: never available in the United States
Insulin glulisine: Apidra		PPAR-γ activators (glitazones)
Short-acting preparations		Rosiglitazone: Avandia, withdrawn from European market; restricted use in the United States
Regular human insulin: Humulin-R and Novolin-R		Pioglitazone: Actos
Intermediate-acting preparations		Troglitazone: Rezulin, withdrawn from the market
NPH, isophane: Humulin-N and Novolin-N		**Incretin Mimetics and Enhancers**
Lente (insulin zinc suspension): no longer available in the United States		Incretin Mimetics (GLP-1 receptor agonists)
Long-acting preparations		Exenatide: Byetta
Protamine zinc insulin: no longer available in the United States		Liraglutide: Victoza
Ultralente insulin: no longer available in the United States		Exenatide-QW: pending approval
Insulin glargine: Lantus		Taspoglutide: withdrawn from development
Insulin detemir: Levemir		Albiglutide: Syncria, in development
Premixed preparations		Incretin enhancers (DPP-4 inhibitors)
70% NPH/30% regular: Humulin 70/30 and Novolin 70/30		Sitagliptin: Januvia
50% NPH/50% regular: Humulin 50/50		Saxagliptin: Onglyza
75% Intermediate/25% lispro: Humalog Mix 75/25		Vildagliptin: Galvus, not available in the United States
50% Intermediate/50% lispro: Humalog Mix 50/50		Alogliptin: in development
70% Intermediate/30% aspart: Novolog Mix 70/30		Linagliptin: in development
30% Intermediate/70% aspart: in development		**Other Classes**
High-concentration preparations		α-Glucosidase inhibitors
U500 Regular		Acarbose: Precose
Inhaled preparations		Miglitol: Glyset
Inhaled insulin powder: Exubera, withdrawn from the market		Voglibose: not available in the United States
Technosphere insulin: Afrezza, pending approval		Amylin analogues
Insulin Secretagogues		Pramlintide: Symlin
Sulfonylureas		Bile acid sequestrants
Tolbutamide: Orinase, now generic		Colesevelam: Welchol
Chlorpropamide: Diabinese, now generic		Dopamine agonists
Tolazamide: Tolinase, now generic		Bromocriptine-QR: Cycloset
Acetohexamide: Dymelor, now generic		SGLT-2 inhibitors
Glipizide: Glucotrol, now generic		Dapagliflozin: in development
Glipizide-GITS: Glucotrol-XL, now generic		Remogliflozin: in development
Glyburide: Diabeta and Micronase, now generic		Canagliflozin: in development
Glyburide (micronized): Glynase, now generic		**Combination Products**
Glimepiride: Amaryl, now generic		Glyburide-metformin: Glucovance
Gliclazide: Diamicron, now generic (not available in the United States)		Glipizide-metformin: Metaglip
Glinides		Rosiglitazone-metformin: Avandamet, withdrawn from the European market; restricted use in the United States
Repaglinide: Prandin		Rosiglitazone-glimepiride: Avandaryl, withdrawn from the European market; restricted use in the United States
Nateglinide: Starlix		Pioglitazone-metformin: ActoPlus Met
Insulin Sensitizers		Pioglitazone-glimepiride: Duetact
		Sitagliptin-metformin: Janumet

FIGURE 8-32. Glucose-lowering agents.

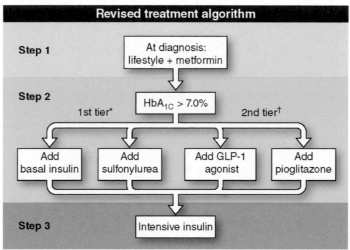

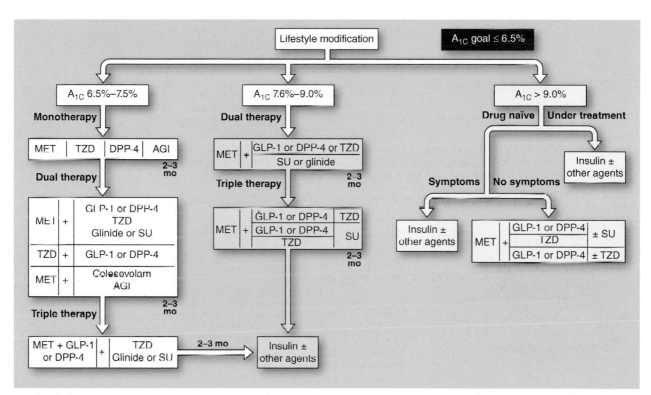

FIGURE 8-33. 2009 ADA/EASD consensus algorithm. The ADA/ EASD 2009 consensus algorithm commences with lifestyle together with metformin and adds additional drugs when a target of A$_{1C}$ of 7% is not reached. It breaks the additions at Step 2 into two tiers: those with a larger body of evidence and those with less well-established evidence, although that distinction may be blurring (adapted from Nathan et al. [71]).

FIGURE 8-34. 2009 AACE/ACE treatment guidelines. The AACE/ ACE 2009 treatment guidelines use a target of A$_{1C}$ of 6.5%, commences with lifestyle alone, and adds different drugs and combinations in different groups contingent on prevailing A$_{1C}$ (adapted from Rodbard et al. [72]).

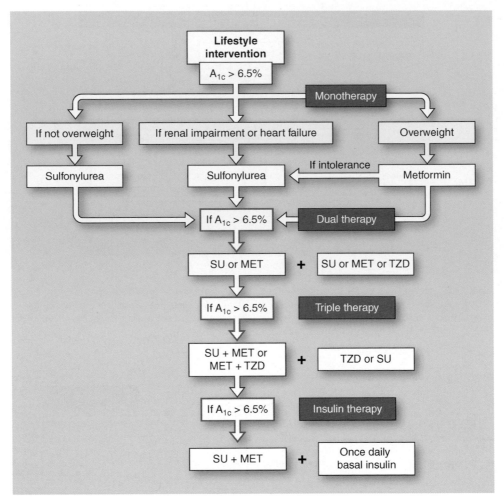

FIGURE 8-35. IDF type 2 diabetes mellitus treatment algorithm. The IDF treatment algorithm starts out with a target of A_{1c} of 6.5%, but raises the target later on as therapy becomes more complex. It commences with lifestyle alone and adds different drugs and combinations in different groups of patients (adapted from IDF [73]).

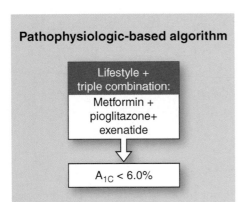

FIGURE 8-36. Pathophysiologic-based algorithm. DeFronzo's so-called "pathophysiologic-based algorithm" uses lifestyle plus triple combination therapy from the outset, the notion being that all three drugs used (metformin, pioglitazone, and exenatide) work on different components of the pathways leading to type 2 diabetes, and that the early introduction of such a combination is best able to correct the fundamental defects (adapted from DeFronzo [8]).

References

1. Cowie CC, Rust KF, Ford ES, *et al.*: Full accounting of diabetes and pre-diabetes in the U.S. population in 1988–1994 and 2005–2006. *Diabetes Care* 2009, 32:287–294.

2. Ong KL, Cheung BMY, Wong LYF, *et al.*: Prevalence, treatment, and control of diagnosed diabetes in the U.S National Health and Nutrition Examination Survey 1999–2004. *Ann Epidemiol* 2008, 18:222–229.

3. Gregg EW, Cadwell BL, Cheng YJ, *et al.*: Trends in the prevalence and ratio of diagnosed to undiagnosed diabetes according to obesity levels in the U.S. *Diabetes Care* 2004, 27:2806–2812.

4. Wee CC, Hamel MB, Huang A, *et al.*: Obesity and undiagnosed diabetes in the U.S. *Diabetes Care* 2008, 31:1813–1815.

5. Selvin E, Coresh J, Brancati FL: The burden and treatment of diabetes in elderly individuals in the U.S. *Diabetes Care* 2006, 29:2415–2419.

6. Centers for Disease Control and Prevention: National Diabetes Fact Sheet 2007. Available at: http://www.cdc.gov/diabetes/pubs/estimates07.htm#1. Accessed March 5, 2010.

7. American Diabetes Association Position Statement: Diagnosis and classification of diabetes mellitus. *Diabetes Care* 2010, 33(Suppl 1):S62–S67.

8. DeFronzo RA: Banting lecture 2009. From the triumvirate to the ominous octet: a new paradigm for the treatment of type 2 diabetes. *Diabetes* 2009, 58:773–795.

9. Boden G, Chen X: Effects of fat on glucose uptake and utilization in patients with non-insulin-dependent diabetes. *J Clin Invest* 1995, 96:1261–1268.

10. Groop LC, Bonadonna RC, DelPrato, S *et al.*: Glucose and free fatty acid metabolism in non-insulin-dependent diabetes mellitus. Evidence for multiple sites of insulin resistance. *J Clin Invest* 1989, 84:205–213.

11. Lewis GF, Carpentier A, Vranic M, Giacca A: Resistance to insulin's acute direct hepatic effect in suppressing steady-state glucose production in individuals with type 2 diabetes. *Diabetes* 1999, 48:570–576.

12. Shepard PR, Kahn BB: Mechanisms of disease: glucose transporters and insulin action—implications for insulin resistance and diabetes mellitus. *N Engl J Med* 1999, 341:248–257.

13. Weyer C, Tataranni PA, Bogardus C, *et al.*: Insulin resistance and insulin secretory dysfunction are independent predictors of worsening of glucose tolerance during each stage of type 2 diabetes development. *Diabetes Care* 2000, 24:89–94.

14. Kahn S: The importance of β-cell failure in the development and progression of type 2 diabetes. *J Clin Endocrinol Metab* 2001, 86:4047–4058.

15. Weyer C, Bogardus C, Mott D, *et al.*: The natural history of insulin secretory dysfunction and insulin resistance in the pathogenesis of type 2 diabetes mellitus. *J Clin Invest* 1999, 104:787–794.

16. Nguyen NT, Magno CP, Lane KT, *et al.*: Association of hypertension, diabetes, dyslipidemia, and metabolic syndrome with obesity: findings from the National Health and Nutrition Examination Survey, 1999 to 2004. *J Am Coll Surg* 2008, 207:928–934.

17. Hu F, Manson J, Stamfer M, *et al.*: Diet, lifestyle, and the risk of type 2 diabetes in women. *N Engl J Med* 2001, 345:790–797.

18. Wei M, Schweitner H, Blair S: The association between physical activity, physical fitness, and type 2 diabetes mellitus. *Compr Ther* 2000, 26:176–182.

19. American Diabetes Association: Position statement. Screening for type 2 diabetes. *Diabetes Care* 2004, 27(Suppl 1):S11–S14.

20. International Expert Committee Report on the Role of the A1C Assay in the Diagnosis of Diabetes. *Diabetes Care* 2009, 32:1327–1334.

21. National Diabetes Statistics, 2007. NIH Publication No. 08–3892. June 2008. Available at: http://diabetes.niddk.nih.gov/dm/pubs/statistics/.

22. Geiss LS, Herman WH, Smith PJ: Mortality in non-insulin dependent diabetes. In *Diabetes in America*, edn 2. National Diabetes Data Group, Bethesda, MD: National Institute of Health; NIH pub no. 95–1468, 1995, 233–257.

23. Malmberg K, Yusuf S, Gerstein HC, *et al.*: Impact of diabetes on long-term prognosis in patients with unstable angina and non-Q-wave myocardial infarction: results of the OASIS (Organization to Assess Strategies for Ischemic Syndromes) Registry. *Circulation* 2000, 102:1014–1019.

24. Haffner SM, Lehto S, Rönnemaa T, *et al.*: Mortality from coronary heart disease in subjects with type 2 diabetes and in non-diabetic subjects with and without prior myocardial infarction. *N Engl J Med* 1998, 339:229–234.

25. Ginsberg HN: Insulin resistance and cardiovascular disease. *J Clin Invest* 2000, 106:453–458.

26. Hsueh WA, Law RE: Cardiovascular risk continuum: implications of insulin resistance and diabetes. *Am J Med* 1998, 105:4S–14S.

27. Adler AI, Stratton IM, Neil HA, *et al.*: Association of systolic blood pressure with macrovascular complications of type 2 diabetes (UKPDS: 36) *BMJ* 2000, 321:412–419.

28. Meigs JB, Mittleman MSA, Nathan DM, *et al.*: Hyperinsulinemia, hyperglycemia and impaired homeostasis. The Framingham Offspring Study. *JAMA* 2000, 283:221–228.

29. Cooper ME, Bonnet F, Oldfield M, Jandeleit-Dahm K: Mechanisms of diabetic vasculopathy: an overview. *Am J Hypertens* 2001, 14:475–486.

30. Brownlee M: Biochemistry and molecular cell biology of diabetic complications. *Nature* 2001, 414:813–820.

31. Stamler J, Vaccaro O, Neaton JD, Wentworth D: Diabetes, other risk factors, and 12-yr cardiovascular mortality for men screened in the Multiple Risk Factor Intervention Trial. *Diabetes Care* 1993, 16:434–444.

32. Turner RC, Millns H, Neil HA, *et al.*: Risk factors for coronary artery disease in non-insulin dependent diabetes mellitus: United Kingdom Prospective Diabetes Study (UKPDS: 23). *BMJ* 1998, 316:823–828.

33. The Diabetes Control and Complications Trial Research Group: The effect of intensive treatment of diabetes on the development and progression of long-term complications in insulin-dependent diabetes mellitus. *N Engl J Med* 1993, 329:977–986.

34. The Diabetes Complications and Control/Epidemiology of Diabetes Interventions and Complications Research Group: Retinopathy and nephropathy in patients with type 1 diabetes four years after a trial of intensive therapy. *N Engl J Med* 2000, 342:381–389.

35. The Diabetes Control and Complications (DCCT) Research Group: Effect of intensive therapy on the development and progression of diabetic nephropathy in the Diabetes Control and Complications Trial. *Kidney Int* 1995, 47:1703–1720.

36. United Kingdom Prospective Diabetes Study Group: Effect of intensive blood glucose control with sulfonylurea or insulin compared with conventional treatment and risk of complications in patients with type 2 diabetes. *Lancet* 1998, 352:837–853.

37. Ohkubo Y, Kishikawa H, Araki E, *et al.*: Intensive insulin therapy prevents the progression of diabetic microvascular complications in Japanese patients with non-insulin-dependent diabetes mellitus: a randomized prospective 6-year study. *Diabetes Res Clin Pract* 1995, 28:103–117.

38. Reichard P, Pihl M, Rosenqvist U, Sule J: Complications in IDDM are caused by elevated blood glucose level: the Stockholm Diabetes Intervention Study (SDIS) at 10-year follow up. *Diabetologia* 1996, 39:1483–1488.

39. Stratton IM, Adler AI, Neil HAW, *et al.* for the UK Prospective Diabetes Study Group: Association of glycemia with macrovascular and microvascular complications of type 2 diabetes (UKPDS 35): prospective observational study. *BMJ* 2000, 321:405–412.

40. Holman RR, Paul SK, Bethel MA, *et al.*: 10-year follow-up of intensive glucose control in type 2 diabetes. *N Engl J Med* 2008, 359:1577–1589.

41. Lachin JM, Genuth S, Nathan DM, *et al.*: DCCT/EDIC Research Group. Effect of glycemic exposure on the risk of microvascular complications in the diabetes control and complications trial-revisited. *Diabetes* 2008, 57:995–1001.

42. Nathan DM, Cleary PA, Backlund JY, *et al.*: The Diabetes Control and Complications Trial/Epidemiology of Diabetes Interventions and Complications (DCCT/EDIC) Study Research Group. Intensive Diabetes treatment and cardiovascular disease in patients with type 1 diabetes. *N Engl J Med* 2005, 22:2643–2653.

43. The ADVANCE Collaborative Group: Intensive blood glucose control and vascular outcomes in patients with Type 2 diabetes. *N Engl J Med* 2008, 358:2560–2572.

44. The Action to Control Cardiovascular Risk in Diabetes (ACCORD) Study Group: Effects of intensive glucose lowering in type 2 diabetes. *N Engl J Med* 2008, 358:2545–2559.

45. Duckworth W, Abraira C, Moritz T, *et al.* for the VADT Investigators: Glucose control and vascular complications in veterans with type 2 diabetes. *N Eng J Med* 2009, 360:129–139.

46. Turnbull FM, Abraira C, Anderson RJ, *et al.*: Intensive glucose control and macrovascular outcomes in type 2 diabetes. *Diabetologia* 2009, 52:2288–2298.

47. Skyler JS, Bergenstal R, Bonow RO, *et al.*: Intensive glycemic control and the prevention of cardiovascular events: implications of the ACCORD, ADVANCE, and VADT diabetes trials. A position statement of the American Diabetes Association and a scientific statement of the American College of Cardiology Foundation and the American Heart Association. *Diabetes Care* 2009, 32:187–192, *Circulation* 2009, 119:351–357, and *J Am Coll Cardiol* 2009, 53:298–304.

48. American Diabetes Association: Standards of medical care in diabetes—2010. *Diabetes Care* 2010, 33:S11–S61.

49. AACE Diabetes Mellitus Clinical Practice Guidelines Task Force: American Association of Clinical Endocrinologists medical guidelines for clinical practice for the management of diabetes mellitus. *Endocr Pract* 2007,13(Suppl 1):1–68.

50. Heart Outcomes Prevention Evaluation Study Investigators: Effects of ramipril on cardiovascular and microvascular outcomes in people with diabetes mellitus: results of the HOPE study and MICRO-HOPE substudy. *Lancet* 2000, 355:253–259.

51. Hansson L, Zanchetti A, Carruthers SG, *et al.*: Effects of intensive blood-pressure lowering and low-dose aspirin in patients with hypertension: principal results of the Hypertension Optimal Treatment (HOT) randomised trial. HOT Study Group. *Lancet* 1998, 351:1755–1762.

52. Collins R, Armitage J, Parish S, *et al.*, Heart Protection Study Collaborative Group: MRC/BHF Heart Protection Study of cholesterol-lowering with simvastatin in 5963 people with diabetes: a randomised placebo-controlled trial. *Lancet* 2003, 361:2005–2016.

53. Colhoun HM, Betteridge DJ, Durrington PN, *et al.*, CARDS investigators: Primary prevention of cardiovascular disease with atorvastatin in type 2 diabetes in the Collaborative Atorvastatin Diabetes Study (CARDS): multicentre randomised placebo-controlled trial. *Lancet* 2004, 364:685–696.

54. Cannon CP, Braunwald E, McCabe CH, *et al.*: Intensive versus moderate lipid lowering with statins after acute coronary syndromes. *N Engl J Med* 2004, 350:1495–1504.

55. Expert Panel on Detection, Evaluation, and Treatment of High Blood Cholesterol in Adults (Adult Treatment Panel III): Executive summary of the third report of the National Cholesterol Education Program Expert Panel on detection, evaluation, and treatment of high blood cholesterol in adults. *JAMA* 2001, 285:2486–2497.

56. Gaede P, Vedel P, Larsen N, *et al.*: Multifactorial intervention and cardiovascular disease in patients with type 2 diabetes. *N Engl J Med* 2003, 348:383–393.

57. Gaede P, Lund-Andersen H, Parving HH, *et al.*: Effect of a multifactorial intervention on mortality in type 2 diabetes. *N Engl J Med* 2008, 358:580–591.

58. Riddle MC, Rosenstock J, Gerich J, Insulin Glargine 4002 Study Investigators: The treat-to-target trial: randomized addition of glargine or human NPH insulin to oral therapy of type 2 diabetic patients. *Diabetes Care* 2003, 26:3080–3086.

59. Holman RR, Thorne KI, Farmer AJ, *et al.*, 4-T Study Group: Addition of biphasic, prandial, or basal insulin to oral therapy in type 2 diabetes. *N Engl J Med* 2007, 357:1716–1730.

60. Holman RR, Farmer AJ, Davies MJ, *et al.*, 4-T Study Group: Three-year efficacy of complex insulin regimens in type 2 diabetes. *N Engl J Med* 2009, 361:1736–1747.

61. Drucker DJ: Enhancing incretin action for the treatment of type 2 diabetes. *Diabetes Care* 2003, 26:2929–2940.

62. Palalau AI, Tahrani AA, Piya MK, Barnett AH: DPP-4 inhibitors in clinical practice. *Postgrad Med* 2009, 121:70–100.

63. Kendall DM, Cuddihy RM, Bergenstal RM: Clinical application of incretin-based therapy: therapeutic potential, patient selection and clinical use. *Am J Med* 2009, 122(Suppl 6):S37–S50.

64. Lovshin JA, Drucker DJ: Incretin-based therapies for type 2 diabetes mellitus. *Nat Rev Endocrinol* 2009, 5:262–269.

65. Chia CW, Egan JM: Incretin-based therapies in type 2 diabetes mellitus. *J Clin Endocrinol Metab* 2008, 93:3703–3716.

66. Fonseca VA, Handelsman Y, Staels B: Colesevelam lowers glucose and lipid levels in type 2 diabetes: the clinical evidence. *Diabetes Obes Metab* 2010, 12:384–392.

67. Pijl H, Ohasi H, Marsuda M, *et al.*: Bromocriptine: a novel approach to the treatment of type 2 diabetes. *Diabetes Care* 2000, 23:1154–1161.

68. Gaziano JM, Cincotta AH, O'Connor CM, *et al.*: Randomized clinical trial of quick-release bromocriptine among patients with type 2 diabetes on overall safety and cardiovascular outcomes. *Diabetes Care* 2010, 33:1503–1508.

69. Edelman S, Maier H, Wilhelm K: Pramlintide in the treatment of diabetes mellitus. *BioDrugs* 2008, 22:375–386.

70. Riddle M, Pencek R, Charenkavanich S, *et al.*: Randomized comparison of pramlintide or mealtime insulin added to basal insulin treatment for patients with type 2 diabetes. *Diabetes Care* 2009, 32:1577–1582.

71. Nathan DM, Buse JB, Davidson MB, *et al.*: Medical management of hyperglycemia in type 2 diabetes: a consensus algorithm for the initiation and adjustment of therapy: a consensus statement of the American Diabetes Association and the European Association for the Study of Diabetes. *Diabetes Care* 2009, 32:193–203.

72. Rodbard HW, Jellinger PS, Davidson JA, *et al.*: Statement by an American Association of Clinical Endocrinologists/American College of Endocrinology consensus panel on type 2 diabetes mellitus: an algorithm for glycemic control. *Endocr Pract* 2009, 15:540–559.

73. International Diabetes Federation: *Global Guideline for Type 2 Diabetes.* Brussels: International Diabetes Federation; 2005. Available at http://www.idf.org/node/1285?unode=B7462CCB-3A4C-472C-80E4-710074D74AD3.

9

Diabetes and Pregnancy

Lois Jovanovič

Hyperglycemia during pregnancy is the most common metabolic problem of pregnancy today [1]. The prevalence of hyperglycemia during pregnancy may be as high as 13% [0.1% of the pregnant population per year have type 1 diabetes, 2–3% have type 2 diabetes, and up to 12% of the population have gestational diabetes mellitus (GDM)] [2]. Although all types of diabetes increase the risk of complications to the mother and the fetus, it is most important to distinguish among the types because each has a different impact on the course of pregnancy and the development of the fetus. Pregestational diabetes mellitus (type 1 or type 2) is more serious because it is present before pregnancy; thus, its effect begins at fertilization and implantation and continues throughout pregnancy and thereafter. In particular, organogenesis may be disrupted, leading to a high risk of early abortion [3], severe congenital defects [4], and retarded growth [5]. Maternal manifestations are also more serious, especially in the presence of vascular complications such as retinopathy or nephropathy [6]. GDM usually appears in the second half of pregnancy and affects mainly fetal growth rate [7]. The offspring of mothers with GDM have a higher risk of subsequent obesity and slower systemic and psychosocial development and probably other long term metabolic effects [8, 9].

Historically, few women with pregestational diabetes lived to childbearing age before the advent of insulin therapy. Until insulin became commercially available in 1924, less than 100 pregnancies were reported in diabetic women, and most likely these women had type 2, and not type 1, diabetes. Even with this assumption, these cases of diabetes and pregnancy were associated with a greater than 90% infant mortality rate and a 30% maternal mortality rate [10]. As late as 1980, some physicians were still counseling diabetic women to avoid pregnancy [11]. This philosophy was justified because of the poor obstetric history in 30–50% of diabetic women. Infant mortality rates finally began to improve after 1980, when treatment strategies stressed better control of maternal plasma glucose levels and after self-monitoring of blood glucose and hemoglobin A_{1c} became available to enable better metabolic control in persons with diabetes [12]. As the pathophysiology of pregnancy complicated by diabetes has been elucidated and as management programs have achieved and maintained near normoglycemia throughout pregnancy complicated by types 1 and 2 diabetes and GDM, perinatal mortality rates have become comparable with those of the general population [13]. The Pedersen [14] hypothesis links maternal hyperglycemia-induced fetal hyperinsulinemia to morbidity of the infant. Fetal hyperinsulinemia may cause increased fetal body mass (macrosomia) and, subsequently, a difficult delivery, or cause inhibition of pulmonary maturation of surfactant and, therefore, respiratory distress of the neonate. The fetus may also have decreased serum potassium levels caused by the elevated insulin and glucose levels that may induce fatal cardiac arrhythmias. Neonatal hypoglycemia may cause permanent neurologic damage.

The literature since the advent of insulin has documented that programs of near-normal glycemia are associated with improved outcome [15]. Therefore, treatment strategies have been developed to minimize the fetal exposure to either sustained or intermittent periods of hyperglycemia [16]. The maternal postprandial glucose level has been shown to be the most important variable to affect the subsequent risk of neonatal macrosomia [17]. When the postprandial glucose levels are blunted 1 h after beginning a meal, the risk of macrosomia is minimized [18].

J.S. Skyler (ed.), *Atlas of Diabetes: Fourth Edition*,
DOI 10.1007/978-1-4614-1028-7_9, © Springer Science+Business Media, LLC 2012

There is an increased prevalence of congenital anomalies and spontaneous abortions in women with types 1 and 2 diabetes who are in poor glycemic control during the period of fetal organogenesis, which is nearly complete by 7 weeks postconception [19]. It has also been reported that some women with GDM are also at risk for bearing a malformed infant because they most probably had undiagnosed (and thus untreated) type 2 diabetes during the time of organogenesis. Because women may not know they are pregnant during the critical time period for organ formation, prepregnancy counseling and planning are essential for all pregestational diabetic women of childbearing age [20, 21].

For the past 30 years, the classification, diagnosis, and treatment of GDM have been based on the recommendations of the International Workshop – Conference on Gestational Diabetes Mellitus [22]. As of 1997, four such international meetings had been held, and their recommendations were adopted by major medical institutions in Europe and America (American College of Obstetrics and Gynecology, American Diabetes Association, European Association for the Study of Diabetes, World Health Organization). Despite decades of debate on the optimal screening and diagnostic criteria, there still remains divided opinion as to the best means to diagnose GDM. A recent multinational, multicenter study analyzed 25,505 pregnant women who underwent 75-g oral glucose tolerance testing at 24–28 weeks of gestation to determine whether maternal hyperglycemia less severe than that in diabetes mellitus is associated with increased risks of adverse pregnancy outcomes. Results indicated a strong, continuous association of maternal glucose levels below those diagnostic of diabetes with increased birth weight and increased cordblood serum C-peptide levels. [23, 24].

Since 1980, the inception of "tight glycemia control" achieved by "intensive conventional therapy," including self-monitoring of blood glucose, has become an integral part of the treatment program for pregnancies complicated by hyperglycemia. As early as 1954, Pedersen [10] observed that "the common maternal, fetal, and neonatal complications of a pregnancy complicated by diabetes could be diminished by carefully supervised regulation of maternal metabolism." There is now a wealth of literature and experience to justify intensive approaches toward achieving normoglycemia in pregnancy. It is time to invest energy to simplify and disseminate these systems.

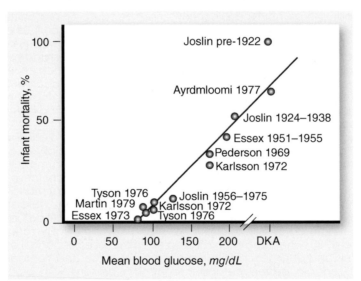

FIGURE 9-1. Literature review of the relationship between mean maternal glucose concentrations and infant mortality. Before the advent of insulin, an infant of a diabetic mother rarely survived. Before 1922, the fewer than 100 reported cases of survival are probably the offspring of type 2 rather than type 1 diabetic women [10]. A review of the major studies over the years since insulin became commercially available and when intensive glucose control systems were developed reveals that as the mean maternal blood glucose concentrations decrease, the percent infant mortality decreases [25]. A linear regression line drawn through the points on this graph indicates that at a mean maternal glucose level of 84 mg/dL, there would be no increased risk of infant mortality over the risk in the general population (adapted from Jovanovič and Peterson [26]).

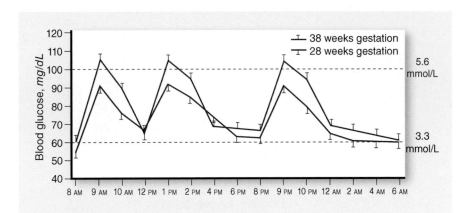

Figure 9-2. The report by Parretti et al. [27] on the blood glucose levels in normal, healthy pregnant women shows that the overall daily mean fasting glucose level is 56 mg/dL and the peak postprandial response occurs at 1 h after the meal. This peak level never exceeds 105.2 mg/dL. The calculated mean glucose concentration in their population was 85 mg/dL, close to the projected mean glucose concentration derived from the literature review [26].

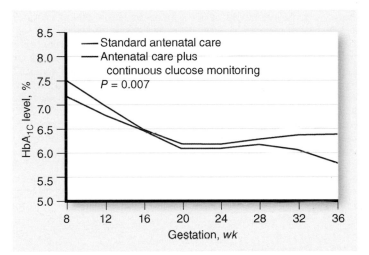

Figure 9-3. This study was designed to evaluate the effectiveness of continuous glucose monitoring during pregnancy on maternal glycemic control, infant birth weight, and risk of macrosomia in women with type 1 and type 2 diabetes [27]. Two secondary care multidisciplinary obstetric clinics for diabetes in the UK participated in this prospective, open-label randomized controlled trial. Seventy-one women with type 1 diabetes (*n*=46) and type 2 diabetes (*n*=25) allocated to antenatal care plus continuous glucose monitoring (*n*=38) or to standard antenatal care (*n*=33). Continuous glucose monitoring was used as an educational tool to inform sharp decision-making and future therapeutic changes at intervals of 4–6 weeks during pregnancy. All other aspects of antenatal care were equal between the groups. The primary outcome was maternal glycemic control during the second and third trimesters as measured by the A_{1c} levels every 4 weeks. Secondary outcomes were birth weight and risk of macrosomia using birth weight SD scores and customized birth weight centiles. Statistical analyses were done on an intention-to-treat basis. Women randomized to continuous glucose monitoring had lower mean A_{1c} levels from 32 to 36 weeks' gestation compared with women randomized to standard antenatal care: 5.8% (SD, 0.6) vs. 6.4% (SD, 0.7). Compared with infants of mothers in the control arm, infants of mothers in the intervention arm had decreased mean birth weight SD scores (0.9 vs. 1.6; effect size, 0.7 SD; 95% CI, 0.0–1.3), decreased median customized birth weight centiles (69 vs. 93%), and a reduced risk of macrosomia (OR, 0.36; 95% CI, 0.13–0.98). Continuous glucose monitoring during pregnancy is associated with improved glycemic control in the third trimester, lower birth weight, and reduced risk of macrosomia (adapted from Murphy et al. [28]).

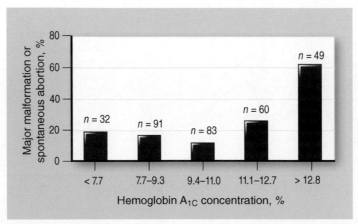

Figure 9-4. Combined prevalence of major malformation and spontaneous abortion according to the glycosylated hemoglobin (A_{1C}) concentration during the first trimester of pregnancy. In women with preexisting diabetes (pregestational diabetes), pregnancy should be deferred until the patient is under good glycemic control and has been thoroughly evaluated for complications of diabetes. Prepregnancy counseling should begin at the onset of puberty, with the need for abstinence or effective contraception clearly explained and understood [20]. A_{1C} values provide the best assessment of the degree of chronic glycemic control, reflecting the average blood glucose concentration during the preceding 6–8 weeks. As a result, measurement of A_{1C} can, in early pregnancy, estimate the level of glycemic control during the period of fetal organogenesis [21, 25, 29]. There are two important consequences in this regard (1) A_{1C} values early in pregnancy are correlated with the rates of spontaneous abortion and major congenital malformations and (2) normalizing blood glucose concentrations before and early in pregnancy can reduce the risks of spontaneous abortion and congenital malformations nearly to that of the general population [5, 21, 30]. One report compared 110 women who were already 6–30 weeks pregnant at the time of referral with 84 women recruited before conception and then put on a daily glucose-monitoring regimen [21]. The mean blood glucose concentration was between 60 and 140 mg/dL (3.3 and 7.8 mmol/L) in 50% of the latter women. The incidence of anomalies was 1.2% in the women recruited before conception vs. 10.9% in those first seen during pregnancy. Very similar findings were noted in another study: 1.4 vs. 10.4% incidence of congenital abnormalities [30]. Major congenital malformations (specifically, caudal regression, 252 times more common in infants of diabetic mothers; situs inversus, 84 times common than in the normal population; and renal and cardiac defects, six and four times more common, respectively, than in the infants of diabetic mothers compared with the normal population), which either require surgical correction or significantly affect the health of the child, are more common in infants of mothers with poorly controlled diabetes [19]. There is also a substantial increase in spontaneous abortions in women who enter pregnancy in poor metabolic control as reflected by an elevated hemoglobin A_{1C} level [3]. The teratogenicity of glucose appears to be the major factor before the seventh gestational week [19].

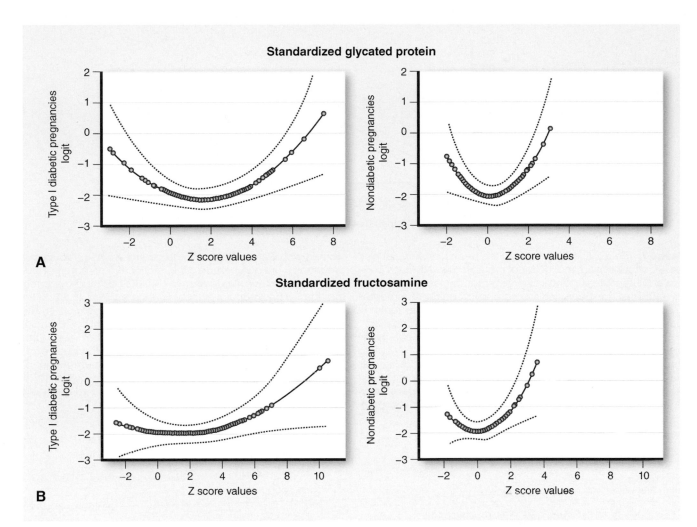

Standardized glycated protein

Standardized fructosamine

Figure 9-5. (A) Logit plots of pregnancy loss vs. standardized glycated protein values in type 1 diabetic and nondiabetic pregnancy. **(B)** Logit plots of pregnancy loss vs. standardized fructosamine values in type 1 diabetic and nondiabetic pregnancy. *Dashed lines* represent the fifth and 95th percentile CIs (adapted from Jovanovič et al. [31]).

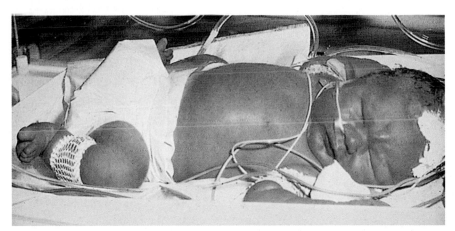

Figure 9-6. Diabetic fetopathy. The most common and significant neonatal complication clearly associated with diabetes in pregnancy is macrosomia: an oversized baby with a birth weight greater than the 90th percentile for gestational age and gender or a birth weight greater than 2 SD above the normal mean birth weight. This infant was macrosomic, weighed 4,583 g, was delivered 1 month prematurely, had all of the signs of an infant of a diabetic mother (hypoglycemia, hypocalcemia, hyperbilirubinemia), and died of respiratory distress 2 days after this photograph was taken.

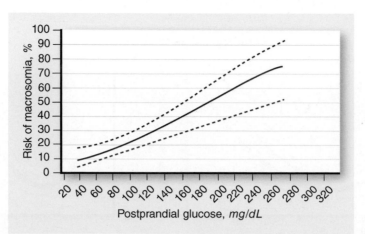

Figure 9-7. The relationship between the peak postprandial glucose concentration and the risk of macrosomia. Although controversial, the rate of complications in pregnancies complicated by diabetes has been tied to metabolic control of maternal glucose [5, 15, 17, 21, 25, 29]. Perhaps the debate remains because many of the reports claim that neonatal complications occur despite excellent metabolic control, but these reports fail to measure postprandial glucose levels [17, 18]. Postprandial glucose control has been suggested as key to neonatal outcome for pregnant women with either type 1 or gestational diabetes [17, 32]. The Diabetes in Early Pregnancy (DIEP) study was a multicenter trial of type 1 diabetic pregnant women who were compared with control women throughout pregnancy. This group studied the relationship of maternal glucose levels and risk of macrosomia [17]. The DIEP study reported that the 1-h postprandial glucose levels predicted 28.5% of the macrosomic infants born to diabetic mothers. This figure shows that the risk of macrosomia is a continuum. Any postprandial peak increases the risk of macrosomia above that seen in the normal population (10% risk). In addition, when the peak postprandial response is greater than 120 mg/dL, then the risk of macrosomia rises rapidly (adapted from Jovanovic et al. [17]). The lines represent the mean postprandial glucose level (bold line) ± SD (dotted lines).

Stepwise Logistic Regression of Maternal Metabolic Factors and Estimates of Neonatal Body Composition*		
	r^2	$*\Delta*r^2$
Birthweight		
Insulin sensitivity index[†]	0.28	—
Maternal weight gain	0.48	0.20
Fat-free mass		
Insulin sensitivity index[†]	0.33	—
Maternal weight gain	0.53	0.20
Fat mass		
Insulin sensitivity[‡]	0.15	—
Parity	0.29	0.14
Neonatal sex	0.39	0.10
Insulin sensitivity index[†]	0.46	0.07

*In 16 neonates of women with normal glucose tolerance (n = 6) or gestational diabetes (n = 10).

[†]Late pregnancy.

[‡]Pregravid.

FIGURE 9-8. Stepwise logistic regression of maternal metabolic factors and estimates of neonatal body composition. Catalano et al. [7] evaluated the relationship of various aspects of maternal carbohydrate metabolism and estimates of neonatal body composition. They evaluated 16 infants of women who participated in a long-term study of alterations in glucose metabolism. The results of a stepwise logistic regression of maternal carbohydrate metabolism factors showed that maternal weight gain played the most significant role (adapted from Catalano et al. [7]).

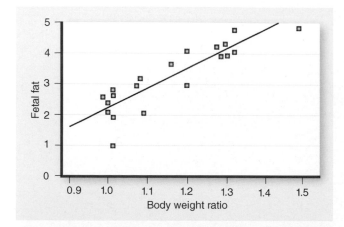

Figure 9-9. Relationship between fetal fat and subsequent birth weight, as measured by ponderal index or body weight ratio. Using magnetic resonance imaging (MRI), Jovanovic et al. [32] also found that the mother's adiposity was a predictor of the baby's birth weight. The relationship of fetal fat, as determined by the mean of two points of maximal thickness of the fetal abdominal wall subcutaneous fat on the MRI taken at 36 weeks of gestation compared with the infant birth weight ratio was highly significant ($P<0.001$; $r=0.88$) (adapted from Jovanovič et al. [33]).

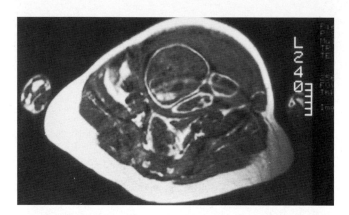

Figure 9-10. Magnetic resonance image of the fetus of a diabetic woman in excellent glucose control. This image was taken at the level of the maternal umbilicus at 38 weeks of gestation [33]. The mother had gestational diabetes mellitus and maintained excellent glucose control with preprandial glucose concentrations of 70–90 mg/dL; all of her blood glucose levels at 1 h after the meal were less than 120 mg/dL. This infant weighed 3,300 g at birth and was normal for percent body fat (from Jovanovič et al. [33], with permission).

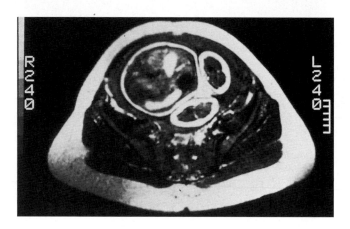

Figure 9-11. Magnetic resonance image of the fetus of a diabetic woman in poor glucose control. This image was taken at the level of the maternal umbilicus at 38 weeks of gestational age. As can be seen, this fetus not only has increased subcutaneous fat but also already has accrual of visceral fat [33]. This mother had no antenatal care and presented to the emergency room with a urinary tract infection. She was found to have severe hyperglycemia. Her glucose concentration on admission was 396 mg/dL, probably indicative that she had undiagnosed type 2 diabetes. This fetus weighed 4,340 g at birth, had 50% of its neonatal weight composed of fat, and had all of the signs of an infant of a diabetic mother (from Jovanovič et al. [33], with permission).

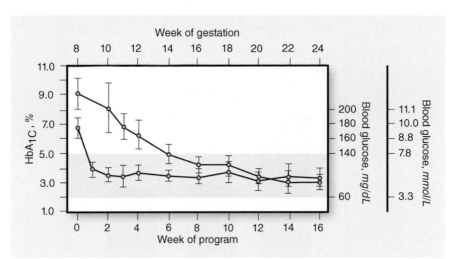

FIGURE 9-12. The time course for normalization of maternal glycosylated hemoglobin level in relationship to the normalization of maternal glucose concentrations. One of the first reports of a significant improvement in the outcome of type 1 diabetic pregnancies was published by Jovanovic et al. [29] in 1980. This report showed that when maternal blood glucose levels were normalized by the eighth gestational week, the birth weights of the infants were also normalized. This figure shows the time course for the normalization of glycosylated hemoglobin (HbA$_{1C}$) and blood glucose for ten pregnant women with type 1 diabetes. *Purple circles* represent the mean ± SD HbA$_{1C}$, and *blue circles* represent mean ± SD blood glucose concentrations (each time point is based on eight to ten glucose determinations obtained from all ten patients over 2-week intervals). The *shaded area* is the normal range for both HbA$_{1C}$ and blood glucose concentrations in the third trimester. All ten women had normal infants at term (adapted from Jovanovič et al. [29]).

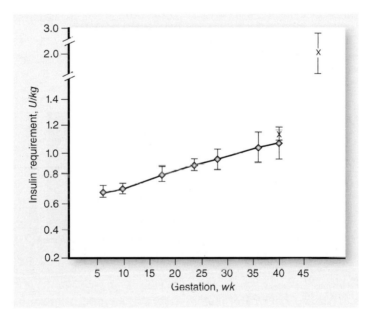

FIGURE 9-13. The insulin requirement throughout pregnancy in type 1 diabetic women. In a larger study of type 1 diabetic women who were maintained with normoglycemia from the sixth gestational week onward, there was a smooth increase in the insulin requirement throughout pregnancy. Fifty-three infants born to 52 type 1 diabetic women were all normal at birth. The insulin requirement of the woman who delivered twins was double that of the other 51 women. This increased need for insulin was manifested from the sixth gestational week onward. The *cross sign* shows the mean daily dosage of insulin during weeks 34–37 of gestation (adapted from Jovanovič et al. [15]). The cross sign in the right upper corner represents one twin pregnancy who manifested with twice the insulin requirement from week 6 to term.

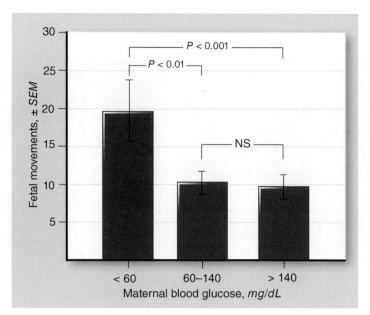

Figure 9-14. The relationship between fetal movements and maternal glucose concentrations. In this same population of diabetic women whose glucose control was documented in the study shown in Figure 9-13, the assessment of fetal well-being using the parameter of fetal movements associated with heart rate (HR) acceleration is shown here. The *bars* show comparison of fetal movements with accelerations with maternal blood-glucose concentrations less than 60 mg/dL, with mater-nal blood-glucose concentrations of 60–140 mg/dL, and with maternal blood-glucose concentrations greater than 140 mg/ dL. It can be seen that the fetuses had significantly more movements with HR acceleration when the blood glucose concentrations were low. It appears, therefore, that transient, mild hypoglycemia is well tolerated by fetuses and may actually be preferred by them. *NS* not significant, *SEM* standard error of the mean (adapted from Holden et al. [34]).

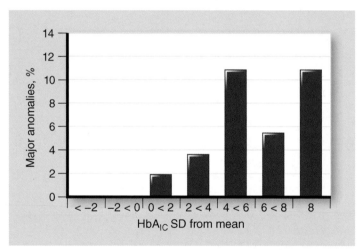

Figure 9-15. Malformations relate to glucose, not type of insulin. In a multinational, multicenter, retrospective study to determine the rate of major congenital anomalies in offspring of a large group of women with diabetes mellitus treated with insulin lispro (Humalog), mothers with diabetes diagnosed before conception were treated with insulin lispro for at least 1 month before conception and during at least the first trimester of pregnancy [35]. In 533 pregnancies, resulting in 542 offspring (500 live births, 31 spontaneous and 7 elective abortions, and 4 stillbirths), the rate of major congenital anomalies was 5.4% (95% CI [3.45%, 7.44%]) for offspring of mothers with diabetes treated with insulin lispro before and during pregnancy. Because current published rates of major anomalies in infants born to mothers with diabetes treated with insulin are between 2.1 and 10.9%, these findings suggest that the anomaly rate with insulin lispro treatment is similar to published major congenital anomaly rates for other insulin treatments (adapted from Wyatt et al. [35]).

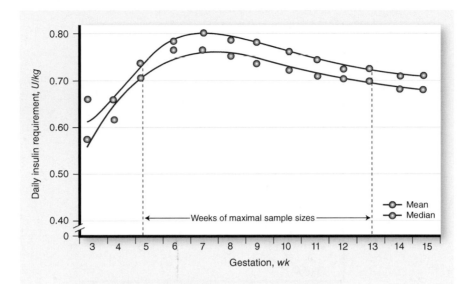

Figure 9-16. The declining insulin requirement in the first trimester of type 1 diabetic pregnant women. In the Diabetes in Early Pregnancy Study, the insulin requirement in the first trimester was studied. The daily insulin dosage (expressed as either a weekly mean or median in units per kg from weeks 3–8) increased, but there was an insulin dosage decrease in the late first trimester. The *purple circles* represent the mean dosage of 346 type 1 diabetic women who had healthy infants. The *blue circles* represent the median dosage of these same patients (adapted from Jovanovič et al. [36]).

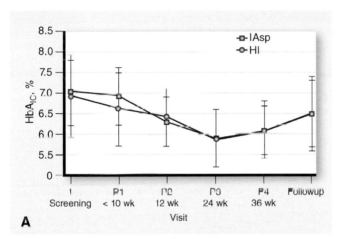

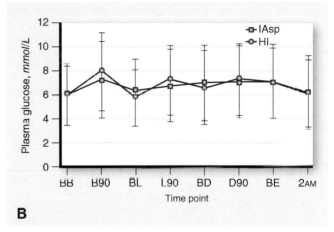

Figure 9-17. (A) Mean A_{1c} (%) by treatment group during pregnancy and at the follow up (6 weeks postpartum) visit. Data at visit P1 only includes data for subjects pregnant after screening. Data are means±SD. **(B)** Mean 8-point plasma glucose profile (mmol/l +SD) by treatment group at visit P2 (12 weeks of gestation). *B90* 90 min after breakfast, *BB* before breakfast, *BD* before dinner, *BE* bedtime, *BL* before lunch, *D90* 90 min after dinner, *L90* 90 min after lunch (adapted from Mathiesen et al. [37]). *IAsp* insulin aspart, *HI* human insulin.

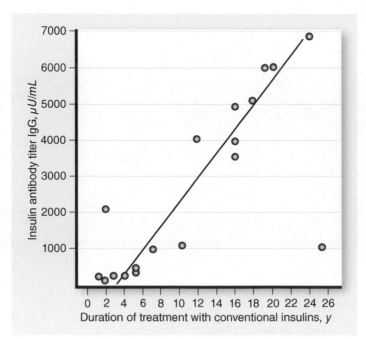

FIGURE 9-18. The relationship between anti-insulin antibody levels and duration of treatment with animal insulin. Although maternal glucose is the most likely causal agent of neonatal macrosomia, some have suggested that neonatal morbidity is secondary to the variability of maternal serum glucose and presence of antibodies to insulin. Placental transfer of insulin bound to immunoglobulin G (IgG) has also been associated with fetal macrosomia in mothers with near-normal glycemic control during gestation. Menon et al. [38] reported that antibody-bound insulin transferred to the fetus was proportional to the concentration of antibody-bound insulin measured in the mother. Also, the amount of antibody-bound insulin transferred to the fetus correlated directly with macrosomia in the infant and was independent of maternal blood glucose levels. By contrast, researchers found that only improved glucose control, as evidenced by lower postprandial glucose excursions but not lower insulin antibody levels, correlated with lower fetal weight [39]. They showed that insulin antibodies to exogenous insulin do not influence infant birth weight or insulin dosage. They did report, however, that there is a relationship between duration of treatment with conventional insulin and IgG antibody titer, as shown here (adapted from Jovanovič et al. [40]).

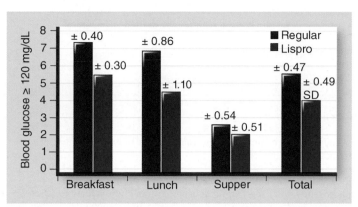

Figure 9-19. The postprandial glucose concentrations of diabetic women treated with insulin lispro compared with the postprandial glucose concentrations of diabetic women treated with human insulin during pregnancy. Our group reported that insulin lispro, an analog of human insulin with a peak insulin action achieved within 1 h after injection, significantly improves the postprandial glucose concentrations in pregnant diabetic patients. Jovanovič et al. [41] showed that the postprandial glucose level is significantly lower ($P<0.01$) throughout pregnancy in insulin-requiring gestational diabetic women treated with insulin lispro compared with gestational diabetic women treated with human insulin (adapted from Jovanovic et al. [41]).

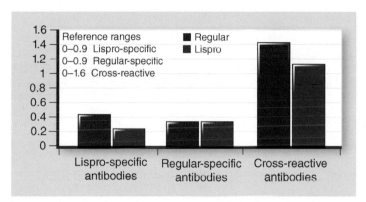

Figure 9-20. Insulin antibody findings. The antibody levels were no different in the women treated with insulin lispro compared with human insulin. In addition, lispro was not detected in the cord blood of the infants whose mothers were treated with lispro. A clinical trial [42] has shown the safety and efficacy of insulin aspart for the treatment of gestational diabetes. In this study, similar to the lispro study, insulin aspart proved to lower the postprandial glucose concentrations better than the concentrations achieved with human regular insulin, and the insulin appeared not to be immunogenic. Because of the importance of blunting the postprandial peak glucose concentration and the lack of immunogenicity of rapid-acting insulin analogs, the treatment of choice in pregnancy is now to suggest that these insulins be used in pregnancies complicated by diabetes (adapted from Jovanovič et al. [41]).

Insulin dosage regimen for diabetic pregnancy

□ 1. Pregnancy NPH plus rapid-acting insulin schedule   Patient weight in kg =   Date & Time:

"Big I" = total daily units of insulin

Circle One: Gestational weeks =

0-12	13-28	29-34	35-40	OTHER
k = 0.7	0.8	0.9	1.0	

Calculate desired units of insulin from above line.

"Big I" = _____ (k units X weight kg)/24 hours

"Big I" = Basal insulin requirement + Bolus (meal-related) insulin requirement

Basal = ½ "Big I," Bolus = ½ "Big I"

Basal: Divide so that 1/6 of "Big I" is NPH given before breakfast, 1/6 of "Big I" is NPH given before dinner, and 1/6 of "Big I" is NPH given before bedtime.

Bolus: Divide so that 1/6 of "Big I" is rapid-acting insulin given before breakfast, 1/6 of "Big I" is rapid-acting insulin given before lunch, and 1/6 of "Big I" is rapid-acting insulin given before dinner. The rapid-acting insulin is then titrated based on the blood glucose.

0800 Pre-breakfast: NPH = 1/6 "Big I" = _____ _____.

Check yesterday's pre-dinner BS:

If yesterday's pre-dinner BS < 60, then decrease today's AM NPH by 2 units.

If yesterday's pre-dinner BS 61-90, no change in today's AM NPH.

If yesterday's pre-dinner BS > 91, then increase today's AM NPH by 2 units.

Do not feed the patient until the blood sugar is below 120 mg/dL.

Rapid-acting insulin = 1/6 "Big I" = _____ to be adjusted according to the following scale:

Pre-breakfast BS < 60 = _____ = (1/6 "Big I" dose) – 3% of the "Big I."

61-90 = _____ = 1/6 "Big I" dose.

91-120 = _____ = (1/6 "Big I" dose) + 3% of the "Big I."

> 121 = _____ = (1/6 "Big I" dose) + 6% of the "Big I."

If today's BS 1 hour after breakfast is < 110, then decrease tomorrow's pre-breakfast rapid insulin by 2 units.

If today's BS 1 hour after breakfast is 111-120, no change in tomorrow's pre-breakfast rapid insulin.

If today's BS 1 hour after breakfast is > 121, then increase tomorrow's pre-breakfast rapid insulin by 2 units.

1200 Pre-lunch: Rapid-acting insulin is 1/6 "Big I" = _____ to be adjusted according to the following scale:

Do not feed the patient until the blood sugar is below 120 mg/dL.

Pre-lunch BS < 60 = _____ = (1/6 "Big I" dose) – 3% of "Big I."

61-90 = _____ = 1/6 "Big I" dose

91-120 = _____ = (1/6 "Big I" dose) + 3% of "Big I."

>121 = _____ = (1/6 "Big I" dose) + 6% of "Big I."

If today's BS 1 hour after lunch is < 110, then decrease tomorrow's pre-lunch rapid insulin by 2 units.

If today's BS 1 hour after lunch is 111-120, no change in tomorrow's pre-lunch rapid insulin.

If today's BS 1 hour after lunch is > 121, then increase tomorrow's pre-lunch rapid insulin by 2 units.

1700 Pre-dinner: NPH = 1/6 "Big I" = _____.

Rapid-acting insulin is 1/6 "Big I" = _____ to be adjusted according to the following scale:

If yesterday's pre-bedtime BS < 60, then decrease today's dinner NPH by 2 units.

If yesterday's pre-bedtime BS 61-90, no change in today's dinner NPH.

If yesterday's pre-bedtime BS > 91, then increase today's dinner NPH by 2 units.

Do not feed the patient until the blood sugar is Below 120 mg/dL.

Pre-dinner BS < 60 = _____ = (1/6 "Big I" dose) – 3% of "Big I."

61-90 = _____ = 1/6 "Big I" dose

91-120 = _____ = (1/6 "Big I" dose) + 3% of "Big I."

>121 = _____ = (1/6 "Big I" dose) + 6% of "Big I."

If today's BS 1 hour after dinner is < 110, then decrease tomorrow's dinner rapid insulin by 2 units.

If today's BS 1 hour after dinner is 111-120, no change in tomorrow's dinner rapid insulin.

If today's BS 1 hour after dinner is > 121, then increase tomorrow's dinner rapid insulin by 2 units.

2400 Bedtime NPH: Give 1/6 "Big I" = _____ _____.

If today's pre-breakfast BS is < 60, then decrease today's bedtime NPH by 2 units.

If today's pre-breakfast BS is 61-90, no change in today's bedtime NPH.

If today's pre-breakfast BS is > 91, then check the 3 AM BS and, if it is <70 (regardless of today's pre-breakfast BS), decrease today's bedtime NPH by 2 units.

If today's pre-breakfast BS is > 91, and the 3 AM BS > 70, increase today's bedtime NPH by 2 units.

Also, if the 3 AM BS is > 91, then call the doctor for 3 AM rapid insulin scale equal to the pre-lunch rapid scale.

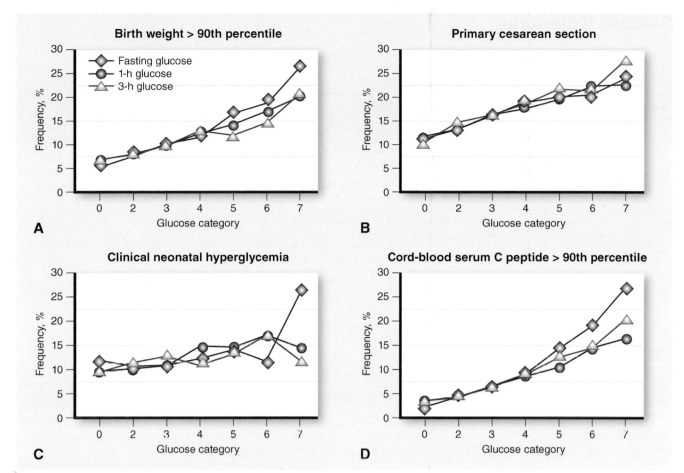

Figure 9-22. Frequency across glucose categories of primary outcomes, including birth weight more than 90th percentile (**A**); primary cesarean section (**B**); clinical neonatal hypoglycemia (**C**); and cord-blood serum C-peptide higher than 90th percentile (**D**) A recent multinational, multicenter study analyzed 25,505 pregnant women who underwent 75-g oral glucose tolerance testing at 24–23 weeks of gestation to determine whether maternal hyperglycemia less severe than that in diabetes mellitus is associated with increased risks of adverse pregnancy outcomes. Results indicated a strong, continuous association of maternal glucose levels below those diagnostic of diabetes with increased birth weight and increased cord-blood serum C-peptide levels (adapted from HAPO Study Cooperative Research Group et al. [23]).

Figure 9-21. Insulin dosage regimen for pregnancy complicated by diabetes. This treatment algorithm has proven to achieve normal glycemia in pregestational diabetic women. The insulin doses are divided into frequent injections to provide the basal and the meal-related insulin needs. The smooth increase in the total daily insulin requirement throughout pregnancy is calculated based on gestational week and maternal pregnant weight. The insulin requirement at 0–12 weeks of gestation is 0.7 U/kg/day (with careful monitoring of the blood glucose levels to prevent hypoglycemia from occurring if there is a decline in dosage during weeks 9–12). During weeks 13–28 of gestation, the dosage is 0.8 U/kg/day; during weeks 29–34, the insulin requirement is 0.9 U/kg/day. At term, the insulin requirement is 1.0 U/kg/day [15]. *BS* blood sugar, *NPH* neutral protamine Hagedorn (adapted from Jovanovič and Peterson [43]).

Glucose Categories

Category number	Fasting plasma glucose level	One-hour plasma glucose level	Two-hour plasma glucose level
1	< 75 mg/dL (4.2 mmol/L)	≤ 105 mg/dL (5.8 mmol/L)	≤ 90 mg/dL (5.0 mmol/L)
2	75–79 mg/dL (4.2–4.4 mmol/L)	106–132 mg/dL (5.9–7.3 mmol/L)	91–108 mg/dL (5.1–6.0 mmol/L)
3	80–84 mg/dL (4.5–4.7 mmol/L)	133–155 mg/dL (7.4–8.6 mmol/L)	109–125 mg/dL (6.1–6.9 mmol/L)
4	85–89 mg/dL (4.8–4.9 mmol/L)	156–171 mg/dL (8.7–9.5 mmol/L)	126–139 mg/dL (7.0–7.7 mmol/L)
5	90–94 mg/dL (5.0–5.2 mmol/L)	172–193 mg/dL (9.6–10.7 mmol/L)	140–157 mg/dL (7.8–8.7 mmol/L)
6	95–99 mg/dL (5.3–4.4 mmol/L)	194–211 mg/dL (10.8–11.7 mmol/L)	158–177 mg/dL (8.8–9.8 mmol/L)
7	≥ 100 mg/dL (5.6 mmol/L)	≥ 212 mg/dL (11.8 mmol/L)	≥ 178 mg/dL (9.9 mmol/L)

Outcome	Standard group (n = 100)	Ultrasound group (n = 99)	P value
Gestational age at delivery, wk	39.3 ± 1.3	39.0 ± 1.9	0.2
Induction, %	23.0	23.2	0.5
Cesarean delivery, %	15.0	18.2	0.5
Birth weight, g	3271.2 ± 500	3306.1 ± 558	0.4
SGA, %	13.0	12.1	0.5
LGA, %	10.0	12.1	0.4
Neonatal BMI, kg/m2	13.1 ± 1.2	12.8 ± 1.5	0.2
Sum of skinfolds, mm*	13.2 ± 3.2	14.1 ± 3.4	0.07
Hypoglycemia (< 40 mg/dL), %	16.0	17.0	0.5
Intravenous glucose, %	11	9.1	0.4
Cord blood insulin, μU/mL†	9.1 ± 6.2	8.8 ± 6.82	0.8
Transfer to NICU, %	15.0	14.1	0.5

*Sum of skinfold measured at four locations on the body (subscapular, iliac crest, triceps, and thigh).
†Missing in four infants of women who did not complete the study.
BMI—body mass index; LGA—large for gestational age; NICU—neonatal intensive care unit; SGA—small for gestational age.

Outcome	Glyburide (n = 201)	Insulin (n = 203)	P value
Neonatal features			
Large size for gestational age, n (%)	24 (12)	26 (13)	0.76
Birth weight, g	3256 ± 543	3194 ± 598	0.28
Ponderal index > 2.85, n (%)*	18 (9)	24 (12)	0.33
Macrosomia, n (%)	14 (7)	9 (4)	0.26
Metabolic outcomes			
Cord serum insulin, μU/mL†	15 ± 13	15 ± 21	0.84
Intravenous glucose therapy, n (%)	28 (14)	22 (11)	0.36
Hypoglycemia, n (%)	18 (9)	12 (6)	0.25
Hypocalcemia, n (%)	2 (1)	2 (1)	0.99
Hyperbilirubinemia, n (%)	12 (6)	8 (4)	0.36
Polycythemia, n (%)	4 (2)	6 (3)	0.52
Lung complications, n (%)	16 (8)	12 (6)	0.43
Respiratory support, n (%)	4 (2)	6 (3)	0.52
Admission for neonatal intensive care unit, n (%)	12 (6)	14 (7)	0.68
Congenital anomaly	5 (2)	4 (2)	0.74
Perinatal mortality, n (%)‡			
Stillbirth	1 (0.5)	1 (0.5)	0.99
Neonatal death	1 (0.5)	1 (0.5)	0.99

Plus-minus values are mean ± SD.
*The ponderal index was calculated as 100 times the weight in grams divided by the cube of the length in centimeters.
†To convert values for insulin to picomoles per liter, multiply by 6.0.
‡Numbers include infants with congenital abnormalities.

Figure 9-23. **(A)** Guidelines for management of pregnancies complicated by gestational diabetes mellitus (GDM) generally call for normalization of maternal glucose concentrations. This strategy requires frequent glucose monitoring with initiation of insulin therapy if the blood glucose concentrations increase above the target levels. Management of women with GDM with the use of fetal ultrasonography has been shown to safe and can identify those who are at risk of delivering neonates who are large for gestational age if insulin therapy is withheld. Two trials testing the fetal growth-based approach in a predominately Latino population [44, 45] demonstrated low rates of macrosomic infants when the fetus' abdominal circumference on ultrasonography remained below the 75th percentile during pregnancy. Recently, a third study [46] reported the management of women with GDM based predominantly on monthly fetal growth ultrasound examinations with an approach based solely on maternal glycemia. Women with GDM who attained fasting capillary glucose (FCG) below 120 mg/dL and 2 h postprandial capillary glucose (2 h-CG) below 200 mg/dL after 1 week of diet were randomized to management based on maternal glycemia alone (standard) or glycemia plus ultrasound. In the standard group, insulin was initiated if FCG was repeatedly above 90 mg/dL or 2 h-CG was above 120 mg/dL. In the ultrasound group, thresholds were 120 and 200 mg/dL, respectively, or a fetal abdominal circumference above the 75th percentile (AC > p75). Outcome criteria were rates of cesarean section, small-for-gestational-age (SGA) or large-for-gestational-age (LGA) infants, neonatal hypoglycemia (<40 mg/dL), and neonatal care admission. As seen here, in the ultrasound group, AC > p75 was the sole indication for insulin. The ultrasound-based strategy, compared with the maternal glycemia-only strategy, resulted in a different treatment assignment in 34% of women. Rates of cesarean section (19 vs. 18.2%), LGA (10 vs. 12.1%), SGA (13 vs. 12.1%), hypoglycemia (16 vs. 17.0%), and admission (15 vs. 14.1%) did not differ significantly. The authors concluded that GDM management based on fetal growth combined with high glycemic criteria provides outcomes equivalent to management based on strict glycemic criteria alone. Inclusion of fetal growth might provide the opportunity to reduce glucose testing in low-risk pregnancies. **(B)** Women with gestational diabetes mellitus are rarely treated with a sulfonylurea drug, because of concern about teratogenicity and neonatal hypoglycemia. There is little information about the efficacy of these drugs in this group of women. Recently, however, there was a randomized trial [47] of 404 women with singleton pregnancies and gestational diabetes that required treatment. The women were randomly assigned between 11 and 33 weeks of gestation to receive glyburide or insulin according to an intensified treatment protocol. The primary end point was achievement of the desired level of glycemic control. Secondary end points included maternal and neonatal complications. As can be seen by in this figure, the mean pretreatment blood glucose concentration and glucose during treatment as measured at home was not significantly different in the glyburide group compared with the insulin group. Eight women in the glyburide group (4%) required insulin therapy. There were no significant differences between the glyburide and insulin groups in the percentage of infants who were large for gestational age, who had macrosomia, defined as a birth weight of 4,000 g or more, who had lung complications, who had hypoglycemia, or who were admitted to a neonatal intensive care unit. The cord-serum insulin concentrations were similar in the two groups, and glyburide was not detected in the cord serum of any infant in the glyburide group. The authors concluded that in women with gestational diabetes, glyburide is a clinically effective alternative to insulin therapy. Further studies are necessary, however, before glyburide can be safely prescribed in clinical practice. *BMI* body mass index, *NICU* neonatal intensive care unit.

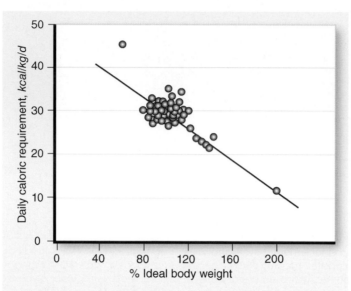

Figure 9-24. The caloric needs for pregnant women based on their ideal body weight. The main goal of treatment of women with gestational diabetes mellitus (GDM) is to prevent adverse effects to the mother and infant. Normalization of glucose levels is a proven factor to achieve this goal. In addition, postprandial glucose levels are more closely associated with macrosomia than are fasting levels. Women with GDM must follow an individually tailored diet prepared by a dietitian who also takes into account the amount, time, and type of insulin injection (if necessary). The diet must satisfy the minimum daily nutritional requirements for all pregnant women. The caloric intake must be compatible with the state of pregnancy and ensure the proper weight gain according to the patient's ideal weight before and during pregnancy. In this figure, the caloric needs of pregnancy are related to maternal body weight. The *closed circles* show that for a woman who is of normal body weight (80–120% ideal body weight), the caloric requirement is 30 kcal/kg/day (present pregnant weight). For overweight women, fewer calories are needed. Most overweight women are 130% above ideal body weight, and they require 24 kcal/kg/day. Morbidly obese women (>150% above ideal body weight) may require as few as 12 kcal/kg/day (present pregnant weight) [48] (adapted from Jovanovič [49]).

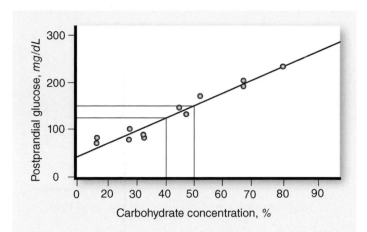

Figure 9-25. The relationship between carbohydrate concentration, the meal plan, and the peak postprandial response. The calories are divided into frequent small feedings with the caveat that breakfast needs to be the smallest meal of the day, with less than 33% carbohydrate. This degree of carbohydrate restriction is necessary because the hypercortisolemia seen normally in early waking hours is potentiated in pregnancy. After the cortisol levels wane, then the other meals can be composed of 40% carbohydrate. This figure clearly shows that when the carbohydrate concentration in lunch and dinner is greater than 40%, then the peak postprandial glucose level is greater than 120 mg/dL or that level reported to be associated with a rapidly increasing risk of neonatal macrosomia [17] (adapted from Peterson and Jovanovič [50]).

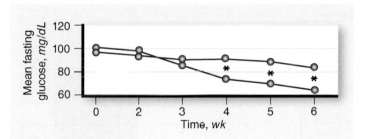

Figure 9-26. Weekly fasting glucose concentrations during a cardiovascular training program compared with no exercise program in women with gestational diabetes mellitus (GDM). An arm exercise has been shown to be a safe and effective mode of therapy for treating these women. Our group documented that women with GDM can train using arm ergometry and that a program of this kind of cardiovascular conditioning exercise results in lower levels of glycemia than a program of diet alone. The effects of exercise on fasting glucose concentrations became apparent after 4 weeks of training (asterisks) (adapted from Jovanovič et al. [31]).

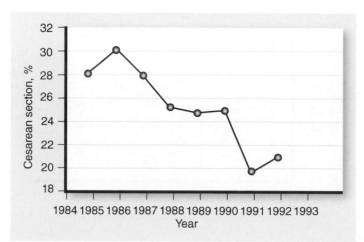

Figure 9-27. The decrease in the cesarean section rate in Santa Barbara County concomitant with the introduction of a program of universal screening and treatment of hyperglycemia in pregnancy. When the glucose level cannot be maintained within recommended limits (90 mg/dL before meals and no higher than 120 mg/dL at 1 h after meals) by diet and exercise, then insulin treatment is needed. Rapid-acting insulin analogs can improve glycemic levels, and their use is increasing in most leading centers in the USA and Europe. Our experience in Santa Barbara County Health Care Service [52] with a program of universal screening and treatment of postprandial glucose by targeting the blood glucose level to be less than 120 mg/dL (with diet, exercise, and initiation of insulin when blood glucose levels are elevated) has shown that the birth weight is normalized. This degree of intensive care for all gestational diabetic women results in more than $2,000 saved per pregnancy by avoiding cesarean sections necessitated to deliver macrosomic infants and neonatal intensive care admissions of sick infants (adapted from Jovanovič and Bevier [53]).

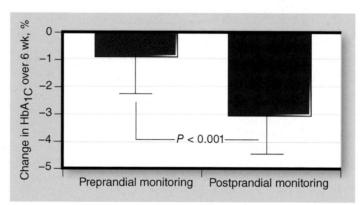

Figure 9-28. The glycosylated hemoglobin levels after 6 weeks of monitoring only preprandial glucose concentrations in women with gestational diabetes mellitus (GDM) needing insulin therapy compared with the glycosylated hemoglobin levels achieved in a matched population of women who were also monitoring postprandial glucose concentrations. de Veciana et al. [18] have also shown that when insulin-requiring women with GDM measure their preprandial glucose levels alone, the prevalence of macrosomia is 42%. When the postprandial glucose levels are measured and the treatment designed to maintain the levels at lower than 120 mg/dL, the prevalence of macrosomia was decreased to 12%. With only 6 weeks of treatment designed to blunt the postprandial glucose levels, the glycosylated hemoglobin level was significantly lower than in the group of gestational diabetes patients who were only monitoring glucose preprandially.

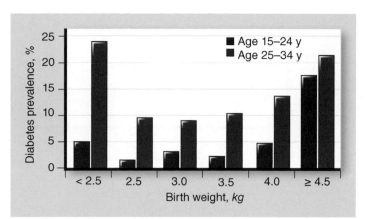

FIGURE 9-29. Relationship of birth weight to the risk of subsequent diabetes. Women who have had gestational diabetes mellitus previously should be advised to undergo repeated oral glucose tolerance tests once yearly and maintain a healthy lifestyle with regular exercise and normal body weight. They should seek consultation before their next pregnancy [22]. The follow-up of the offspring of diabetic mothers should include careful measurement of growth and development and concern for glucose intolerance during childhood. Children of diabetic mothers are at higher risk of obesity and glucose intolerance. Evidence is accumulating that good metabolic control in the mother during pregnancy can decrease this risk. There appears to be a U-shaped curve that relates birth weight to the risk of subsequent diabetes. Both at the low and high birth weights, it appears that the infants have a lack of pancreatic reserve of insulin; thus, as they grow and develop, they cannot increase their insulin secretion sufficiently to maintain glucose homeostasis (adapted from McCance et al. [53]).

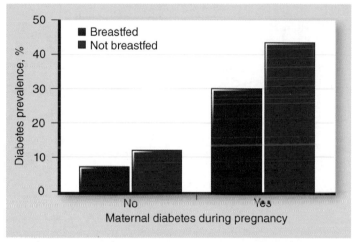

FIGURE 9-30. Predictors of subsequent diabetes in the offspring in Pima Indians. Pettitt and Knowler [9] reported that there is a long-term consequence of the intrauterine environment. When they adjusted for age, gender, birth weight, presence of diabetes in either parent, and whether or not the child was breastfed for at least 2 months after birth, the strongest predictors of subsequent diabetes in the child was the presence of maternal diabetes and not being breastfed. The *blue bars* represent the children who were not breastfed; the *purple bars* represent the children who were breastfed. Thus, it is clear that the intrauterine environment must be normalized and sufficient nutrition must be provided (but not overnutrition). Maintaining the nutritional status of the child after birth is paramount in decreasing the rapidly increasing rate of diabetes (adapted from Pettitt and Knowler [9]).

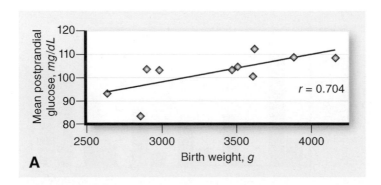

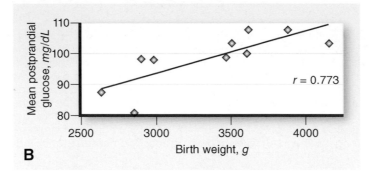

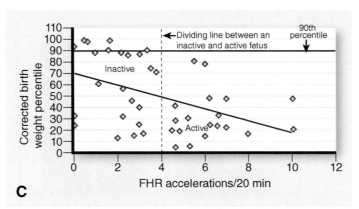

FIGURE 9-31. The Fidgety Fetus Hypothesis study was designed to determine whether some offspring of women with diabetes are intrinsically more active than others in utero and whether those who are active can normalize their birth weight despite maternal hyperglycemia. Phase I of the study assessed maternal perception of fetal movements in a population of 10 women with diabetes. To improve fetal monitoring techniques, phase 2 analyzed fetal movements using the Card Guard home fetal monitoring device (CG 900P; Lifewatch, Rosemont, IL) in a population of 13 women with gestational diabetes mellitus (GDM). Phase 3 applied the observations of fetal movements to a larger population by conducting a retrospective analysis of fetal monitoring (HP 8041A) from 46 women with GDM to examine the relationship between fetal heart rate (FHR) accelerations and percentile birth weight, corrected for gestational age. Phase 1 confirmed that there is little variability in fetal movements (i.e., fetal kicks did not significantly deviate from one another on a day-to-day basis). In phase 2, the fetal monitoring strips illustrated that the active fetuses (defined as ≥4 FHR accelerations in a 20-min period) were always active, and the inactive fetuses were always inactive. The mean birth weight percentile, corrected for gestational age, in the active group, was 37 vs. 63% in the inactive group (P=0.05). In phase 3, the fetal monitoring strips showed an inverse correlation between

the mean number of FHR accelerations and the birth weight of the fetus, corrected for gestational age. The mean birth weight percentile in the active group was 37 vs. 62% in the inactive group (P=0.0017). The fetus appears to play a role in determining its own density. Increased fetal activity may minimize the impact of hyperglycemia on subsequent birth weight. The inactive fetus appears to be at higher risk for glucose-mediate macrosomia. (**A**) Phase 1 unadjusted mean postprandial glucose vs. birth weight. *Diamonds* indicate each woman's unadjusted mean 1-h postprandial glucose value derived from the diaries. (**B**) Phase 1 adjusted mean postprandial glucose vs. birth weight. *Diamonds* indicate each woman's adjusted mean 1-h postprandial glucose value. Dividing the mean number of fetal kicks per day by a factor of 10 and subtracting the result from the mean maternal 1-h postprandial glucose concentration adjusted the glucose values from the patients' diaries. (**C**) Corrected birth weight percentile vs. FHR acceleration/20 min. *Diamonds* indicate birth weight percentile corrected for gestational age. *Inactive* and *active* refer to fetus activity. An inactive fetus has less than 4 FHR accelerations/20-min period and an active fetus has ≥4 FHR accelerations/20-min period. *Dashed line* represents the dividing line between an inactive and active fetus. *Solid bold line* represents a birth weight in the 90th percentile (adapted from Zisser et al. [54]).

References

1. American Diabetes Association: Clinical practice recommendations 2001: gestational diabetes. *Diabetes Care* 2001, 24(suppl):S77–S79.

2. Hod M, Diamant YZ: Diabetes in pregnancy. Norbert Freinkel Memorial Issue. *Isr J Med Sci* 1991, 27:421–540.

3. Mills JL, Simpson JL, Driscoll SG, Jovanovič L, *et al.*: Incidence of spontaneous abortion among normal women and insulin dependent diabetic women whose pregnancies were identified within 21 days of conception. *N Engl J Med* 1988, 319:1617–1623.

4. Mills JL, Knopp RH, Simpson JL, Jovanovič L, *et al.*: Lack of relation of increased malformation roles in infants of diabetic mothers to glycemic control during organogenesis. *N Engl J Med* 1988, 318:671–676.

5. Petersen M, Pedersen SA, Greisen G, *et al.*: Early growth delay in diabetic pregnancy: relation to psychomotor development at age 4. *Br Med J* 1988, 296:598–600.

6. van Dijk DJ, Axer-Siegel R, Erman A, Hod M: Diabetic vascular complications and pregnancy. *Diabetes Rev* 1995, 3:632.

7. Catalano PM, Drago NM, Amini S: Maternal carbohydrate metabolism and its relationship to fetal growth and body composition. *Am J Obstet Gynecol* 1995, 172:1464–1470.

8. Hod M, Diamant YZ: The offspring of a diabetic mother—short- and long-range implications. *Isr J Med Sci* 1992, 28:81–86.

9. Pettitt DJ, Knowler WC: Long-term effects of the intrauterine environment, birth weight, and breast-feeding in Pima Indians. *Diabetes Care* 1998, 21:B138–B141.

10. Pedersen J: Fetal mortality in diabetes in relation to management during the latter part of pregnancy. *Acta Endocrinol* 1954, 15:282–294.

11. Freinkel N: Banting Lecture 1980: of pregnancy and progeny. *Diabetes* 1980, 29:1023–1035.

12. Jovanovič L, Peterson CM: Moment in history: turning point in blood glucose monitoring of diet and insulin dosing. *Trans Am Soc Artif Intern Organs* 1990, 36:799.

13. Buchanan TA, Unterman T, Metzger BE: The medical management of diabetes in pregnancy. *Clin Perinatol* 1985, 12:625–650.

14. Pedersen J, Pedersen LM: Diabetes mellitus and pregnancy: the hyperglycemia, hyperinsulinemia theory and the weight of the newborn baby. In *Proceedings of the 7th Congress of the International Diabetes Federation*. Edited by Rodriguez RR, Vallance-Owen J. Amsterdam: Excerpta Medica; 1971:678.

15. Jovanovič L, Druzin M, Peterson CM: Effect of euglycemia on the outcome of pregnancy in insulin-dependent diabetics as compared to normal controls. *Am J Med* 1981, 71:921–927.

16. Jovanovič L, Peterson CM: Rationale for prevention and treatment of glucose-mediated macrosomia: a protocol for gestational diabetes. *Endocrinol Pract* 1996, 2:118.

17. Jovanovič L, Peterson CM, Reed GF, *et al.*: Maternal postprandial glucose levels and infant birth weight: the Diabetes in Early Pregnancy Study. The National Institute of Child Health and Human Development—Diabetes in Early Pregnancy Study. *Am J Obstet Gynecol* 1991, 164:103–111.

18. de Veciana M, Major CA, Morgan MA, *et al.*: Postprandial versus preprandial blood glucose monitoring in women with gestational diabetes mellitus requiring insulin therapy. *N Engl J Med* 1995, 333:1237–1241.

19. Mills JL, Baker L, Goldman A: Malformations in infants of diabetic mothers occur before the seventh gestational week: implications for treatment. *Diabetes* 1979, 23:292–293.

20. Steel JM, Johnstone FD, Hepburn DA, Smith AF: Can prepregnancy care of diabetic women reduce the risk of abnormal babies? *Br Med J* 1990, 301:1070–1074.

21. Kitzmiller JL, Gavin LA, Gin GD, Jovanovič L, *et al.*: Preconception care of diabetes: glycemic control prevents congenital anomalies. *JAMA* 1991, 265:731–736.

22. Metzger BE, Coustan DR: Proceedings of the Fourth International Workshop-Conference on Gestational Diabetes Mellitus. *Diabetes Care* 1998, 21(suppl):B1–B167.

23. HAPO Study Cooperative Research Group, Metzger BE, Lowe LP, *et al.*: Hyperglycemia and adverse pregnancy outcomes. *N Engl J Med* 2008, 358:1991–2002.

24. International Association of Diabetes and Pregnancy Study Groups Consensus Panel: International Association of Diabetes and Pregnancy Study Groups recommendations on the diagnosis and classification of hyperglycemia in pregnancy. *Diabetes Care* 2010, 33:676–691.

25. Ylinen K, Aula P, Stenman UH, *et al.*: Risk of minor and major fetal malformations in diabetics with high hemoglobin A_{1C} values in early pregnancy. *Br Med J* 1984, 289:345–346.

26. Jovanovič L, Peterson CM: Management of the pregnant diabetic woman. *Diabetes Care* 1980, 3:63–68.

27. Parretti E, Mecacci F, Papini M, *et al.*: Third trimester maternal glucose levels from diurnal profiles in non-diabetic pregnancies: correlation with sonographic parameters of fetal growth. *Diabetes Care* 2001, 24:1317–1323.

28. Murphy HR, Rayman G, Lewis, et al. Effectiveness of continuous glucose monitoring in pregnant women with diabetes: randomized clinical trial. *Br Med J* 2008, 337:a1680.

29. Jovanovič L, Saxena BB, Dawood MY, *et al.*: Feasibility of maintaining euglycemia in insulin-dependent diabetic women. *Am J Med* 1980, 68:105–112.

30. Greene MF, Hare JW, Cloherty JP, *et al.*: First-trimester hemoglobin A1 and risk for major malformation and spontaneous abortion in diabetic pregnancy. *Teratology* 1989, 39:225–231.

31. Jovanovič L, Knopp RH, Kim H, *et al.*: Elevated pregnancy losses at high and low extremes of maternal glucose in early normal and diabetic pregnancy: evidence for a protective adaptation in diabetes. *Diabetes Care* 2005, 28:1113–1117.

32. Jovanovic L: *Medical Management of Pregnancy Complicated by Diabetes*. Alexandria: American Diabetes Association; 1993, revised 1995, 2000, and 2009.

33. Jovanovič L, Crues J, Durak E, Peterson CM: Magnetic resonance imaging in pregnancies complicated by gestational diabetes predicts infant birth weight ratio and neonatal morbidity. *Am J Perinatol* 1993, 10:432–437.

34. Holden KP, Jovanovič L, Druzin ML, Peterson CM: Increased fetal activity with low maternal blood glucose levels in pregnancies complicated by diabetes. *Am J Perinatol* 1984, 1:161–164.

35. Wyatt JW, Frias JL, Hoyme HE, Jovanovič L, *et al.*: Congenital anomaly rate in offspring of pre-gestational diabetic women treated with insulin lispro during pregnancy. *Diabetic Med* 2004, 21:2001–2007.

36. Jovanovič L, Knopp RH, Brown A, *et al.*: Declining insulin requirements in the late first trimester of diabetic pregnancy. *Diabetes Care* 2001, 24:1130–1136.

37. Mathiesen ER, Kinsley B, Amiel SA, *et al.*: Maternal glycemic control and hypoglycemia in type 1 diabetic pregnancy. *Diabetes Care* 2007, 30:771–776.

38. Menon RK, Cohen RM, Sperling MA, *et al.*: Transplacental passage of insulin in pregnant women with insulin-dependent diabetes mellitus. Its role in fetal macrosomia. *N Engl J Med* 1990, 323:309–315.

39. Jovanovič L, Kitzmiller JL, Peterson CM: Randomized trial of human versus animal species insulin in diabetic pregnant

women: improved glycemic control, not fewer antibodies to insulin, influences birth weight. *Am J Obstet Gynecol* 1992, 167:1325–1330.

40. Jovanovič L, Mills JL, Peterson CM: Anti-insulin titers do not influence control or insulin requirements in early pregnancy. *Diabetes Care* 1984, 7:68

41. Jovanovič L, Ilic S, Pettitt DJ, *et al.*: The metabolic and immunologic effects of insulin lispro in gestational diabetes. *Diabetes Care* 1999, 22:1422–1427.

42. Pettitt DJ, Ospina P, Kolaczynski JW, Jovanovič L: Comparison of an insulin analog, insulin aspart, and regular human insulin with no insulin in gestational diabetes mellitus. *Diabetes Care* 2003, 26:183–186.

43. Jovanovič L, Peterson CM: The art and science of maintenance of normoglycemia in pregnancies complicated by type 1 diabetes mellitus. *Endocrinol Pract* 1996, 2:130.

44. Buchanan TA, Kjos SL, Montoro MN, *et al.*: Use of fetal ultrasound to select metabolic therapy for pregnancies complicated by mild gestational diabetes. *Diabetes Care* 1994, 17:275–283.

45. Kjos SL, Schaefer-Graf U, Sardesi S, *et al.*: A randomized controlled trial using glycemic plus fetal ultrasound parameters versus glycemic parameters to determine insulin therapy in gestational diabetes with fasting hyperglycemia. *Diabetes Care* 2001, 24:1904–1910.

46. Schaefer-Graf UM, Kjos SL, Fauzan OH, *et al.*: A randomized trial evaluating a predominantly fetal growth-based strategy to guide management of gestational diabetes in Caucasian women. *Diabetes Care* 2004, 27:297–302.

47. Langer O, Conway DL, Berkus MD, *et al.*: A comparison of glyburide and insulin in women with gestational diabetes mellitus. *N Engl J Med* 2000, 343:1134–1138.

48. Jovanovič L: Nutritional management of the obese gestational diabetic woman [guest editorial]. *J Am Coll Nutr* 1992, 11:246–250.

49. Jovanovič L: Time to reassess the optimal dietary prescription for women with gestational diabetes [editorial]. *Am J Clin Nutr* 1999, 70:3–4.

50. Peterson CM, Jovanovič L: Percentage of carbohydrate and glycemia response to breakfast, lunch, and dinner in women with gestational diabetes. *Diabetes* 1991, 40(suppl):172.

51. Jovanovič L, Durak EP, Peterson CM: Randomized trial of diet versus diet plus cardiovascular conditioning on glucose levels in gestational diabetes. *Am J Obstet Gynecol* 1989, 161:415–419.

52. Jovanovič L, Bevier W: The Santa Barbara County Health Care Services Program: birth weight change concomitant with screening for and treatment of glucose-intolerance of pregnancy: a potential cost-effective intervention. *Am J Perinatol* 1997, 14:221–228.

53. McCance DR, Pettitt DJ, Hanson RL, *et al.*: Birth weight and non-insulin dependent diabetes: thrifty genotype, thrifty phenotype, or surviving small baby genotype? *Br Med J* 1994, 308:942–945.

54. Zisser H, Jovanovič L, Thorsell A, *et al.*: The fidgety fetus hypothesis: fetal activity is an additional variable in determining birth weight of offspring of women with diabetes. *Diabetes Care* 2006, 29:63–67.

Mechanisms of Hyperglycemic Damage in Diabetes

Ferdinando Giacco and Michael Brownlee

All forms of diabetes are characterized by hyperglycemia, a relative or absolute lack of insulin action, and the development of diabetes-specific pathology in the retina, renal glomerulus, and peripheral nerve. Diabetes is also associated with accelerated atherosclerotic disease, which affects arteries that supply the heart, brain, and lower extremities. As a consequence of its disease-specific pathology, in the developed world diabetes mellitus is now the leading cause of new blindness in working-age people and the leading cause of end-stage renal disease (ESRD). More than 60% of diabetic patients are affected by neuropathy, which includes distal symmetrical polyneuropathy (DSPN), mononeuropathies, and a variety of autonomic neuropathies that cause erectile dysfunction, urinary incontinence, gastroparesis, and nocturnal diarrhea. Diabetic accelerated lower extremity arterial disease in conjunction with neuropathy accounts for more than 50% of all nontraumatic amputations in the USA [1]. Diabetes and insulin resistance increase cardiovascular disease risk three- to eightfold. Thus, over 30% of patients hospitalized with acute myocardial infarction have diabetes and 35% have impaired glucose tolerance [2]. Finally, new blood vessel growth in response to ischemia is impaired in diabetes, resulting in decreased collateral vessel formation in ischemic hearts and in non-healing foot ulcers [3]. Overall, diabetic microvascular complications are caused by prolonged exposure to high glucose levels. This finding has been established by large-scale prospective studies for both type 1 and type 2 diabetes by the Diabetes Control and Complications Trial/Epidemiology of Diabetes Interventions and Complications (DCCT/EDIC) [4] and the UK Prospective Diabetes Study (UKPDS) [5]. In contrast, hyperglycemia appears to play less of a role in the pathogenesis of diabetic macrovascular complications, in which the consequences of pathway-selective insulin resistance make a significant contribution.

This chapter reviews the mechanisms of hyperglycemia-induced damage in diabetes. The discussion includes the specificity of target organ damage, the five major mechanisms of hyperglycemia-induced damage and their common activating mechanism, the roles of insulin resistance, genetic determinants for the susceptibility of complications, and the unaltered rate of microvascular complication progression after significant improvement in control of hyperglycemia (hyperglycemic memory).

J.S. Skyler (ed.), Atlas of Diabetes: Fourth Edition,
DOI 10.1007/978-1-4614-1028-7_10, © Springer Science+Business Media, LLC 2012

Specificity of Target Organ Damage

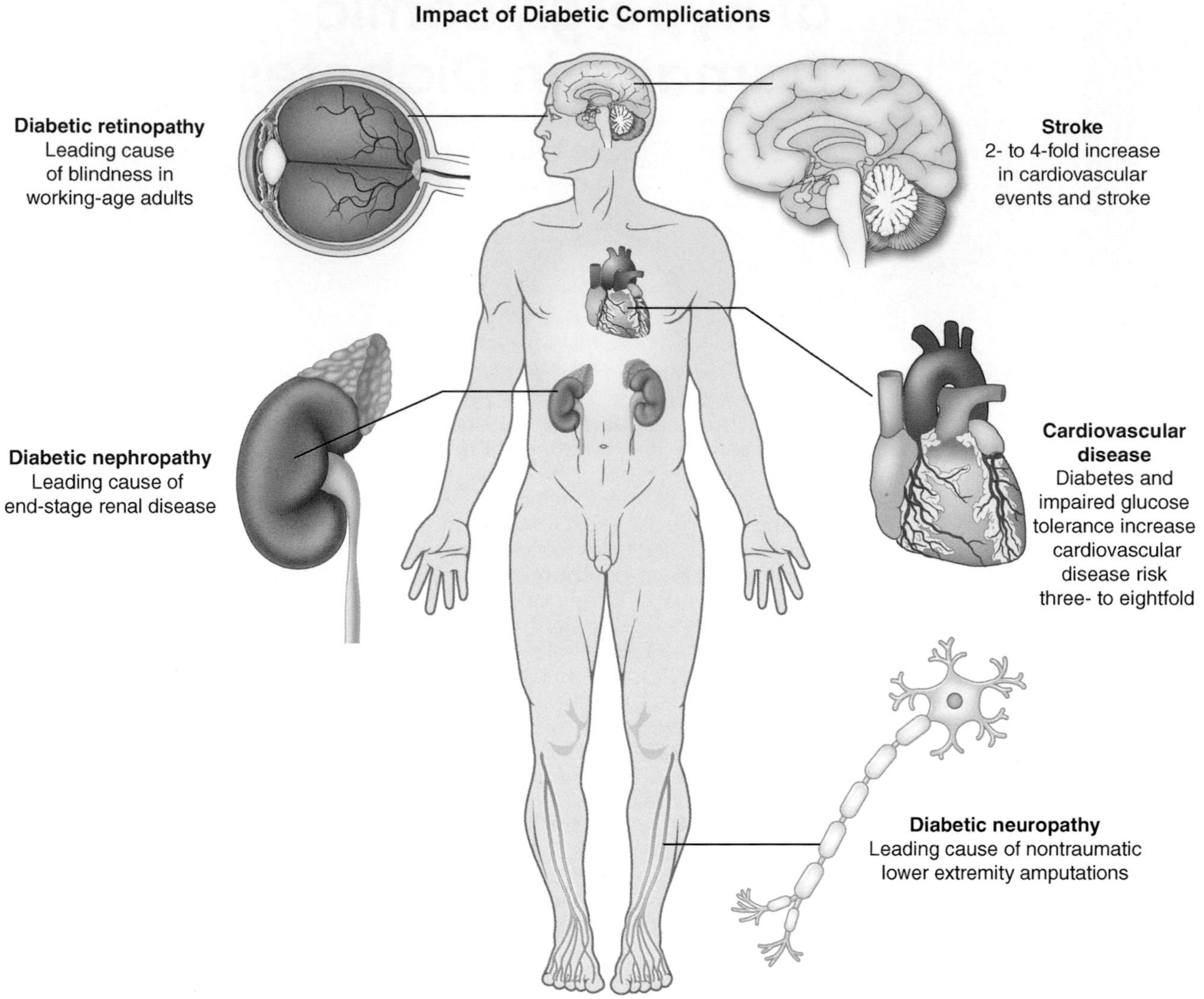

Impact of Diabetic Complications

Diabetic retinopathy
Leading cause
of blindness in
working-age adults

Stroke
2- to 4-fold increase
in cardiovascular
events and stroke

Diabetic nephropathy
Leading cause of
end-stage renal disease

Cardiovascular disease
Diabetes and
impaired glucose
tolerance increase
cardiovascular
disease risk
three- to eightfold

Diabetic neuropathy
Leading cause of nontraumatic
lower extremity amputations

Figure 10-1. Impact of diabetic complications. Diabetes mellitus is the leading cause of new blindness in working-age people and the leading cause of ESRD. More than 60% of diabetic patients are affected by neuropathy, which includes DSPN, mononeuropathies, and a variety of autonomic neuropathies that cause erectile dysfunction, urinary incontinence, gastroparesis, and nocturnal diarrhea. Diabetic neuropathy, in conjunction with accelerated lower extremity arterial disease, accounts for more than 50% of all nontraumatic amputations in the USA. Diabetes and impaired glucose tolerance increase cardiovascular disease risk three- to eightfold [1].

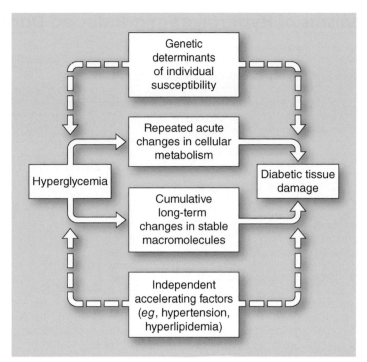

Figure 10-2. Mechanisms by which hyperglycemia and independent risk factors interact to cause chronic microvascular diabetic complications. One group of mechanisms involves repeated acute changes in cellular metabolism that are reversible when euglycemia is restored. Another group of mechanisms involves cumulative changes in long-living macromolecules that persist despite the restoration of euglycemia. These mechanisms are influenced by genetic determinants of susceptibility or resistance to hyperglycemic damage and by independent risk factors, such as hypertension and dyslipidemia [1] (adapted from Brownlee [6]).

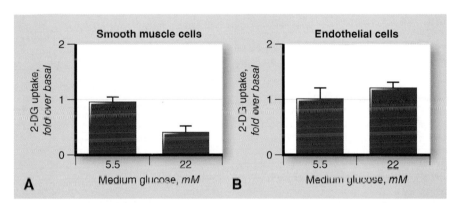

Figure 10-3. Target specificity of hyperglycemic damage. The targeting of specific cell types by generalized hyperglycemia reflects the failure of those cells to downregulate their uptake of glucose when extracellular glucose concentrations are elevated. **(A)** Cells that are not directly susceptible to direct hyperglycemic damage (e.g., vascular smooth muscle) show an inverse relationship between extracellular glucose concentra-tions and glucose transport, measured as 2-deoxyglucose uptake (2-DG). **(B)** Vascular endothelial cells, a major target of hyperglycemic damage, show no significant change in glucose transport rate when the glucose concentration is elevated, resulting in intracellular hyperglycemia. Thus, intracellular hyperglycemia appears to be the major determinant of tissue damage [7] (adapted from Kaiser et al. [7]).

Five Major Mechanisms of Hyperglycemia-Induced Damage

Mechanisms of Hyperglycemia-induced Damage
Increased flux of glucose and other sugars through the polyol pathway
Increased intracellular formation of AGEs
Increased expression of the receptor for advanced glycation end products and its activating ligands
Activation of PKC isoforms
Overactivity of the hexosamine pathway
AGEs—advanced glycation end products; PKC—protein kinase C.

FIGURE 10-4. Mechanisms of hyperglycemia-induced damage. There are nearly 20,000 publications that implicate five major mechanisms by which hyperglycemia causes diabetic complications, shown here. However, the results of clinical studies in which one of these pathways has been blocked pharmacologically have been disappointing, which led to the hypothesis, first proposed in 2000, that all five mechanisms are activated by a single upstream event: mitochondrial overproduction of the reactive oxygen species (ROS) superoxide caused by intracellular hyperglycemia. This provides a unifying hypothesis for understanding the pathogenesis of diabetic microvascular complications [6].

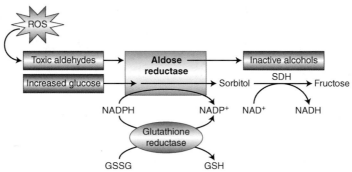

FIGURE 10-5. Hyperglycemia-induced increased polyol pathway flux. The polyol pathway involves the enzyme aldose reductase, which can utilize as substrates a number of toxic aldehydes generated during normal metabolism and by reactive oxygen species. When intracellular hyperglycemia is present, the classical representation holds that glucose is converted to sorbitol by aldose reductase. Sorbitol is then oxidized to fructose by the enzyme sorbitol dehydrogenase (SDH), with nicotinamide adenine dinucleotide (NAD$^+$) being reduced to its reduced form, NADH. Aldose reductase is found in tissues, such as nerve, retina, lens, glomerulus, and blood-vessel wall. A reduction of glucose to sorbitol by NADPH consumes the latter. Since NADPH is a cofactor required to regenerate reduced glutathione (GSH), an important scavenger of ROS, this could induce or exacerbate intracellular oxidative stress. Indeed, overexpression of human aldose reductase increased atherosclerosis in diabetic mice and reduced the expression of genes that regulate the regeneration of GSH. Reduced GSH is depleted in the lens of transgenic mice that overexpress aldose reductase and in diabetic rat lens compared to nondiabetic lens [8]. Glucose itself does not appear to be the substrate for aldose reductase in diabetic cells, however. The K_m (the concentration of substrate needed for half-maximal enzyme activity) of aldose reductase for glucose is 100 mM [9] while the intracellular concentration of glucose in diabetic endothelial cells is 30 nmol/mg protein [10]. Although the aldehyde form of glucose is a much better substrate for aldose reductase than are the ring forms [11], with a K_m of 0.66 µM for the aldehyde form of glucose, the aldehyde form of glucose represents only 0.002% of the total glucose [12]. Glycolytic metabolites of glucose, such as glyceraldehyde 3-phosphate, which is elevated in cells with intracellular hyperglycemia, may be the physiologically relevant substrate, since aldose reductase has a much higher affinity for this glycolytic metabolite. *NADP$^+$* nicotinamide adenine dinucleotide phosphate, *GSSG* glutathione disulfide, *NAD$^+$* nicotinamide adenine dinucleotide, *SDH* sorbitol dehydrogenase.

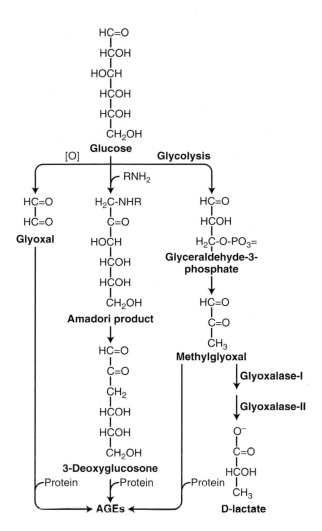

Figure 10-6. AGE formation. AGEs are formed by the reaction of glucose and other glycating compounds (e.g., dicarbonyls such as 3-deoxyglucosone, methylglyoxal, and glyoxal) with proteins and, to a lesser extent, nucleic acids. The reactions proceed through a series of stages, which are initially reversible and yield early glycation products, but eventually undergo irreversible changes that markedly impair the structural, enzymatic, or signaling functions of the glycated proteins. AGE can arise intracellularly from the auto-oxidation of glucose to glyoxal, the decomposition of an Amadori product to 3-deoxyglucosone, or the fragmentation of glyceraldehyde-3-phosphate to yield methylglyoxal. All of these reactive intracellular dicarbonyls react readily with uncharged amino groups of intracellular and extracellular proteins to form AGE. Methylglyoxal is the major intracellular AGE precursor [13].

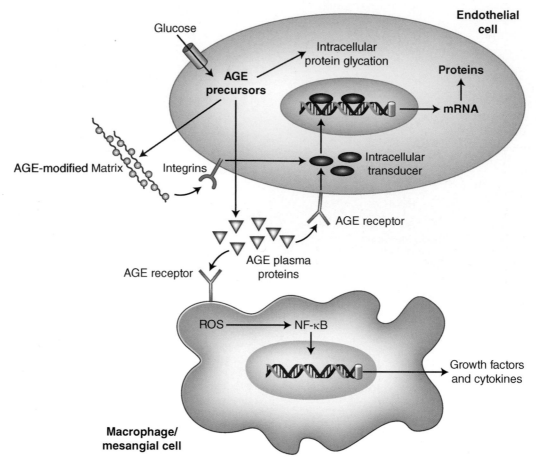

FIGURE 10-7. General mechanisms of AGE-induced damage. The intracellular production of AGE precursors can damage cells by three general mechanisms. First, intracellular proteins modified by AGE have altered functions that affect processes, such as gene transcription and protein degradation. Second, extracellular matrix components modified by AGE precursors interact abnormally with other matrix components and with matrix receptors (integrins) that are expressed on the surface of cells. Finally, plasma proteins modified by AGE precursors bind to AGE receptors on cells, such as macrophages; binding induces the production of ROS, which in turn activates the pleiotropic transcription factor, nuclear factor-kappa B (NF-κB), causing multiple pathological changes in gene expression. It has been demonstrated that AGE modification of intracellular protein can be involved in diabetic retinopathy. AGE formation alters the functional properties of several important matrix molecules. Collagen was the first matrix protein in which glucose-derived AGEs were shown to form covalent, intermolecular bonds. These AGE-induced cross-links alter tissue function, notably in blood vessels. AGEs decrease the elasticity in arteries from diabetic rats, even after vascular tone is abolished, and increase fluid filtration across the carotid artery. AGE formation on the extracellular matrix also interferes with the ways in which cells interact with the matrix. For example, the methylglyoxal modification of type IV collagen's cell-binding domains decreases endothelial-cell adhesion and inhibits angiogenesis [1].

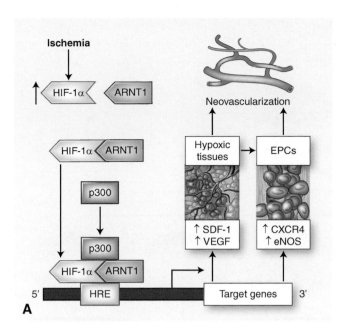

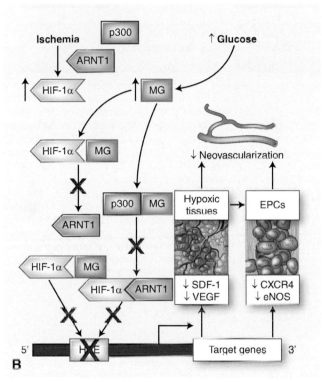

FIGURE 10-8. Effect of methylglyoxal (MG) AGE formation on hypoxia-inducible factor-1α (HIF1α)-mediated transcription and neovascularization in response to ischemia. Clinically, diabetes is associated with poor outcomes following acute vascular occlusive events, which results in part from a failure to form adequate compensatory microvasculature in response to ischemia. AGEs play a central role in this failure. High glucose induces a decrease in transactivation by the transcription factor HIF-1α, which mediates hypoxia-stimulated chemokine and vascular endothelial growth factor (VEGF) production by hypoxic tissue, as well as chemokine receptor and endothelial nitric oxide synthase (eNOS) expression in endothelial precursor cells in the bone marrow. Decreased HIF-1α functional activity is specifically caused by impaired HIF-1α–aryl hydrocarbon receptor nuclear translocator protein (ARNT-1) association and impaired binding of the coactivator p300. Hyperglycemia-induced covalent modification of HIF-1α and p300 by the dicarbonyl metabolite MG is responsible for this decreased association [14, 15]. *EPCs* endothelial progenitor cells, *HRE* hypoxia-responsive element, *SDF-1* stromal cell-derived factor-1.

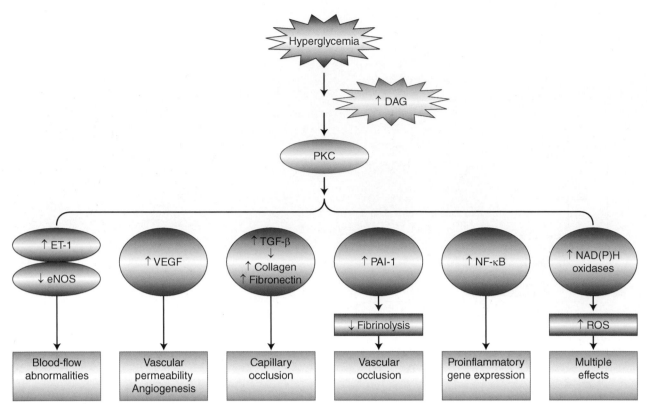

FIGURE 10-9. Hyperglycemia-induced increased PKC activation. PKC is a family of at least 11 isoforms that are widely distributed in mammalian tissues. The enzyme phosphorylates various target proteins. The activity of the classic isoforms is dependent on both Ca²⁺ ions and phosphatidylserine, and is greatly enhanced by diacylglycerol (DAG). The persistent and excessive activation of several PKC isoforms operates as a another common pathway-mediating tissue injury induced by hyperglycemia and associated biochemical and metabolic abnormalities. This results from enhanced de novo synthesis of DAG from glucose from the glycolytic intermediate triose phosphate and from the phospholipase cleavage of cell membrane lipids. Hyperglycemia primarily activates the β and δ isoforms of PKC, in cultured vascular cells and in the retina and glomeruli of diabetic animals, but increases in other isoforms have also been found, such as PKC-α, -ε, and -β isoforms in the retina, and PKC-α and -δ in the glomerulus of diabetic rats. In early experimental diabetes, the activation of PKC-β isoforms has been shown to mediate the diabetes-related decreases in retinal and renal blood flow, perhaps by depressing the production of the vasodilator nitric oxide (NO) by endothelial nitric oxide synthetase (eNOS) or increasing endothelin-1 (ET-1), a potent vasoconstrictor. The increased endothelial-cell permeability induced by high glucose in cultured cells is mediated by the activation of PKC-α-induced vascular endothelial cell growth factor (VEGF) production. PKC activation also causes the accumulation of microvascular matrix protein by inducing the expression of transforming growth factor-β1 (TGF-β1), fibronectin, and type IV collagen in both cultured mesangial cells and in glomeruli, as well as by overexpression of the fibrinolytic inhibitor, plasminogen activator inhibitor-1 (PAI-1). The activation of PKC can also activate the proinflammatory transcription factor NF-κB [16]. *ET-1* endothelin-1.

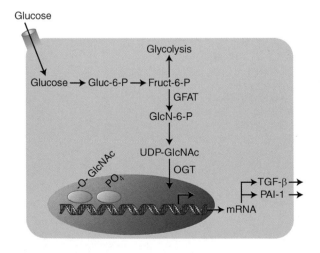

FIGURE 10-10. Hyperglycemia-induced increased hexosamine pathway flux. Hyperglycemia also contributes to the pathogenesis of diabetic complications by shunting glucose into the hexosamine pathway. In this pathway, fructose 6-phosphate (fruct-6-P) is diverted from glycolysis to provide substrate for the rate-limiting enzyme of this pathway, glutamine:fructose-6-phosphate amidotransferase (GFAT). GFAT converts fruct-6-P to glucosamine 6-phosphate, which is then converted to UDP-*N*-acetylglucosamine (UDP-GlcNAc) and is used by specific *O*-linked *N*-acetylglucosamine (*O*-GlcNAc) transferases for posttranslational modification of specific serine and threonine residues on cytoplasmic and nuclear proteins. The inhibition of GFAT blocks hyperglycemia-induced increases in the transcription of both TGF-β and PAI [17]. *OGT* GlcNAc transferase, *Gluc-6-P* glucose 6-phosphate.

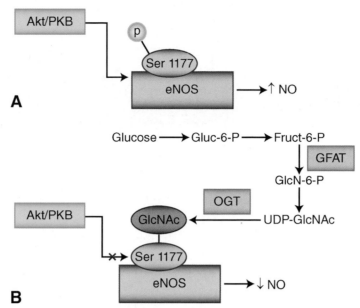

FIGURE 10-11. Effect of hyperglycemia-induced increased hexosamine pathway flux on endothelial cell function. eNOS is activated by the phosphorylation of serine 1177 by the protein kinase Akt/protein kinase B (PKB). (**A**) In aortic endothelial cells, hyperglycemia inhibits eNOS activity by 70%. The hyperglycemia-associated inhibition of eNOS is accompanied by a twofold increase in the *O*-GlcNAc modification of eNOS and a reciprocal decrease in O-linked serine phosphorylation at residue 1177. (**B**) Chronic impairment of eNOS activity by this mechanism may partly explain the accelerated atherosclerosis of diabetes [18].

Hyperglycemia-induced Damage: A Unifying Mechanism

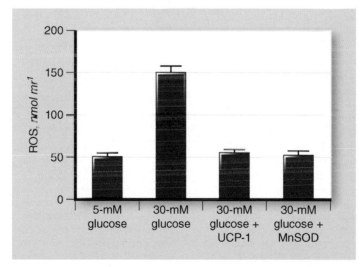

FIGURE 10-12. Intracellular hyperglycemia causes increased ROS production by the mitochondrial electron transport chain. Intracellular hyperglycemia increases ROS formation in aortic endothelial cells. However, hyperglycemia does not increase ROS when either the voltage gradient across the mitochondrial membrane is collapsed by uncoupling protein-1 overexpression (UCP-1) or when the superoxide produced is degraded by the mitochondrial isoform of manganese superoxide dismutase (MnSOD). Thus, intracellular hyperglycemia causes increased ROS production through the mitochondrial electron transport chain [19] (adapted from Nishikawa et al. [19]).

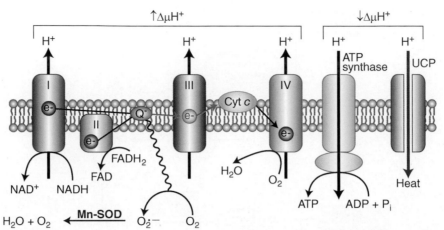

Figure 10-13. Production of superoxide by mitochondrial electron transport chain. In euglycemic conditions in endothelial cells, electron transfer through Complexes I, III, and IV extrude protons outward into the intermembrane space, generating a proton gradient that drives adenosine triphosphate (ATP) synthase (Complex V) as protons pass back through the inner membrane into the mitochondrial matrix. In contrast, in diabetic cells with high glucose inside, more glucose-derived pyruvate is oxidized in the tricarboxylic acid cycle, which increases the flux of electron donors (NADH and flavin adenine dinucleotide [FADH$_2$]) into the electron transport chain. As a result, the voltage gradient across the mitochondrial membrane increases until a critical threshold is reached. At this point, electron transfer inside Complex III is blocked, causing the electrons to back up to coenzyme Q, which donates the electrons one at a time to molecular oxygen, thereby generating superoxide. MnSOD degrades this oxygen-free radical to hydrogen peroxide, which is then converted to H$_2$O and O$_2$ by other enzymes [6]. *ADP* adenosine diphosphate, *FAD* flavin adenine dinucleotide, *NAD$^+$* nicotinamide adenine dinucleotide, *UCP* uncoupling protein.

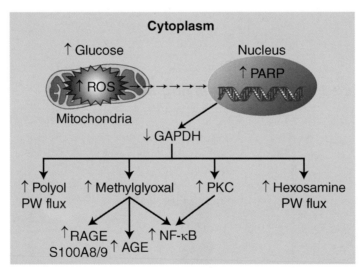

Figure 10-14. Hyperglycemia-induced mitochondrial overproduction of ROS activates all five major pathways of diabetic cellular damage. In cell types that develop intracellular hyperglycemia, the activity of the key glycolytic enzyme glyceraldehyde 3-phosphate dehydrogenase (GAPDH) is reduced. Hyperglycemia-induced ROS inhibit GAPDH activity by causing DNA double-strand breaks. This activates the nuclear DNA-repair enzyme poly(ADP-ribose) polymerase (PARP), which then modifies GAPDH with polymers of ADP-ribose. GAPDH is commonly thought to reside exclusively in the cytosol. However, it normally shuttles in and out of the nucleus, where it plays a critical role in DNA repair [20]. When GAPDH activity is inhibited, the levels of all the glycolytic intermediates that are upstream of GAPDH increase. These are then shunted into the five pathways (PWs) described earlier, resulting in increased polyol pathway flux, increased formation of methylglyoxal-derived AGEs that increase the expression of RAGE and endogenous RAGE ligands [21], activation of PKC, and increased flux through the hexosamine pathway [20].

Role of Insulin Resistance

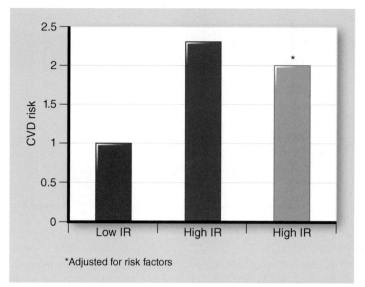

FIGURE 10-15. Insulin resistance (IR) and atherosclerosis. IR occurs in the majority of patients with type 2 diabetes and in two-thirds of subjects with impaired glucose tolerance. Both these groups have a significantly higher risk of developing cardiovascular disease (CVD). In order to isolate the effects of IR from those of hyperglycemia and diabetes, several studies have evaluated subjects with normal glucose tolerance. In nonobese subjects without diabetes, IR predicted the development of CVD independently of other known risk factors.

In another group of subjects without diabetes or impaired glucose tolerance, those in the highest quintile of IR had an approximately twofold increase in CVD risk compared with those in the lowest quintile after adjusting for 11 known cardiovascular risk factors, including low-density lipoprotein, triglycerides, high-density lipoprotein, systolic blood pressure, and smoking [22]. These data indicate that IR itself promotes atherogenesis in the absence of hyperglycemia (adapted from Hanley et al. [22]).

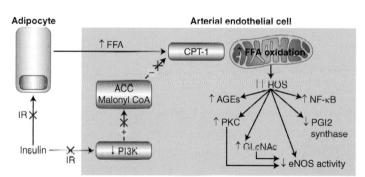

FIGURE 10-16. Insulin resistance causes fatty acid-induced ROS production, which activates proatherogenic pathways in arterial endothelium. IR in adipocytes increases the release of free fatty acids (FFAs) from stored triglycerides and inhibits the production of malonyl CoA by acetyl CoA carboxylase (ACC), which normally inhibits CPT-1 transfer of fatty acids into the mitochondria. This increased oxidation of FFAs in insulin-resistant aortic endothelial cells causes increased the production of superoxide by the mitochondrial electron transport chain. By activating the same mechanisms as hyperglycemia-induced ROS, FFA-induced overproduction of superoxide activates a variety of proinflammatory signals and also inactivates two important antiatherogenic enzymes: prostacyclin synthase and eNOS [23]. *CPT-1* carnitine palmitoyltransferase I, *PGI₂* prostacyclin (adapted from Brownlee [6]).

Genetics of Complications

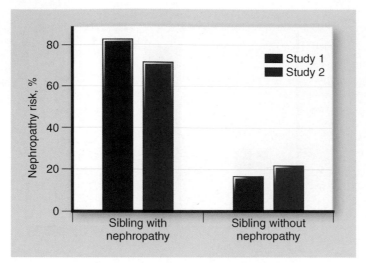

FIGURE 10-17. Familial clustering of diabetes complications. In two studies of families that have two or more siblings with type 1 diabetes mellitus, if one diabetic sibling had advanced diabetic nephropathy, the other diabetic sibling had a nephropathy risk of 83% and 72%, respectively. By contrast, the risk was only 17% or 22%, respectively, if the index patient did not have diabetic nephropathy or retinopathy [24, 25]. Similar results have been obtained with other diabetic microvascular complications.

Genetic Polymorphisms and the Risk of Diabetic Complications
HLA-DQB10201/0302 alleles
Aldose reducta se
Sorbitol dehydrogenase
Promoter of erythropoietin gene
Transcription factors and signaling molecules: *HNF1B1/TCF2, NRP1, PRKCB1, SMAD3* , and *USF1*
Components of the extracellular matrix and its degradation: *COL4A1, LAMA4,LAMC1 MMP9,* and *TIMP3*
Growth factors or growth factors receptors: *IGF1, TGFBR2,* and *TGFBR3*
Genes likely to be important in kidney function: *AGRT1, AQP1, BCL2, CAT, GPX1, LPL* , and *p22phox*
Multiple superoxide dismutase 1 variants

FIGURE 10-18. Summary of genetic polymorphisms associated with the risk of various diabetic complications. Numerous associations have been made between various genetic polymorphisms and the risk of various diabetic complications. Those include the *HLA-DQB10201/0302* alleles, polymorphisms of the aldose reductase gene and sorbitol dehydrogenase, and polymorphisms of the erythropoietin gene promoter. A study of type 1 diabetes among families of European descent showed a positive linkage and an association with diabetic nephropathy of simple tandem repeat polymorphisms and single nucleotide polymorphisms in 20 genes: five genes code for transcription factors and signaling molecules (*HNF1B1/TCF2, NRP1, PRKCB1, SMAD3,* and *USF1*); three genes code for components of the extracellular matrix (*COL4A1, LAMA4,* and *LAMC1*) and two involved in its degradation (*MMP9* and *TIMP3*); three genes code for growth factors or growth factor receptors (*IGF1, TGFBR2,* and *TGFBR3*); and other genes that are likely to be important in kidney function (*AGRT1, AQP1, BCL2, CAT, GPX1, LPL,* and *p22phox*). The DCCT/EDIC trial reported familial clustering and an association of multiple superoxide dismutase 1 variants with the development and progression of diabetic nephropathy [1].

Microvascular Complications Occur and Progress at the Same Rate for Years After Significant Improvement in Control of Hyperglycemia ("Hyperglycemic Memory")

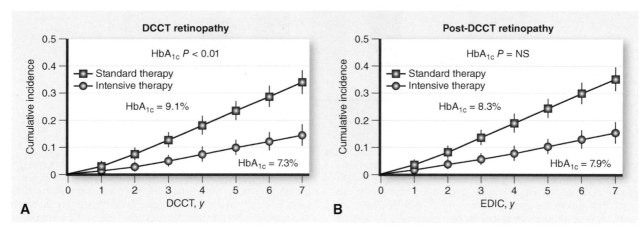

FIGURE 10-19. Hyperglycemic memory. In 1993, the results of the landmark DCCT study showed that, in people with short-duration type 1 diabetes, intensive glycemic control dramatically reduced the occurrence and severity of diabetic microvascular complications (**A**). The post-DCCT hemoglobin A_{1c} (HbA_{1c}) values for both groups soon became statistically identical and remained so during the 14 years of follow-up in the ongoing EDIC study (**B**). Surprisingly, the effects of a 6.5-year difference in HbA_{1c} during the DCCT on the rate of incidence of retinopathy and nephropathy have persisted [26]. This phenomenon has been given the name *glycemic memory*. *NS* not significant (adapted from Diabetes Control and Complications Trial/ Epidemiology of Diabetes Interventions and Complications Research Group [26]).

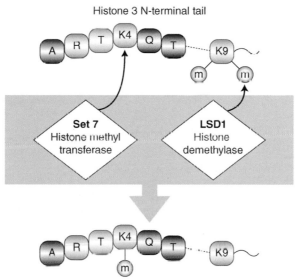

FIGURE 10-20. Short-term hyperglycemic memory in arterial cells (I). Posttranslational modifications of histones cause chromatin remodeling and changes in levels of gene expression. Since these modifications do not involve differences in DNA sequence, they are called "epigenetic." One of the best understood histone modifications is methylation. Hyperglycemia affects two histone-3 methylations in the NF-κB p65 promoter, both of which increase expression of this gene. One is the methylation of lysine 4 (*H3K4*), which results from the recruitment of a specific histone methyltransferase enzyme (Set 7) by hyperglycemia-induced ROS. The other is demethylation of lysine 9 in histone 3 (*H3K9*). This also occurs as a result of hyperglycemia-induced ROS, which recruits the specific histone demethylase LSD1 [27]. Similar epigenetic changes have been seen in lymphocytes from patients with type 1 diabetes [28] and in vascular smooth muscle cells derived from db/db mice [29, 30].

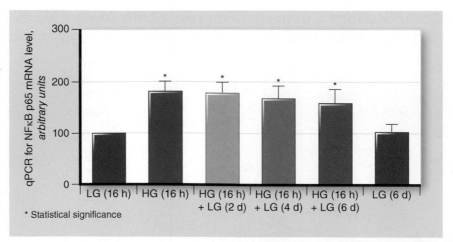

Figure 10-21. Short-term hyperglycemic memory in arterial cells (II). Transient hyperglycemia, at a level sufficient to increase mitochondrial ROS production, induces long-lasting activating epigenetic changes in the proximal promoter of the NF-κB subunit p65 in human aortic endothelial cells (16-h exposure). These epigenetic changes cause sustained increases in p65 gene expression and in the expression of p65-dependent proinflammatory genes. Both the epigenetic and gene-expression changes persist for at least 6 days of subsequent normal glycemia in cultured cells and in mice. These results highlight the dramatic and long-lasting effects that short-term hyperglycemic spikes can have on vascular cells and suggest that transient spikes of hyperglycemia may be an HbA_{1c}-independent risk factor for diabetic complications [31] (adapted from El-Osta et al. [31]).

References

1. Giacco F, Brownlee M: *Textbook of Diabetes*, 4th edn. Hoboken, NJ: Wiley; 2010.

2. Norhammar A, Tenerz A, Nilsson G, et al.: Glucose metabolism in patients with acute myocardial infarction and no previous diagnosis of diabetes mellitus: a prospective study. *Lancet* 2002, 359:2140–2144.

3. Abaci A, Oğuzhan A, Kahraman S, et al.: Effect of diabetes mellitus on formation of coronary collateral vessels. *Circulation* 1999, 99:2239–2242.

4. Diabetes Control and Complications Trial Research Group: The effect of intensive treatment of diabetes on the development and progression of long-term complications in insulin-dependent diabetes mellitus. *N Engl J Med* 1993, 329:977–986.

5. UK Prospective Diabetes Study (UKPDS) Group: Intensive blood-glucose control with sulphonylureas or insulin compared with conventional treatment and risk of complications in patients with type 2 diabetes (UKPDS 33). *Lancet* 1998, 352:837–853.

6. Brownlee M: The pathobiology of diabetic complications: a unifying mechanism. *Diabetes* 2005, 54:1615–1625.

7. Kaiser N, Sasson S, Feener EP, et al.: Differential regulation of glucose transport and transporters by glucose in vascular endothelial and smooth muscle cells. *Diabetes* 1993, 42:80–89.

8. Ramasamy R, Goldberg IJ: Aldose reductase and cardiovascular diseases, creating human-like diabetic complications in an experimental model. *Circ Res* 2010, 106:1449–1458.

9. Bohren KM, Grimshaw CE, Gabbay KH: Catalytic effectiveness of human aldose reductase. Critical role of C-terminal domain. *J Biol Chem* 1992, 267:20965–20970.

10. Zhang JZ, Gao L, Widness M, et al.: Captopril inhibits glucose accumulation in retinal cells in diabetes. *Invest Ophthalmol Vis Sci* 2003, 44:4001–4005.

11. Inagaki K, Miwa I, Okuda J: Affinity purification and glucose specificity of aldose reductase from bovine lens. *Arch Biochem Biophys* 1982, 216:337–344.

12. Bunn HF, Higgins PJ: Reaction of monosaccharides with proteins: possible evolutionary significance. *Science* 1981, 213:222–224.

13. Ahmed N, Thornalley PJ: Advanced glycation endproducts: what is their relevance to diabetic complications? *Diabetes Obes Metab* 2007, 9:233–245.

14. Thangarajah H, Yao D, Chang EI, et al.: The molecular basis for impaired hypoxia-induced VEGF expression in diabetic tissues. *Proc Natl Acad Sci U S A* 2009, 106:13505–13510.

15. Ceradini DJ, Yao D, Grogan RH, et al.: Decreasing intracellular superoxide corrects defective ischemia-induced new vessel formation in diabetic mice. *J Biol Chem* 2008, 283: 10930–10938.

16. Geraldes P, King GL: Activation of protein kinase C isoforms and its impact on diabetic complications. *Circ Res* 2010, 106:1319–1331.

17. Brownlee M: Biochemistry and molecular cell biology of diabetic complications. *Nature* 2001, 414:813–820.

18. Du XL, Edelstein D, Dimmeler S, et al.: Hyperglycemia inhibits endothelial nitric oxide synthase activity by posttranslational modification at the Akt site. *J Clin Invest* 2001, 108:1341–1348.

19. Nishikawa T, Edelstein D, Du XL, et al.: Normalizing mitochondrial superoxide production blocks three pathways of hyperglycaemic damage. *Nature* 2000, 404:787–790.

20. Du X, Matsumura T, Edelstein D, et al.: Inhibition of GAPDH activity by poly(ADP-ribose) polymerase activates three major pathways of hyperglycemic damage in endothelial cells. *J Clin Invest* 2003, 112:1049–1057.

21. Yao D, Brownlee M: Hyperglycemia-induced reactive oxygen species increase expression of the receptor for advanced glycation end products (RAGE) and RAGE ligands. *Diabetes* 2010, 59:249–255.

22. Hanley AJ, Williams K, Stern MP, Haffner SM: Homeostasis model assessment of insulin resistance in relation to the incidence of

cardiovascular disease: the San Antonio Heart Study. *Diabetes Care* 2002, 25:1177–1184.

23. Du X, Edelstein D, Obici S, *et al.*: Insulin resistance reduces arterial prostacyclin synthase and eNOS activities by increasing endothelial fatty acid oxidation. *J Clin Invest* 2006, 116: 1071–1080.

24. Seaquist ER, Goetz FC, Rich S, Barbosa J: Familial clustering of diabetic kidney disease. Evidence for genetic susceptibility to diabetic nephropathy. *N Engl J Med* 1989, 320:1161–1165.

25. Quinn M, Angelico MC, Warram JH, Krolewski AS: Familial factors determine the development of diabetic nephropathy in patients with IDDM. *Diabetologia* 1996, 39:940–945.

26. Diabetes Control and Complications Trial/Epidemiology of Diabetes Interventions and Complications Research Group: Retinopathy and nephropathy in patients with type 1 diabetes four years after a trial of intensive therapy. *N Engl J Med* 2000, 342: 381–389.

27. Brasacchio D, Okabe J, Tikellis C, *et al.*: Hyperglycemia induces a dynamic cooperativity of histone methylase and demethy-lase enzymes associated with gene-activating epigenetic marks that co-exist on the lysine tail. *Diabetes* 2009, 58:1229–1236.

28. Miao F, Smith DD, Zhang L, *et al.*: Lymphocytes from patients with type 1 diabetes display a distinct profile of chromatin histone H3 lysine 9 demethylation: an epigenetic study in diabetes. *Diabetes* 2008, 57:3189–3198.

29. Reddy MA, Villeneuve LM, Wang M, *et al.*: Role of the lysine-specific demethylase 1 in the proinflammatory phenotype of vascular smooth muscle cells of diabetic mice. *Circ Res* 2008, 103:615–623.

30. Villeneuve LM, Reddy MA, Lanting LL, *et al.*: Epigenetic histone H3 lysine 9 methylation in metabolic memory and inflammatory phenotype of vascular smooth muscle cells in diabetes. *Proc Natl Acad Sci U S A* 2008, 105:9047–9052.

31. El-Osta A, Brasacchio D, Yao D, *et al.*: Transient high glucose causes persistent epigenetic changes and altered gene expression during subsequent normoglycemia. *J Exp Med* 2008, 205:2409–2417.

11

Management and Prevention of Diabetic Complications

Sunder Mudaliar and Robert R. Henry

Type 2 diabetes is a chronic disease characterized by insulin resistance, impaired insulin secretion, and hyperglycemia. The long-term complications of diabetic retinopathy, nephropathy, neuropathy, and accelerated atherosclerosis lead to significant morbidity in the form of preventable blindness, end-stage renal disease (ESRD), limb amputations, and premature cardiovascular disease (CVD) [1]. Although patients with diabetes suffer from the morbidity of their microvascular complications, the majority of them ultimately die from the complications of macrovascular coronary artery disease (CAD).

A pathophysiologic hallmark of type 2 diabetes is insulin resistance, which has genetic and acquired components [2]. Glucose intolerance and hyperglycemia supervene only when the pancreatic β cell is unable to maintain compensatory hyperinsulinemia to overcome tissue resistance to insulin action [3]. In addition to having hyperglycemia and insulin resistance, nearly 80% of those who have diabetes are obese and have a host of other metabolic abnormalities, including dyslipidemia [increased small, dense, low-density lipoprotein (LDL) cholesterol, decreased high-density lipoprotein (HDL) cholesterol, and raised triglyceride levels], hypertension, and abnormalities of coagulation and the fibrinolytic system. This cluster of metabolic abnormalities, which has been termed the *metabolic syndrome* [4] or the *cardiovascular dysmetabolic syndrome* [5], is associated with a higher incidence of cardiovascular morbidity and mortality [6].

The major cause of tissue damage in diabetes is vascular disease in the micro- and macrovasculature [7, 8]. Four major molecular mechanisms have been implicated in glucose-mediated vascular damage. These include increased polyol pathway flux, increased flux through the hexosamine pathway, increased formation of diacylglycerol with subsequent activation of specific protein kinase C isoforms, and accelerated nonenzymatic formation of advanced glycation end products (AGEs). Recent evidence seems to suggest that each of these mechanisms is triggered by a single hyperglycemia-induced process of overproduction of superoxide by the mitochondrial electron transport chain [8]. The net result of these changes induced by hyperglycemia in diabetes is overproduction of potentially damaging reactive oxygen species and upregulation of cytokines and tissue growth factors. In insulin-resistant patients with type 2 diabetes, in addition to hyperglycemia, insulin resistance also plays a major role in the induction of macrovascular abnormalities and atherosclerotic CVD [4, 5].

The development of diabetic complications is no longer inevitable. Results from the UK Prospective Diabetes Study (UKPDS) clearly demonstrate that tight glucose and blood pressure (BP) control in patients with type 2 diabetes prevents the development of, and delays the progression of, microvascular complications and possibly macrovascular disease [9–11]. In addition, results from the UKPDS and other studies have shown that treatment of concomitant risk factors, such as lipids and BP, and the use of aspirin have favorable effects on cardiovascular complications in patients with type 2 diabetes [12]. However, the ultimate goal in the management of diabetes is the prevention of diabetes. Recent results from the Diabetes Prevention Program have shown that with intensive lifestyle modification, it is possible to delay or prevent the onset of type 2 diabetes in high-risk individuals [13].

J.S. Skyler (ed.), *Atlas of Diabetes: Fourth Edition*,
DOI 10.1007/978-1-4614-1028-7_11, © Springer Science+Business Media, LLC 2012

Complications of Diabetes

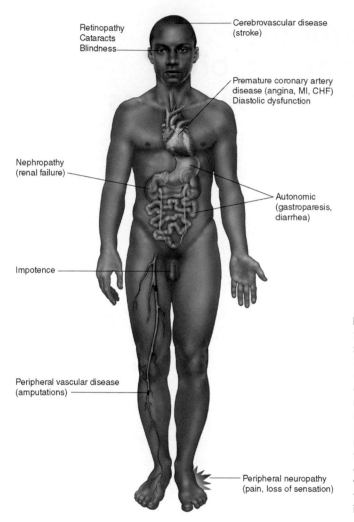

Retinopathy
Cataracts
Blindness

Cerebrovascular disease
(stroke)

Premature coronary artery
disease (angina, MI, CHF)
Diastolic dysfunction

Nephropathy
(renal failure)

Autonomic
(gastroparesis,
diarrhea)

Impotence

Peripheral vascular disease
(amputations)

Peripheral neuropathy
(pain, loss of sensation)

Figure 11-1. Clinical manifestations of diabetes. The complications of diabetes are protean and encompass nearly all organ systems. Diabetes is currently the leading cause of adult-onset blindness in the USA and it accounts for more than one-third of new cases of ESRD. Accelerated lower extremity arterial disease in diabetics with neuropathy is responsible for 50% of all nontraumatic amputations, and the death rate for CVD in diabetes patients is at least 2.5 times that in nondiabetic patients [1]. Heart disease appears earlier in type 2 diabetes and is more often fatal. Throughout their lives, diabetic individuals suffer from the microvascular complications of blindness, ESRD, and neuropathy, and, sooner rather than later, most patients with diabetes ultimately die from the complications of macrovascular CVD. *CHF* congestive heart failure, *MI* myocardial infarction.

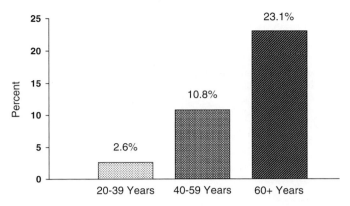

Estimated Prevalence of Diagnosed and Undiagnosed Diabetes in the US (2007)

Figure 11-2. Epidemiology of diabetes and its complications. Diabetes mellitus is an important clinical and public health problem in the USA. In 2007, nearly 23.6 million people – 7.8% of the population – were estimated to have diabetes. Of these, 17.9 million people were diagnosed and 5.7 million people were undiagnosed. In a recent study in newly screened people with diabetes, 19% had preexisting CVD, 97% were overweight or obese, 86% had hypertension, 75% had dyslipidemia, and 20% had microalbuminuria. Moreover, of those with hypertension, 35% were not prescribed drugs and 42% were suboptimally treated. Of participants with dyslipidemia, 68% were not prescribed medications and 22% were poorly controlled. Using the Framingham Risk Score, the median 10-year CVD risk was 38.6% in men and 24.6% in women [1, 14].

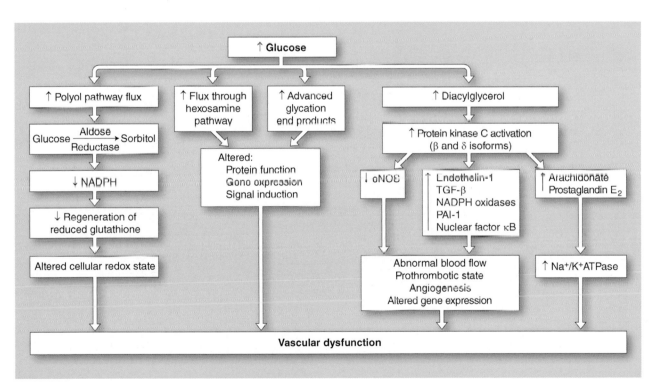

Figure 11-3. Possible cellular and molecular mechanisms of vascular disease in diabetes. Hyperglycemia in diabetes causes damage to many tissues, including the retina, kidneys, nerves, heart, brain, and skin. A major cause of tissue damage is vascular disease, which affects the micro- and macrovasculature. Hyperglycemia-induced mechanisms that induce vascular damage include increased polyol pathway flux, increased flux through the hexosamine pathway, increased formation of diacylglycerol and the subsequent activation of specific protein kinase C isoforms, and the accelerated nonenzymatic formation of AGEs. Each of these mechanisms contributes to vascular dysfunction through a number of mechanisms, including the production of vasodilatory prostaglandins, overproduction of potentially damaging reactive oxygen species, and upregulation of cytokines and growth factors. *eNOS* endothelial nitric oxide synthase, *NADPH* nicotinamide adenine dinucleotide phosphate, *PAI-1* plasminogen activator inhibitor-1, *TGF-β* transforming growth factor-β (adapted from King [7] and Brownlee [8]).

Diabetic Retinopathy

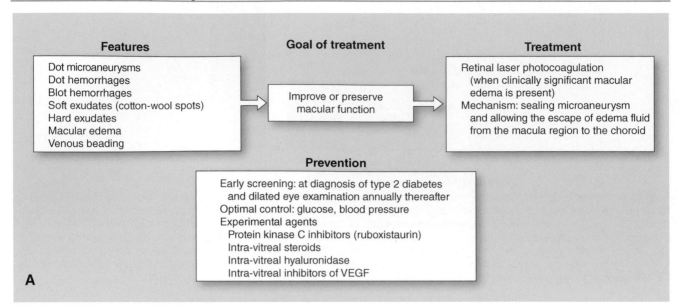

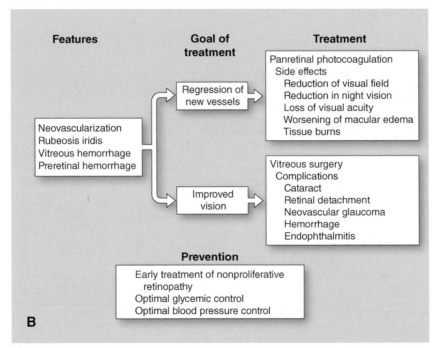

Figure 11-4. Clinical features and management of diabetic retinopathy. Diabetes is the leading cause of new blindness in adults. Retinopathy is present in a considerable proportion of patients who have type 2 diabetes at the time of diagnosis. After 15 or more years of disease, the risk of any retinopathy is approximately 78%, with approximately one-third of patients having macular edema and approximately one-sixth of patients having proliferative retinopathy [15]. Diabetic retinopathy may be classified as nonproliferative diabetic retinopathy (NPDR) or proliferative diabetic retinopathy (PDR). **(A)** NPDR is characterized by structural abnormalities of the retinal vessels (primarily the capillaries, but also the venules and arterioles), varying degrees of retinal nonperfusion, retinal edema, lipid exudates, and intraretinal hemorrhage. NPDR may be mild, moderate, or severe. **(B)** PDR is predicted by the presence of extensive areas of hemorrhages, microaneurysms, venous beading, or intraretinal microvascular abnormalities (tortuous dilated vessels adjacent to nonperfused areas of the retina). For patients with mild, moderate, or severe NPDR, the risk of developing PDR is 5%, 12–24%, and 50%, respectively [15]. All patients with type 2 diabetes should have a dilated eye examination at the time of diagnosis and annually, or more often, thereafter [16]. Preventing retinopathy is best accomplished by maintaining near-normal glycemia. After NPDR develops, intensive attempts should be made to optimize glucose and BP control, and clinically significant macular edema (i.e., retinal edema that threatens the fovea) should be treated with focal or grid photocoagulation, which reduces the risk of moderate visual loss by approximately 50%. Panretinal photocoagulation may be beneficial in PDR, along with measures to optimize glucose and BP control [15]. The UKPDS has confirmed that intensive blood glucose and BP control reduces the risk of retinopathy progression [9–11]. *VEGF* vascular endothelial growth factor.

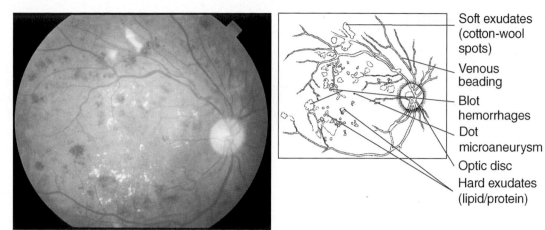

FIGURE 11-5. NPDR. The characteristic features of NPDR include dot aneurysms (hypercellular, saccular outpouchings of the capillary wall), blot hemorrhages resulting from vascular occlusion, cotton-wool spots (retinal nerve-fiber infarcts caused by ischemia), hard exudates (lipid and protein exudates caused by excessive vascular permeability), and venous beading (abnormal appearance of retinal veins with localized swellings and constrictions resembling sausage links) (courtesy of Dr. M. Goldbaum, UCSD/VA San Diego Health Care System, San Diego, CA).

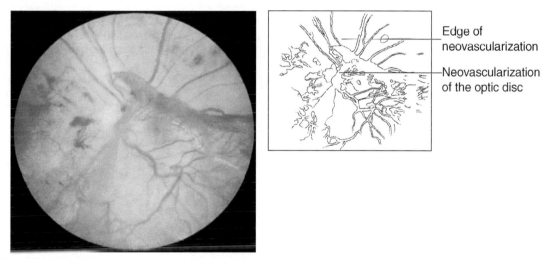

FIGURE 11-6. Classical features of PDR. The development of neovascularization is pathognomonic of this stage. The presence of new vessels on the optic nerve head or on more than one-fourth of the disc area, together with preretinal or vitreous hemorrhages, is indicative of high-risk PDR and is an absolute indication for panretinal photocoagulation, it technically possible (courtesy of Dr. M. Goldbaum, UCSD/VA San Diego Health Care System, San Diego, CA).

Diabetic Nephropathy

Urinary Albumin Excretion Rate

	Urinary AER, 24-h collection, *mg*	Timed collection, *µg/min*	Spot collection, *µg/mg creatinine*
Normal	< 30	< 20	< 30
Microalbuminuria	30–299	20–199	30–299
Miacroalbuminuria (overt neuropathy)	300 or greater	200 or greater	300 or greater

FIGURE 11-7. Urinary albumin excretion rate (AER). The incidence of ESRD in type 2 diabetes ranges from 4% to 20%. Because type 2 diabetes is ten times or more prevalent than type 1 diabetes, the incidence of ESRD is approximately the same in both types of diabetes [1]. In the USA, diabetic nephropathy accounts for about 40% of new cases of ESRD and, in 2001, the total annual medical costs incurred by all payers in managing diabetic nephropathy was 16.8 billion for all patients with diabetes [17].

A patient who does not have diabetes with normal kidneys excretes less than 30 mg of albumin every 24 h (20 µm/min) into the urine and, in a spot urine collection, has an albumin:creatinine ratio of less than 30 (mg of albumin/mg of creatinine). Microalbuminuria is present at the diagnosis in 3–30% of patients with type 2 diabetes. Without specific interventions, 20–40% of type 2 diabetes patients with microalbuminuria progress to overt nephropathy. However, 20 years after the onset of overt nephropathy, only approximately 20% have progressed to ESRD [18]. There is substantial evidence that the onset of microalbuminuria and progression of nephropathy correlate closely with poor glycemic control and, more importantly, that improved glycemic and BP control reduces the onset and progression of microalbuminuria and nephropathy [9–11, 19]. Screening for microalbuminuria should be performed at the time of diagnosis and annually thereafter by a random/spot urine albumin and creatinine measurement. (This test has good correlation with 24-h albumin measurements.) Because the urine AER is variable, two of three specimens collected within a 3- to 6-month period should be abnormal before a patient is considered to have crossed a diagnostic threshold. Exercise within the preceding 24 h, fever, heart failure, marked hyperglycemia, and marked hypertension may elevate the urine AER over borderline values [18].

Stages of Diabetic Nephropathy in Type 2 Diabetes

Asymptomatic	Renal insufficiency	End-stage renal disease
Normal GFR/creatinine	Decreasing GFR	Uremia
Hypertension	Increasing creatinine	Greatly increased creatinine
Microalbuminuria (30–300 mg/d)	Proteinuria > 500 mg/d	Greatly decreased GFR (< 15 mL/min)

FIGURE 11-8. Stages of diabetic nephropathy in type 2 diabetes. The natural history of nephropathy in type 2 diabetes is not as clear as it is in type 1 diabetes, for which five stages of nephropathy have been described: (1) an early stage of increased glomerular filtration, progressing through, (2) a stage of early glomerular lesions with glomerular basement thickening and mesangial matrix expansion, and on to (3) incipient diabetic nephropathy with microalbuminuria (urinary albumin 30–300 mg/day). Ultimately, (4) clinical nephropathy with overt proteinuria over 500 mg/day and a declining glomerular filtration rate (GFR) develop and culminate in, (5) ESRD. The early stages of nephropathy have not yet been well-documented in type 2 diabetes (data from Friedman [20]).

Measures to Prevent or Retard Diabetic Nephropathy

Optimal glycemic control: HbA$_{IC}$ < 7% (caution in the elderly and in those with multiple co-morbid conditions)

Adequate BP control: < 130/80 mm Hg (caution in those with autonomic neuropathy)

ACE inhibitors and ARBs (when microalbuminuria is present with urinary albumin 30–300 mg/d)

Dietary protein restriction (when overt neuropathy is present with urinary protein > 500 mg/d or when there is a strong family history of neuropathy)

Experimental

Aminoguanidine (inhibits AGE formation)

Protein kinase C inhibitors

Renin inhibitor (aliskiren)

Figure 11-9. Measures to prevent or retard diabetic nephropathy. In the UKPDS, tight glycemic control (with a median hemoglobin A$_{1c}$ [HbA$_{1c}$] of <7%) and BP control (with a mean BP of 144/82 mmHg) were associated with reductions in the progression of microalbuminuria [9–11]. More recently, in the Microalbuminuria, Cardiovascular, and Renal Outcomes-Heart Outcomes Prevention Evaluation (MICRO-HOPE) study [21], 3,577 subjects with type 2 diabetes were randomized to placebo or 10 mg/day of ramipril, an angiotensin-converting enzyme inhibitor. The study was stopped 6 months early (after 4.5 years) because ramipril had consistent benefits in not only reducing the risk of overt nephropathy by 16%, but also was associated with significant reductions in the risk of MI, stroke, cardiovascular mortality, and all-cause mortality by approximately 30%. *ACE* angiotensin-converting enzyme, *ARBs* angiotensin receptor blockers.

Diabetic Neuropathy

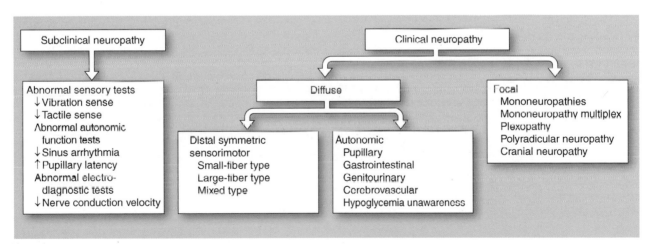

Figure 11-10. Clinical features of diabetic neuropathy. Diabetic neuropathy is one of the most common complications of diabetes. Its clinical manifestations cause much suffering among diabetic patients. Acute hyperglycemia decreases nerve function and chronic hyperglycemia is characterized by a progressive loss of nerve fibers, a loss that can be assessed noninvasively by several tests of nerve function, including quantitative sensory tests, autonomic function tests, and electrophysiologic testing [22].

Clinical Features of Distal Sensorimotor Diabetic Neuropathy

Large fiber type	Small fiber type
Unsteady gait	Pain predominates
Absent reflexes	Variable reflexes
Decreased vibration/position sense	Variable position/vibration sense
Charcot's joints available	Variable presence of Charcot's joints
Mimics posterior column lesions	Ultimately leads to sensory loss

Figure 11-11. Distal sensorimotor diabetic neuropathy.

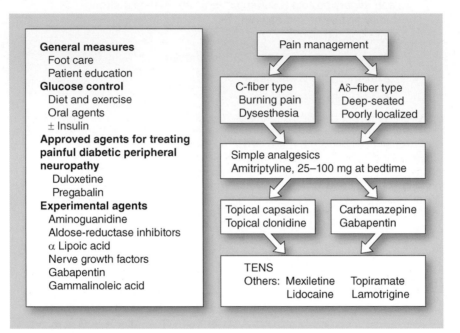

Figure 11-12. Management of peripheral diabetic neuropathy. The pathophysiologic mechanisms underlying decreased nerve function and nerve fiber loss in diabetics still are not fully understood but may include the formation of sorbitol by aldose reductase and the formation of AGEs [22]. Similar to other diabetic complications, the progression of neuropathy is related to glycemic control. Chronic sensory neuropathy with moderate or severe sensory loss involving large-fiber sensation (touch, vibration, and joint position sense) or small-fiber sensation (pain and temperature sense) is associated with a high risk of ulceration. Current approaches to the prevention and treatment of diabetic neuropathy include measures to optimize glucose control, measures for pain control (duloxetine and pregabalin are approved for the treatment of painful diabetic neuropathy) and the use of aldose reductase inhibitors, which appear to slow the progression of neuropathy rather than provide symptomatic relief [23]. *TENS* transcutaneous electrical nerve stimulation.

Diabetic Foot Disease

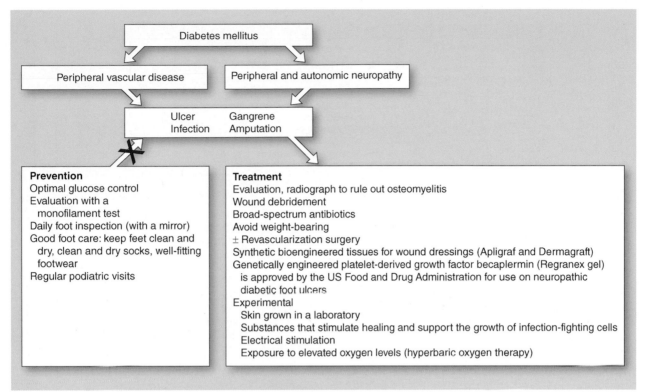

FIGURE 11-13. Clinical features and management of diabetic foot disease. Diabetic foot lesions are a major cause of hospitalization, with approximately 20% of all patients with diabetes entering the hospital due to foot problems. Nearly 55,000 lower extremity amputations are performed on diabetic individuals each year in the USA, accounting for 50% of all nontraumatic amputations [24]. Diabetic foot lesions are the result of a combination of peripheral and autonomic neuropathy and peripheral vascular disease (ischemia). The cascade of events begins with foot ulcers, infection, and gangrene, ultimately resulting in amputation. Management of diabetic foot ulcers should be aggressive and should include a detailed evaluation of the ulcer and the foot, radiography to exclude osteomyelitis, broad-spectrum antibiotics, wound debridement (If indicated), and avoidance of weight bearing. Topical application of antibacterial agents and platelet-derived growth factors may be useful adjunctive measures. Preventive measures include optimal glycemic control; daily foot inspections (with the aid of a mirror); good foot care (keeping the feet clean and dry); wearing clean socks and appropriate, well-fitting shoes; and regular podiatric visits. Good patient education and a team approach are the keys to the prevention and treatment of diabetic foot disease.

Diabetic individuals are particularly prone to foot deformities and the development of cocked-up toes, which results in pressure at the tips of the toes and under the first metatarsal head, leading to ulceration and infection. The ideal treatment is prophylactic surgery to straighten the toes. If this is not feasible, special shoes with a cushioned insole to protect the toes and metatarsal head should be worn. All patients with diabetes should have the protective sensory function in their feet evaluated with a 10 g Semmes–Weinstein monofilament. If a patient cannot consistently feel a 10-g monofilament, protective sensory function has been lost and the patient is at a high risk of developing foot ulcers [25].

Diabetic Male Sexual Dysfunction

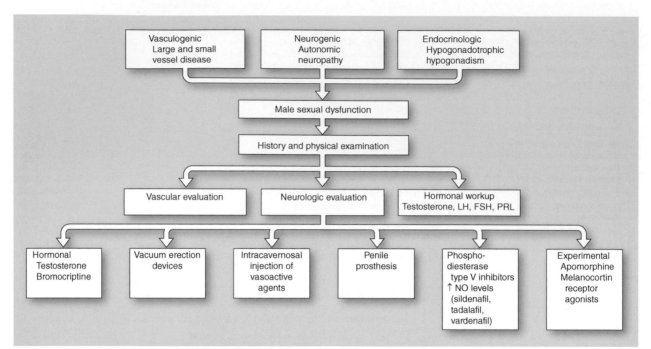

Figure 11-14. Evaluation and management of diabetic male sexual dysfunction. The prevalence of erectile dysfunction in diabetic men ranges from 35% to 75%, significantly higher than that in the general population [26]. Its onset is insidious and may occur early in diabetes. The major underlying abnormalities are vascular (cavernosal artery insufficiency, corporal veno-occlusive dysfunction) and neurologic (autonomic neuropathy). The role of hormonal abnormalities is controversial. All diabetic men with erectile dysfunction require a detailed endocrinologic workup [luteinizing hormone (LH), follicle-stimulating hormone (FSH) prolactin (PRL), and testosterone levels] and, in select cases, vascular evaluation (intracavernosal injection test, visual sexual stimulation, and penile duplex ultrasonography) and neurologic evaluation (nocturnal penile tumescence test, cavernosal electrical activity potential, somatosensory-evoked potentials, and sacral latency test). Treatment options include hormonal therapy, if indicated (testosterone replacement in hypogonadism, bromocriptine or surgery for prolactinomas, discontinuation of medications causing hyperprolactinemia); vacuum erection devices; intracavernosal injection of vasoactive agents; penile prostheses (in selected cases); and the recently introduced phosphodiesterase V inhibitors sildenafil, vardenafil, and tadalafil, which act by increasing nitric oxide (NO) levels.

Cardiovascular Disease in Diabetes

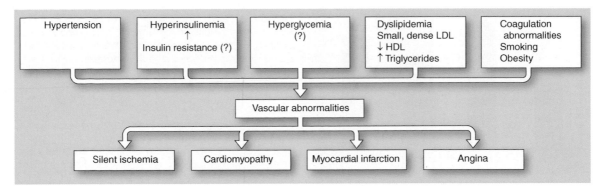

FIGURE 11-15. Pathogenesis and clinical features of heart disease in diabetes. The risk for CVD in patients with diabetes is two to four times that in nondiabetic persons [1]. At the time of diagnosis of type 2 diabetes, nearly 20% of patients have preexisting CAD [14]. Numerous risk factors contribute to macrovascular dysfunction in type 2 diabetes. Some conditions appear to be related to the insulin resistance and hyperinsulinemia that is characteristic of the early stages of type 2 diabetes before the onset of pancreatic β-cell exhaustion and overt hyperglycemia, and include the various components of the cardiovascular dysmetabolic syndrome (i.e., hypertension, central obesity, dyslipidemia, glucose intolerance, and coagulation abnormalities) [5]. Heart disease in diabetics may result in silent myocardial ischemia or manifest as angina, MI, or CHF (diabetic cardiomyopathy).

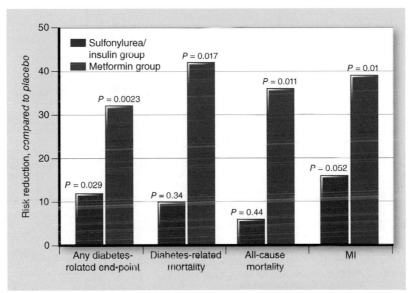

FIGURE 11-16. Results: The UKPDS. The UKPDS was a large study in which 5,102 subjects with newly diagnosed type 2 diabetes were followed for an average of 10 years to determine whether intensive glucose lowering reduces cardiovascular and microvascular complications and to determine the benefits and disadvantages of sulfonylureas, metformin, and insulin [9, 10]. The UKPDS results demonstrated that although microvascular complications are decreased by nearly 25% by lowering HbA$_{1c}$ to a median of 7% (compared with 7.9% in the conventional group), there was no significant effect on cardiovascular complications, with only a nonsignificant 16% reduction in the risk of combined fatal or nonfatal MI. However, an epidemiologic analysis showed a continuous association between the risk of cardiovascular complications and glycemia such that for every percentage point decrease in HbA$_{1c}$ (e.g., 9–8%), there was a 25% reduction in diabetes-related deaths, a 7% reduction in all-cause mortality, and an 18% reduction in fatal or nonfatal MI.

In the subgroup of obese diabetic subjects treated with metformin, intensive glucose lowering with a median HbA$_{1c}$ of 7.4% (compared with 8.0% in the conventional group) was associated with significantly decreased risks of diabetes-related deaths, all-cause mortality, and MI [10]. However, in a surprise outcome, in obese subjects with diabetes in this substudy, who had metformin added to the existing sulfonylurea treatment, there was a significant increase in all-cause and diabetes-related mortality and no beneficial effects on cardiovascular or microvascular outcomes. In the UKPDS, reassuringly, tight BP control (144/82 vs. 154/87 mmHg) was associated with significant reductions in virtually all cardiovascular and microvascular outcomes [11].

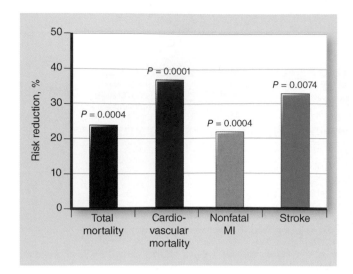

Figure 11-17. Microalbuminuria, Cardiovascular, and Renal Outcomes-Heart Outcomes Prevention Evaluation (MICRO-HOPE) study results. In contrast to the UKPDS, which studied patients with newly diagnosed diabetes, the landmark MICRO-HOPE study randomized 3,577 patients with long-standing (mean about 12 years' duration) type 2 diabetes to treatment with placebo or ramipril (an angiotensin-converting enzyme inhibitor) [21]. The study was stopped 6 months early (after 4.5 years) because 10 mg/day of ramipril significantly lowered the risk of all the measured cardiovascular outcomes, including fatal and nonfatal MI, stroke, nephropathy, and all-cause and cardiovascular mortality by 22% to 37%. The cardiovascular benefit in this study was greater than that attributable to the small decrease in BP seen in this study and also additive to those of baseline therapeutic agents, which included aspirin, lipid-lowering agents, and other BP-lowering drugs.

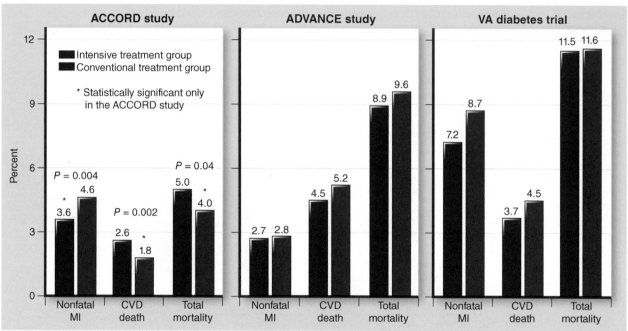

Figure 11-18. Comparison of diabetes studies: Action to Control Cardiovascular Risk in Diabetes (ACCORD), Action in Diabetes and Vascular Disease: Preterax and Diamicron MR Controlled Evaluation (ADVANCE), and Veterans Affairs (VA). Although intensive glucose control significantly reduces microvascular complications in patients with diabetes, there is as yet no clear evidence that it improves macrovascular CVD outcomes. Data from recent studies (the ACCORD study, the ADVANCE study, and the VA Diabetes Trial) showed that intensive glycemic control (HbA$_{1c}$ 6.3–6.9% vs. 7–8.5%) had no significant effect on CVD outcomes. In the ACCORD study, in the intensively treated group, there was slightly increased cardiovascular and all-cause mortality, especially in older patients with long-standing type 2 diabetes and preexisting CVD [27–29]. Based on these studies, the American Diabetes Association recommends an HbA$_{1c}$ target of less than 7%, provided this can be achieved without hypoglycemia and other adverse side effects of antidiabetic treatment [19]. Less-stringent HbA$_{1c}$ goals may be appropriate in older patients with advanced micro- and macrovascular complications, other comorbid conditions, and a history of severe hypoglycemia with treatment. In all patients, treatment should begin early and include intensive efforts to promote a healthy lifestyle and aggressively control cholesterol, blood pressure, and other CVD risk factors.

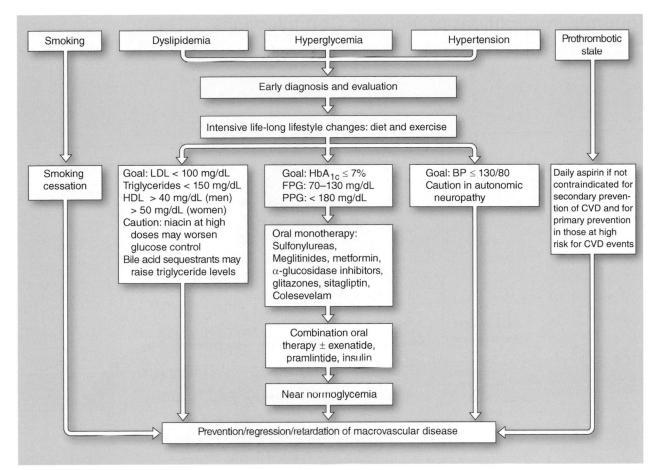

FIGURE 11-19. Multifactorial approach to the management of CVD in diabetes. Multiple risk factors contribute to accelerated atherosclerosis and premature CAD in patients with diabetes. The cornerstone of prevention is aggressive intervention to identify and favorably modify established risk factors, including hyperglycemia, hyperlipidemia, and hypertension. Due to the extremely high risk of macrovascular disease in diabetes, the National Cholesterol Education Program has recently designated diabetes as a "CAD risk equivalent" [4]. Therefore, in patients with diabetes, the target LDL cholesterol level should be less than 100 mg/dL, the target HDL cholesterol goal should be above 40 mg/dL in men and 50 mg/dL in women, and the triglyceride goal should be less than 150 mg/dL [30]. Unless contraindicated, all eligible patients with diabetes should take aspirin daily [19, 31]. The importance of lifestyle changes and strict adherence to dietary and exercise recommendations should be emphasized at all times. The success of a focused, multifactorial intervention approach with continued patient education and motivation, as well as strict targets, was demonstrated in the recently concluded steno-2 study. In this study, patients in the group assigned to intensive multifactorial intervention not only achieved significantly better glycemic control, bp, and lipid parameters, but also had a significantly lower risk of cardiovascular and microvascular events by approximately 50% [32]. *FPG* fasting plasma glucose, *PPG* postprandial glucose.

Economic Implications of Diabetic Complications

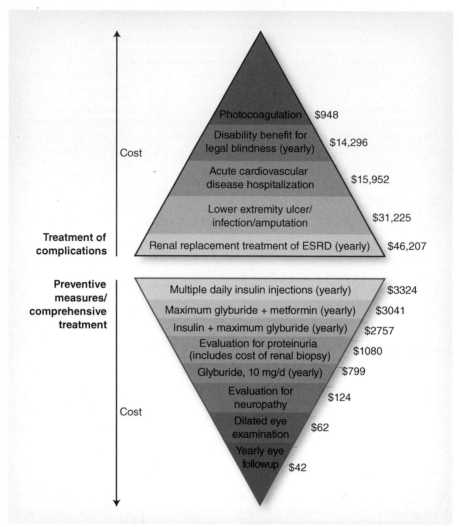

FIGURE 11-20. Dollar cost of diabetic complications: Prevention versus treatment. The annual expense of treating diabetes and its complications in the USA (most of which is for treatment of type 2 diabetes) is estimated at about $174 billion [17]. Not only is type 2 diabetes costly, but it also causes excessive morbidity and mortality. Analysis of data has shown that preventing this disease is not only preferable to treatment, but is also more cost-effective. This figure compares the cost of comprehensive treatment of diabetes with medications and preventive measures with the monumental costs of treating disease complications, such as retinopathy, nephropathy, neuropathy, foot disease, and CVD. It has been estimated that comprehensive treatment of type 2 diabetes with hemoglobin A_{1c} values maintained at 7.2% will reduce the cumulative incidence of blindness by 72%, ESRD by 87%, and lower extremity amputation by 67%. CVD risk is increased by 3%, and life expectancy is increased by 1.39 years. The estimated incremental cost per quality-adjusted life year gained is $16,002. This efficiency of treating type 2 diabetes is similar to that for screening and treating hypertension and is in the range of interventions considered to be cost-effective. Treatment is more cost-effective for those with earlier onset of diabetes, minorities, and those with higher hemoglobin A_{1c} under standard care (data from Eastman et al. [33]).

Future Directions: Prevention of Type 2 Diabetes

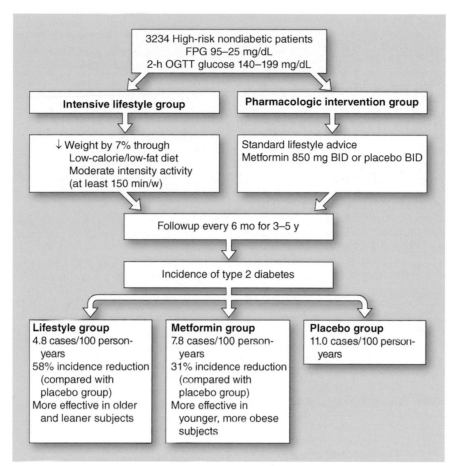

FIGURE 11-21. Prevention of type 2 diabetes. It is now clear that type 2 diabetes is not a milder form of diabetes. Its complications can be the same as or more severe than those of type 1 diabetes. Moreover, these complications occur early during the natural course of the disease, even before the disease's clinical onset.

Results from several large randomized studies, including the UKPDS, have confirmed that treatment of hyperglycemia, hypertension, and hyperlipidemia may prevent or retard the progression of diabetic complications [9–12].

However, even with early intervention and intensive treatment, type 2 diabetes has significant morbidity and high costs. Ultimately, preventing or delaying the onset of diabetes may be more cost-effective than treatment [13]. Impaired glucose tolerance (IGT) with fasting plasma glucose (110–125 mg/dL) or 2-h postoral glucose tolerance test (OGTT) glucose (140–199 mg/dL) has been shown to be a strong risk factor for the development of type 2 diabetes and a possible risk factor for CAD. Data suggest that at this stage of IGT, patients are at high risk for diabetes and CAD but have not yet developed end-organ disease.

The Diabetes Prevention Program (DPP), which was supported by the National Institutes of Health, was designed to determine if it is possible to prevent or delay the progression to type 2 diabetes through lifestyle changes or pharmacologic intervention in high-risk patients with IGT [13]. The DPP study randomized 3,234 high-risk subjects with IGT to either an intensive lifestyle intervention arm or pharmacologic or placebo treatment with standard lifestyle advice. The study was stopped 1 year early (average follow up 2.8 years) due to a significant reduction in the incidence of diabetes in the lifestyle arm of the study. Subjects randomized to a low-calorie and low-fat diet combined with moderate-intensity physical activity lost an average of 5.6 kg and had a 58% reduction in the incidence of diabetes over 2.8 years. However, pharmacologic treatment with metformin 850 mg twice daily (BID) resulted in only a 31% reduction in the incidence of diabetes compared with placebo.

In the recent past, several randomized controlled trials have demonstrated that individuals at high risk for developing diabetes [those with impaired fasting glucose (fasting plasma glucose 100–125 mg/dL) and IGT (plasma glucose after 75 gm of glucose between 140–199 mg/dL)] can significantly decrease their chances of developing diabetes with the help of interventions, like intensive lifestyle modification, and use of the pharmacologic agents, like metformin, acarbose, orlistat, and thiazolidinediones. These interventions have been shown to decrease incident diabetes by 25–60% [19].

References

1. http://diabetes.niddk.nih.gov/DM/PUBS/statistics/ Accessed September 5, 2009.

2. De Fronzo RA: Lilly Lecture 1987: The triumvirate: β cell, muscle, liver. A collusion responsible for NIDDM. *Diabetes* 1988, 37:667–687.

3. Pratley RE, Weyer C: The role of impaired early insulin secretion in the pathogenesis of type II diabetes mellitus. *Diabetologia* 2001, 44:929–945.

4. Reaven GM: Insulin resistance, the insulin resistance syndrome, and cardiovascular disease. *Panminerva Med* 2005, 47:201–210.

5. Fagan TC, Deedwania PC: The cardiovascular dysmetabolic syndrome. *Am J Med* 1998, 105:77 S–82 S.

6. Wilson PW, D'Agostino RB, Parise H, *et al.*: Metabolic syndrome as a precursor of cardiovascular disease and type 2 diabetes mellitus. *Circulation* 2005, 112:3066–3072.

7. Brownlee M. The pathobiology of diabetic complications: a unifying mechanism. *Diabetes* 2005, 54:1615–1625.

8. Brownlee M: Biochemistry and molecular cell biology of diabetic complications. *Nature* 2001, 414:813–820.

9. UK Prospective Diabetes Study Group: Intensive blood-glucose control with sulfonylurea or insulin compared with conventional treatment and risk of complications in patients with type 2 diabetes (UKPDS 33). *Lancet* 1998, 352:837–853.

10. UK Prospective Diabetes Study Group: Effect of intensive blood-glucose control with metformin on complications in overweight patients with type 2 diabetes (UKPDS 34). *Lancet* 1998, 352:854–865.

11. UK Prospective Diabetes Study Group: Tight blood pressure control and risk of macrovascular and microvascular complications in type 2 diabetes: UKPDS 38. *BMJ* 1998, 7160:703–713.

12. Buse JB, Ginsberg HN, Bakris GL, *et al.*: American Heart Association; American Diabetes Association. Primary prevention of cardiovascular diseases in people with diabetes mellitus: a scientific statement from the American Heart Association and the American Diabetes Association. *Circulation* 2007, 115:114–126.

13. Diabetes Prevention Program Research Group: Reduction in the incidence of type 2 diabetes with lifestyle intervention or metformin. *N Engl J Med* 2002, 346:393–403.

14. Echouffo-Tcheugui JB, Sargeant LA, Prevost AT, *et al.*: How much might cardiovascular disease risk be reduced by intensive therapy in people with screen-detected diabetes? *Diabet Med* 2008, 25:1433–1439.

15. Fong DS, Aiello LP, Ferris FL 3 rd, *et al.*: Diabetic retinopathy. *Diabetes Care* 2004, 27:2540–2553. .

16. American Diabetes Association: Position statement: diabetic retinopathy. *Diabetes Care* 2004, 27:S84–S87.

17. Gordois A, Scuffham P, Shearer A, Oglesby A: The health care costs of diabetic nephropathy in the United States and the United Kingdom. *J Diabetes Complicat* 2004, 18:18–26.

18. American Diabetes Association: Position statement: diabetic nephropathy. *Diabetes Care* 2004, 27:S79–S83.

19. American Diabetes Association: Clinical practice recommendations 2009. *Diabetes Care* 2011, 34:1–61.

20. Friedman E: Renal syndromes in diabetes. *Endocrinol Metab Clin North Am* 1996, 25:293–324.

21. Heart Outcomes Prevention Evaluation Study Investigators: Effects of ramipril on cardiovascular and microvascular outcomes in people with diabetes mellitus: results of the HOPE study and MICRO-HOPE substudy. *Lancet* 2000, 355:253–259.

22. Harati Y: Diabetic neuropathies: unanswered questions. *Neurol Clin* 2007, 25:303–317.

23. Vinik A, Ullal J, Parson HK, *et al.*: Diabetic neuropathies: clinical manifestations and current treatment options. *Nat Clin Pract Endocrinol Metab* 2006, 2:269–281.

24. Frykberg RG, Zgonis T, Armstrong DG, *et al.*: Diabetic foot disorders. A clinical practice guideline (2006 revision). *J Foot Ankle Surg* 2000, 39(Suppl 5):S1–S60.

25. American Diabetes Association: Position statement: preventive foot care in diabetes. *Diabetes Care* 2004, 27:S63–S64.

26. Hidalgo-Tamola J, Chitaley K: Review type 2 diabetes mellitus and erectile dysfunction. *J Sex Med* 2009, 6:916–926.

27. Action to Control Cardiovascular Risk in Diabetes Study Group, Gerstein HC, Miller ME, *et al.*: Effects of intensive glucose lowering in type 2 diabetes. *N Engl J Med* 2008, 358:2545–2559.

28. ADVANCE Collaborative Group, Patel A, MacMahon S, *et al.*: Intensive blood glucose control and vascular outcomes in patients with type 2 diabetes. *N Engl J Med* 2008, 358: 2560–2572.

29. Duckworth W, Abraira C, Moritz T, *et al.*: VADT investigators. Glucose control and vascular complications in veterans with type 2 diabetes. *N Engl J Med* 2009, 360:129–139.

30. American Diabetes Association: Position statement: management of dyslipidemia in adults with diabetes mellitus. *Diabetes Care* 2004, 27:S68–S71.

31. American Diabetes Association: Position statement: aspirin therapy in diabetes. *Diabetes Care* 2004, 27:S72–S73.

32. Gaede P, Vedel P, Larsen N, *et al.*: Multifactorial intervention and cardiovascular disease in patients with type 2 diabetes. *N Engl J Med* 2003, 348:383–393.

33. Eastman RC, Javitt JC, Herman WH, *et al.*: Model of complications in NIDDM: Analysis of the health benefits and cost-effectiveness of treating NIDDM with the goal of normoglycemia. *Diabetes Care* 1997, 20:735–744.

12

Eye Complications of Diabetes

Lloyd Paul Aiello, Paolo S. Silva, and Jennifer K. Sun

Diabetic retinopathy is a well-characterized, sight-threatening, chronic, ocular disorder that eventually develops, to some degree, in nearly all patients with diabetes mellitus. With experienced ophthalmic evaluation, diabetic retinopathy can be detected in its early stages. Existing therapies are remarkably effective at preventing some types of visual loss when administered at the appropriate time in the disease process. In addition, improved systemic glycemic control is associated with a delay in onset and slowing of progression of diabetic retinopathy. Nevertheless, diabetic retinopathy is the leading cause of new cases of legal blindness, as well as of severe and moderate visual loss among Americans between the ages of 20 and 74 years. The pathologic changes associated with diabetic retinopathy are similar in types 1 and 2 diabetes mellitus, although there is a higher risk of more frequent and severe ocular complications in type 1 diabetes [1]. However, because more patients have type 2 than type 1 disease, patients with type 2 disease account for a higher proportion of those with visual loss.

Most visual loss associated with diabetes results from either new vessel growth on the retina [proliferative diabetic retinopathy (PDR)] or increased retinal vascular permeability [diabetic macular edema (DME)]. The clinical stage associated with the greatest risk of severe visual loss is termed *high-risk PDR*, while the stage with the greatest risk of moderate visual loss is termed *clinically significant macular edema* (CSME). In the USA, an estimated 700,000 persons have PDR, 130,000 have high-risk PDR, 500,000 have macular edema, and 325,000 have CSME [2–5]. An estimated 63,000 cases of PDR, 29,000 of high-risk PDR, 80,000 of macular edema, and 56,000 of CSME, as well as 5,000 new cases of legal blindness occur yearly as a result of diabetic retinopathy [1, 6]. Blindness has been estimated to be 25 times more common in persons with diabetes than in those without the disease [7, 8].

Estimates of the medical and economic impact of retinopathy-associated morbidity have been performed using computer simulations. The models predict that if patients with type 1 disease receive treatment as recommended in the clinical trials in the absence of good glycemic control, a savings of $624 million and 173,540 person-years of sight would be realized [3, 4]. The Diabetes Control and Complication Trial (DCCT) showed that the rate of development of any retinopathy and, once present, the rate of retinopathy progression were significantly reduced after 3 years of intensive insulin therapy [9, 10]. Subsequent studies have confirmed a continuing benefit of intensive insulin therapy [11]. Applying DCCT intensive insulin therapy to all persons with insulin-dependent diabetes mellitus in the USA would result in a gain of 920,000 person-years of sight, although the costs of intensive therapy are three times that of conventional therapy [12, 13].

An understanding of the pathogenesis, natural history, and available treatment options for patients with diabetic retinopathy is critical for all health-care providers because current therapeutic options can be remarkably effective at preventing severe visual loss when administered in an appropriate and timely manner. Indeed, with appropriate medical and ophthalmologic care, over 90% of severe visual loss resulting from PDR can be prevented [14, 15].

J.S. Skyler (ed.), *Atlas of Diabetes: Fourth Edition*,
DOI 10.1007/978-1-4614-1028-7_12, © Springer Science+Business Media, LLC 2012

Anatomy, Symptoms, and Pathology

Overall, the International Classification of Diabetic Retinopathy and Diabetic Macular Edema simplifies descriptions of the categories of diabetic retinopathy, but is not a replacement for ETDRS levels of diabetic retinopathy in large-scale clinical trials or studies in which precise retinopathy classification is required.

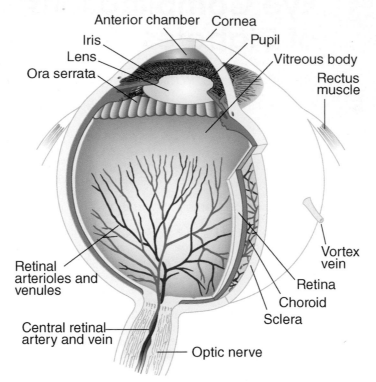

Figure 12-1. Normal ocular anatomy. This schematic cross-section shows the normal anatomy of the human eye. Diabetes can affect almost all ocular structures (see Fig. 12.2). However, the characteristic and most common changes occur in the retina and are termed *diabetic retinopathy*. Most of the severe sight-threatening complications involve either pathologic growth of vessels (neovascularization) in the retina or increased retinal vessel permeability [15]. These conditions are termed *PDR* and *DME*, respectively. Neovascularization also can arise at the iris, potentially leading to neovascular glaucoma.

Ocular Structures Affected by Diabetes	
Ocular Structure	**Diabetes associated Pathology**
Lids, nerves, and muscles	Palsy of cranial nerves III, IV, or VI
Cornea	Reduced sensitivity
	Increased susceptibility to corneal erosions
	Increased susceptibility to infection (corneal ulcers)
Anterior chamber	Hyphema (blood)
	Shallowing with longer disease duration
Iris	Neovascularization
	Depigmentation
Lens	Increased susceptibility to cataract
Vitreous	Vitreous hemorrhage
	Early posterior vitreous detachment
	Asteroid hyalosis
Retina	Retinal hemorrhage
	Microaneurysm
	VB
	IRMAs
	Capillary loss
	Neovascularization
	Edema
	Lipid deposits
Optic disc	Neovascularization
	Diabetic papillopathy (swelling)
Sclera and other tissues	Delayed wound healing

FIGURE 12-2. Diabetes can affect most structures of the human eye [16]. Diabetes-induced ischemia of cranial nerves III, IV, and VI can result in drooping of the lids, ocular motility abnormalities, or both as a result of impaired innervation of the ocular muscles. Corneal erosions, corneal ulcers, cataracts, and delayed wound healing also reflect the general diabetic state. However, most vision loss associated with diabetes arises from complications involving neovascularization of the retina (or iris) or increased vasopermeability of the retinal vasculature. *IRMAs* intraretinal microvascular abnormalities, *VB* venous beading.

Clinical Presentations of Diabetic Eye Complications	
Diabetes-associated Pathology	**Clinical Symptoms**
Palsy of cranial nerves III, IV, and VI	Diplopia (binocular)
	Ptosis
	Anisocoria
	"Blurred vision"
Reduced corneal sensitivity or corneal erosions or corneal infections	Ocular pain
	Ocular discharge
	Corneal opacification
	Decreased vision
Hyphema	Decreased vision
	Blood layering in anterior chamber
Angle closure glaucoma	Ocular pain
	"Halos" around light
	Decreased vision
Iris neovascularization	Ocular pain
	Decreased vision
	Blood layering in anterior chamber
Cataract	Decreased vision
	Glare with bright light
Vitreous hemorrhage	"Spots," "cobwebs," "lines" in vision (floaters)
	Decreased vision
Macular edema	Moderately decreased vision
	Image distortion
Proliferative diabetic retinopathy	Symptoms associated with vitreous hemorrhage and macular edema
Retina detachment	Photopsia
	Floaters
	Scotoma
	Decreased vision
	Image distortion
Diabetic papillopathy	Visual field change

FIGURE 12-3. Clinical presentations associated with diabetic eye complications. Each of the numerous diabetes-associated ocular pathologies can present with a diverse array of symptoms. Only a partial list is presented here. It is important to realize that serious diabetic eye disease may exist without any discernible symptoms. This fact underscores the essential need for regular, routine, life-long follow-up regardless of the presence or absence of visual symptoms.

Ocular Pathology Associated with Retinopathy Progression	
Disease Stage	Common Pathologic Changes
Preclinical stages	Alterations in cellular biochemistry
	Alterations in retinal blood flow
	Loss of retinal pericytes
	Thickening of basement membranes
Early stages Mild NPDR	Retinal vascular microaneurysms and blot hemorrhages
	Increased retinal vascular permeability
	Cotton wool spots
Middle stages	Venous caliber changes or beading
Moderate NPDR	IRMAs
Severe NPDR	Retinal capillary loss
Very severe NPDR	Retinal ischemia
	Extensive intraretinal hemorrhages a nd microaneurysms
Advanced stage	Neovascularization of the disc
PDR	NVE
	NVI
	Neovascular glaucoma
	Pre-retinal and vitreous hemorrhage
	Retinal traction, retinal tears, and retinal detachment

FIGURE 12-4. Ocular pathology associated with progression of diabetic retinopathy. Diabetic retinopathy generally progresses through well-characterized stages. Each stage is associated with typical pathologic changes. Some degree of clinically apparent retinopathy occurs in nearly all patients with diabetes of 20 or more years' duration, although preclinical alterations in blood flow, pericyte number, and basement membrane thickness can occur much earlier [17]. The clinical stages before the development of neovascularization are termed *nonproliferative diabetic retinopathy* (NPDR). NPDR is subdivided into mild, moderate, severe, or very severe categories, depending on the type and extent of clinical pathology present. Increased vascular permeability can occur at this or any later stage. As the disease progresses, a gradual loss of the retinal microvasculature results in retinal ischemia. Venous caliber abnormalities, IRMAs, and more severe vascular leakage are common reflections of this increasing retinal nonperfusion (see Fig. 12.8). Once ischemia-induced neovascularization occurs, the disease is referred to as PDR (see Fig. 12.10). Neovascularization can arise at the optic disc (neovascularization of the disc) or elsewhere in the retina [called *neovascularization elsewhere* (NVE)]. The new vessels are fragile and prone to bleeding, resulting in vitreous hemorrhage. With time, the neovascularization tends to undergo fibrosis and contraction, resulting in retinal traction, retinal tears, vitreous hemorrhage, and retinal detachment (see Fig. 12.14). New vessels also can arise on the iris, resulting in neovascular glaucoma (see Fig. 12.15). *NVI* neovascularization of the iris (adapted from Aiello et al. [15]).

International Clinical Diabetic Retinopathy and Diabetic Macular Edema Scale	
Level of Diabetic Retinopathy	Findings
No apparent retinopathy	No abnormalities
Mild NPDR	Microaneurysms only
Moderate NPDR	More than microaneuysms, but less than severe NPDR
Severe NPDR	Any of the following: > 20 intraretinal hemorrhages in each four retinal quadrants; definite VB in two or more retinal quadrants; prominent IRMA in one or more retinal quadrants; and no PDR
PDR	
Level of DME	Findings
DME apparently absent	No apparent retinal thickening or hard exudates (HE) in posterior pole
DME apparently present	Mild DME: Some retinal thickening or HE in posterior pole, but distant from center of the macula
	Moderate DME: Retinal thickening or HE approaching the center, but not involving the center
	Severe DME: Retinal thickening or HE involving the center of the macula

FIGURE 12-5. International Clinical Diabetic Retinopathy and Diabetic Macular Edema scale. To simplify classification and standardize communications between health-care providers worldwide, in 2001 the American Academy of Ophthalmology initiated a project to establish a consensus International Classification of Diabetic Retinopathy and Diabetic Macular Edema [18, 19]. The consensus panel relied on evidence-based studies including the Early Treatment Diabetic Retinopathy Study (ETDRS) and the Wisconsin Epidemiologic Study of Diabetic Patients.

Nonproliferative Diabetic Retinopathy

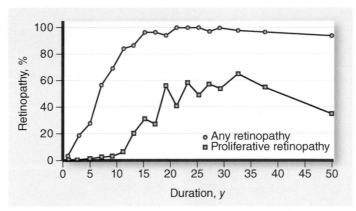

Figure 12-6. Incidence prevalence of diabetic retinopathy by duration of diabetes. The percentage of patients developing either any diabetic retinopathy or PDR is presented as a function of the duration of type 1 diabetes in years. Note that almost all patients have some evidence of diabetic retinopathy once the duration of diabetes exceeds 15 years. In addition, the incidence prevalence of PDR is negligible within 5 years of the onset of diabetes, although nearly 60% of patients eventually will develop PDR. These observations serve as the foundation for clinical care recommendations concerning the appropriate timing of initial ophthalmologic evaluation, as detailed in Fig. 12.7 (adapted from Krolewski et al. [20]).

Initial Ophthalmologic Examination Schedule		
Age at Onset of Diabetes Mellitus	**Recommended First Examination**	**Minimum Routine Followup***
29 years or younger	Within 3–5 years after diagnosis of diabetes	Yearly
	Once patient is 10 years of age or older	
30 years or older	At time of diagnosis of diabetes	Yearly
Pregnancy	Prior to conception and during the first trimester	Physician discretion pending results of first-trimester examination

*Abnormal findings necessitate more frequent followup.

Figure 12-7. Schedule for initial ophthalmologic examination. Only approximately 25% of patients with type 1 diabetes will have any retinopathy after 5 years, although most eventually will develop the disease (see Fig. 12.6) [21]. The prevalence of PDR is less than 2% at 5 years. For patients with type 2 disease, however, the onset date of diabetes frequently is not known precisely; thus, more severe disease can be observed soon after diagnosis. Up to 3% of patients first diagnosed after age 30 may have CSME or high-risk PDR at the initial diagnosis of diabetes [22]. Thus, in patients over 10 years of age, the initial ophthalmic examination is recommended beginning 5 years after the diagnosis of type 1 diabetes mellitus and on diagnosis of type 2 diabetes mellitus [15]. The onset of vision-threatening retinopathy is rare in children before puberty, regardless of the duration of diabetes; however, if diabetes is diagnosed between 10 and 30 years of age, significant retinopathy may arise within 6 years [2]. Puberty can accelerate the progression of retinopathy. Thus, the initial ophthalmic evaluation is recommended within 3–5 years of diagnosis, once the patient is 10 years of age or older [15, 23]. The onset of puberty is occurring progressively earlier and, consequently, the timing of the initial evaluation of children is under periodic review. Diabetic retinopathy also can become particularly aggressive during pregnancy in women with diabetes [24]. Ideally, patients with diabetes who are planning pregnancy should have an eye examination within 1 year of conception. Pregnant women should have a comprehensive eye examination in the first trimester of pregnancy. Close follow-up throughout pregnancy is indicated, with subsequent examinations determined by the findings present at the first-trimester examination. This guideline does not apply to women who develop gestational diabetes because they are not at increased risk of developing diabetic retinopathy (adapted from Aiello et al. [15]).

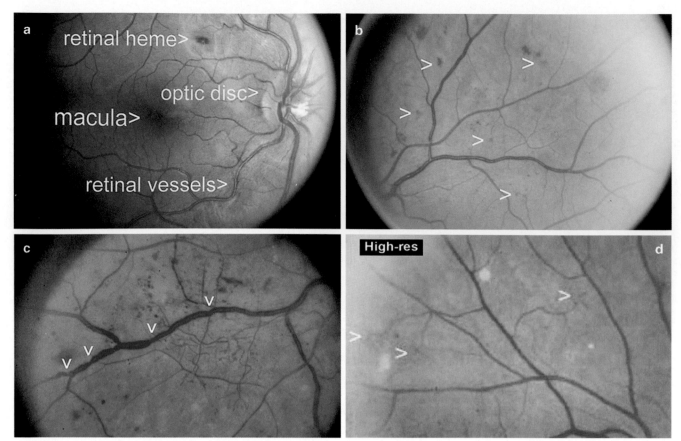

Figure 12-8. Characteristic findings in NPDR. The classic findings associated with NPDR are demonstrated. (**A**) The central region of the human retina is called the macula and is responsible for detailed vision. This patient's right eye has minimal diabetic retinopathy and the retina is normal except for a single retinal hemorrhage (retinal heme). The optic disc is located nasal to the macula and the retinal vessels emanate from the optic disc and surround the macula. (**B**) Retinal blot hemorrhages (*arrow heads*) and microaneurysms, which are saccular dilations of the vessel wall, are shown. These lesions often are two of the earliest clinically observed abnormalities. The patient has severe NPDR when hemorrhages and microaneurysms of this extent or greater in all four quadrants of the retina are observed. (**C**) Venous caliber changes are referred to as *VB*.

This finding often represents more advanced retinopathy, as is evident in this photograph (*arrow heads*). Two or more retinal quadrants of any VB (not necessarily as pronounced as shown) signify severe NPDR. (**D**) *Arrow heads* show IRMAs. IRMAs are abnormalities within the retina and may be a harbinger of early retinal neovascularization. IRMAs often are associated with more advanced NPDR and only one or more retinal quadrants of IRMAs of this or greater extent represent severe NPDR. Note that the clinical findings associated with severe NPDR therefore may be quite subtle. Any two or more of the findings associated with severe NPDR place the patient in the "very severe" category of NPDR [(**B**–**D**) from the Early Treatment Diabetic Retinopathy Study Research Group [25], with permission].

Proliferative Diabetic Retinopathy and Macular Edema

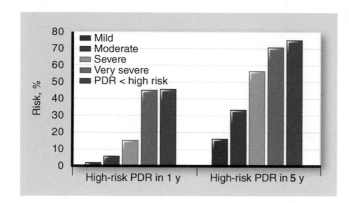

FIGURE 12-9. Progression from NPDR to PDR. The progression to high-risk PDR becomes more likely as the severity of NPDR increases. Demonstrated is the likelihood of developing high-risk PDR (see Fig. 12.10) within 1 or 5 years for patients with mild, moderate, severe, and very severe levels of NPDR or PDR with less than high-risk characteristics (HRCs). High-risk PDR in 1 is associated with the greatest incidence of severe and irreversible visual loss. Each increase in NPDR severity level is associated with an increase in the progression to the sight-threatening proliferative stage of the disease. The known progression rates permit the determination of appropriate intervals between follow-up ocular evaluations for patients with differing levels of diabetic retinopathy. Typically, follow-up ocular evaluations are performed as follows: annually for no retinopathy, every 6–12 months for mild to moderate NPDR, every 3–4 months for severe to very severe NPDR, and every 2–3 months for PDR that is less than high risk [15] (adapted from the Early Treatment Diabetic Retinopathy Study Research Group [26]).

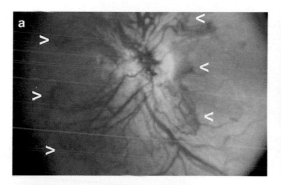

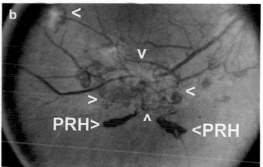

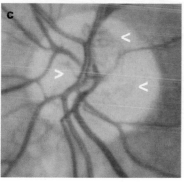

FIGURE 12-10. Characteristic clinical manifestations of PDR. When any neovascularization is present, diabetic retinopathy is termed PDR. The extent and location of neovascularization determine whether the PDR is considered to be high risk or less than high risk. Neovascularization at the optic disc (NVD), larger areas of vessels, and the presence of concurrent vitreous hemorrhages are the critical findings. Without laser photocoagulation, patients with high-risk PDR have a 28% risk of severe visual loss (<5/200 maintained for at least 4 months, which is worse than legally blind) within 2 years. This risk compares with a 7% risk of severe visual loss after 2 years for patients with PDR without the HRCs [27, 28]. (**A**) Extensive NVD is shown. (**B**) Extensive neovascularization at an area remote (>1,500 m) from the optic disc, referred to as NVE, is shown. Preretinal hemorrhage (PRH) also is present. (**C**) NVD approximately equal to one third to one fourth of the disc area is shown. The following are risk factors: the presence of any neovascularization within the eye; NVD; preretinal (or vitreous) hemorrhage; and large areas of neovascularization. NVD equal to or greater than that shown in (**C**) is considered to be large. NVE greater than or equal to half of the disc area is considered to be large. When three or more of the risk factors listed previously are present, the patient has PDR with HRCs (PDR-HRCs). Thus, the patient in (**A**) has PDR-HRC because neovascularization is present, located at the disc, and large in extent. The patient in (**B**) also has PDR-HRC because neovascularization is present, the extent of NVE is large, and PRH is present. (**C**) represents the minimal amount of NVD required for PDR-HRC [(**B, C**) from the Early Treatment Diabetic Retinopathy Study Research Group [25, with permission].

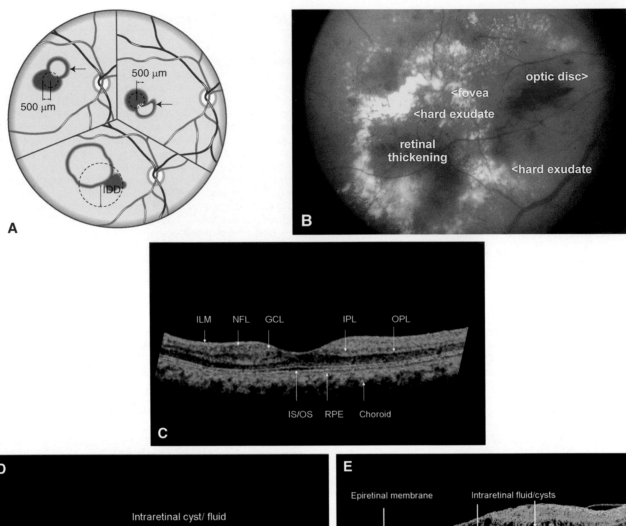

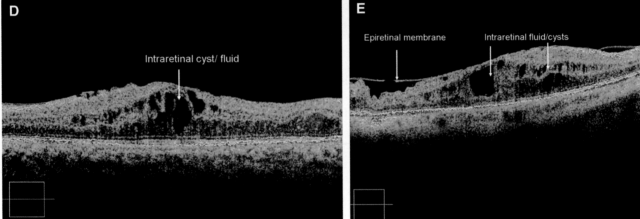

FIGURE 12-11. Clinical manifestations of DME. Increased permeability of the retinal microvasculature can result in transudation of serum and other blood components into the substance of the retina, often with the deposition of lipid in the form of hard exudates. Retinal edema, most commonly in the central retina or macula, results. Macular edema may be present at any level of diabetic retinopathy and is defined as retinal thickening within 3,000 μm of the center of the macula (fovea). Macular edema that meets predetermined criteria for extent or location is termed *CSME* [26, 29]. (**A**) Situations in which macular edema (*white*) is of sufficient extent and correct location to be termed CSME are provided. Specifically, edema qualifies as CSME when it is at or within 500 μm of the fovea; associated with hard exudates (*arrows*) that are at or within 500 μm of the fovea; or one disc area in size or greater, with any part of the edema at or within 1,500 μm of the fovea. (**B**) CSME owing to extensive hard exudate and thickening involving the fovea and surrounding retina is shown. (**C**) In addition to these clinical findings of macular edema, retinal imaging with optical coherence tomography (OCT) provides in vivo retinal images that approximate histologic sections. The availability of these images have aided in the identification of subtle retinal edema previously undetectable on clinical examination. (**D**) This OCT image shows CSME involving the fovea. (**E**) These OCT images show an epiretinal membrane with accompanying retinal edema. *1DD* one-disk diameter, *GCL* ganglion cell layer, *ILM* internal limiting membrane, *IPL* inner plexiform layer, *IS/OS* inner/outer photoreceptor segments, *NFL* nerve fiber layer, *OPL* outer plexiform layer, *RPE* retinal pigment epithelium [(**A**) adapted from Cavallerano [30]; (**B–D**) courtesy of Beetham Eye Institute Image Library].

Complications and Causes of Visual Loss

Causes of Visual Loss in Diabetic Retinopathy	
Complications Threatening Vision	Common Therapeutic Approach
Clinically significant macular edema	Focal and/or grid laser photocoagulation surgery, if unresponsive possible intravitreous steroid (although efficacy and side effects are currently under evaluation by clinical trial)
Macular capillary nonperfusion	No currently effective therapy
High-risk proliferative diabetic retinopathy	Scatter PRP laser surgery
Vitreous hemorrhage	Careful observation or vitrectomy
Traction, rhegmatogenous retinal detachment, or both	Vitrectomy
Traction distorting the macula	Careful observation or vitrectomy
Fibrovascular tissues obscuring the retina	Careful observation or vitrectomy
Neovascular glaucoma	PRP, cryotherapy plus intraocular pressure management, or both

PRP—panretinal photocoagulation.

FIGURE 12-12. Results of diabetic retinopathy. Diabetic retinopathy can result in permanent visual loss by several mechanisms. Long-standing CSME induces moderate visual loss from edema in the foveal region (see Fig. 12.11). If extensive capillary closure occurs in the macular region, vision can be permanently affected from the loss of blood supply to the fovea (see Fig. 12.13). Untreated high-risk PDR primarily causes severe visual loss either by vitreous hemorrhage or retinal traction. Vitreous hemorrhage can reduce vision markedly owing to obscuration of the visual axis by blood (see Fig. 12.13). However, because the blood itself is relatively benign, vision will be recovered (in the absence of other ocular damage) once the hemorrhage clears spontaneously or, when not resolving, after vitrectomy surgery (see Fig. 12.20). By contrast, neovascularization eventually tends to undergo a scarring process with fibrosis and contraction, resulting in retinal traction (see Fig. 12.14). Such traction can cause visual loss by distorting the macula; tearing the retina; or precipitating retinal detachment, further vitreous hemorrhage, or both. Rarely, fibrovascular tissue itself may obscure the visual axis (see Fig. 12.13). If NVI occurs, neovascular glaucoma may result and lead to permanent visual loss (see Fig. 12.15) (adapted from Aiello et al. [15]).

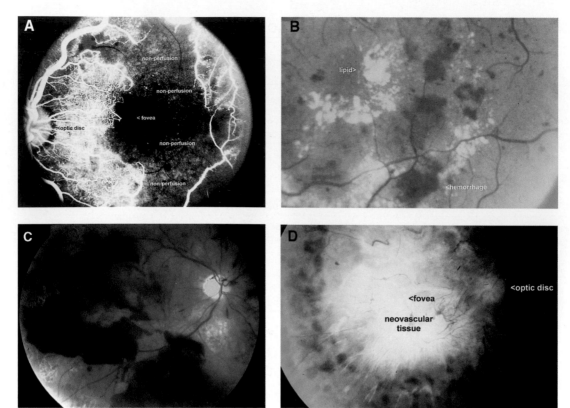

FIGURE 12-13. Ophthalmic complications associated with visual loss in diabetic retinopathy. Visual loss associated with diabetic retinopathy can arise from multiple complications of the disease. If the characteristic progressive capillary loss eventually involves a large portion of the central macula, then visual acuity is compromised. (**A**) Fluorescein angiogram showing extensive macular capillary nonperfusion. Fluorescent dye (fluorescein) was injected into the patient's antecubital vein and photographs were taken of the retina as the dye was passing through the retinal vessels. This technique, called *fluorescein angiography*, allows excellent visualization of the retinal vasculature. In this instance, the dye in the retinal vessels appears white, and the photograph shows nearly complete loss of the retinal vasculature perfusion in the macular region. These anatomic changes and their visual sequelae are irreversible. (**B**) Extensive retinal vascular leakage into the macular region with retinal thickening, lipid deposits, and retinal hemorrhage. This patient has severe macular edema, with associated visual loss. (**C**) Blood in the vitreous, a condition termed *vitreous hemorrhage* or *PRH*, is shown here. PRH refers specifically to blood immediately in front of the retina, whereas vitreous hemorrhage may be anywhere in the vitreous cavity. Vitreous hemorrhages are common in diabetic retinopathy owing to the fragility of new vessels and traction often exerted on these vessels by progressive retinal fibrosis. Although the hemorrhages usually clear spontaneously, surgical intervention may be required if they persist (see Fig. 12.20). Not only can vitreous hemorrhage obscure the patient's vision but also the ophthalmologist's view of the retina, which may necessitate evaluation of the retinal anatomy using ultrasonography if the hemorrhage is severe (see Fig. 12.14). (**D**) A rare form of visual loss in diabetes in which a sheet of neovascular tissue obscures the visual axis. Removal of the tissue by vitrectomy surgery often can restore useful vision (see Fig. 12.20) [(**A**, **B**, and **D**) courtesy of the Wilmer Ophthalmological Institute].

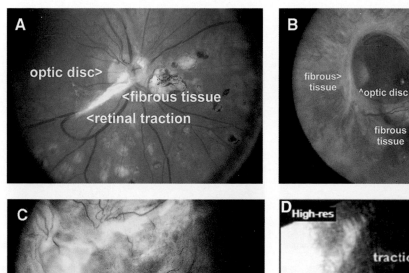

FIGURE 12-14. Ophthalmic complications associated with retinal traction in diabetic retinopathy. Some of the most severe visual losses associated with diabetic retinopathy result from the complications of traction exerted on the retina by fibrosing neovascular tissue. Initially, the traction can result in localized retinal detachment that, when distant from the critical areas of the retina, has little visual significance. (**A**) A localized traction retinal detachment from the optic disc to an inferior retinal vessel is shown. Note the elevation and distortion of the retinal vessel at the area of traction. As seen here, the detachment does not threaten the macula but should be examined carefully at regular intervals for progression toward the fovea. (**B**) More extensive fibrovascular tissue and traction along the vascular arcades of the retina surrounding the macula is shown. This configuration is typical of retinal traction in diabetic retinopathy because of the predilection for fibrovascular tissues to form along the vascular arcades. This configuration has been termed "wolf-jaw" owing to its apparent imminent "bite" on the macula. (**C**) A nearly total retinal detachment with extensive fibrovascular proliferation is shown. Large retinal detachments also may occur when the tractional forces are sufficient to tear a hole in the retina, allowing vitreous fluid to pass into the subretinal space (rhegmatogenous detachment). If vitreous hemorrhage obscures the view of the retina, ultrasonography is indicated to monitor ocular status. (**D**) Ultrasonography of vitreous hemorrhage (VH), retinal traction, and traction retinal detachment. When traction retinal detachment threatens the macula, vitrectomy surgery usually is indicated (see Fig. 12.20) [(**D**) courtesy of R. Calderon, OD].

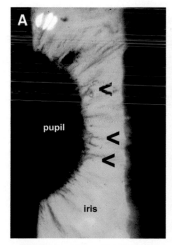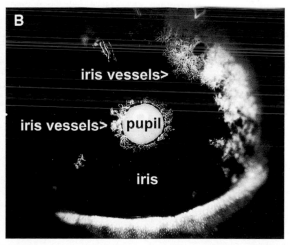

FIGURE 12-15. Neovascularization of the iris. In PDR, neovascularization can occur not only on the retina but also on the iris. NVI is sometimes referred to as *rubeosis iridis*. If the neovascularization progresses to the base of the iris, the normal outflow channels for the aqueous fluid from the anterior chamber can become occluded and the intraocular pressure can increase dramatically. This condition, called *neovascular glaucoma*, can result in severe and permanent visual loss. Treatment involves prompt scatter laser photocoagulation as done for PDR (see Fig. 12.14). (**A**) NVI is shown, with the iris vessels marked by *arrow heads*. (**B**) Iris neovascularization using fluorescein angiography is shown (see Fig. 12.13a). Fluorescein dye in the iris vessels (*white*) demonstrates the extent of the neovascularization on the iris.

Treatment

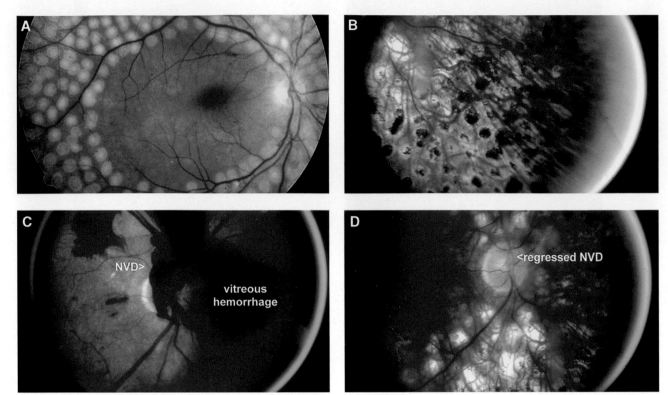

FIGURE 12-16. Panretinal laser photocoagulation for PDR. The primary therapy for PDR is scatter (panretinal) laser photocoagulation. However, cryotherapy or vitrectomy with endophotocoagulation may be effective when photocoagulation is not feasible. Treatment entails using a laser to place multiple burns throughout the midperiphery of the retina in an attempt to reduce the risk of visual loss. In general, prompt treatment is advised for patients with high-risk PDR. Some patients with PDR that is less than high-risk or with severe or very severe NPDR also may benefit from panretinal photocoagulation, depending on factors such as type of diabetes, medical status, access to care, compliance with follow-up, status and progression of the fellow eye, and family history [26, 31]. (**A**) The clinical appearance of the retina shortly after panretinal photocoagulation in PDR is shown. The 500-mm-diameter retinal burns appear moderately white in intensity and one-half burn width apart. Laser burns are not placed over the retinal vessels, optic disc, or within the macular region. A total of 1,200–1,800 retinal burns generally are applied over two to three sessions occurring a few days to weeks apart. The procedure is done on an outpatient basis and generally requires only topical anesthesia. (**B**) Panretinal photocoagulation scars as they appear months to years after their application are shown. Note the areas of increased retinal pigmentation, atrophy, and spreading of the area of each retinal scar. (**C**) Shown are PDR, neovascularization of the disk, and vitreous hemorrhage before laser panretinal photocoagulation. (**D**) The same patient 2 years after panretinal photocoagulation is shown. Note the resolution of the vitreous hemorrhage and regression of the neovascularization with only a small, fibrotic, nonperfused remnant of the original neovascular frond at the optic disc. Such remnants often do not regress completely and usually do not threaten vision. [(**B–D**) from The American Academy of Ophthalmology, Diabetes 2000, Diabetic Retinopathy Course, with permission)].

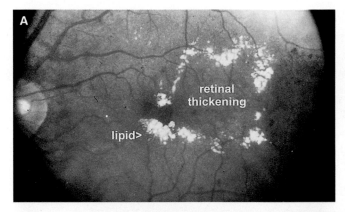

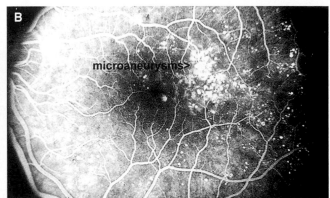

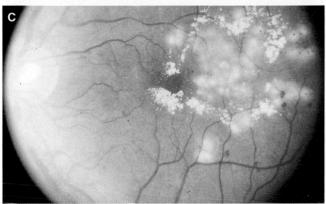

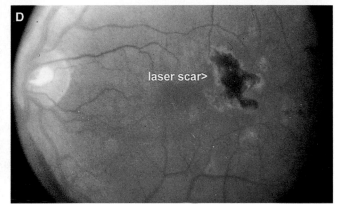

Figure 12-17. Focal laser photocoagulation for clinically significant DME. The primary therapy for clinically significant DME is focal laser photocoagulation. The treatment entails placing light 50–100-mm-diameter burns focally over leaking microaneurysms or in a grid pattern if retinal leakage is diffuse. Once the need for the treatment is determined clinically, fluorescein angiography often is used to identify the type of leakage and specific microaneurysms for treatment. If the treatment is successful, resolution of the macular edema may be expected 3 or more months after therapy. The treatment may be reapplied if the edema persists or recurs. (**A**) Circinate lipid deposits, CSME, and reduced visual acuity are shown. (**B**) This fluorescein angiogram demonstrates multiple microaneurysms in the area of thickening within the circinate ring. (**C**) The clinical appearance of the retina immediately after focal laser photocoagulation to the leaking microaneurysms is shown. The retinal burns applied in this case are more intense than is optimal. (**D**) Shown is the clinical appearance of the eye several months after laser therapy. The lipid and edema have resolved, and no thickening of the retina is present. Likewise, visual acuity has improved. The residual scarring of the retina is heavier than desired owing to the intensity of the initial laser burns (from the American Academy of Ophthalmology Diabetes 2000 Program, with permission).

Therapeutic Efficacy in the Treatment of Diabetic Retinopathy		
Indication	Treatment	Efficacy
Clinically significant macular edema	Focal laser photocoagulation	50% reduction in moderate visual loss* after 3 y
High-risk proliferative diabetic retinopathy (PDR)	Scatter photocoagulation	60% reduction in severe visual loss[†] after 3 y
Development of high-risk PDR	Scatter photocoagulation	87% reduction in severe visual loss[†] after 3 y
		97% reduction in bilateral severe visual loss[†] after 3 y
		90% reduction in legal blindness after 5 y
Severe PDR and severe vitreous hemorrhage[‡]	Vitrectomy	60% increased chance of 20/40 or better after 2 y
Severe PDR and vision 10/200 or better[‡]	Vitrectomy	34% increased chance of 20/40 or better after 2 y
No diabetic retinopathy	Intensive glycemic control	76% reduction in onset of retinopathy
Nonproliferative diabetic retinopathy	Intensive glycemic control	63% reduction in retinopathy progression
		47% reduction in severe nonproliferative diabetic retinopathy and PDR
		26% reduction in development of macular edema
		51% reduction in need for laser treatment

*Moderate visual loss is defined as at least doubling of visual angle (eg, 20/40 to 20/80)

[†]Severe visual loss is defined as best corrected acuity of 5/200 or worse on two consecutive visits 4 mo apart.

[‡]For patients with type 1 diabetes only; no benefit was observed in the group having type 2 diabetes.

Figure 12-18. Therapeutic efficacy of diabetic retinopathy. The only patient-initiated efforts proven to reduce the risk of visual loss include maintenance of optimal glycemic control and insistence on routine ophthalmologic evaluation [10, 32]. Once visually significant complications of diabetes have arisen, the mainstay of therapy is laser photocoagulation. Scatter (pan-retinal) photocoagulation for the treatment of PDR is remarkably effective in preventing severe visual loss when patients who are at risk receive therapy in an appropriate and timely manner. Indeed, with appropriate medical and ophthalmologic care, over 95% of visual loss resulting from diabetic retinopathy can be prevented [14]. Focal photocoagulation for the treatment of CSME is somewhat less effective, although half of moderate visual loss can be prevented in this manner. If the application of laser photocoagulation is not possible or is ineffective, pars plana vitrectomy surgery also is useful in preventing visual impairment (see Fig. 12.20). Recently, steroids (especially triamcinolone) have been injected into the vitreous to reduce macular edema that is otherwise unresponsive to laser photocoagulation. Although many patients may have a reduction in edema following such a treatment, the extent to which the edema resolves, the improvement of visual acuity, the need for reinjection, and risks of known complications including cataract and severe glaucoma have not been fully elucidated to date. Rigorous clinical trials are currently underway to address these issues and to determine the appropriate role of this therapy in the treatment of patients with DME (adapted from Aiello et al. [15]).

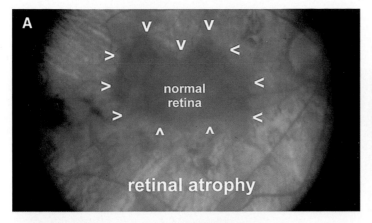

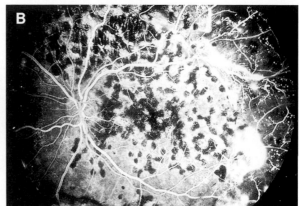

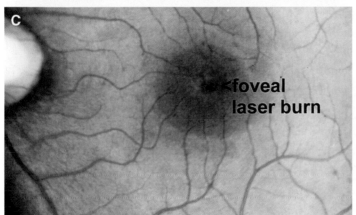

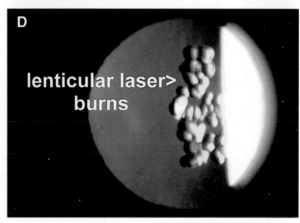

FIGURE 12-19. Side effects and complications of laser photocoagulation. Although laser photocoagulation is remarkably effective at preventing the visual loss associated with diabetic retinopathy, the therapy itself is inherently destructive. Each retinal laser burn destroys a portion of previously viable retina in an attempt to maintain better visual function than would be achieved without treatment. Thus, the therapy itself is associated with unavoidable side effects, most notably the constriction of peripheral visual field and reduced night vision. These symptoms result from the selective destruction of the retinal midperiphery that subserves these functions. Unexpected complications also can arise from laser photocoagulation. (**A**) Note the appearance of the retina several years after excessive laser panretinal photocoagulation; the atrophy resulting from individual laser scars has spread to the point at which confluent loss of the peripheral retina occurs. Only the central aspect of the macula (*arrow heads*) remains intact. As expected, this patient has severe constriction of the visual field and significant difficulty with night vision. (**B**) This fluorescein angiogram shows panretinal photocoagulation mistakenly applied directly through the macula. The dark laser scars in this macular area, which is critical for detailed vision, cause permanent blind spots in the center of vision and reduced visual acuity. (**C**) A single laser burn mistakenly applied to the fovea is shown. This area of retina subserves central vision, accounting for the large central blind spot and poorly detailed vision experienced by this patient, who now is legally blind. (**D**) Laser photocoagulation focused too far anteriorly may result in vaporization of the crystalline lens, as observed in this retroilluminated photograph of the human lens. Visual loss associated with this rare complication can be corrected by cataract surgery. [(**B–D**) courtesy of the Wilmer Ophthalmological Institute].

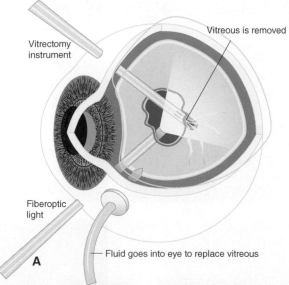

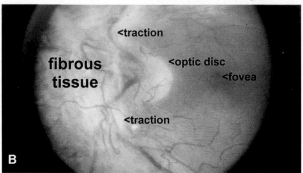

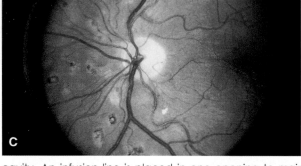

Figure 12-20. Pars plana vitrectomy surgery. Instances occur when high-risk PDR is not amenable to laser photocoagulation and may arise as a result of the following: advanced disease, poor retinal visualization (i.e., severe vitreous hemorrhage or cataract), active neovascularization despite complete laser treatment, traction–macular detachment, or combined traction–rhegmatogenous retinal detachment. In such cases, pars plana vitrectomy surgery may offer a therapeutic option. Vitrectomy surgery has the potential for serious complications, including profound visual loss and permanent pain and blindness. Thus, surgery should be undertaken only after careful consideration of the potential risks and benefits [33]. Vitrectomy performed by an experienced vitreoretinal surgeon, however, often can maintain vision in patients who otherwise almost certainly would have severe visual loss. (**A**) This schematic representation is of the pars plana vitrectomy procedure. Three openings are made from the outside of the eye into the vitreous cavity. An infusion line is placed in one opening to maintain pressure within the eye during surgery. The other two openings are used for the variety of instruments that can manipulate the vitreous and retina. Fiberoptic instruments allow for illumination and the surgery is monitored by visualization through the pupil using an operating microscope. (**B**) PDR and extensive fibrovascular neovascularization before vitrectomy surgery is shown. Note the fibrous tissue surrounding the optic disc that is exerting traction on the major superior and inferior retinal vessels, dragging them nasally. (**C**) The same retina after vitrectomy surgery. Note the removal of the fibrous tissue that had surrounded the optic disc with return of the major retinal vessels to a more normal anatomic position after removal of the traction [(**A**) from "For my patient: retinal detachment and vitreous surgery," The Retina Research Fund; (**B**, **C**) from the American Academy of Ophthalmology Diabetic Retinopathy Vitrectomy Study course, with permission].

Systemic Factors Potentially Affecting Diabetic Retinopathy	
Glycemic control	Pregnancy
Hypertension	Smoking
Renal disease	Anemia
Dyslipidemia	

Figure 12-21. Systemic factors affecting retinopathy. Although great emphasis is placed on the clinical evaluation of the retina and the adherence to rigorous treatment algorithms, concomitant systemic disorders can exert significant influence on the development, progression, and ultimate outcome of diabetic eye disease. Optimized control of systemic disorders can improve the visual prognosis of the patient with diabetes [11]. Such care often involves an intensive, multifaceted, health-care team approach to the treatment of patients with diabetes [34]. A list of systemic disorders potentially affecting diabetic retinopathy is presented; these disorders should be managed carefully.

Growth Factors and Potential Novel Therapies

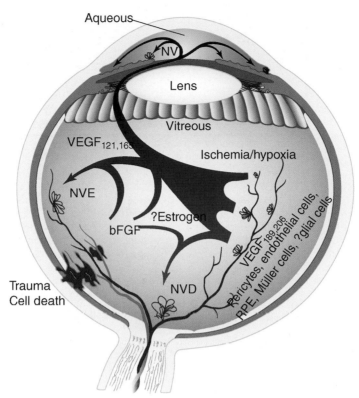

FIGURE 12-22. Model of growth factor action in diabetic retinopathy. For the past 50 years, investigators have recognized that numerous ischemic retinopathies result in retinal neovascularization and vascular leakage similar to that observed in diabetic retinopathy. These findings have suggested that common inciting events and mediating factors may be responsible for these complications. The potential role of growth factors in mediating retinal neovascularization was first suggested by Michaelson in 1948 and later refined by numerous investigators [35]. A schematic representation of the growth factor model of intraocular neovascularization is shown. Damage to the retinal tissues, probably caused by capillary loss and subsequent hypoxia in the case of diabetes, results in the release of growth factors from the retina. These growth factors are secreted by a variety of retinal cell types and may act locally to produce neovascularization and vascular permeability or may diffuse through the vitreous cavity to induce these complications at distant sites. The presence of two or more growth factors may actually augment the induction of neovascular activity, as is the case with basic fibroblast growth factor (bFGF) and vascular endothelial growth factor (VEGF). In addition, the growth factors may diffuse down a concentration gradient from the vitreous cavity into the aqueous cavity, where they are eventually cleared through the trabecular meshwork at the base of the iris. This diffusion path would account for the neovascularization observed at the iris. Numerous growth factors have been implicated in this process. Molecules that probably contribute to the neovascularization in diabetic retinopathy include VEGF, growth hormone, insulin-like growth factor-1, and bFGF. Of these, VEGF is thought to be the major mediator of intraocular neovascularization and vasopermeability, although many factors are likely to contribute to such complex processes. The relative growth factor concentrations and angiogenic potency are represented by arrow width (adapted from Aiello et al. [36]).

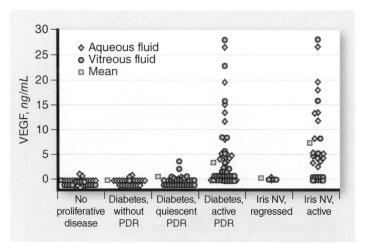

Figure 12-23. Angiogenic growth factors increase when neovascularization is present. For a growth factor to mediate intraocular neovascularization in diabetic retinopathy, it should be present at elevated concentrations during or shortly before the onset of active neovascularization. Demonstrated are the results of a study in which intraocular fluids were obtained from 136 patients with diabetes who were undergoing intraocular surgery. The concentration of VEGF in the intraocular fluids was evaluated and the results plotted by extent of retinopathy. Concentrations of VEGF were low in patients who did not have diabetes or who had diabetes, but no PDR. However, when patients had active neovascularization either of the retina or iris, concentrations of VEGF were greatly elevated. Once neovascularization had become quiescent, concentrations of vascular endothelial factor returned to baseline. The study also demonstrated the predicted concentration gradient between the vitreous and aqueous cavities and a 75% decrease in VEGF levels after successful laser panretinal photocoagulation. *NV* neovascularization (adapted from Aiello et al. [37]).

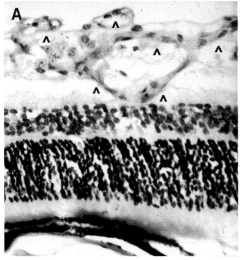

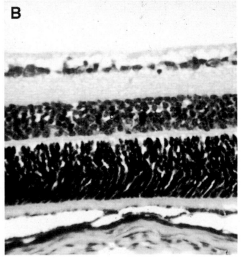

Figure 12-24. Inhibition of VEGF suppresses retinal neovascularization in animals. If VEGF is responsible for a significant portion of the neovascular response in ischemic retinopathies, then inhibition of this molecule should result in the suppression of retinal neovascularization. Several investigators have now evaluated this causal relationship. Inhibition of VEGF using different techniques has resulted in the suppression of retinal and iris neovascularization in murine and primate models [38–40]. Demonstrated are the results from one of these studies using the chimeric receptor antagonists in a murine model of ischemia-induced retinopathy [38, 41]. When these inhibitors of VEGF are injected into the neonatal eye at the time when the retinas become hypoxic, the suppression of subsequent retinal neovascularization occurs in 95–100% of animals. The magnitude of inhibition is approximately 50%. (**A**) A histologic cross-section of a neonatal mouse retina that received an intraocular injection of an inactive control compound is shown. The *arrow heads* show the extensive inner retinal neovascularization. (**B**) The corresponding area of retina in the contralateral eye of the same animal that received an active inhibitor of VEGF is shown. Note the suppression of inner retinal neovascularization and normal appearance of the retina by light microscopic examination without evidence of retinal toxicity. These data suggest that growth factor inhibitors eventually may prove useful as novel therapies for diabetic retinopathy and macular edema. Such therapeutic approaches theoretically would eliminate the side effects inherent in the retinal-destructive treatments in use today (see Figs. 12.16 and 12.19) (from Aiello [42], with permission).

Novel Therapeutic Approaches Under Investigation for Diabetic Retinopathy		
Prevention	Intervention	Restoration
Antihyperglycemics*	*Anti-permeability*	Medical approaches
ARI*	Intravitreous steroids, PKC inhibitors*, antihistamines*, anti-AGE*	Stem cell utilization
Anti-AGE*	*Anti-angiogenesis*	Gene therapy
PKC inhibitors	GH/IGF-1 inhibitors*, PKC inhibitors*, angiostatin/endostatin, ribozymes, aptamers* (*eg*, Macugen), antiobodies* (*eg*, Lucentis; Novartis, Basel, Switzerland), chimeric receptors, PEDF	Surgical approaches
Preservation of function	*Anti-proliferation*	Retinal transplantation
Antioxidants*	Anti-integrins, metalloproteinases*	Ocular transplantation
Hemostabilization	*Vitreal lysis**	Artificial visual prosthetics*
Neuroprotection		

Compounds in or pending clinical trials.

Figure 12-25. Novel therapeutic approaches for diabetic retinopathy. The possibility of preventing visual loss from diabetes in a nondestructive manner utilizing a pharmacologic approach has become the focus of intensive investigations. Multiple approaches have been proposed and inhibition of VEGF has recently been proven to be highly effective in preserving vision loss from diabetic eye complications. Preliminary results of several clinical trials have recently been published, which support the efficacy of VEGF inhibition in improving visual outcome in patients with center-involved DME. A partial list of other approaches under investigation is presented. Anti-VEGF therapy including Pegaptanib (Macugen, OSI Pharmaceuticals, Melville, NY), Bevacizumab (Avastin, Genentech Inc., San Francisco, CA), and Ranibizumab (Lucentis, Genentech Inc., San Francisco, CA), have been shown to be effective for chor-oidal neovascularization from age-related macular degeneration, and clinical trials in diabetic patients have also demonstrated a beneficial effect for DME. There may be beneficial effects on reducing retinopathy progression as well, although these data are not conclusive at this time. The 2-year results of a randomized clinical trial comparing focal laser to intravitreal triamcinolone (IVT) has shown that IVT appears to be effective in rapidly reducing DME, although its long-term benefit on visual acuity and retinal thickness is inferior to focal laser. IVT treatment is associated with a substantial increase in ocular complications such as cataracts and glaucoma, and these have resulted in a substantial decline in its use clinically [43]. *AGE* advanced glycation end product, *ARI* aldose reductase inhibitor, *IGF-1* insulin-like growth factor-1, *GH* growth hormone, *PEDF* pigment-epithelium derived factor, *PKC* protein kinase C.

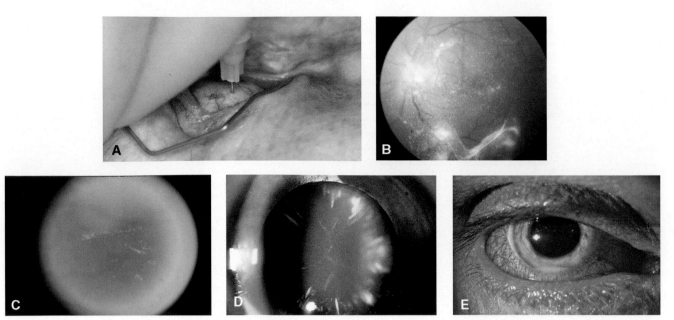

Figure 12-26. Intravitreal injections. The novel pharmacologic agents are delivered as an intravitreal injection and performed on a repetitive basis dependent on the response to treatment. (**A**) Intravitreal injections are usually performed as an office procedure with gauge 27 or 30 needle inserted through the pars plana and the medication is delivered directly into the vitreous cavity. Currently commercially available pharmacologic agents are used off-label for the indication of diabetic macular edema and include triamcinolone acetonide and anti-VEGF agents; Ranibizumab and Bevacizumab. (**B**) Injected triamcinolone acetonide and (**C**) rarely silicone oil droplets may be visible immediately after an injection, with patients reporting floaters immediately after injection that may persist for more than 3 months. (**D**) The most common complication following corticosteroid injections is the development or worsening of a cataract. The cumulative incidence of cataract surgery in patients treated with 4 mg of triamcinolone is 83% compared to 13% in patients treated with focal laser over 3 years. Severe complications related to intravitreal injections although rare may significantly compromise visual recovery if not identified appropriately. (**E**) Endophthalmitis.

Figure 12-27. Comparison of IVT to focal laser. The efficacy and safety of IVT compared to focal laser was evaluated in a 2-year prospective multicenter randomized clinical trial [43]. The trial directly compared intraocular preservative-free triamcinolone acetonide to focal laser. The study had three treatment arms and eyes were randomized either to focal laser, 1 mg IVT, or 4 mg IVT. Retreatment for new or persistent DME was performed at 4-month intervals and the primary outcome was measured at 2 years. A total of 840 eyes with center-involving DME and reduced visual acuity (VA) were enrolled. (**A**) A graph of VA results of the trial over time is presented. At 4 months, it was observed that 4-mg IVT-treated eyes had greater improvement in best corrected visual acuity (BCVA) compared to focal/grid laser and the 1-mg IVT group was no different from the laser group. At 1 year, there were no significant differences in VA between all three groups. Beginning at 16 months and extending to the primary outcome at 2 years, the laser group had a greater improvement in BCVA than the IVT groups, both of which showed a loss of ETDRS letters and were not statistically different from each other. (**B**) Results for macular thickness paralleled the trend seen in vision. (**C**) This representative case highlights the findings of the study. A 55-year-old man with type 2 diabetes presented with reduced visual acuity with moderate NPDR and center involved DME in both eyes. OCT shows marked retinal thickening, intraretinal cysts, and subretinal fluid. He was randomized to IVT oculus dexter and focal laser oculus sinister. (d) This case emphasizes the observed clinical effects of IVT compared to focal laser. In the IVT-treated eye, there is an initial rapid reduction in macular thickness paralleled by an improvement in VA at 4 months. At 1 year, the vision returns to baseline. Beginning at 16 months and continuing into the 24th month, despite retreatment there is recurrence of the macular edema and loss of five letters compared to baseline. In the laser-treated eye, there is a slow gradual response first evident at 1 year and continued improvement into the 24th month. There was no recurrence of the macular edema and the patient had an improvement in visual acuity of greater than15 letters. Long-term final visual acuity and macular thickness was better and improvement was sustained in the eye receiving focal laser. In the eye treated with IVT, cataract developed, which required surgery and intraocular pressure increased sufficiently to necessitate glaucoma medications [(a, b) adapted from ref. [43]; (c, d) courtesy of Beetham Eye Institute Image Library].

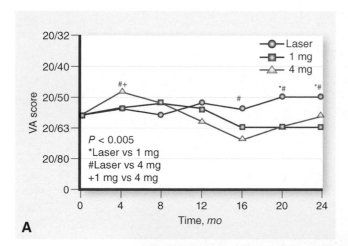

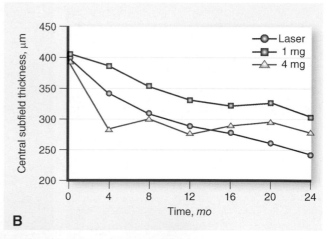

A

20/32
20/40
20/50
20/63
20/80
0

VA score

○ Laser
■ 1 mg
△ 4 mg

#+

#

*#

*#

P < 0.005
*Laser vs 1 mg
#Laser vs 4 mg
+1 mg vs 4 mg

0   4   8   12   16   20   24
Time, mo

B

450
400
350
300
250
200

Central subfield thickness, μm

○ Laser
■ 1 mg
△ 4 mg

0   4   8   12   16   20   24
Time, mo

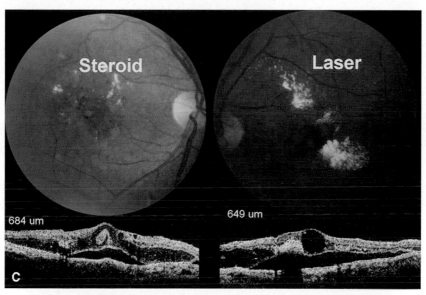

C

Steroid   Laser

684 um   649 um

D

	Steroid(OD)	Focal (OS)	
Baseline 20/63 684 um			20/125 649 um
4 mo 20/50 351 um			20/125 766 um
12 mo 20/63 264 um			20/100 228 um
16 mo 20/200 389 um			20/100 229 um
24 mo 20/80 260 um			20/63 217 um

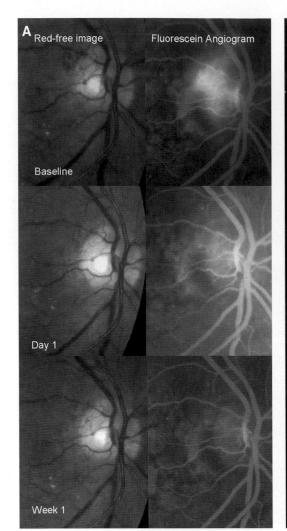

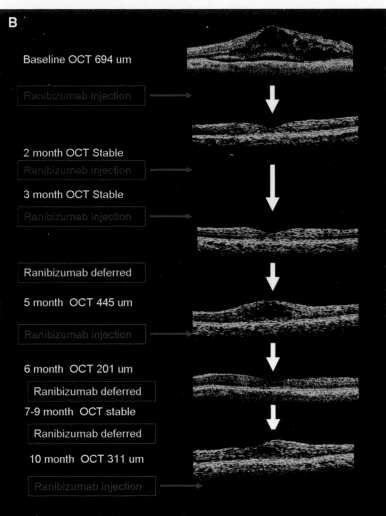

Figure 12-28. Pharmacologic treatment of retinal complications of diabetes. The pharmacologic treatment of DME and proliferative retinopathy has ushered in a new paradigm in the treatment of retinal complications of diabetes. Anti-VEGF agents have been shown to be exquisitely effective in inducing temporary regression of retinal neovascularization [38]. (**A**) An intravitreal injection of bevacizumab has been shown to induce a marked regression of retinal neovascularization beginning as early as 1 day after injection with further regression after 1 week. (**B**) This patient received repeated intravitreal ranibizumab injections that led to regression of DME. It is important to note that many patients with DME will require repeated injections due to the recurrence of the retinal thickening once the effect has worn off [(**A**) from Avery et al. [47], with permission, and (**B**) courtesy of Beetham Eye Institute Image Library).

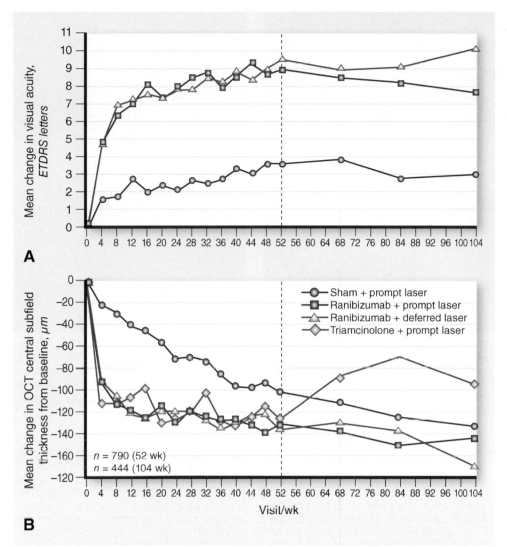

Figure 12-29. Anti-VEGF agents for the treatment of DME. The repeated intravitreal administration of anti-VEGF agents has been shown to be more effective than the standard focal/grid laser alone in the treatment of DME in results from multiple controlled randomized clinical trials [48–50]. The DRCR.net website published the 1-year results of a phase III trial that evaluated the safety and efficacy of intravitreal 0.5-mg ranibizumab or 4-mg triamcinolone treatments combined with focal/grid laser compared with focal/grid laser alone for the treatment of DME [50]. Patients were randomized into four treatment arms: 0.5 mg intravitreal ranibizumab with prompt laser treatment (n=187); 0.5 mg intravitreal ranibizumab with laser treatment deferred for at least 24 weeks (n=188); focal/grid laser alone with sham injection (n=293); and 4 mg intravitreal triamcinolone with prompt laser treatment (n=186). Retreatment followed an algorithm facilitated by a web-based, real-time data-entry system that resulted in over 95% compliance with the complex treatment algorithm. (**A**) For the 1-year primary outcome, the mean change in the visual acuity letter score from baseline was significantly greater in the ranibizumab with prompt laser group (+9, P=0.001) and ranibizumab with deferred laser group (+9, P=0.001), but not in the triamcinolone with prompt laser group (+4, P=0.31) compared with the sham injections with prompt laser group (+3). In the two ranibizumab groups compared with the sham+prompt laser group, a greater proportion of eyes had substantial improvement of 10 letters or more (50% and 47% vs. 28%) and 15 letters or more (30% and 28% vs. 15%) and a lower proportion of eyes had substantial worsening of 10 letters or more (4% and 3% vs. 13%) and 15 letters or more (2% and 2% vs.8%). The preliminary 2-year outcomes available for 57% of the study cohort generally mirrored the 1-year primary outcome results. (**B**) The OCT results generally paralleled the overall visual acuity results and were more favorable for the ranibizumab groups. The study reported a favorable safety profile for intravitreal ranibizumab with 0.08% incidence of endophthalmitis and no significant increase in the cardiovascular events compared to controls. Subgroup analysis showed that ranibizumab injection may potentially have beneficial effects in delaying the progression of retinopathy. Among patients with NPDR severe or worse, ranibizumab groups showed a trend toward a reduction in two-level retinopathy progression and an increase in two-level retinopathy regression. This association was also observed using clinical surrogates of retinopathy progression to proliferative disease; both the ranibizumab and triamcinolone groups showed a statistically significant reduction in the incidence of vitreous hemorrhage and the need for panretinal laser photocoagulation compared to sham-focal/grid laser group (3%, P=0.002 and 3%, P=0.02, respectively, vs. 8%) (adapted from Elman et al. [51]).

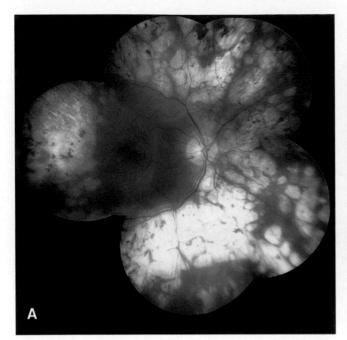

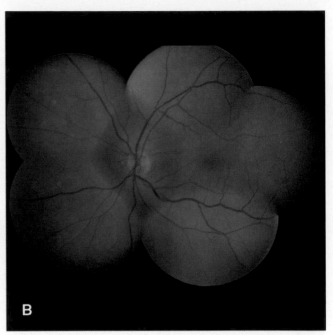

A

B

FIGURE 12-30. Joslin Diabetes Center study of type 1 diabetes results. Joslin Diabetes Center initiated the 50-Year Medal Program to recognize patients who survived 50 years or more with type 1 diabetes. In this cohort of patients, nearly half had either no or mild NPDR [52]. This investigation hopes to identify risk factors or protective mechanism that may explain the marked difference in outcomes represented by these two patients. The 50-year medalists include (**A**) a medalist with PDR (61 years of diabetes) and (**B**) a medalist with mild non-proliferative retinopathy (63 years of diabetes) [(**A, B**) from Keenan et al. [52], courtesy of Beetham Eye Institute Image Library].

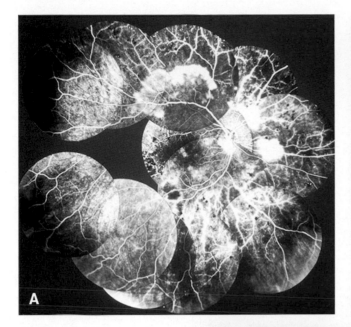

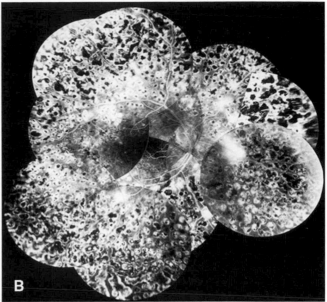

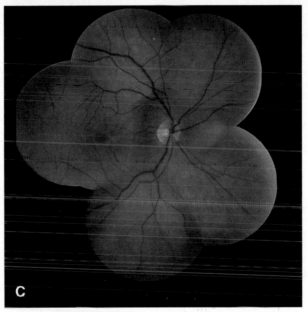

FIGURE 12-31. Treatment for PDR. The treatment for PDR has evolved considerably over the past 40 years. Currently, with adherence to evidence-based recommendations set forth by the major clinical trials in diabetic retinopathy, the risk for severe visual loss per person can be reduced to less than 2%. (**A**) Active PDR with extensive retinal neovascularization and ischemia threatening vision is shown. (**B**) Treatment with panretinal photocoagulation-inducing regression of the neovascular process and preventing visual loss is shown. (**C**) In the future, it is hoped that for patients with diabetes, we might be able to preserve vision at a stage such as shown here, without clinical evidence of retinopathy [(**A**, **B**) courtesy of Lloyd M. Aiello; (**C**) from Beetham Eye Institute Image Library].

Acknowledgments The excellent technical and editorial assistance of Jerry D. Cavallerano, OD, PhD, is gratefully acknowledged. Portions of this chapter are adapted from Aiello et al. [15] and the American Academy of Ophthalmology, Diabetes 2000, Diabetic Retinopathy course.

References

1. Klein R, BE Klein, Moss SE: Visual impairment in diabetes. Ophthalmology 1984, 91:1–9.2.

2. Klein R, Klein BE, Moss SE, Cruickshanks KJ: The Wisconsin Epidemiologic Study of Diabetic Retinopathy. XV. The long-term incidence of macular edema. Ophthalmology 1995, 102:7–16.

3. Javitt JC, Aiello LP, Bassi LJ, et al.: Detecting and treating retinopathy in patients with type I diabetes mellitus. Savings associated with improved implementation of current guidelines. American Academy of Ophthalmology. Ophthalmology 1991, 98:1565–1573.

4. Javitt JC, Aiello LP, Chiang Y, et al.: Preventive eye care in people with diabetes is cost-saving to the federal government. Implications for health-care reform. Diabetes Care 1994, 17:909–917.

5. Javitt JC, Aiello LP: Cost-effectiveness of detecting and treating diabetic retinopathy [see comments]. Ann Intern Med 1996, 124:164–169.

6. Javitt, JC, Canner JK, Sommer A: Cost effectiveness of current approaches to the control of retinopathy in type 1 diabetics. Ophthalmology 1989, 96:255–264.

7. Kahn HA, Hiller R: Blindness caused by diabetic retinopathy. Am J Ophthalmol 1974, 78:58–67.

8. Palmberg PF: Diabetic retinopathy. Diabetes 1977, 26:703–709.

9. The Diabetes Control and Complications Trial Research Group: The effect of intensive treatment of diabetes on the development and progression of long-term complications in insulin-dependent diabetes mellitus [see comments]. N Engl J Med 1993, 329:977–986.

10. The relationship of glycemic exposure (HbA$_{1c}$) to the risk of development and progression of retinopathy in the Diabetes Control and Complications Trial. Diabetes 1995, 44:968–983.

11. Retinopathy and nephropathy in patients with type 1 diabetes four years after a trial of intensive therapy. Am J Ophthalmol 2000, 129:704–705.

12. Lifetime benefits and costs of intensive therapy as practiced in the Diabetes control and complications trial. The Diabetes Control and Complications Trial Research Group [see comments]. JAMA 1996, 276:1409–1415; published erratum, JAMA 1997, 278:25.

13. Resource utilization and costs of care in the Diabetes Control and Complications Trial. Diabetes Care 1995, 18:1468–1478.

14. Ferris FL: How effective are treatments for diabetic retinopathy? JAMA 1993, 269:1290–1291.

15. Aiello LP, Gardner TW, King GL, et al.: Diabetic retinopathy: technical review. Diabetes Care 1998, 21:143–156.

16. National Diabetes Data Group: Diabetes in America. Washington, DC: US Government Printing Office; 1995.

17. Bursell SE, Clermont AC, Kinsley BT, et al.: Retinal blood flow changes in patients with insulin-dependent diabetes mellitus and no diabetic retinopathy. Am J Physiol 1996, 270:R61–R70.

18. Wilkinson CP, Ferris FL III, Klein RE, et al.: Proposed international clinical diabetic retinopathy and diabetic macular edema disease severity scales. Ophthalmology 2003, 110:1677–1682.

19. Chew EY: A simplified diabetic retinopathy scale. Ophthalmology 2003, 110:1675–1676.

20. Krolewski AS, Warram JH, Rand LI, et al.: Risk of proliferative diabetic retinopathy in juvenile-onset type 1 diabetes: a 40-yr follow-up study. Diabetes Care 1984, 9:443–452.

21. Klein R, Klein BE, Moss SE, et al.: The Wisconsin epidemiologic study of diabetic retinopathy. II. Prevalence and risk of diabetic retinopathy when age at diagnosis is less than 30 years. Arch Ophthalmol 1984, 102:520–536.

22. Klein R, Moss SE, Klein BE, et al.: New management concepts for timely diagnosis of diabetic retinopathy treatable by photocoagulation. Diabetes Care 1987, 10:633–638.

23. American Academy of Pediatrics: Screening for retinopathy in the pediatric patient with type 1 diabetes mellitus. Pediatrics 1998, 101:313–314.

24. Klein BE, Moss SE, Klein R: Effect of pregnancy on progression of diabetic retinopathy. Diabetes Care 1990, 13:34–40.

25. The Early Treatment Diabetic Retinopathy Study Research Group: Grading diabetic retinopathy from stereoscopic color fundus photographs: an extension of the modified Airlie House classification. ETDRS report number 10. Ophthalmology 1991, 98:786–806.

26. The Early Treatment Diabetic Retinopathy Study Research Group: Early photocoagulation for diabetic retinopathy. ETDRS report number 9. Ophthalmology 1991, 98:766–785.

27. The Diabetic Retinopathy Study Research Group: Photocoagulation treatment of proliferative diabetic retinopathy. Clinical application of Diabetic Retinopathy Study (DRS) findings, DRS Report Number 8. Ophthalmology 1981, 88:583–600.

28. The Diabetic Retinopathy Study Research Group: Indications for photocoagulation treatment of diabetic retinopathy: Diabetic Retinopathy Study Report no. 14. Int Ophthalmol Clin 1987, 27:239–253.

29. The Early Treatment Diabetic Retinopathy Study Research Group: Photocoagulation for diabetic macular edema. Early Treatment Diabetic Retinopathy Study report number 1. Arch Ophthalmol 1985, 103:1796–1806.

30. Cavallerano J: Diabetic retinopathy. Clin Eye Vis Care 1990, 2:4–14.

31. Ferris F: Early photocoagulation in patients with either type 1 or type 2 diabetes. Trans Am Ophthalmol Soc 1996, 94:505–537.

32. The Diabetes Control and Complications Trial Research Group: The effect of intensive diabetes treatment on the progression of diabetic retinopathy in insulin-dependent diabetes mellitus: the Diabetes Control and Complications Trial. Arch Ophthalmol 1995, 113:36–51.

33. The Diabetic Retinopathy Vitrectomy Study Research Group: Early vitrectomy for severe proliferative diabetic retinopathy in eyes with useful vision. Clinical application of results of a randomized trial: Diabetic Retinopathy Vitrectomy Study Report 4. Ophthalmology 1988, 95:1321–1334.

34. Aiello LP, Cahill MT, Wong JS: Systemic considerations in the management of diabetic retinopathy. Am J Ophthalmol 2001, 132:760–776.

35. Michaelson IC: The mode of development of the vascular system of the retina, with some observations on its significance for certain retinal diseases. Trans Ophthalmol Soc UK 1948, 68:137–180.

36. Aiello LP, Northrup JM, Keyt BA: Hypoxic regulation of vascular endothelial growth factor in retinal cells. Arch Ophthalmol 1995, 113:1538–1544.

37. Aiello LP, Avery RL, Arrigg PG, et al.: Vascular endothelial growth factor in ocular fluid of patients with diabetic retinopathy and other retinal disorders [see comments]. N Engl J Med 1994, 331:1480–1487.

38. Aiello LP, Pierce EA, Foley ED, *et al.*: Suppression of retinal neovascularization in vivo by inhibition of vascular endothelial growth factor (VEGF) using soluble VEGF-receptor chimeric proteins. *Proc Natl Acad Sci U S A* 1995, 92:10457–10461.

39. Adamis AP, Shima DT, Tolentino MJ, *et al.*: Inhibition of vascular endothelial growth factor prevents retinal ischemia-associated iris neovascularization in a nonhuman primate. *Arch Ophthalmol* 1996, 114:66–71.

40. Robinson GS, Pierce EA, Rook SL, *et al.*: Oligodeoxynucleotides inhibit retinal neovascularization in a murine model of proliferative retinopathy. *Proc Natl Acad Sci U S A* 1996, 93:4851–4856.

41. Smith LE, Wesolowski E, McLellan A, *et al.*: Oxygen-induced retinopathy in the mouse. *Invest Ophthalmol Vis Sci* 1994, 35:101–111.

42. Aiello LP: Vascular endothelial growth factor. 20th-century mechanisms, 21st-century therapies. *Invest Ophthalmol Vis Sci* 1997, 38:1647–1652.

43. A randomized trial comparing intravitreal triamcinolone acetonide and focal/grid photocoagulation for diabetic macular edema. *Ophthalmology* 2008,115:1447–1449.

44. Giuliari G: Images in clinical medicine. Intravitreal triamcinolone for diabetic macular edema. *N Engl J Med* 2010, 363:2351.

45. Clark WL, Callejo S, Rosa R, Clayman H: *Atlas of Ophthalmology*. New York; Springer: 2002.

46. Davis J, Palestine A, Mildvan D: Ophthalmic manifestations. In *Atlas of Infectious Diseases*. New York: Springer; 2008.

47. Avery RL, Pearlman J, Pieramici DJ, *et al.*: Intravitreal bevacizumab (Avastin) in the treatment of proliferative diabetic retinopathy. *Ophthalmology* 2006, 113:1695.e1–1695.e15.

48. Nguyen QD, Shah SM, Heier JS, *et al.*: Primary end point (six months) results of the Ranibizumab for Edema of the Macula in Diabetes (READ-2) Study. *Ophthalmology* 2009, 116:2175–2181.

49. Michaelides M, Kaines A, Hamilton RD, *et al.*: A prospective randomized trial of intravitreal bevacizumab or laser therapy in the management of diabetic macular edema (BOLT) study 12-month data: report 2. *Ophthalmology* 2010, 117:1078–1086.

50. Diabetic Retinopathy Clinical Research Network, Elman MJ, Aiello LP, *et al.*: Randomized trial evaluating ranibizumab plus prompt or deferred laser or triamcinolone plus prompt laser for diabetic macular edema. *Ophthalmology* 2010, 117: 1064–1077.

51. Elman MJ, Aiello LP, Beck RW *et al.*: Randomized trial evaluating ranibizumab plus prompt or deferred laser or triamcinolone plus prompt laser for diabetic macular edema. *Ophthalmology* 2010,117:1064–1077.

52. Keenan HA, Costacou T, Sun JK, *et al.*: Clinical factors associated with resistance to microvascular complications in diabetic patients of extreme disease duration: the 50-year medalist study. *Diabetes Care* 2007, 30:1995–1997.

13

Diabetes and the Kidney

Robert C. Stanton

Diabetic nephropathy is a serious public health concern because it has become the major cause of end-stage renal disease (ESRD) in the USA (see Fig. 13.1a). Considering that chronic kidney disease is associated with multiple comorbidities (e.g., anemia and secondary hyperparathyroidism) [1, 2]; a significantly shortened life span, which is directly associated with the degree of albuminuria in diabetic nephropathy [3, 4]; a dramatic increase in cardiovascular disease, which is directly associated with even low levels of albuminuria [5]; and very large personal and societal financial costs [6], early diagnosis and treatment are critical because early intervention may dramatically slow the progression of diabetic nephropathy. For example, the Epidemiology of Diabetes Interventions and Complications (EDIC) study in type 1 diabetic patients showed that early aggressive management of blood sugar continues to have a significant impact on slowing progression, even if blood sugar control worsens over time [7]. Moreover, studies have shown that early aggressive multifactorial management of factors, such as blood sugar, blood pressure, and urine protein, can slow progression dramatically [8, 9]. Thus, early diagnosis and management are essential.

Diabetic nephropathy is characterized primarily by the clinical presentation of decreased glomerular filtration rate (GFR) and/or microalbuminuria, which may progress slowly to frank proteinuria and a gradual decline in GFR, eventually leading to renal failure. Although it has been thought that albuminuria always precedes decreased GFR, it is now clear that decreased GFR due to diabetes may occur in the absence of microalbuminuria [10]. Approximately 20–40% of patients with type 1 diabetes and 10–30% of those with type 2 diabetes develop diabetic nephropathy (decreased GFR and/or microalbuminuria). Of those patients, 10–20% progress to ESRD. Because at this point we do not know who is going to progress, all patients with diabetic nephropathy should be treated as if they will progress. Although only a minority of patients with diabetes mellitus develop renal failure, the number of cases of diabetic nephropathy is increasing every year mostly because of the epidemic increase in the number of patients with type 2 diabetes mellitus.

In the past 20 years, much has been learned about the possible causes of diabetic nephropathy. This understanding has led to the development and use of specific approaches that have been effective in significantly slowing the progression to renal failure, especially medications that block the renin-angiotensin-aldosterone pathway and more stringent blood pressure guidelines. Although effective, these therapies are not cures. Thus, there is an ongoing effort to further identify (1) the risk factors and mechanisms leading to the development of diabetic nephropathy, (2) who is at risk for progression, and (3) the mechanisms underlying progression to renal failure. This chapter presents an overview of the demographics, diagnosis, and natural history as well as current ideas about the pathogenesis underlying the development and progression of diabetic nephropathy. An understanding of these mechanisms has provided specific directions for the development of new, effective treatments that hold promise for the development of new clinically applicable therapies. Although there likely are differences in the pathogenesis of type 1 and type 2 diabetic nephropathy, currently the mechanistic studies and approaches to treatment have more similarities than differences. Thus, this chapter does not differentiate between the nephropathy of type 1 diabetes mellitus and that of type 2 diabetes mellitus.

J.S. Skyler (ed.), *Atlas of Diabetes: Fourth Edition*,
DOI 10.1007/978-1-4614-1028-7_13, © Springer Science+Business Media, LLC 2012

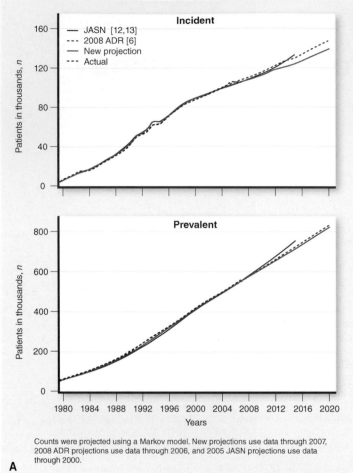

Counts were projected using a Markov model. New projections use data through 2007, 2008 ADR projections use data through 2006, and 2005 JASN projections use data through 2000.

A

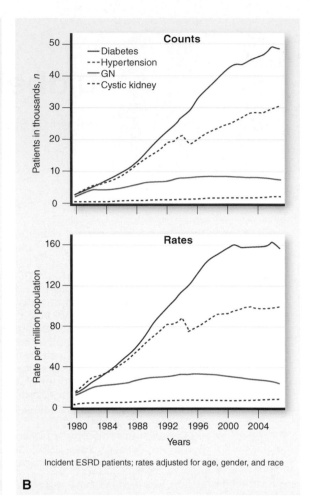

Incident ESRD patients; rates adjusted for age, gender, and race

B

FIGURE 13-1. Demographics of ESRD for all patients with ESRD. (**A**) To appreciate the impact of chronic kidney disease, it is most accurate to look at the epidemic rise in ESRD (which includes all dialysis and kidney-transplant patients). The 2009 annual data report (ADR) from the US Renal Data System (USRDS) presents data from 2007 showing that there are approximately 369,000 dialysis patients and 159,000 transplant recipients in the USA. Of course, there are millions more with chronic kidney disease. As shown here, there has been an epidemic rise in ESRD over the past 30 years. Diabetic nephropathy occurs in about 20–40% of patients with type 1 diabetes mellitus and 10–30% of those with type 2 diabetes mellitus. It is a significant cause of morbidity in these patients; that is primarily due to a very significant increased prevalence of cardiovascular disease [12]. Indeed there is a very strong positive correlation of kidney disease with cardiovascular disease that leads to significant increases in hospitalizations and medical care costs. (**B**) The major causes of ESRD in the USA are diabetes, hypertension, and glomerulonephritis (GN), and since the late 1980s, diabetes has been the leading cause [11]. The 2009 USRDS report shows that diabetes is by far the most common cause of new cases of ESRD. *JASN* Journal of the American Society of Nephrology (adapted from the USRDS [6]). If current ESRD trends continue, it is predicted that the rapid growth in the ESRD population will outstrip the resources needed to care for this population [13].

PREVALENCE AND INCIDENCE OF END-STAGE RENAL DISEASE BY CAUSE		
Cause	**Prevalence**	**Incidence**
Diabetes mellitus	192,388	47,778
Hypertension	125,953	30,402
Glomerulonephritis	79,592	7436

Figure 13-2. Prevalence and incidence of ESRD by the top three causes in 2007 [11]. The prevalence shown here is the total number of patients with ESRD in 2007; the incidence is the number of new patients with ESRD in 2007.

Diagnosis of Diabetic Nephropathy

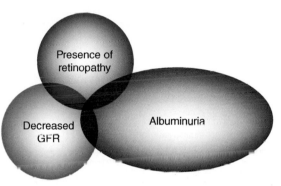

Figure 13-3. Diagnosis of diabetic nephropathy. Patients with very early diabetic nephropathy may have increased GFRs and renal hypertrophy, but this stage is usually not detected clinically. It had been thought that the hallmark of the diagnosis of diabetic nephropathy is albuminuria; however, as previously noted, the first sign of diabetic nephropathy may be decreased GFR and/or microalbuminuria [10]. Thus, to diagnose kidney disease in diabetic patients, it is important to measure serum creatinine and to use a formula, such as the Modification of Diet in Renal Disease (MDRD) equation [14], to estimate GFR as well as to check for albuminuria. Typically, microalbuminuria progresses to frank proteinuria over a period of years. The rate of progression and loss of GFR are based on several factors, which are discussed later in this chapter. Thus, increased GFR and increased kidney size are additional signs of early diabetic nephropathy. There are clear associations between diabetic nephropathy and two other diagnostically important factors: (1) the duration of diabetes in type 1 patients and (2) preexisting retinopathy. It is unusual for diabetic nephropathy to appear in patients who have had type 1 diabetes for less than 5 years. Most patients (as many as 90%) with diabetic nephropathy also have retinopathy [15]. Thus, either a short duration of type 1 diabetes or no evidence of retinopathy in a patient with evidence of renal dysfunction should lead the clinician to consider other renal diseases. Importantly, patients with type 2 diabetes may have diabetic nephropathy at the time of diagnosis, as the duration of diabetes is unknown in type 2 diabetes [16].

Reasons to Consider Other Renal Diseases in Patients with Diabetes Mellitus

Absence of albuminuria

Diabetes mellitus present for < 5 y in type 1 patients

Rapidly increasing serum creatine

Presence of active urinary sediment

Very high levels of urine protein

FIGURE 13-4. Reasons to consider other renal diseases in patients with diabetes mellitus. The most common nondiabetic kidney diseases that occur in patients with diabetes are hypertension and IgA nephropathy (for which there is no reliable treatment other than blood pressure control and lowering urine protein excretion). It is not critical to do a biopsy to document whether a diabetic patient has hypertension or IgA nephropathy because the treatment plan would not change. However, if certain other signs are present, then a further workup for another renal disease is indicated because there may be an effective treatment to prevent ESRD. Signs that should stimulate a search for other kidney diseases are as follows: (1) Worsening renal function in a patient with type 1 diabetes mellitus for less than 5 years should prompt the physician to consider other causes of renal failure. Typically, the decrease in GFR occurs over years. If a patient has a decreasing creatinine clearance or increasing serum creatinine that occurs over weeks to months, other renal diseases should be considered. (2) The presence of an active urinary sediment (i.e., the presence of elements, such as red blood cells, white blood cells, or red blood cell casts) should lead the physician to consider other renal diseases. Most patients with diabetic nephropathy have a relatively inactive urinary sediment; however, as many as 25–30% may have hematuria [17]. Nevertheless, the finding of an active urine sediment should alert the physician to consider other renal diseases. (3) A rapid increase in urine protein levels or very high levels of proteinuria may reflect another kidney disease.

Microalbuminuria and Macroalbuminuria

Definition of microalbuminuria

> 30 mg/24 h or > 20 μg/min

Albumin/creatinine ratio of > 30 mg/g

Definition of frank albuminuria or macroalbuminuria

> 300 mg/24 h or > 200 μg/min

Common causesof transient increases in albuminuria

Exercise

Pregnancy

Poor glycemic control

Congestive heart failure

Hypertension

Urinary tract infection

FIGURE 13-5. Detection of albuminuria. All diabetic patients should be routinely screened for the presence of microalbuminuria because it is a marker of kidney disease and a risk factor for progression of both kidney disease and cardiovascular disease [5, 18]. Although a timed urine collection is an effective way to determine albumin excretion accurately, it is neither convenient nor cost-effective. Many studies have shown that the albumin/creatinine ratio, obtained by measuring a spot urine sample for albumin and creatinine, is a highly accurate method for screening and following patients with diabetes mellitus [19]. It is important to note that dipsticks used for determining protein in the urine are not sensitive enough to measure low level increases in urine albumin level. The dipstick may give a false negative in up to 50% of diabetic patients with microalbuminuria. Thus, direct laboratory measurement of albumin is required to detect microalbuminuria. A spot measurement of albumin alone is affected by the urine volume, but normalizing to the amount of creatinine in the urine eliminates this concern. A value greater than 30 mg/g indicates microalbuminuria.

In determining the presence of microalbuminuria, one must consider causes of transient increases in albuminuria as noted above. Whereas macroalbuminuria (>300 mg/g) almost always reflects progressive nephropathy and therefore increased attention should be given to treatment (see Fig. 13.17). Thus, repeat measurements of albumin excretion in patients with microalbuminuria are recommended before labeling a patient with a diagnosis of diabetic nephropathy.

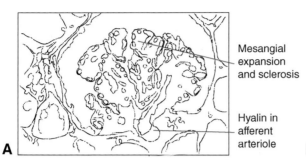

Mesangial expansion and sclerosis

Hyalin in afferent arteriole

A

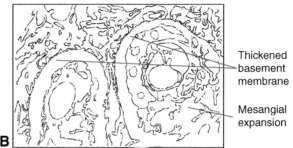

Thickened basement membrane

Mesangial expansion

B

FIGURE 13-6. Pathology of diabetic nephropathy. Typical changes of diabetic nephropathy are seen on light micrograph (**A**) and electron micrograph (**B**) [20]. (**A**) Shows nodular sclerosis, mesangial expansion, and hyalin deposition in the afferent arteriole. (**B**) Shows two capillary loops. The capillary loop on the right shows basement membrane thickening and mesangial expansion. Although these changes are typical of diabetic nephropathy, they are not pathognomonic. Two other diseases also must be considered in a patient with these renal biopsy findings: light chain deposition disease and amyloidosis. It is possible to differentiate among these diseases by specific stains and history (courtesy of Dr. Helmut Rennke, Boston, MA).

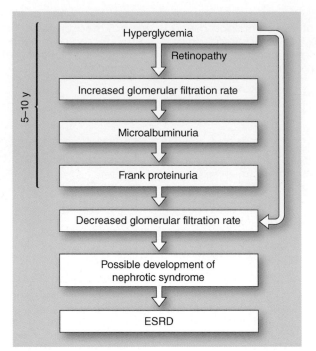

Figure 13-7. Natural history of diabetic nephropathy. The rate of progression of kidney disease after a patient with diabetes mellitus develops microalbuminuria is not entirely clear. Indeed, a study in type 1 diabetes has shown that microalbuminuria might regress to normal [21]. An important area of research is the determination of who will progress and who do not. Because at this time we do not know who will progress, it is necessary to treat any diabetic patient with microalbuminuria and/or decreased GFR as if he or she will progress. This schematic shows the likely progression in an idealized patient. A patient who is going to develop renal failure usually has detectable retinopathy and shows evidence of renal failure 5–10 years after the diagnosis of diabetes mellitus. Interestingly, if the patient has not developed diabetic nephropathy after 15–20 years of diabetes, the likelihood of his or her developing renal disease with progression to renal failure is greatly reduced [22]. The reasons for progression are multifactorial. The following figures demonstrate the possible causes of the development of diabetic nephropathy and the reasons for its progression.

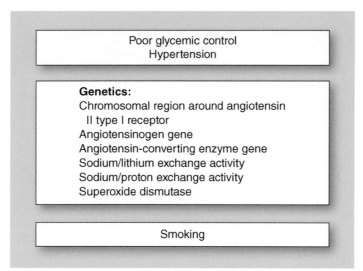

FIGURE 13-8. Risk factors for the development of diabetic nephropathy. Poor glycemic control and hypertension have been shown to increase the likelihood of developing diabetic nephropathy [8, 23, 24]. Both these factors are independently correlated with the development of diabetic nephropathy. Patients with poor glycemic control also are more likely than those with good glycemic control to have hypertension [25]. In addition, there has been a concerted effort to detect specific genes that predispose patients to the development of diabetic nephropathy. The existence of such genes is supported by several findings. A family history of diabetic nephropathy increases the likelihood of developing nephropathy [26]. In addition, certain genetically similar groups are more susceptible than others to nephropathy. For example, members of the Pima Indian tribe in Arizona have a high rate of development of type 2 diabetes, and more than 60% of those above age 45 with type 2 diabetes have developed nephropathy, a percentage much higher than average [27]. Specific genes listed in this figure have been suggested to be associated with the development of nephropathy [28–30]. Smoking, probably because of its deleterious effects on vascular endothelial cells, also has been shown to increase the likelihood of developing diabetic nephropathy in patients with type 1 and in those with type 2 diabetes mellitus [31].

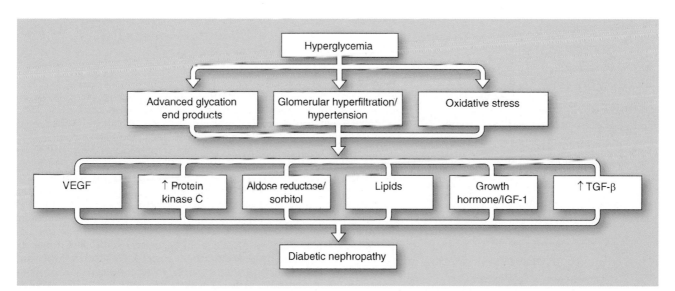

FIGURE 13-9. Suggested mechanisms underlying the development and progression of diabetic nephropathy. Several mechanisms have been proposed to be responsible for the development of diabetic nephropathy. None of these are mutually exclusive, and it is likely that interactions among many of these factors contribute to diabetic nephropathy. An understanding of these mechanisms is essential for producing appropriate therapies to prevent both the development and progression of diabetic nephropathy. A number of existing therapies, as well as treatments currently in development or in clinical trials, are based on altering one or more of the mechanisms shown in this figure. The ensuing figures provide a brief review of each of these mechanisms. *IGF-1* insulin-like growth factor-1, *TGF-β* transforming growth factor-β, *VEGF* vascular endothelial growth factor.

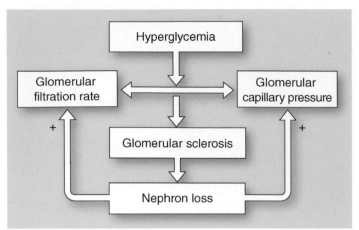

Figure 13-10. Glomerular hyperfiltration. Glomerular hyperfiltration is a hallmark of diabetic nephropathy. GFRs ≥ 150 mL/min are seen in early diabetic nephropathy. Zatz et al. [32] were the first to show that intervention directed at decreasing hyperfiltration significantly slowed the progression of diabetic nephropathy in rats. The hypothesis is that the increased GFR is associated with increased pressure in the glomerular capillary tuft. This glomerular hypertension then leads to glomerular sclerosis and loss of functioning nephrons. Although the total GFR eventually decreases when enough nephrons undergo sclerosis, the hypothesis suggests that the filtration and, thus, the pressure in the remaining functioning glomeruli are high because the filtered load delivered to the kidney is the same as it was when there were more functioning glomeruli. Much research supports this general hypothesis. More importantly, efforts to use interventions that lead specifically to a reduction in glomerular capillary pressure (e.g., angiotensin-converting enzyme inhibitors and angiotensin receptor blockers) are now mainstays of treatment for diabetic nephropathy. An extension of this hypothesis was suggested by Brenner and Mackenzie [33], who proposed that one predisposing factor for the progression of renal disease and possibly for the development of diabetic nephropathy is the number of glomeruli one has at birth. That is, the presence of fewer glomeruli would lead to relative glomerular hyperfiltration/hypertension, which would predispose to development of kidney disease.

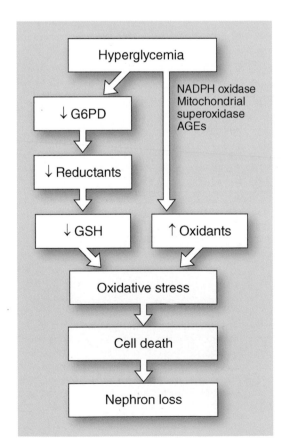

Figure 13-11. Oxidative stress. Many studies in both humans and animals have determined that patients with diabetes have evidence of increased oxidant stress [34]. Intracellular oxidant levels increase because of an imbalance between processes that produce oxidants and those that lower the oxidant level (called reductants or antioxidants). Intracellular oxidants may increase as a result of intracellular production of oxidants or by exposure to extracellular oxidants. Hyperglycemia may increase the level of intracellular oxidants by stimulating processes that produce oxidants, such as NADPH oxidase [35] and increased mitochondrial production of superoxide [36]. Studies also have shown that hyperglycemia may lead to decreased antioxidant function [34, 37, 38]. Thus, hyperglycemia causes a dysfunctional cellular response that leads to cell damage and cell death. Increased oxidants may cause defects in several intracellular events and cause cell death [36]. In addition, increased oxidants lead to increased activity of protein kinase C, thus linking two pathophysiologic mechanisms. Indeed, Brownlee [36] proposed a unifying mechanism (see Fig. 13.15b) whereby increased mitochondrial superoxide production leads to inhibition of a glycolytic enzyme, resulting in activation of many pathophysiologic processes associated with development and progression of diabetic complications. To date, antioxidant studies have not been too promising. These disappointing results likely are a result of the lack of specific targeting of the exact cellular defect leading to increased oxidant levels. New approaches to treatment are aimed at targeting specific cellular defects rather than using a general antioxidant. *AGEs* advanced glycation end products, *G6PD* glucose-6-phosphate dehydrogenase, *GSH* reduced glutathione.

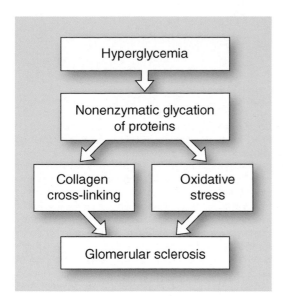

Figure 13-12. Advanced glycation end products (AGEs). AGEs are proteins that have reacted nonenzymatically with glucose. Although they exist normally, the number of AGEs increases significantly in patients with diabetes (and with normal aging). AGEs have been implicated in the development of complications of diabetes [39]. In particular, AGE production leads to increased oxidant stress. AGEs also may cause collagen cross-linking and, by binding to specific receptors, may lead to intracellular increases in intracellular oxidants. Administration of AGEs to animals may cause several changes that are seen with diabetes, including glomerular sclerosis [40]. Accumulation of AGEs parallels the severity of diabetic nephropathy [41]. Clinical trials have been done using an inhibitor of the formation of AGEs, aminoguanidine, to determine whether this drug can help patients with established nephropathy and also help prevent diabetic nephropathy [42]. The results to date have not been promising. A newer drug aimed at AGEs, pyridoxamine, has shown some efficacy, but more research is needed [43].

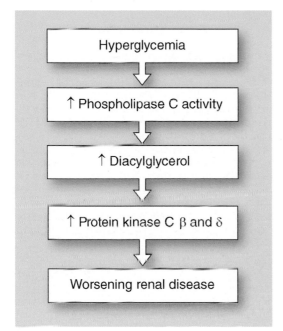

Figure 13-13. Protein kinase C (PKC). PKC is a serine/threonine kinase shown to play important roles in normal cell growth, cancerous cell growth, and several other intracellular processes. Work by Koya and King [44] has shown that hyperglycemia leads to activation of PKC. More detailed work has demonstrated that specific isoforms of PKC are specifically activated by hyperglycemia. The prevention of PKC activation may reduce mesangial expansion and prevent the progression of renal disease. The deleterious effects of PKC on the kidney may be the result of stimulation of the production of the cytokine TGF-β (see Fig. 13.14). In particular, PKC β has been suggested to play an important pathophysiologic role in the development of vascular, retinal, and other complications of diabetes mellitus. Ishii et al. [45] showed in diabetic rats that an inhibitor that specifically blocks PKC greatly reduced the increase in renal TGF-β and also reduced the increase in other proteins associated with sclerosis. This suggests that PKC inhibitors may play an important role in future treatments for diabetic nephropathy. Studies to date with the PKC inhibitor ruboxistaurin for the kidney are intriguing, but more clinical studies are needed [46].

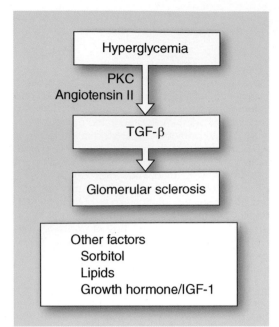

Figure 13-14. Transforming growth factor-β (TGF-β). TGF-β is a cytokine that can stimulate some cells to grow and inhibit the growth of other cells. Ziyadeh [47] provided a strong body of work supporting the hypothesis that TGF-β is an important mediator of the lesions seen in diabetic nephropathy. The suggestion that TGF-β plays a role in the pathogenesis of diabetic nephropathy is supported by the following evidence: (1) patients with diabetic nephropathy have increased levels of TGF-β; (2) TGF-β can cause glomerular sclerosis in animal models of diabetic nephropathy; and (3) neutralizing antibodies to TGF-β have prevented the development of diabetic nephropathy in an animal model. An interesting speculation is that increased activity of PKC leads to increased expression of TGF-β. Thus, hyperglycemia might be the initiating point that leads to increased oxidative stress, which leads to increased activity of PKC, which leads to increased expression of TGF-β. In addition, hyperglycemia leads to the production of advanced glycation end products. Thus, all these mechanisms, separately and together, contribute to the development and progression of diabetic nephropathy. An ongoing National Institutes of Health study is using the antifibrosis drug pirfenidone, which also inhibits TGF-β [48].

Other factors have been implicated as well. Aldose reductase activity and the production of sorbitol have been implicated in diabetic complications [49]. Sorbitol is produced by the reduction of glucose by aldose reductase. Sorbitol is osmotically active; thus, increased sorbitol may lead to cell swelling and cell death. In addition, the action of aldose reductase leads to the loss of intracellular antioxidants, thereby increasing oxidative stress. Although increased aldose reductase activity may play a significant role in the pathogenesis of other diabetic complications, to date it has not been shown to play an important role in diabetic nephropathy. Studies using an inhibitor of aldose reductase, sorbinil, have been disappointing. Epidemiologic studies also have implicated increased lipids as possible mediators. Although it is likely that increased lipids are associated with progression of diabetic nephropathy, the mechanism underlying this association has not been well-defined [50]. VEGF, which has been shown to be a major factor in diabetic retinopathy, also may play a role in glomerular dysfunction and development of increased urine albumin [51]. Moreover, a body of research suggests that growth hormone/IGF-1 may play an important role in the pathogenesis of diabetic nephropathy. A study showed a strong, positive correlation between urinary levels of growth hormone and IGF-1 and the development of microalbuminuria and increased kidney size in patients with type 1 diabetes mellitus [52]. Lastly, studies using the glycosaminoglycan sulodexide initially were intriguing [53], but to date clinical trials have been inconclusive.

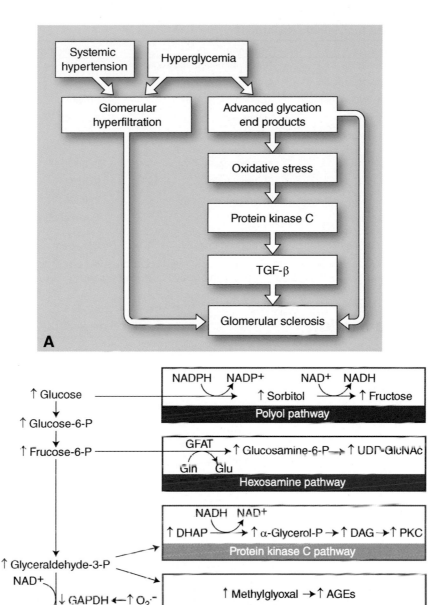

Figure 13-15. Possible connections between various mechanisms that may contribute to diabetic nephropathy. (**A**) This model suggests that controlling blood sugar is of paramount importance. Research from the Diabetes Control and Complications Trial (DCCT) strongly supports this idea [7, 11]. Nevertheless, after there is evidence of diabetic nephropathy, many of these mechanisms may occur independent (to some extent) of the current blood glucose control. For example, if nephron loss has occurred, then glomerular hyperfiltration/hypertension continue, even in the presence of tight control of blood sugar. Other mechanisms shown in the figure also may become somewhat autonomous after initial damage to the glomerulus. Thus, tight control of blood sugar and other interventions that block mechanisms shown in this figure probably are needed to prevent the progression of diabetic nephropathy. Likely, a mixture of all of these mechanisms leads to diabetic nephropathy. (**B**) Brownlee [36] suggested a model that links these mechanisms based on mitochondrial overproduction of superoxide. In this model, superoxide inhibits GAPDH and the subsequent upstream accumulation of metabolic intermediates leads to activation of many processes associated with the pathogenesis of diabetic nephropathy. This interesting model also provides a testable hypothesis for treatment that is currently ongoing. *ACE* angiotension-converting enzyme, *DAG* diacylglycerol, *DHAP* dihydroxyacetone phosphate, *GFAT* glutamine:fructose-6-phosphate aminotransferase, *UDP* uridine diphosphate.

Treatment for Diabetic Nephropathy

Mechanism	Treatment	Efficacy in humans
Hyperglycemia	Tight control of blood sugar	Proven
Systemic hypertension	Antihypertensive agents	Proven
Glomerular hypertension	ACE inhibitors/ARB	Proven
Lipids/cholesterol	Statins/diet	Possible
Advanced glycation end products	Pyridoxamine	In trials
Oxidative stress	Antioxidants	In trials
Increased PKC	Ruboxistaurin	In trials
TGF-β	Pirfenidone	In trials
Increased aldose reductase/sorbitol	Sorbinil	Questionable
Growth hormone/IGF-1	No obvious therapy	Unknown

FIGURE 13-16. The efficacy in humans of various treatments for diabetic nephropathy, listed according to mechanism. As previously noted, a combined therapeutic approach probably is the most beneficial. *ARBs* angiotensin receptor blockers.

Treatment and Prevention

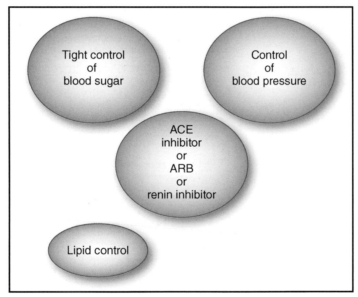

FIGURE 13-17. Treatment and prevention of diabetic nephropathy. The mainstay of prevention is tight control of blood sugar and control of hypertension. The DCCT Research Group clearly showed that control of blood sugar is very beneficial in preventing both the onset and the progression of type 1 diabetic nephropathy [7, 11]. This is entirely consistent with the information presented previously suggesting that hyperglycemia may be the predominant mechanism leading to the activation of the other proposed mechanisms. Research also supports the importance of blood sugar control in type 2 diabetes [54]. In addition, many studies clearly have indicated that hypertension both predisposes to and worsens diabetic nephropathy [23]. Thus, before microalbuminuria has developed, all patients should be urged to monitor their blood sugar closely and to control their blood pressure. The current recommendation is to aim for a blood pressure lower than 130/80 mmHg or lower than 125/75 mmHg if the urine protein/creatinine ratio is greater than 1.0 g/g (equivalent to 1 g of protein excretion per 24 h). At this point, there is no compelling evidence for treating all diabetic patients with ACE inhibitors or ARBs to prevent the development of diabetic nephropathy.

If the first indication of diabetic nephropathy is decreased GFR, then the main therapeutic goals are blood sugar control and blood pressure control. At this point, there is no compelling evidence that ACE inhibitors or ARBs are more effective than other antihypertensives in the absence of microalbuminuria. When microalbuminuria develops, in addition to tight control of blood glucose and control of hypertension all patients should receive an ACE inhibitor or ARB [55, 56]. Indeed, patients who have excellent blood sugar and blood pressure control and persistent microalbuminuria or macroalbuminuria should be on an ACE inhibitor or ARB to lower the urine albumin level. ACE inhibitors and ARBs, although not a cure, clearly have been shown to slow the progression of diabetic nephropathy. These drugs reduce the levels of angiotensin II, leading to a decrease in glomerular filtration and pressure. This effect may or may not be the main mechanism by which these drugs work. For example, in addition to its vasoactive properties, angiotensin II is also a growth factor. Thus, it has been proposed that ACE inhibitors also work by inhibiting the growth-promoting effects of angiotensin II [57]. The angiotensin II receptor-blocking drugs are useful alone or as an alternative

in patients who develop a cough while taking an ACE inhibitor. Also, recently, a renin inhibitor, aliskiren, became available [58]. The specific use of this medication at this time likely is as an additional agent if urine protein targets have not been achieved with ACE inhibitors or ARBs, although a recent trial suggested otherwise.

Other recommended treatments are adherence to a low-protein diet and control of lipids. A low-protein diet probably acts similarly to ACE inhibitors by decreasing intraglomerular pressure. In practical terms, it is somewhat difficult to achieve a low enough intake of protein because the diet is rather bland. Moreover, there are limited data on the success of a low-protein diet (especially, in type 2 patients). Typically, dietary counseling is important for blood sugar management, salt intake, caloric intake, and avoidance of a high-protein diet (e.g., >2–3 g/kg per day). However, the specific utility of a low-protein diet (<0.8 g/kg per day) is questionable. A recent 5-year study comparing a low-protein diet with a normal-protein diet showed no benefit in patients with diabetic nephropathy [59]. Moreover, as many studies have found, it is extremely difficult to adhere to a low-protein diet.

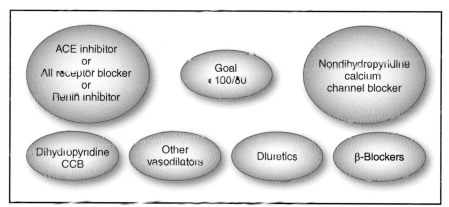

FIGURE 13-10. Antihypertensive agents. In addition to dietary modifications and medications that block renin or angiotensin, other antihypertensive agents play important roles in the treatment of hypertension in diabetic nephropathy. Of particular interest are the calcium channel blockers (CCBs). Specifically, the nondihydropyridine CCBs (e.g., diltiazem and verapamil) offer benefits similar to those provided by ACE inhibitor drugs in both reducing blood pressure and slowing the progression of renal disease [60]. Dihydropyridine CCBs (e.g., nifedipine and amlodipine) also are very effective in treating hypertension, but alone they do not offer the same lowering effects on urine albumin levels observed with the ACE inhibitor and ARB drugs

and the nondihydropyridines. Various combinations of antihypertensive agents also have been evaluated and may offer further benefits. The combination of a nondihydropyridine and an ACE inhibitor/ARB may be more effective than either drug alone in slowing the progression of diabetic nephropathy [60]. Thus, in treating hypertension and kidney disease, there are two goals: blood pressure control and lowering of urine albumin level. The selection of a specific medicine depends on which goal needs to be focused on. Other antihypertensive agents also may be used in patients with diabetic nephropathy, such as diuretics, β-blockers, and vasodilators. All angiotensin II.

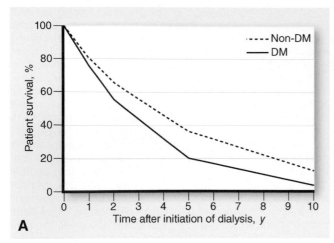

A

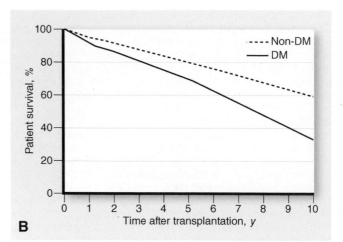

B

Figure 13-19. Survival estimates for patients on dialysis. As noted in Figure 13-1, diabetic nephropathy is the leading cause of ESRD in the USA. In addition, the rate of increase in ESRD resulting from diabetes is significantly greater than that for the other leading causes of renal failure. Most of this increase reflects an aging population in which type 2 diabetes mellitus (DM) is prevalent. A review covers the general issues of ESRD in the diabetic population [24]. Probably because of the many comorbid conditions present in diabetic patients, diabetic patients on dialysis (**A**) or post transplantation (**B**) have a lower rate of survival than do nondiabetic ESRD patients [24]. It is not clear whether the mode of dialysis has any effects, positive or negative, on morbidity or mortality, although most ESRD diabetic patients are treated by hemodialysis [24]. The decision to use hemodialysis versus peritoneal dialysis should be made on consideration of factors, such as lifestyle, the overall health of the patient, and comorbid conditions (e.g., vision impairment). The use of peritoneal dialysis may simplify or complicate glucose management. Because peritoneal dialysate contains varying concentrations of glucose (1.5, 2.5, and 4.25%), glucose control may be significantly affected when dialysate exchanges occur. This problem is minimized by injecting insulin directly into the dialysate solution. This insulin delivery method may be used not only to counteract the effects of the acute exposure to the high glucose concentrations, but also as a way to provide a constant level of insulin, which may help maintain a reasonably stable blood glucose level throughout the day. This method of insulin delivery is effective for overall blood glucose maintenance only for patients who do fluid exchanges during the day. Many patients prefer to do peritoneal dialysis by repeated nighttime exchanges using a machine that cycles the fluid in and out of the abdomen. During the day, these patients have no fluid exchanges. The insulin injected in each bag at night is dosed to maintain a steady glucose concentration through the night, and the patient follows a standard schedule of subcutaneous injections throughout the day (data from the USRDS [6]).

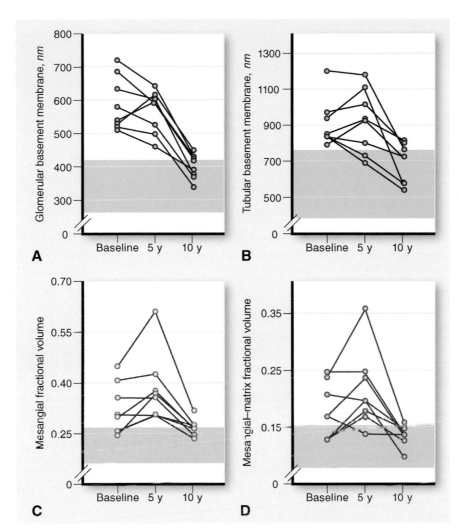

FIGURE 13-20. Kidney and pancreas transplantation. Kidney or kidney/pancreas transplantation generally is the preferred therapy for patients with ESRD. Survival rates after transplantation are higher than those for patients who remain on dialysis (see Fig. 13.19). Diabetic nephropathy recurs in most kidney-transplant recipients, although it usually is many years before diabetic nephropathy is severe enough to cause loss of the transplant (**A–D**). Thus, loss of the transplant because of the recurrence of diabetic nephropathy is rare. Pancreas transplantation usually is done only in conjunction with a kidney transplant. It has been believed that because blood glucose levels can be controlled with insulin pancreas trans-plantation alone offers too many risks compared with its benefits. The biggest risks relate to immunosuppression and the increased risk of life-threatening infections. In addition, there has been little evidence showing that early pancreas trans-plantation would affect the progression of diabetic nephropathy. An intriguing study by Fioretto et al. [61] shows, however, that pancreas transplantation alone may cause actual reversal in the lesions of diabetic nephropathy. But this apparent improvement only became evident after 5 years of normo-glycemia. This finding may increase interest in pancreas trans-plantation as a way to prevent the development of diabetic nephropathy (adapted from Fioretto et al. [61]).

Screen: Measure serum creatinine at least annually to estimate the GFR, regardless of the degree of urine albumin excretion (see *Guidelines for Specialty Consultation/Referral*).

Obtain estimated GFR (eGFR) using the MDRD equation.

If eGFR is < 60 mL/min, evaluate for complications of kidney disease (anemia, hyperparathyroidism, and vitamin D deficiency) Consider a referral to a nephrologist to:

Assess cause(s) of impaired kidney function, including assessing for nondiabetes kidney disease.

Maximize therapies aimed at slowing the progression of kidney disease (*eg*, blood pressure control and reduction of the urine protein level) Treat complications of kidney disease.

Screen for micro/macro albuminuria by checking the urine albumin/creatinine (A/C) ratio as follows:
Type I patients within 5 y of diagnosis, then yearly

Type 2 patients at diagnosis (after glucose has been stabilized), then yearly

Annually in all patients up to age 70 y

As clinically indicated in patients > age 70 y

Micro/macro albuminuria is recognized as a major independent risk factor for CAD in patients with diabetes.

Albuminuria may be measured with a spot or timed urine collection. Spot urine is preferred for simplicity. Continue the use of routine urinalysis, as clinically indicated.

Treatment:

If A/C ratio < 30 mcg/mg or timed urine < 30 mg/24 h

Recheck in I y

If A/C ratio 30–300 mcg/mg or timed urine 30–300 mg/24 h

Confirm the presence of microalbuminuria with at least 2 of 3 positive collections done within 3–6 mo. In the process, rule out confounding factors that cause a false-positive, such as UTI, pregnancy, excessive exercise, menses, or severe hypoglycemic event. Consider testing first morning urine.

Consider consulting with the nephrology team for blood pressure control, successive increases in microalbumin, and other issues (*ie*, GFR < 60 mL/min)

Once confirmed:

Evaluate BP and initiate/modify aggressive blood pressure treatment to achieve a BP of < 130/80 mmHg

Recommend patient self-monitor BP with a portable cuff and maintain a record/log. The monitoring schedule should be determined with the healthcare provider and is based on patient circumstance.

Strive to improve glycemic control with an optimal goal AIC of < 7% or as otherwise clinically indicated for individual patients.

Refer to a diabetes educator for glucose management.

Initiate/modify the ACE inhibitor or angiotensin II antagonist treatment if microalbuminuria persists.

Check K+ and creatinine 1–2 wk after making changes.

Repeat the A/C ratio at least every 6 mo; consider an increase in frequency when changes in medication are made.
If A/C ratio > 300 mcg/mg (>300 mg/24 h) or proteinuria (positive dipstick for protein or ≥ 30 mg/dL):

Follow all guidelines as stated for A/C ratio 30–300 mcg/mg.

Consider BP goal of < 125/75 mmHg.

Consult with nephrologist if:

1) Rapid a rise in serum creatinine, abnormal sediment, or sudden increase in proteinuria.

2) eGFR < 60 mL/min; estimated GFR is calculated by using the serum creatinine level and applying it to an accepted formula (*eg*, MDRD equation).

3) Need to refine the treatment program to prevent further deterioration.

4) Problems with ACE inhibitors, difficulties in the management of high BP, or hyperkalemia.

5) Etiology of nephropathy is questionable.

6) Management of hyperphosphatemia presents difficulties.

7) Anemia due to renal disease.

Consider reducing protein in the diet.

Figure 13-21. Screening and treatment recommendations for proteinuria. The current recommendations for treating proteinuria at the Joslin Diabetes Center in Boston, Massachusetts, are based on the level of proteinuria. The physicians at the Joslin Diabetes Center believe that a collaborative model of care is best for the patient with diabetes. Thus, patients with early diabetic nephropathy are cared for primarily by an endocrinologist in consultation with a nephrologist. When a patient nears ESRD, much of his or her care transfers to the nephrologist, but other caregivers (e.g., endocrinologist, ophthalmologist, dietitian) continue to work collaboratively to care for the patient. *A/C* albumin/creatinine, *BP* blood pressure, *CAD* coronary artery disease, *eGFR* estimated GFR, *UTI* urinary tract infection.

References

1. Mehdi U, Toto RD: Anemia, diabetes, and chronic kidney disease. *Diabetes Care* 2009, 32:1320–1326.

2. Tomasello S: Secondary hyperparathyroidism and chronic kidney disease. *Diabetes Spectr* 2008, 21:19–25.

3. Adler AI, Stevens RJ, Manley SE, *et al.*: Development and progression of nephropathy in type 2 diabetes: the United Kingdom Prospective Diabetes Study (UKPDS 64). *Kidney Int* 2003, 63:225–232.

4. Allen KV, Walker JD: Microalbuminuria and mortality in long-duration type 1 diabetes. *Diabetes Care* 2003, 26:2389–2391.

5. Gerstein HC, Mann JF, Yi Q, *et al.*: Albuminuria and risk of cardiovascular events, death, and heart failure in diabetic and nondiabetic individuals. *JAMA* 2001, 286:421–426.

6. US Renal Data System: *USRDS 2009 Annual Data Report: Atlas of Chronic Kidney Disease and End-Stage Renal Disease in the United States.* Bethesda, MD: National Institutes of Health, National Institute of Diabetes and Digestive and Kidney Diseases; 2009.

7. Writing Team for the Diabetes Control and Complications Trial/Epidemiology of Diabetes Interventions and Complications Research Group: Sustained effect of intensive treatment of type 1 diabetes mellitus on development and progression of diabetic nephropathy: the Epidemiology of Diabetes Interventions and Complications (EDIC) study. *JAMA* 2003, 290:2159–2167.

8. Joss N, Ferguson C, Brown C, *et al.*: Intensified treatment of patients with type 2 diabetes mellitus and overt nephropathy. *QJM* 2004, 97:219–227.

9. Katakura M, Naka M, Kondo T, *et al.*: Development, worsening, and improvement of diabetic microangiopathy in older people: six-year prospective study of patients under intensive diabetes control. *J Am Geriatr Soc* 2007, 55:541–547.

10. Perkins BA, Ficociello LH, Roshan B, *et al.*: In patients with type 1 diabetes and new onset micro-albuminuria the development of advanced chronic kidney disease may not require progression to proteinuria. *Kidney Int* 2010, 77:57–64.

11. The effect of intensive treatment of diabetes on the development and progression of long-term complications in insulin-dependent diabetes mellitus. The Diabetes Control and Complications Trial Research Group. *N Engl J Med* 1993, 329:977–986.

12. Foley RN, Murray AM, Li S, *et al.*: Chronic kidney disease and the risk for cardiovascular disease, renal replacement, and death in the United States Medicare population, 1998 to 1999. *J Am Soc Nephrol* 2005, 16:489–495.

13. Gilbertson DT, Liu J, Xue JL, *et al.*: Projecting the number of patients with end-stage renal disease in the United States to the year 2015. *J Am Soc Nephrol* 2005, 16:3736–3741.

14. Stevens LA, Levey AS: Current status and future perspectives for CKD testing. *Am J Kidney Dis* 2009, 53:S17–S26.

15. Stephenson JM, Fuller JH, Viberti GC, *et al.*: Blood pressure, retinopathy and urinary albumin excretion in IDDM: the EURODIAB IDDM Complications Study. *Diabetologia* 1995, 38:599–603.

16. Zimmet P: Preventing diabetic complications: a primary care perspective. *Diabetes Res Clin Pract* 2009, 84:107–116.

17. Chihara J, Takebayashi S, Taguchi T, *et al.*: Glomerulonephritis in diabetic patients and its effect on the prognosis. *Nephron* 1986, 43:45–49.

18. Araki S, Haneda M, Koya D, *et al.*: Clinical impact of reducing microalbuminuria in patients with type 2 diabetes mellitus. *Diabetes Res Clin Pract* 2008, 82(suppl 1):S54–S58.

19. Warram J, Krolewski A: Use of the albumin/creatinine ratio in patient care and clinical studies. In *The Kidney and Hypertension in Diabetes Mellitus.* Edited by Mogensen CE. London: Kluwer Academic Publishers; 1998:85–96.

20. Tisher C, Hostetter T: Diabetic nephropathy. In *Diabetic Nephropathy.* Edited by Tisher C, Brenner B. Philadelphia: JB Lippincott; 1994:1387–1412.

21. Perkins BA, Krolewski AS: Early nephropathy in type 1 diabetes: a new perspective on who will and who will not progress. *Curr Diab Rep* 2005, 5:455–463.

22. Parving HH, Hommel E, Mathiesen E, *et al.*: Prevalence of microalbuminuria, arterial hypertension, retinopathy and neuropathy in patients with insulin dependent diabetes. *Br Med J (Clin Res Ed)* 1988, 296:156–160.

23. Bakris GL: The importance of blood pressure control in the patient with diabetes. *Am J Med* 2004, 116(suppl 5A): 30S–38S.

24. Williams ME, Stanton RC: Diabetes and the kidney. In *Chronic Kidney Disease, Dialysis, and Transplantation,* edn 3. Edited by Himmelfarb J, Sayegh M. Philadelphia: Elsevier; 2010, In press.

25. Krolewski AS, Fogarty DG, Warram JH: Hypertension and nephropathy in diabetes mellitus: what is inherited and what is acquired? *Diabetes Res Clin Pract* 1998, 39(suppl):S1–S14.

26. Quinn M, Angelico MC, Warram JH, Krolewski AS: Familial factors determine the development of diabetic nephropathy in patients with IDDM. *Diabetologia* 1996, 39:940–945.

27. Nelson RG, Newman JM, Knowler WC, *et al.*: Incidence of end-stage renal disease in type 2 (non-insulin-dependent) diabetes mellitus in Pima Indians. *Diabetologia* 1988, 31:730–736.

28. Al Kateb H, Boright AP, Mirea L, *et al.*: Multiple superoxide dismutase 1/splicing factor serine alanine 15 variants are associated with the development and progression of diabetic nephropathy: the Diabetes Control and Complications Trial/Epidemiology of Diabetes Interventions and Complications Genetics study. *Diabetes* 2008, 57:218–228.

29. Dronavalli S, Duka I, Bakris GL: The pathogenesis of diabetic nephropathy. *Nat Clin Pract Endocrinol Metab* 2008, 4:444–452.

30. Mollsten A, Lajer M, Jorsal A, Tarnow L: The endothelial nitric oxide synthase gene and risk of diabetic nephropathy and development of cardiovascular disease in type 1 diabetes. *Mol Genet Metab* 2009, 97:80–84.

31. Biesenbach G, Grafinger P, Janko O, Zazgornik J: Influence of cigarette-smoking on the progression of clinical diabetic nephropathy in type 2 diabetic patients. *Clin Nephrol* 1997, 48:146–150.

32. Zatz R, Dunn BR, Meyer TW, *et al.*: Prevention of diabetic glomerulopathy by pharmacological amelioration of glomerular capillary hypertension. *J Clin Invest* 1986, 77:1925–1930.

33. Brenner BM, Mackenzie HS: Nephron mass as a risk factor for progression of renal disease. *Kidney Int Suppl* 1997, 63:S124–S127.

34. Forbes JM, Coughlan MT, Cooper ME: Oxidative stress as a major culprit in kidney disease in diabetes. *Diabetes* 2008, 57:1446–1454.

35. Tojo A, Asaba K, Onozato ML: Suppressing renal NADPH oxidase to treat diabetic nephropathy. *Expert Opin Ther Targets* 2007, 11:1011–1018.

36. Brownlee M: The pathobiology of diabetic complications: a unifying mechanism. *Diabetes* 2005, 54:1615–1625.

37. Xu Y, Osborne BW, Stanton RC: Diabetes causes inhibition of glucose-6-phosphate dehydrogenase via activation of PKA, which contributes to oxidative stress in rat kidney cortex. *Am J Physiol Renal Physiol* 2005, 289:F1040–F1047.

38. Zhang Z, Liew CW, Handy DE, *et al.*: High glucose inhibits glucose-6-phosphate dehydrogenase, leading to increased oxidative stress and beta-cell apoptosis. *FASEB J* 2010, 24:1497–1505.

39. Tan AL, Forbes JM, Cooper ME: AGE, RAGE, and ROS in diabetic nephropathy. *Semin Nephrol* 2007, 27:130–143.

40. Vlassara H, Striker LJ, Teichberg S, *et al.*: Advanced glycation end products induce glomerular sclerosis and albuminuria in normal rats. *Proc Natl Acad Sci U S A* 1994, 91:11704–11708.

41. Makita Z, Radoff S, Rayfield EJ, *et al.*: Advanced glycosylation end products in patients with diabetic nephropathy. *N Engl J Med* 1991, 325:836–842.

42. Thornalley PJ: Use of aminoguanidine (Pimagedine) to prevent the formation of advanced glycation endproducts. *Arch Biochem Biophys* 2003, 419:31–40.

43. Williams ME, Bolton WK, Khalifah RG, *et al.*: Effects of pyridoxamine in combined phase 2 studies of patients with type 1 and type 2 diabetes and overt nephropathy. *Am J Nephrol* 2007, 27:605–614.

44. Koya D, King GL: Protein kinase C activation and the development of diabetic complications. *Diabetes* 1998, 47:859–866.

45. Ishii H, Jirousek MR, Koya D, *et al.*: Amelioration of vascular dysfunctions in diabetic rats by an oral PKC beta inhibitor. *Science* 1996, 272:728–731.

46. Tuttle KR: Protein kinase C-beta inhibition for diabetic kidney disease. *Diabetes Res Clin Pract* 2008, 82(suppl 1):S70–S74.

47. Ziyadeh FN: Mediators of diabetic renal disease: the case for tgf-Beta as the major mediator. *J Am Soc Nephrol* 2004, 15(suppl 1):S55–S57.

48. RamachandraRao SP, Zhu Y, Ravasi T, *et al.*: Pirfenidone is renoprotective in diabetic kidney disease. *J Am Soc Nephrol* 2009, 20:1765–1775.

49. Chung SS, Chung SK: Aldose reductase in diabetic microvascular complications. *Curr Drug Targets* 2005, 6:475–486.

50. Rosario RF, Prabhakar S: Lipids and diabetic nephropathy. *Curr Diab Rep* 2006, 6:455–462.

51. Kim NH, Oh JH, Seo JA, *et al.*: Vascular endothelial growth factor (VEGF) and soluble VEGF receptor FLT-1 in diabetic nephropathy. *Kidney Int* 2005, 67:167–177.

52. Flyvbjerg A: The role of growth hormone in the pathogenesis of diabetic kidney disease. *Pediatr Endocrinol Rev* 2004, 1(suppl 3):525–529.

53. Gambaro G, Kinalska I, Oksa A, *et al.*: Oral sulodexide reduces albuminuria in microalbuminuric and macroalbuminuric type 1 and type 2 diabetic patients: the Di.N.A.S. randomized trial. *J Am Soc Nephrol* 2002, 13:1615–1625.

54. Patel A, MacMahon S, Chalmers J, *et al.*: Intensive blood glucose control and vascular outcomes in patients with type 2 diabetes. *N Engl J Med* 2008, 358:2560–2572.

55. Bakris GL, Toto RD, McCullough PA, *et al.*: Effects of different ACE inhibitor combinations on albuminuria: results of the GUARD study. *Kidney Int* 2008, 73:1303–1309.

56. Remuzzi G, Ruggenenti P, Perna A, *et al.*: Continuum of renoprotection with losartan at all stages of type 2 diabetic nephropathy: a post hoc analysis of the RENAAL trial results. *J Am Soc Nephrol* 2004, 15:3117–3125.

57. Wolf G, Ziyadeh FN: The role of angiotensin II in diabetic nephropathy: emphasis on nonhemodynamic mechanisms. *Am J Kidney Dis* 1997, 29:153–163.

58. Pimenta E, Oparil S: Role of aliskiren in cardio-renal protection and use in hypertensives with multiple risk factors. *Vasc Health Risk Manag* 2009, 5:453–463.

59. Koya D, Haneda M, Inomata S, *et al.*: Long-term effect of modification of dietary protein intake on the progression of diabetic nephropathy: a randomised controlled trial. *Diabetologia* 2009, 52:2037–2045.

60. Bakris GL, Weir MR, Secic M, *et al.*: Differential effects of calcium antagonist subclasses on markers of nephropathy progression. *Kidney Int* 2004, 65:1991–2002.

61. Fioretto P, Steffes MW, Sutherland DE, *et al.*: Reversal of lesions of diabetic nephropathy after pancreas transplantation. *N Engl J Med* 1998, 339:69–75.

14

Diabetic Neuropathies

Aaron I. Vinik

Diabetic neuropathy is not a single entity but rather a number of different syndromes, each with a range of clinical and subclinical manifestations. According to the San Antonio Conference [1], the main groups of neurologic disturbance in diabetes mellitus include subclinical neuropathy determined by abnormalities in electrodiagnostic and quantitative sensory testing, diffuse clinical neuropathy with distal symmetric sensorimotor and autonomic syndromes, and focal syndromes. There is reason to add proximal neuropathy as a separate entity based on the nature of the pathology and response to treatment. However, we have found it more appropriate to classify neuropathy into different clinical syndromes based on their pathogenesis because this is what ultimately determines the choice of treatment. We classify neuropathies into somatic and autonomic. There are two types of somatic neuropathy: focal and diffuse. The focal neuropathies include mononeuritis and entrapment syndromes. The diffuse neuropathies include proximal neuropathies and large- and small-fiber distal symmetric polyneuropathies.

Estimates of the prevalence of diabetic neuropathy range from 10 to 90% of the diabetic population, depending on the criteria used to define neuropathy [1–6]. Neurologic complications occur equally in patients with type 1 and type 2 diabetes mellitus, as well as various forms of acquired diabetes.

In this pictorial overview, clinical presentations and therapeutic approaches to common forms of neuropathy are presented and discussed, including distal symmetric, proximal motor, and autonomic neuropathies. Also provided are algorithms for recognition and management of common pain and entrapment syndromes. A global approach is used for recognition of syndromes requiring specialized treatments based on our improved understanding of their etiopathogenesis.

J.S. Skyler (ed.), *Atlas of Diabetes: Fourth Edition*,
DOI 10.1007/978-1-4614-1028-7_14, © Springer Science+Business Media, LLC 2012

Distal Neuropathies

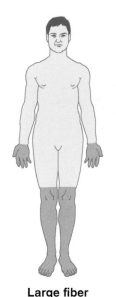
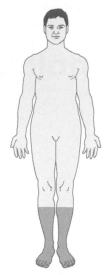
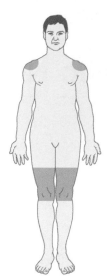
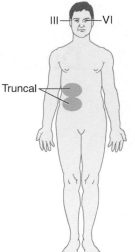
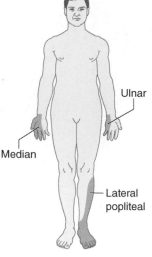

Large fiber neuropathy	Small fiber neuropathy	Proximal motor neuropathy	Acute mono neuropathies	Pressure palsies
Sensory loss: 0→ +++ (touch, vibration)	Sensory loss: 0→ + (thermal, allodynia)	Sensory loss: 0→ +	Sensory loss: 0→ +	Sensory loss in nerve distribution: + → +++
Pain: + → +++	Pain: + → +++	Pain: + → +++	Pain: + → +++	Pain: + → ++
Tendon reflex: N → ↓↓↓	Tendon reflex: N → ↓	Tendon reflex: ↓↓	Tendon reflex: N	Tendon reflex: N
Motor deficit: 0→ +++	Motor deficit: 0	Proximal motor deficit: + → +++	Motor deficit: + → +++	Motor deficit: + → +++

FIGURE 14-1. Schematic representation of different clinical presentations of diabetic neuropathy. The spectra of clinical neuropathic syndromes described in patients with diabetes mellitus include dysfunction of almost every segment of the somatic peripheral and autonomic nervous systems [7]. Each syndrome can be distinguished by its pathophysiologic, therapeutic, and prognostic features. Initial neurologic evaluation should be directed toward detection of the specific part of the nervous system affected by diabetes. Diabetes may damage small fibers, large fibers, or both. Small nerve-fiber dysfunction usually, but not always, occurs early and often is present before objective signs or electrophysiologic evidence of nerve damage is found [8–10]. Small nerve-fiber dysfunction is manifested first in the lower limbs by pain and hyperalgesia. Loss of thermal sensitivity follows, with reduced light touch and pinprick sensation. Large-fiber neuropathies may involve sensory or motor nerves or both. The neuropathies are manifested by reduced vibration (often, the first objective evidence of neuropathy) and position sense, weakness, muscle wasting, and depressed tendon reflexes. Most patients with distal sensory polyneuropathy have a mixed variety, with both large and small nerve-fiber involvement. In the case of distal sensory polyneuropathy, a "glove and stocking" distribution of sensory loss is almost universal [7]. Early in the course of the neuropathic process, multifocal sensory loss may also be found. Diabetic peripheral symmetric polyneuropathy is thought to be a dying-back disorder, with prevailing effects on the axons and consequent demyelination. There is an early functional phase in which metabolic abnormalities are responsible for the clinical symptoms and signs. Later structural changes occur in the nerves so that treatment strategies have been developed to arrest or slow the rate of progression. When neuronal cell death occurs, little can be done to induce recovery. Clearly, all attempts at treating neuropathy should be oriented toward the reversible phase of the disorder (adapted from Vinik [11]).

Peripheral Nerve Components

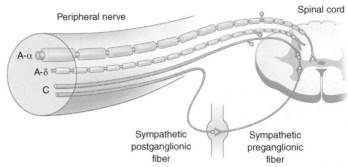

FIGURE 14-2. Cutaneous nerve components. Peripheral nerves are composed of several different types of nerve fibers, each with their own function. The large myelinated α fibers conduct rapidly and subserve motor power, proprioception, and coordination. The thinner yet myelinated A-δ fibers subserve cold thermal detection and deep-seated pain. The thin unmyelinated fibers are responsible for warm detection threshold, heat pain, part of touch sensation, and sympathetic nerve supply to the skin.

Large-Fiber Neuropathy

Clinical Presentation and Management of Large Fiber Neuropathy

Presentation

Impaired vibration present

Pain of A-δ type; deep seated, gnawing

Ataxia

Wasting of small muscles, intrinsic minus feet with hammer toes

Weakess

Increased blood flow (the hot foot)

Risk of Charcot neuroarthropathy

Management

Proper shoes

Orthotics

Tendon lengthening

Foot reconstruction

FIGURE 14-3. Clinical presentation and management of large-fiber neuropathy.

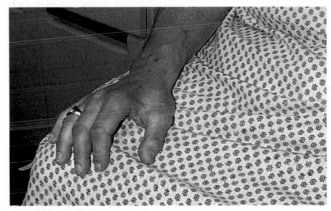

FIGURE 14-4. Wasting of the small muscle of the hand in large-fiber neuropathies. This wasting must not be mistaken for ulnar entrapment, which is amenable to treatment. In large-fiber neuropathies, all peripheral nerves are affected equally and the sensory disturbance is of the "glove and stocking" variety, not confined to the nerve distribution. In ulnar entrapment, the sensory loss involves the ring and little fingers.

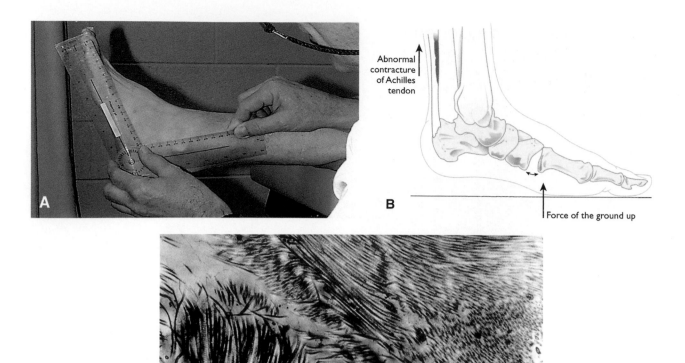

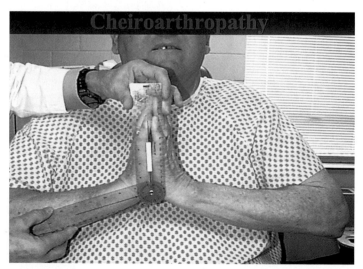

FIGURE 14-5. Wasting of small muscles of the feet in fiber neuropathies. In large-fiber neuropathies, there is wasting of the small muscles of the feet: intrinsic minus feet as well as talipes equinovarus owing to shortening of the Achilles tendon. (**A**) Measurement of the angle of the ankle in full flexion. Using a goniometer, the flexion should be at least 90°. (**B**) Greater than 100° indicates tendo-Achilles shortening, with its impact on increasing midfoot pressure and a breakdown of Lisfranc's joint in the midfoot. (**C**) Electron micrograph of disrupted collagen fibers in the Achilles tendon in a patient with large-nerve neuropathy.

FIGURE 14-6. Upper extremity features of large-fiber neuropathies. This patient is unable to extend his hands at the wrist to beyond 90°, as shown using the goniometer. Note the separation of the small fingers, creating a diamond-shaped open space indicative of cheiroarthropathy. These features accompany large-fiber neuropathies as well as entrapment syndromes. This is not universal and the two conditions may well have different causes.

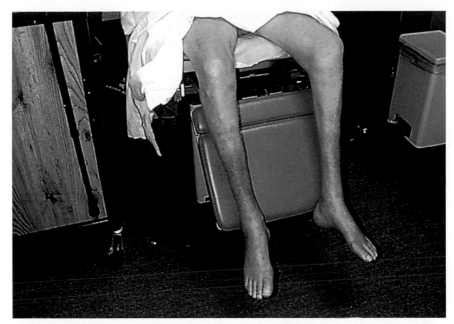

Figure 14-7. Lower extremity features of large-fiber neuropathies. This patient shows a combination of severe muscle wasting of the lower limbs resembling that seen in Charcot–Marie–Tooth disease, the equinus of the feet owing to shortening of the Achilles tendon, and wasting of the proximal muscles of the thigh owing to a combination of a proximal neuropathy and a distal large-fiber neuropathy.

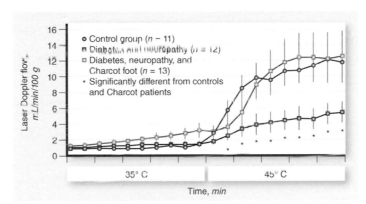

Figure 14-8. Neurovascular dysfunction in neuropathy (adapted from Shapiro et al. [12]).

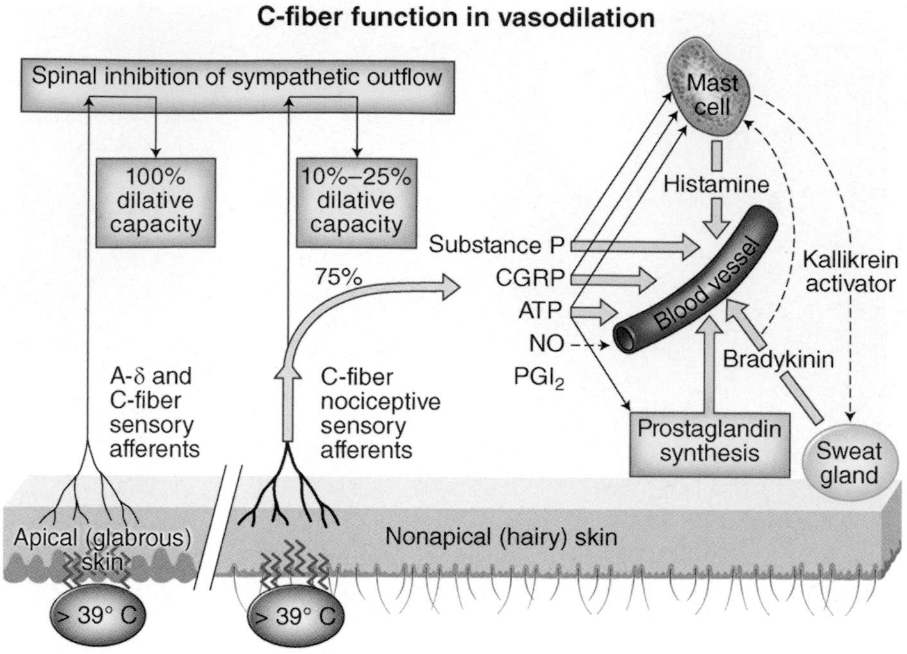

C-fiber function in vasodilation

FIGURE 14-9. Vasodilation and C-fiber function. Factors that control vasodilation in glabrous skin, such as that found on the pads and soles and hairy skin found on the dorsum of the feet and hands, are shown. In glabrous skin, vasodilation is, for the most part, a consequence of relaxation of the sympathetic tone. In hairy skin, C fibers are essential for vasodilation, a process mediated by a variety of neurotransmitters, including the neuropeptides, substance P, and calcitonin gene-related peptide (CGRP), as well as bradykinin. Defective trophic support for skin with reduced levels of neuronal growth factor results in decreased substance P and CGRP, thereby impairing the ability to dilate in response to noxious stimuli and heat. Thus, nutrient delivery is compromised and there is susceptibility to ulceration. *ATP* adenosine triphosphate (adapted from Burnstock and Ralevic [13]; modified by Vinik et al. [14, 15]).

Nerve fibers in skin

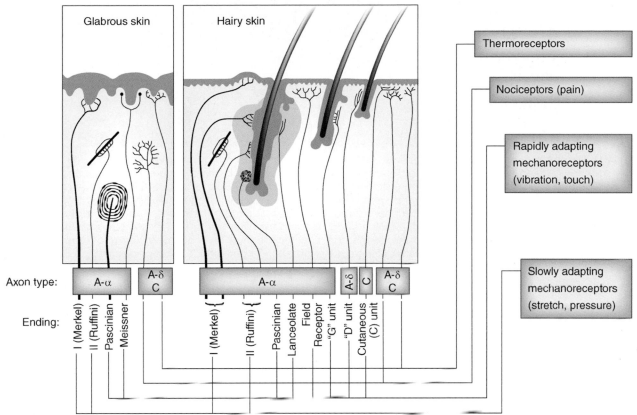

FIGURE 14-10. Different nerve fibers in skin and their different roles in sensory perception and mechanoreceptor function. C-fiber-type pain generally is described as throbbing, shooting, stabbing, sharp, hot, burning, and tender. Touch is misinterpreted as pain (i.e., allodynia) and patients cannot bear contact with bedclothes or other objects. In contrast, A-δ pain often is described as cramping, gnawing, aching, heavy, splitting, tiring and exhausting, sickening, fearful, and punishing and cruel. A patient may say, "I have a toothache in my foot," "there is a dog gnawing at the bones of my feet," or "my feet feel as if they are encased in concrete." These pains derive from different fibers and have a different mechanism of production. The scheme is based on this information, which proves helpful in the management of patients with neuropathic pain. Pain disappears when a loss of C fibers occurs; the loss heralds the phase of hypoalgesia, and hypesthesia, with impairment of warm thermal perception and insensitivity to heat pain. These symptoms are particularly dangerous and are the forerunners of repeated minor injury and the subsequent loss of toes and feet.

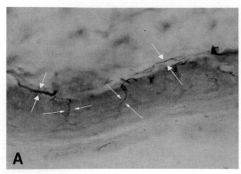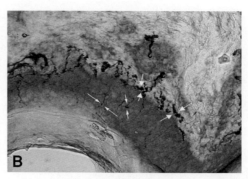

FIGURE 14-11. Photomicrographs of 50-µm sections from skin biopsy specimens taken from the upper thigh of control (**A**) and neuropathic (**B**) patients. The sections were stained with antibody to PCP 9.5 and neuronal antigen, and were evaluated by immunocytochemistry to reveal peripheral, small, unmyelinated neurons. (**A**) Shows straight, uninterrupted, unmyelinated nerve fibers running between the dermis and epidermis in normal skin (*broad arrows*). In addition, there are numerous single, relatively straight fibers projecting into the epidermis of normal skin (*narrow arrows*). (**B**) Demonstrates the changes observed in neuropathic skin, including malformation of the fibers running between the dermis and epidermis, with multiple, irregular swelling (*broad arrows*). The fibers in the epidermis of neuropathic skin are reduced in number compared with normal skin. These changes in skin are characteristic of small-fiber neuropathies and may occur in the absence of any other clinical or laboratory evidence of neuropathy [16].

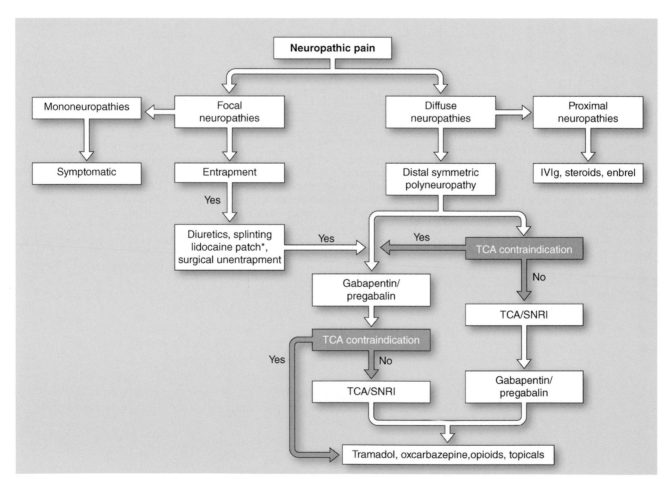

FIGURE 14-12. Treatment algorithm (adapted from Vinik [17]). *TCA* tri-cyclic antidepressant; *SNRI* serotonin–norepinephrine reuptake inhibitor.

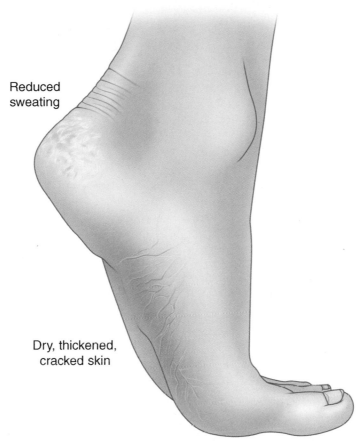

Reduced
sweating

Dry, thickened,
cracked skin

Figure 14-13. Clinical presentation of small-fiber neuropathy. The signs of this disorder include pain (C-fiber type, burning, and superficial), late hypoalgesia, hypoesthesia, impaired warm thermal perception, decreased sweating, and impaired cutaneous blood flow (the cold foot). Risks include foot ulcers, gangrene, and amputations.

Management of C-Fiber Dysfunction

Patients must be instructed on foot care with daily foot inspection (they must have a mirror in the bathroom for inspecting the soles of their feet)

Patients should be provided with a monofilament for self-testing

All diabetic patients should wear padded socks

Shoes must fit well with adequate support and must be inspected for the presence of foreign bodies (*eg*, nails, pins, teeth) before wearing

Patients must exercise care with exposure to heat (*eg*, avoid falling asleep in front of the fireplace)

Emollient creams should be used for the drying and cracking of skin

After bathing, feet should be thoroughly dried and powdered between the toes

Nails should be cut transversely, preferably by a podiatrist

Figure 14-14. Management of C-fiber dysfunction.

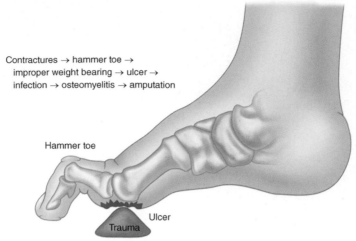

Contractures → hammer toe →
improper weight bearing → ulcer →
infection → osteomyelitis → amputation

Hammer toe

Ulcer

Trauma

FIGURE 14-15. Management of small-fiber neuropathies. In the USA, 65,000 amputations are performed each year. Half of these are attributable to diabetes, and small-fiber neuropathy is implicated in 87% of cases. The combination of decreased pain perception with decreased warm thermal perception and the resulting "hammer toe" deformity that follows intrinsic minus feet lead to blisters on top of the knuckles of toes or ulcers over the heads of metatarsals. These high-pressure points are easily recognized by forced gate analysis scans of the feet. With correct shoes, padded socks, and orthotics, the likelihood of amputation can be reduced by half. Patients should be instructed to protect their feet with padded socks, wear shoes that have adequate support, regularly inspect their feet and shoes, be careful of exposure to heat, and use emollient creams for sympathetic dysfunction.

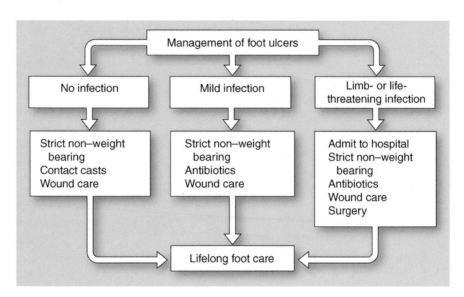

FIGURE 14-16. Management of foot ulcers.

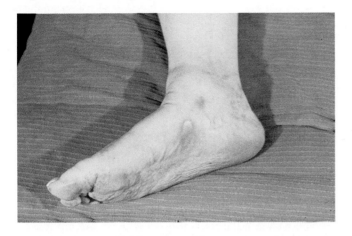

FIGURE 14-17. Hot foot of Charcot neuroarthropathy showing the end result of large-fiber neuropathy. Note the red inflamed foot that is easily mistaken for infection and the collapse of the midfoot.

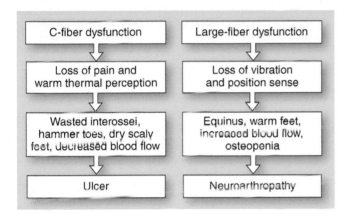

FIGURE 14-18. Prediction of foot ulcers versus neuroarthropathy.

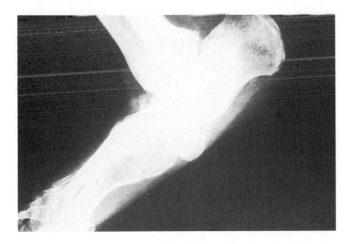

FIGURE 14-19. Radiograph of the foot shown in Figure 14-17. Note the rarefaction and osteopenia of the calcaneus with collapse of the midfoot and loss of architecture of the foot. These results of large-fiber neuropathy and increased blood flow could have been prevented if recognized early enough.

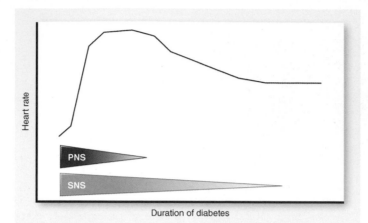

FIGURE 14-20. Model of the effects of autonomic neuropathy on heart rate. The rule in diabetic neuropathy is that the longest fibers are affected early and more severely. In the autonomic nervous system, the longest fibers are those in the vagus [parasympathetic nervous system (PNS)] nerves. Thus, the earliest observations in people with autonomic neuropathy of the cardiovascular system is an increase in heart rate. Later, as the short, efferent fibers of the sympathetic nervous system (SNS) become involved, the heart rate slows down but not to normal. It is indeed a denervated heart. With the loss of the afferent fibers, there also is the loss of pain perception, accounting for the high incidence of painless myocardial infarctions in patients with diabetic neuropathy [18] (adapted from Ewing et al. [19]).

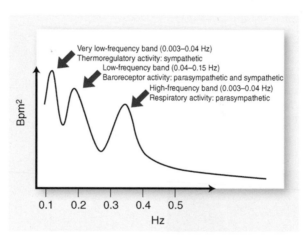

FIGURE 14-21. Respiratory rate (RR) intervals and effects of cardiac autonomic dysfunction. The most sensitive indicator of cardiac autonomic neuropathy is the loss of the normal sinus arrhythmia with breathing. This loss can be measured on an electrocardiogram as loss of the change in the RR interval with deep breathing at six breaths per minute and reflects almost entirely damage to the parasympathetic nervous system. With more sophisticated approaches, computerized spectral analysis of the electrocardiogram tracing allows one to infer the status of the sympathetic nervous system as well. Late in the course of cardiac autonomic neuropathy, the advent of orthostasis (a decrease in blood pressure of >30 mmHg when arising from a lying position) reflects sympathetic nerve damage. Peripheral measures of autonomic function are described in Figs. 14.8 and 14.9 on blood flow in the diabetic foot (adapted from Vinik and Ziegler [20]).

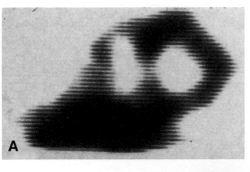

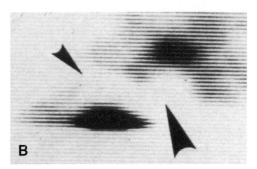

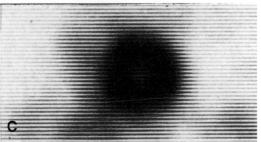

FIGURE 14-22. Segmental loss of sympathetic nerve fibers in the heart, demonstrable using multiple-gated acquisition (**A**), meta-iodobenzylguanidine (**B**), and thallium scans (**C**), does not demonstrate ventricular wall defects. It is now thought that this imbalance in the sympathetic nerve supply of the myocardium is what leads to the irritable foci, which leads to arrhyth-mia and possibly accounts for sudden death in diabetic patients with autonomic neuropathy. This mechanism also is thought to operate in people who have had a myocardial infarction and may be the reason for the effectiveness of β blockade in reducing mortality in patients who have had a myocardial infarction (from Kahn et al. [21], with permission).

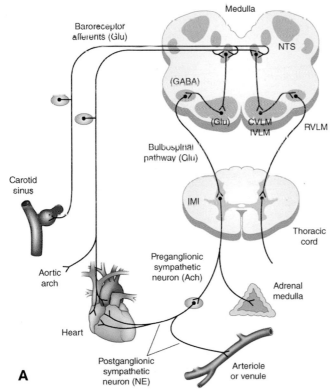

Organizing of the Autonomic Nervous System

Eye
  Abnormal pupillary reaction, with night blindness
Cardiovascular
  Sudden death, silent myocardial infarction
  Orthostasis
  Impaired peripheral vascular reflexes
Respiratory
  Failure of hypoxia-induced respiration
Gut
  Gustatory sweating
  Gastroparesis
  Diarrhea
  Constipation
  Loss of anal sphincter tone and incontinence
Metabolic
  Hypoglycemia unawareness
  Hypoglycemia unresponsiveness
  Hypoglycemia-associated autonomic failure
Genitourinary
  Overflow incontinence
Sexual
  Males: erectile dysfunction
  Females: decreased vaginal lubrication

FIGURE 14-23. Organization of the autonomic nervous system. The organization of the autonomic nervous system is shown in (**A**). Note that diabetes affects the afferent and efferent components of the sympathetic and parasympathetic nervous systems and has diffuse effects throughout the body, shown in (**B**). CVLM and IVLM – paraventricular nuclei of vasomotor center, *GABA* γ-aminobutyric acid, *IML* intermediolateral nucleus, *NTS* solitary tract nucleus, *RVLM* – motor nucleus of vagus.

Gastropathy

Gastric neuromuscular function

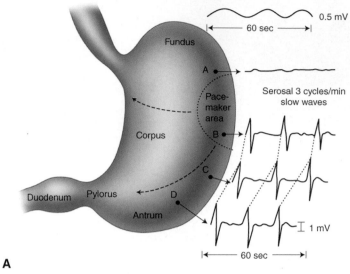

A

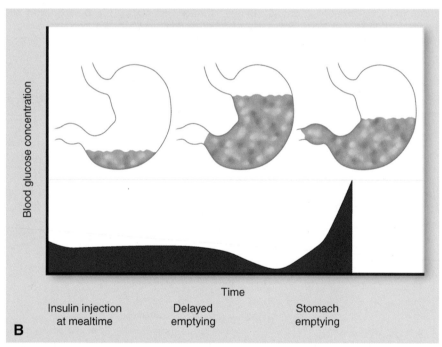

B

| Insulin injection at mealtime | Delayed emptying | Stomach emptying |

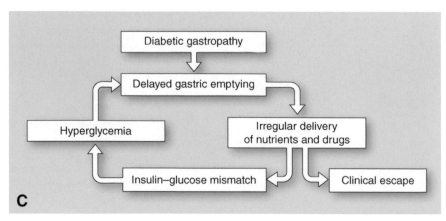

C

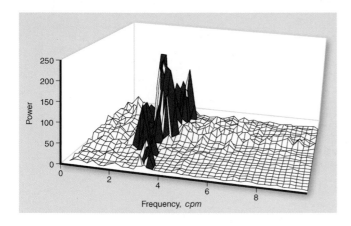

FIGURE 14-25. Normal electrogastrogram. This electrogastrogram was obtained in a normal patient. Note the predominant frequency of 3–6 cpm.

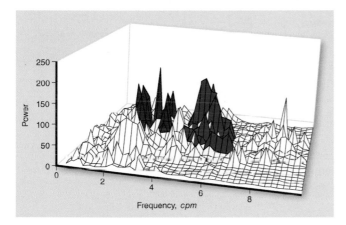

FIGURE 14-26. Electrogastrogram showing hyperglycemia-induced tachygastria. Note two peaks of activity, one at the usual frequency of 3–6 cpm and the major peak at over 6 cpm. Thus, hyperglycemia per se can markedly affect gastric function; many have made the costly error of carrying out gastric-emptying studies when the blood glucose is over 400 mg/dL. Not only does this induce tachygastria, but it may also inhibit the interdigestive myoelectric complex and thus give the erroneous impression of gastroparesis. Gastric pacemaking is being added to the therapeutic armamentarium for severe gastroparesis. New drugs with prokinetic properties and Zelnorm (Novartis; East Hanover, NJ) may be appropriate for functional abnormalities [22].

FIGURE 14-24. Gastropathy. (**A, B**) Gastric neuromuscular function. The stomach is a complex neuromuscular organ. It has a pacemakor that discharges rhythmic electrical impulses that initiate propulsive contractions. It is sensitive to volume, viscosity, osmolarity, caloric density, and the nature of the fuel within. Functional disturbances may occur, such as arrhythmias, tachygastria and bradygastria, pylorospasm, and hypomotility. Organic lesions include gastroparesis, antral dilation and obstruction, inflammation, ulceration, and bezoar formation. Gastric dysfunction should be suspected in patients who have types I and II diabetes; who have had diabetes for over 20 years; who display evidence of distal symmetric polyneuropathy and autonomic neuropathy; in whom there are observations of brittle diabetes with previously well-controlled symptoms; and who have symptoms of early satiety, bloating, and a succussion splash. Anorexia, nausea, vomiting, and dyspepsia are nonspecific and herald other conditions. (**C**) Clinical presentation of gastropathy. Many more patients with gastropathy present with brittle diabetes than do those who present with gastric symptoms. In fact, it has been shown that many of the gastrointestinal symptoms of gastropathy can be nonspecific and do not reflect an abnormality in gastric emptying. The most fertile soil for discovery of those with gastric dysfunction are patients with "difficult-to-control diabetes." The stomach can be regarded as the coarse regulator of blood glucose concentrations, releasing fuel to the small bowel at its own predetermined rate. Therefore, any dysfunction in the bowel would result in a mismatch of fuel delivery and either endogenous or exogenous insulin, thereby creating the apparent pattern of insulin resistance or brittle diabetes. Of interest is how the irregular pattern of delivery applies to drugs used in the treatment of diabetes and may confound the problem. Similar concern applies to other drugs that may fail to reach their absorptive site in the small bowel, leading to clinical escape from the condition being treated. Overzealous adjustment of the insulin dose may result because the real cause may be easily overlooked.

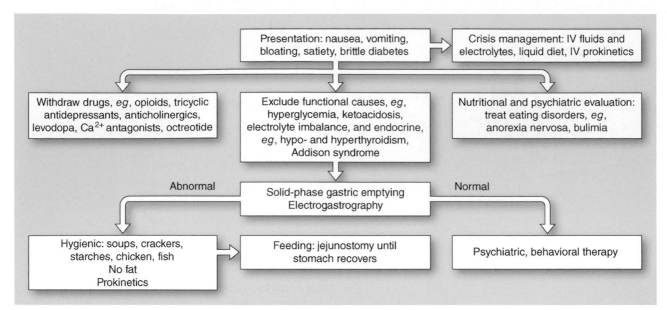

Figure 14-27. Algorithm for the management of gastropathy in patients with diabetes. Prokinetic agents include metoclopramide, erythromycin, and tegaserod [22]. *IV* intravenous.

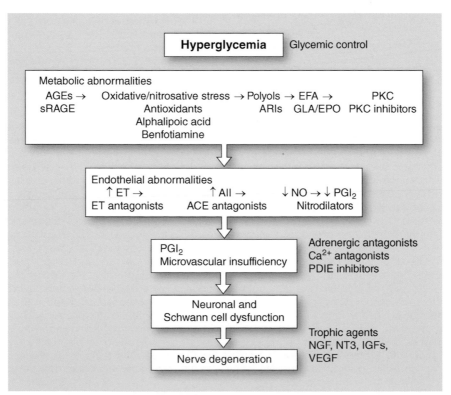

Figure 14-28. Specific interventions in diabetic neuropathy designed to target the major defect. Many of these interventions already have been tested in animal models and currently are in phase 2 and 3 clinical trials in the USA and elsewhere. Some of these interventions are further along and may well be in clinical trials shortly. *ACE* angiotensin-converting enzyme, *AGEs* advanced glycation end products, *AII* angiotensin II, *ARIs* aldose-reductase inhibitors, *Ca²⁺* calcium ion, *EFA* essential fatty acid, *EPO* evening primrose oil, *ET* endothelin, *GLA* g-linolenic acid, *IGFs* insulin-like growth factors, *NGF* neuronal growth factor, *NO* nitric oxide, *NT3* neurotropin 3, *PDIE* phosphodiesterase, *PGI₂* prostaglandin I₂, *PKC* protein kinase C, *rAGE* receptor for AGE, *sRAGE* soluble form of rAGE, *VEGF* vascular endothelial growth factor.

References

1. American Diabetes Association, American Academy of Neurology: Consensus statement: report and recommendations of the San Antonio Conference on Diabetic Neuropathy. *Diabetes Care* 1988, 11:592–597.

2. Vinik AI, Mitchell BD, Leichter SB, *et al.*: Epidemiology of the complications of diabetes. In *Diabetes: Clinical Science and Practice*, Edited by Leslie RDG, Robbins DC. Cambridge, UK: Cambridge University Press; 1995:15, 221.

3. Kjiturnan M, Welborn T, McCann V, *et al.*: Prevalence of diabetic complications in relation to risk factors. *Diabetes* 1986, 35:1332–1339.

4. Young MJ, Boulton AJ, MacLeod AF, *et al.*: A multicenter study of the prevalence of diabetic neuropathy in the United Kingdom hospital clinic population. *Diabetologia* 1993, 36:150–154.

5. Feldman JN, Hirsch SR, Bever BS, *et al.*: Prevalence of diabetic nephropathy at time of treatment for diabetic retinopathy. In *Diabetic Renal-Retinal Syndrome*. Edited by Friedman L'Esperance FA. London: Grune & Stratton; 1982:9.

6. Dyck PJ, Kratz KM, Karnes MS, *et al.*: The prevalence by staged severity of various types of diabetic neuropathy, retinopathy, and nephropathy in a population based cohort: The Rochester Diabetic Neuropathy Study. *Neurology* 1993, 43:817–824.

7. Vinik AI, Holland MT, LeBeau JM, *et al.*: Diabetic neuropathies. *Diabetes Care* 1992, 15:1926–1975.

8. Hanson PH, Schumaker P, Debugne T, Clerin M: Evaluation of somatic and autonomic small fibers neuropathy in diabetes. *Am J Phys Med Rehabil* 1992, 71:44–47.

9. Dyck PJ: Small-fiber neuropathy determination. *Muscle Nerve* 1988, 11:998–999.

10. Jarnal GA, Hansen S, Weir AI, Ballantyne JP: The neurophysiologic investigation of small fiber neuropathies. *Muscle Nerve* 1987, 10:537–545.

11. Shapiro SA, Stansberry KB, Hill MA, *et al.*: Normal blood flow response and vasomotion in the diabetic Charcot foot. *J Diabetes Complications* 1998, 12:147–153.

12. Vinik A: Diabetic neuropathies. *Med Clin North Am* 2004, 88: 947–99, xi.

13. Burnstock C, Ralevic V: New insights into the local regulation of blood flow by perivascular nerves and endothelium. *Br J Plastic Surg* 1994, 47:527–543.

14. Vinik AI, Erbas T, Park T, *et al.*: Methods for evaluation of peripheral neurovascular dysfunction. *Diabetes Technol Ther* 2001, 3:29–50.

15. Vinik AI, Erbas T, Park T, *et al.*: Dermal neurovascular dysfunction in type 2 diabetes. *Diabetes Care* 2001, 24:1468–1475.

16. Pittenger G, Ray M, Burcus N, *et al.*: Intraepidermal nerve fibers are indicators of small fiber neuropathy in both diabetic and non-diabetic patients. *Diabetes Care* 2004, 27:1974–1979.

17. Vinik AI, Maser R, Mitchell B, Freeman R: Autonomic neuropathy. *Diabetes Care* 2003, 26:1553–1579.

18. Vinik A: Neuropathic pain after exclusion of non-diabetic etiologies and stabilization of glycemic control. *JCEM* 2010, 95:4802–4811.

19. Ewing J, Campbell IW, Clarke BF, *et al.*: Heart rate changes in diabetes mellitus. *Lancet* 1981, 1:183–186.

20. Kahn J, Ida B, Vinik A: Stress and cardiovascular function in diabetes. *Diabetes Care* 1985, 12:3–5.

21. Vinik A, Ziegler D: Diabetic cardiovascular autonomic neuropathy. *Circulation* 2007, 115:387–397.

22. Vinik AI, Mehrabyan A, Johnson D: Gastrointestinal disturbances. In *Therapy for Diabetes Mellitus and Related Disorders*, edn 4. Alexandria, VA: American Diabetes Association; 2004:424–439.

23. Johnson B, Nesto R, Pfeifer M, *et al.*: Cardiac abnormalities in diabetic patients with neuropathy. *Diabetes Care* 2004, 27:448–454.

24. Vinik A, Mehrabyan A: Diabetic neuropathies. *Emerg Med* 2004, 36:39–44.

25. Vinik A: Diabetic neuropathy: emerging data on a new therapeutic class. *Johns Hopkins Adv Studies Med* 2004, 4:S421–S427.

26. Vinik A, Mehrabyan A, Colen L, Boulton A: Focal entrapment neuropathies in diabetes. *Diabetes Care* 2004, 27:1783–1787.

27. Pittenger G, Burcus N, McNulty P, *et al.*: Intraepidermal nerve fibers are indicators of small fiber neuropathy in both diabetic and non-diabetic patients. *Diabetes Care* 2004, 27:1974–1979.

28. Vinik A, Mehrabyan A: Diabetic neuropathies. *Med Clin North Am* 2004, 88:947–999.

29. Raskin P, Donofrio P, Vinik A, *et al.*: Topiramate vs placebo in painful diabetic neuropathy: analgesic and metabolic effects. *Neurology* 2004, 63:865–873.

30. Vinik A, Emley M, Megerian J, Gozani S: Median and ulnar nerve conduction measurements in patients with symptoms of diabetic peripheral neuropathy using the NC-Stat System. *Diabetes Technol Ther* 2004, 6:816–824.

31. Vinik A, Emley M, Megerian J, Gozani S: Median and ulnar nerve conduction measurements in patients with symptoms of diabetic peripheral neuropathy using the NC-Stat system. *Diabetes Technol Ther* 2004, 6:816–824.

32. Boulton A, Vinik A, Arezzo J, *et al.*: Diabetic neuropathies, a statement by the American Diabetes Association. *Diabetes Care* 2005, 28:956–962.

33. Witzke K, Vinik A: Diabetic neuropathy in older adults. *Rev Endocr Metab Disord* 2005, 6:117–127.

34. Vinik E, Hayes R, Oglesby A, *et al.*: The development and validation of the Norfolk QOL-DN: a new measure of patients' perception of the effects of diabetes and diabetic neuropathy. *Diabetes Technol Ther* 2005, 7:497–508.

35. Pittenger G, Mehrabyan A, Simmons K, *et al.*: Small fiber neuropathy is associated with metabolic syndrome. *Metab Syndr Relat Disord* 2005, 3:113–121.

36. Vinik AI: Use of antiepileptic drugs in the treatment of chronic painful diabetic neuropathy. *J Clin Endocrinol Metab* 2005, 90:4936–4945.

37. Vinik A, Bril V, Kempler P, *et al.* for the MBBQ Study Group: Treatment of symptomatic diabetic peripheral neuropathy with protein kinase C-beta inhibitor ruboxistaurin, mesylate: results of a phase 2 randomized trial. *Clin Ther* 2005, 27:1164–1180.

38. Donofrio P, Raskin P, Rosenthal N, *et al.* and the CAPSS-141 Study Group: Safety effectiveness of topiramate for the management of painful diabetic neuropathy in an open-label extension study. *Clin Ther* 2005, 27:1420–1431.

39. Vinik A, Bril V, Litchy W, *et al.*: The MBBQ Study Group: sural sensory nerve action potential identifies diabetic peripheral neuropathy responders. *Muscle Nerve* 2005, 32, 619–625.

40. Vinik A, Casellini C: Recent advances in the treatment of diabetic neuropathy. *Curr Opin Endocrinol Diabetes* 2006, 13: 147–153.

41. Vinik A, Ullal J, Parson H, Casellini C: Diabetic neuropathies: clinical manifestations and current treatment options. *Nat Clin Pract Endocrinol Metab* 2006, 2:269–281.

42. Vinik A, Kles K: Pathophysiology and treatment of diabetic peripheral neuropathy: the case for diabetic neurovascular function as an essential component. *Curr Diabetes Rev* 2006, 2:131–145.

43. Vinik A: Diabetic neuropathies: new treatment modalities. *Diabetic Microvasc Compl Today* 2006, 3:23–26.

44. Bourcier ME, Ullal J, Parson HK, *et al.*: Diabetic peripheral neuropathy: how reliable is a homemade 1–6 monofilament for screening? *J Fam Pract* 2006, 55:505–508.

45. Vinik A: Neuropathies in children and adolescents with diabetes: the tip of the iceberg. *Pediatr Diabetes* 2006, 7:301–304.

46. Vinik AI, Tuchman M, Safirstein B, *et al.*: Lamotrigine for treatment of pain associated with diabetic neuropathy: results of two randomized, double-blind placebo-controlled studies. *Pain* 2006, 128:169–179.

47. Vinik AI: Optimizing the management of diabetic neuropathy. *Physician's Weekly* 2006, XXIII:8–10.

48. Cornblath DR, Vinik AI, Feldman E, *et al.*: Surgical decompression for diabetic sensorimotor poly neuropathy. *Diabetes Care* 2007, 30:421–422.

49. Vinik AI, Ziegler D: Diabetic cardiovascular autonomic neuropathy. *Circulation* 2007, 115: 387–397.

50. Casellini CM, Barlow PM, Rice AL, *et al.*: A 6-month, randomized, double-masked, placebo-controlled study evaluating the effects of the protein kinase C-β inhibitor ruboxistaurin on skin microvascular blood flow and other measures of diabetic peripheral neuropathy. *Diabetes Care* 2007, 3:896–902.

51. Vinik AI, Strotmeyer ES, Nakave AA, Patel CV: Diabetic neuropathy in older adults. *Clin Geriatr Med* 2008, 24:407–435.

52. Bourcier ME, Vinik AI: A 41-year-old man with polyarthritis and severe autonomic neuropathy. *Ther Clin Risk Manag* 2008, 4:837–842.

53. Anandacoomaraswamy D, Ullal J, Vinik AI: A 70-year-old male with peripheral neuropathy, ataxia and antigliadin antibodies shows improvement, but not ataxia, after intravenous immunoglobin and gluten-free diet. *J Multidiscipl Healthcare* 2008, 1:93–96.

Obesity Therapy

Steven R. Smith

Obesity is defined as an excess of body fat. It is currently estimated that more than 1.5 billion people worldwide are overweight [1]. According to the National Health and Nutrition Examination Survey (NHANES), at least one-third of Americans are obese. Unfortunately, the tsunami of obesity led to the recent report that bariatric surgery has become the second most common abdominal operation in the USA [2]. These numbers should serve as a call to action for the implementation of obesity therapy in every primary care clinic and in most subspecialty clinics; endocrinology and diabetes care clinics are particularly important. In terms of obesity treatment, there are ample opportunities for secondary "prevention" of weight gain – in both overweight and obese patients – to keep obesity from getting worse, as well as treatment to reduce body weight and to improve health and well-being.

Modest weight loss produces important improvements in weight-related comorbidities and quality of life; in some analyses, it also has economic benefits. Establishing realistic and attainable weight-loss goals can reduce patients' dissatisfaction with the amount of weight they ultimately lose, but attempts to modify unrealistic weight-loss goals are, unfortunately, mostly unsuccessful. Practitioners should be sensitive to their own attitudes and biases and to the patient's background and social milieu. Unfortunately, in comparison to hypertension, hypercholesterolemia and other chronic diseases we have a limited armamentarium of effective treatments. Fortunately, there is an emerging science around not only the biological mechanisms that control body weight, but also the science of obesity therapy. Our understanding of the pathophysiology is nascent. More fundamental research to understand which systems are dysregulated in obese humans is necessary to tailor treatments to individual patients [3]. Until there are great drugs, we have to be diligent to get the "little things right" in the behavioral management of obesity and choose drugs to treat diabetes in a way that does not lead to weight gain and further exacerbation of the problem (obesity) that led to the disease (diabetes). As our fundamental knowledge expands, we will have better, safer drugs. For now, we are left with using the available drugs wisely and surgery as a last resort for those who are at the greatest risk.

J.S. Skyler (ed.), *Atlas of Diabetes: Fourth Edition*,
DOI 10.1007/978-1-4614-1028-7_15, © Springer Science+Business Media, LLC 2012

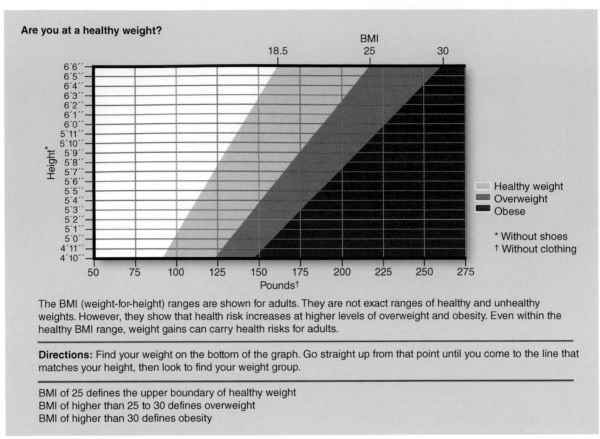

Are you at a healthy weight?

The BMI (weight-for-height) ranges are shown for adults. They are not exact ranges of healthy and unhealthy weights. However, they show that health risk increases at higher levels of overweight and obesity. Even within the healthy BMI range, weight gains can carry health risks for adults.

Directions: Find your weight on the bottom of the graph. Go straight up from that point until you come to the line that matches your height, then look to find your weight group.

BMI of 25 defines the upper boundary of healthy weight
BMI of higher than 25 to 30 defines overweight
BMI of higher than 30 defines obesity

Figure 15-1. Body mass index (BMI) chart. BMI is a measure of body weight and adiposity normalized for a person's height. It can be measured by using the following equations. Metric: BMI=weight (kg)/height (m^2). Imperial: BMI=weight (lb)/height (in^2) × 703.

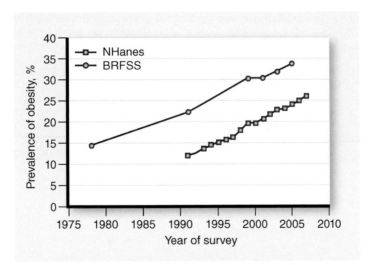

Figure 15-2. Increasing prevalence of obesity in the USA. Shown are changes in the prevalence of obesity among the US adults between 1978 and 2004 in the NHANES and from 1991 to 2007 in the Behavioral Risk Factor Surveillance System (BRFSS). The most recent data from BRFSS supports a continuation of the epidemic: "The results of this report also indicate that the prev- alence of adult obesity in the USA, as measured by BRFSS, con- tinued to increase" [4]. From the epidemiology/population statistics, type 2 diabetes follows obesity with a lag time of about 15 years. Obesity, type 2 diabetes, and associated car- diovascular disease (CVD) will overwhelm our health care sys- tem if the trends continue (adapted from Smith et al. [5]).

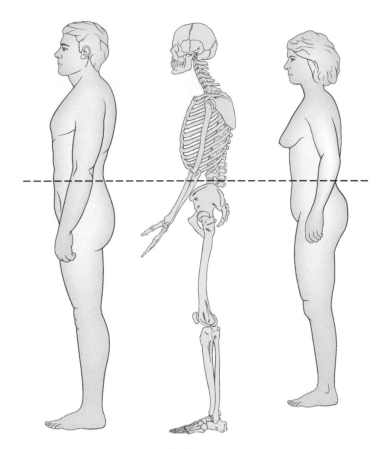

High risk
Men > 102 cm (> 40 in)
Women > 88 cm (> 35 in)

FIGURE 15-3. Measurement of waist circumference. A careful medical evaluation, history of weight-loss attempts and approaches, and a search for secondary and hereditary causes of obesity are essential in treatment planning. Waist circumference is an important risk factor above and beyond BMI. Measuring waist circumference educates the patient and highlights the health risks of central obesity. The US National Institutes of Health (NIH) has recommended waist circumference thresholds of 88 cm in women and 102 cm in men as indicative of increased obesity-related health risks. These cut points for increased risk were established by the National Heart, Lung, and Blood Institute (NHLBI) Obesity Education Initiative Expert Panel on the Identification, Evaluation, and Treatment of Overweight and Obesity in Adults (adapted from NIH [6]).

Classification of Overweight and Obesity by BMI, Waist Circumference, and Associated Disease Risk*				
Category	BMI, kg/m^2	Obesity class	Men ≤ 102 cm (≤ 40 in) or Women ≤ 88 cm (≤ 35 in)	> 102 cm (> 40 in) or > 88 cm (> 35 in)
Underweight	< 18.5		—	—
Normal[†]	18.5–24.9		—	—
Overweight	25.0–29.9		Increased	High
Obesity	30.0–34.9	I	High	Very high
	35.0–39.9	II	Very high	Very high
Extreme obesity	≥ 40	III	Extremely high	Extremely high

*Disease risk for type 2 diabetes, hypertension, and CVD. [†]Increased waist circumference can also be a marker for increased risk even in persons of normal weight.

Figure 15-4. Classification of overweight and obesity. Obesity is associated with an increased risk of several diseases, such as hypertension, diabetes, CVD, and some cancers. BMI, along with waist circumference, should be used to assess risk in patients presenting for obesity treatment. Additional health risk information, such as family history, blood pressure, habitual physical activity, and clinical chemistries, allow further risk prediction. The assessment of obesity comorbidities is crucial to the proper selection of treatments, including pharmacotherapy. Knowing a person's family history may help in understanding the genetic "load" that they bear. If most relatives across several generations are obese, there likely is a strong genetic input to their condition. Similarly, weight at age 18 years can help assess the contribution of the genetic component as weight "tracks" from childhood to adolescence and from adolescence through to adulthood [7]. Although the monogenic obesities (e.g., PC1, MCR4) have no specific therapies now, future work may identify successful strategies, as was the case for leptin deficiency.

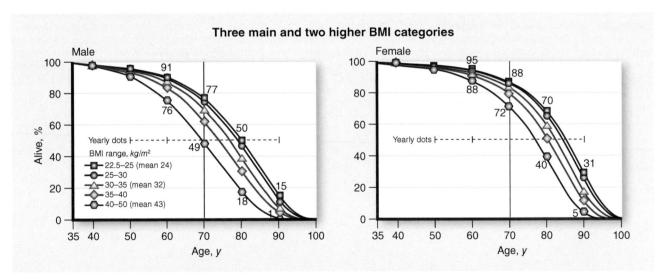

Figure 15-5. BMI and mortality. Obesity is associated with an increase in mortality. Prospective data, starting with the earliest Metropolitan Life insurance tables, demonstrates the increased mortality associated with obesity. For the highest BMI categories, the risk is equivalent to cigarette smoking and reduces life expectancy by an average of 8–9 years (adapted from Whitlock et al. [8]).

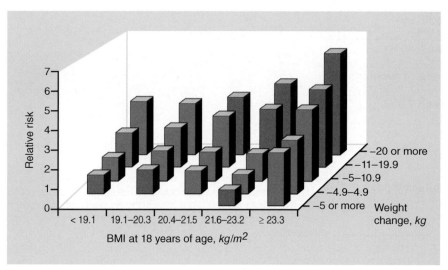

Figure 15-6. Midlife weight gain increases the risk of CVD. Both current body weight and weight gain increase the risk of CVD. Part of our efforts should be directed toward preventing weight gain in the midlife years. This finding is illustrated by the risk of coronary heart disease in the Nurses' Health Study (adapted from Willett et al. [9]).

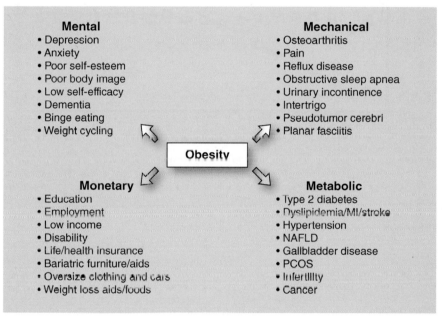

Mental
- Depression
- Anxiety
- Poor self-esteem
- Poor body image
- Low self-efficacy
- Dementia
- Binge eating
- Weight cycling

Mechanical
- Osteoarthritis
- Pain
- Reflux disease
- Obstructive sleep apnea
- Urinary incontinence
- Intertrigo
- Pseudotumor cerebri
- Planar fasciitis

Obesity

Monetary
- Education
- Employment
- Low income
- Disability
- Life/health insurance
- Bariatric furniture/aids
- Oversize clothing and cars
- Weight loss aids/foods

Metabolic
- Type 2 diabetes
- Dyslipidemia/MI/stroke
- Hypertension
- NAFLD
- Gallbladder disease
- PCOS
- Infertility
- Cancer

Figure 15-7. Complications and consequences of obesity. Obesity negatively affects multiple areas of life. This schematic organizes these deleterious effects into four main categories: mental, mechanical, monetary, and metabolic. Each domain has its own field of study and may serve as important areas of reversal with weight-loss therapy. *MI* myocardial infarction; *NAFLD* nonalcoholic fatty liver disease; *PCOS* polycystic ovary disease (adapted from Sharma and Padwal [10]).

Benefits of modest weight loss
Decreased risk of type 2 diabetes
Improved glycemic control in diabetes
Decreased blood pressure
Improved blood lipids
Improved quality of life
Reduced joint pain in osteoarthritis
Improved sleep apnea

FIGURE 15-8. Benefits of modest weight loss. Modest weight loss on the order of 5–10% of body weight is sufficient to produce beneficial effects on metabolism and to prevent diabetes. Rapid weight loss is discouraged and can lead to cholecystitis. In addition, the rapid loss of glycogen and water in the first few weeks of caloric restriction is often misleading.

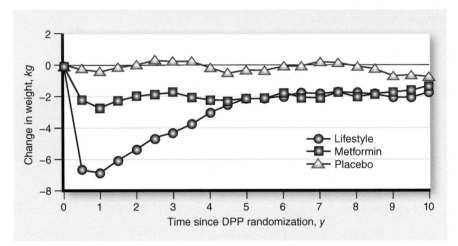

FIGURE 15-9. Weight loss in the Diabetes Prevention Program (DPP). The DPP demonstrated that moderate weight loss can delay or prevent the onset of type 2 diabetes, with a lifestyle intervention for obesity reducing the risk of diabetes by 58%. Lifestyle intervention and treatment with metformin produced modest weight loss in the DPP study. In the main study, there was no lifestyle intervention for metformin-treated patients. As with most weight-loss interventions, body weight increased over time after a successful weight loss (adapted from Knowler et al. [11]).

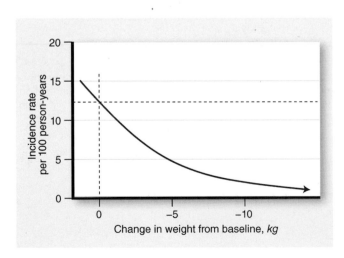

FIGURE 15-10. Weight loss and diabetes prevention in the DPP. The lifestyle arm of the DPP provided both increased physical activity and dietary changes, including caloric restriction. Weight loss, independent of adherence to a low-fat diet and/or exercise, was the only dominant factor in the decreased conversion from impaired glucose tolerance to frank diabetes. The weight change necessary to reduce diabetes risk was modest, with most of the effect seen with a reduction of only 5–10% of body weight (adapted from Hamman et al. [12]).

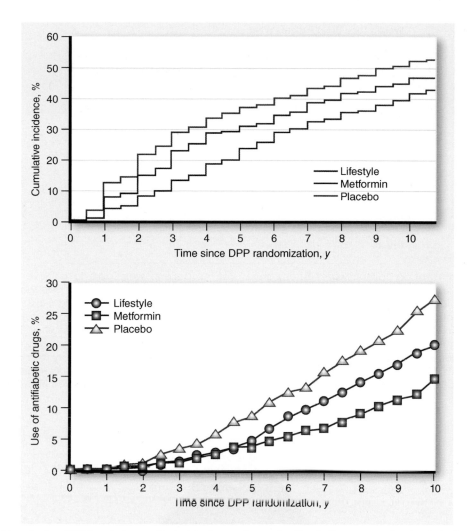

Figure 15-11. Weight loss in the DPP leads to continuing reduction in conversion to diabetes and the use of diabetes drugs. The 10-year follow-up of patients in the DPP leads to a continuing reduction in the conversion to diabetes and use of diabetes drugs (adapted from Knowler et al. [11]).

Weight Loss: What Patients Want		
Weight	Weight, *lb*	Patients that achieve their weight-loss goal, %
Initial	218	—
Disappointed	180	20
Acceptable	163	24
Happy	150	9
Goal	146	0
Dream	135	0

FIGURE 15-12. Weight loss: What do patients want? At any given time, 65% of women are trying to lose weight, a rate that is directly related to satisfaction with body weight [13]. Although it is clear that the amount of weight loss needed to produce medical and metabolic effects is modest, patients have higher expectations. Unfortunately, weight loss of 5–10% of body mass is not what most patients want. In fact, most patients have unrealistic expectations that cannot be met with most treatments. In a survey of patients entering a weight-loss clinic, none of the patients were able to achieve their goal or "dream weight." This reality is important and should be discussed with patients before starting a weight-loss program to manage expectations and prevent disappointment. The exception to this rule is surgery, after which most patients are satisfied with their weight loss. As newer drugs become available, this may change, but for now it is necessary to counsel patients on what degree of weight loss is necessary for improved health rather than cosmetic purposes (adapted from Foster et al. [14]).

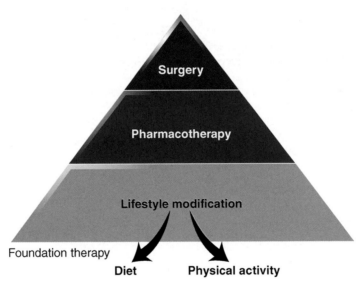

FIGURE 15-13. Approaches to the treatment of obesity. Lifestyle modification is the cornerstone of obesity treatment. Increasing physical activity and modifying diet toward lower energy intake and healthy food choices are keys for any subsequent therapy. Treatments, such as pharmacotherapy and surgery, work alone, but are generally more effective when combined with lifestyle modification [31].

Guidelines for Selecting Obesity Treatment					
	BMI category, *kg/m²*				
Treatment	25–26.9	27–29.9	30–34.9	35–39.9	≥ 40
Diet, exercise, behavior therapy	+	+	+	+	+
Pharmacotherapy	—	With comorbidities	+	+	+
Surgery	—	—	—	With comorbidities	+

Figure 15-14. Guide for selecting obesity treatment. In general, we should match the intensity of the treatment to an individual's health risk and comorbid conditions/functional level. Again, lifestyle modification is the foundation for all other therapies. Weight-loss drugs are generally indicated when BMI is greater than 27 (with comorbidities) or greater than 30 (with or without comorbidities). Surgery is currently recommended only after other treatments have failed and for the highest risk categories (adapted from NIH [6]).

Edmonton Functional Stages of Obesity	
Stage	Description
0	No apparent obesity-related risk factors (*eg*, blood pressure, serum lipids, fasting glucose within normal range), no physical symptoms, no psychopathology, no functional limita tions, and/ or no impairment of well being
1	Presence of obesity -related subclinical risk factors (*eg*, borderline hypertension, impaired fasting glucose, elevated liver enzymes), mild physical symptoms (*eg*, dyspnea on moderate exertion, occasional aches an d pains, fatigue), mild psychopathology, mild functional limitations, and/or mild impairment of well being
2	Presence of established obesity-related chronic disease (*eg*, hypertension, type 2 diabetes, sleep apnea, osteoarthritis, reflux disease, PCOS, anx iety disorder), and moderate limitations in activities of daily living and/or well being
3	Established end -organ damage such as MI, heart failure, diabetic complications, incapacitating osteoarthritis, significant psychopathology, significant functional limitations, and/or impairment of well being
4	Severe (potentially end -stage) disabilities from obesity-related chronic diseases, severe disabling psychopathology, severe functional limitations, and/or severe impairment of well being

Figure 15-15. Edmonton Obesity Staging System. The NHLBI treatment guidelines focus on the BMI and the prevention of comorbidities, such as diabetes and CVD/hypertension. In addition to the system based on the BMI and Waist Circumference NIH Panel for evaluation, obesity can be "staged" based on the presence of comorbidities and their severity. Newer approaches, such as the Edmonton Obesity Staging System, supplement rather than replace the more traditional World Health Organization/NHLBI system for quantifying the diseases and harm associated with obesity (adapted from Sharma and Kushner [15]).

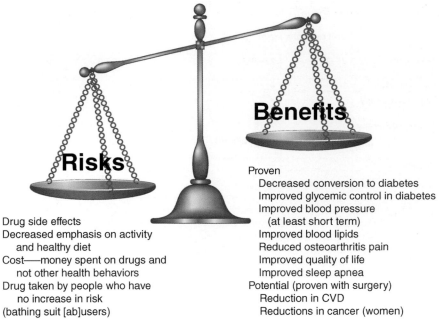

Figure 15-16. Risk–benefit equation. All drugs have risks. In chronic diseases, such as hypertension and hypercholesterolemia, the risk–benefit equation is near balance as the benefits are modest. In obesity, there is particular sensitivity to the risks, which is due to several factors. First, there is a long history of harmful drugs for obesity. Second, in terms of mortality or other "hard" end points, the benefits of modest weight loss are not yet proven. Third, there still is a negative cultural bias against the obese; many people still erroneously believe that obesity is due to gluttony and slothfulness. We should acknowledge this bias and understand how it influences the discussion on the risk–benefit equation. In contrast to the uncertainties of the benefits of drugs, modest weight loss achieved by lifestyle intervention clearly improves intermediate disease risk factors and self-reported measures of functioning and quality of life. This suggests that drugs improve morbidity and mortality.

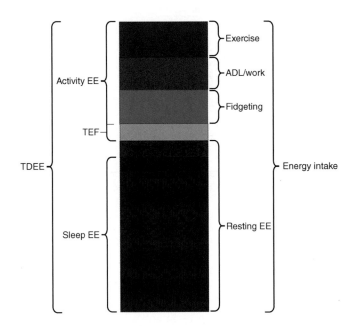

Figure 15-17. Energetics of body-weight regulation. The body consumes energy at rest and in several different activities. On a day-to-day basis, energy balance is tightly regulated, mostly by the feedback inhibition of food intake. Adaptive thermogenesis, the dissipation of energy through increased thermogenesis, is a weak response to overfeeding or increased body weight. Resting energy metabolism is determined largely by lean body mass. Energy expenditure increases after a meal; this is called the *thermic effect of food* (TEF) and is approximately 10% of the calories consumed. Activity energy expenditure includes spontaneous activity (fidgeting), activities of daily living (ADL) and work, and intentional activity that many of us call "exercise." The latter three add up to the activity energy expenditure and all add up to the *total daily energy expenditure* (TDEE) and balance energy intake. *EE* energy expenditure.

Duration of Various Activities to Expend 150 kcal for an Average 70-kg (154-lb) Adult		
Intensity	Activity	Approximate duration, *min*
Moderate	Volleyball, noncompetitive	43
Moderate	Walking, moderate pace (3 mi/h, 20 min/mi)	37
Moderate	Walking, brisk pace (4 mi/h, 15 min/mi)	32
Moderate	Table tennis	32
Moderate	Raking leaves	32
Moderate	Social dancing	29
Moderate	Lawn mowing (powered push mower)	29
Hard	Jogging (5 mi/h, 12 min/mi)	18
Hard	Field hockey	16
Very hard	Running (6 mi/h, 10 min/mi)	13

FIGURE 15-18. Physical activity needed to burn 150 cal. Humans move and consume energy efficiently. It takes only seconds to consume 150 kcal, but a minimum of 13 min to burn an equivalent amount of energy. This difference between energy consumption and expenditure explains why exercise is not a great way to lose weight. For instance, the current record for speed eating is 68 hot dogs in 10 min, which approximates 20,000 cal and 300 g of fat. For a 100-kg person, it would take about 100 h to burn those same calories. The benefits of exercise on other aspects of health are clear, however, and 10,000 steps per day is a reasonable activity goal for most Americans. People with chronic health problems, such as heart disease, diabetes, or obesity, or who are at high risk for these problems should first consult a physician before beginning a new program of physical activity.

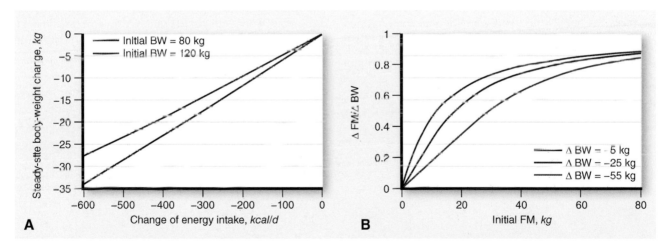

FIGURE 15-19. Models of how diets result in changes in body weight. At one point, it was thought that a pound of body weight equaled 3,500 kcal. However, the energy content of fat and lean tissue differs. Similarly, the amount of body fat at the beginning of a calorie-restricted diet or drug determines how much fat versus lean tissue are lost during weight loss (or gain) (adapted from Hall. ΔBW body-weight loss; ΔFM body-fat mass; BW body weight; FM fat mass [16]).

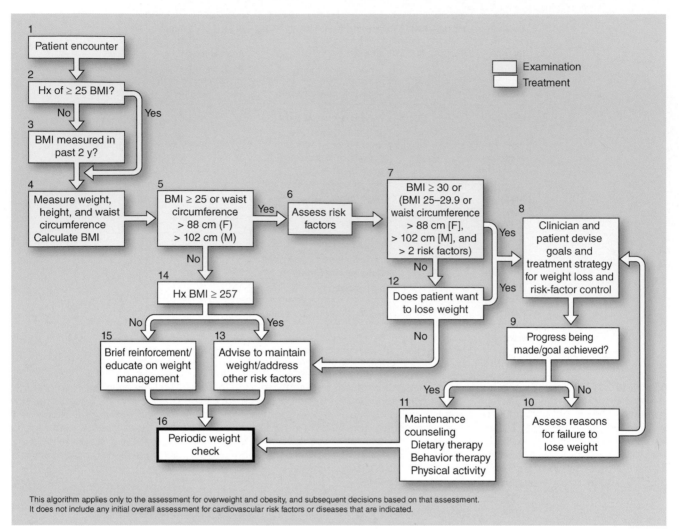

FIGURE 15-20. NHLBI expert panel treatment algorithm. The current NHLBI guidelines include a useful treatment algorithm, as shown. This algorithm applies only to the assessment for overweight and obesity, and subsequent decisions based on that assessment. It does not include any initial overall assessment for cardiovascular risk factors or diseases that are not indicated (adapted from NIH [6]).

Common Myths Surrounding Body Weight and Dieting
Exercise is the most effective means of losing body weight
Some diets are clearly more effective than others
High-protein, high-fat, low-carbohydrate diets uniquely cause weight loss
Most nutritional supplements for weight loss are effective
Nutritional supplements for weight loss are evaluated by the FDA for efficacy
Weight-loss interventions are not worth the effort because no one loses weight and those who do regain weight
Cutting 500 kcal/d from a weight-maintenance diet will result in weight loss at a rate of approximately 1 lb/wk
Weight is lost and gained at a rate of 3500 kcal/lb

FIGURE 15-21. Common myths surrounding body weight and dieting. Some common misconceptions and myths are listed here. *FDA Food and Drug Administration.*

Predictors of Successful Long-Term Weight Loss: National Weight Loss Registry
No similarity in how weight was lost
Great similarity in how weight loss is being maintained
Low-fat diet
Watching total calories
High daily levels of physical activity (average 2621 +/− 2252 kcal/wk)
Frequent self-monitoring

FIGURE 15-22. National Weight Loss Registry: Predictors of long-term successful lifestyle intervention. One thing to keep in mind is that although only a few people are able to lose and maintain weight loss by themselves, there are several features of people who are successful at long-term weight loss. Founded in 1994 by Drs. James Hill and Rena Wing, the National Weight Control Registry collects data from successful losers in order to look at "what works" in the real world. People who have maintained a minimum of 30 lbs of weight loss for a minimum of 1 year have high physical activity levels and consume a low-fat diet. See http://www.nwcr.ws [17, 18].

Behavior-Change (Modification) Techniques
Make sure there is more than one color on your plate (red, green, yellow); avoid brown and white
Put your fork (or other utensil) down between bites
Pause during your meal; talk, laugh, ask questions
Always try to leave some food on your plate
Keep tempting foods out of sight
Shop from a shopping list, buying only what is on the l ist
Remove serving dishes from the table while eating
Leave the table as soon as you are done eating
Serve and eat only one portion at a time
Wait at least 5 min before going back for extra helpings
Store foods in opaque containers, in the freeze r when possible
Go grocery shopping on a full stomach
If you get an urge to eat, wait at least 5 min before eating; the urge may pass
Avoid eating while doing other activities such as reading or watching the television
Do nothing else while eating
Buy foods that you must prepare in order to eat
Have a list of alternative activities handy that you could do anytime you have the urge to eat
Plan out your meals ahead of time
Follow an eating schedule
Keep healthy foods visible
Identify high -risk situations and try to avoid them
Avoid "automatic" eating. Search for patterns in your eating, focusing on certain times of the day you are likely to eat, the amount of food that you eat, the foods that you choose to eat, and the places you eat. Be more conscious of these things, and try to avoid that "automatic" eating Take the time to enjoy the food you are eating; do not rush it

FIGURE 15-23. Behavior-modification tips. As with many other chronic diseases, lifestyle modification is a cornerstone of obesity therapy. A stepped approach is appropriate and works well for other chronic diseases. Behavior modification can be as simple as changing views of food and engaging in specific behaviors that lead to reduced food/energy intake. Although modestly efficacious, these tips are easy to implement and lead to some weight loss. More intensive behavior modification requires a trained coach, dietician, or other practitioner and results in a 5–10% weight loss [19]. Behavioral contracts can be used to clearly identify and target behavioral goals; achieving the goal is increased if the patient is positively reinforced. Motivational interviewing facilitates glycemic control, weight loss, and long-term weight-loss maintenance among women diagnosed with type 2 diabetes [20] (from Smith et al. [5], with permission).

In contrast to successful behavior modification, potentially unsafe over-the-counter (OTC) "supplements" are popular with consumers. Patients continue to seek OTC "neutraceutical" treatments – most of questionable benefit – spending billions of dollars a year with limited benefit. In March 2009, the FDA further expanded its nationwide alert about tainted weight-loss products containing undeclared, active pharmaceutical ingredients. The FDA alert now lists more than 70 weight-loss products that may be harmful. Unsuspecting and desperate consumers fall prey to these potentially unsafe products every day.

Self-monitoring, however, is a key component for successful weight losers. Calorie counting and recording provides feedback on the "energy in" side of the energy balance equation. Activity energy expenditure can be safely increased by walking and a pedometer is a simple way to keep track of steps per day toward a goal of 10,000 steps. An accurate digital scale, along with measuring waist circumference, provides positive feedback on progress toward a realistic goal. Several companies now sell software that helps in the collection and recording of information, such as food intake and daily step counts. These tools are even available for phones and personal digital assistants (PDAs), making them portable and convenient. Patients record their food intake and physical activity using paper forms or electronic hand-held diaries (e.g., PDAs). This information is reviewed with a clinician and used to identify social, environmental, or emotional cues to overeating or inactivity. Patients are also encouraged to keep a record of their daily body weights (or weights that are recorded at regular intervals, e.g., every 3 days). Body weight data is viewed as an indicator of the patient's ability to adhere to the diet and exercise recommendations, which translate

into an energy deficit that causes weight loss. Certain situations or environments become associated with food intake or activity patterns, such as eating popcorn while watching a movie or being sedentary on the weekends. Stimulus control is used to limit the number of stimuli that are associated or "conditioned" with eating behavior and inactivity. Stimulus control recommendations include asking patients to eat at the same time and place in the absence of other stimuli, such as television, slow their rate of eating and put utensils down between bites, eat on small plates and limit portion size, not have second servings, and exercise on a regular schedule. Self-monitoring data can be used to identify situations or stimuli associated with food intake or inactivity.

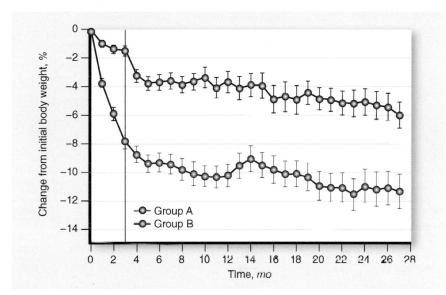

Figure 15-24. Meal replacements. Weight-loss patients are sometimes prescribed a nutritionally adequate calorie-restricted diet under the supervision of a dietitian. Meal plans that are highly structured and include portion-controlled foods or meal replacements are most effective at promoting weight loss. Portion-controlled foods and meal replacements include frozen entrees, nutrition shakes, and bars. These foods are affordable, readily available, and allow patients to easily eat healthy foods that meet the energy requirements of their diets. Meal replacements in the form of portion-controlled drinks, such as Glucerna™ (Abbott Nutrition; Columbus, OH) or Slim Fast™ (Unilever; Englewood Cliffs, NJ), can be used effectively to reduce body weight and improve glycemia [21]. In addition, this strategy can prevent the weight gain seen with drugs, like thiazolidinediones (TZDs) [22]. Results are shown in this figure. Group A represents the patients who were assigned to an energy-restricted diet only and group B consists of patients who had the energy-restricted diet with two meals and two snacks replaced with energy-controlled, nutrient-dense, meal-replacement products.

Stop or Replace Drugs That Cause Weight Gain
Corticosteroids
β blockers
Insulin
Antipsychotics

Figure 15-25. Stop drugs that cause weight gain. It is important to remember stop or replace drugs that cause weight gain, which are listed here. However, weight-loss drugs should not be continued if there is no benefit or if there are side effects. The following guidelines are from the NHLBI Expert Panel on Obesity Diagnosis and Treatment [6].

Weight loss drugs approved by the FDA may only be used as part of a comprehensive weight loss program, including dietary therapy and physical activity, for patients with a BMI of ≥30 with no concomitant obesity-related risk factors or disease, and for patients with a BMI of ≥27 with concomitant obesity-related risk factors or diseases. Weight loss drugs should never be used without concomitant lifestyle modifications. Continual assessment of drug therapy for efficacy and safety is necessary. If the drug is efficacious in helping the patient lose and/or maintain weight loss and there are no serious adverse effects, it can be continued. If not, it should be discontinued

Obesity-Drug Safety		
Year	Drug	Serious adverse events
1893/1949	Thyroid hormone	Hyperthyroidism
1933/1935	Dinitrophenol	Cataracts, neuropathy
1937/1971	Amphetamine	Addiction, psychosis
1965/1972	Aminorex	Pulmonary hypertension
1973/1997	Fenfluramine plus phentemine	Cardiac valvular insufficiency
1960/2000 (USA)*	Phenylpropanolamine	Hemorrhagic stroke
2006/2009	Rimonabant	Depression, suicidal ideation
1997/2010	Sibutramine	CVD
*Phenylpropanolamine is still available in some European countries.		

Figure 15-26. Safety of drugs used to treat obesity. There is a long history of drugs used to treat obesity that cause harm (from Astrup [23], with permission) see also [31].

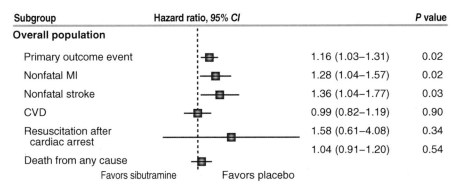

Subgroup	Hazard ratio, 95% CI		P value
Overall population			
Primary outcome event		1.16 (1.03–1.31)	0.02
Nonfatal MI		1.28 (1.04–1.57)	0.02
Nonfatal stroke		1.36 (1.04–1.77)	0.03
CVD		0.99 (0.82–1.19)	0.90
Resuscitation after cardiac arrest		1.58 (0.61–4.08)	0.34
Death from any cause		1.04 (0.91–1.20)	0.54

Favors sibutramine   Favors placebo

Figure 15-27. Sibutramine Cardiovascular Outcomes Trial and increased CVD. Sibutramine is one example of a drug that leads to good weight loss but also increased CVD in high-risk populations. Apart from the effects of a single study of bariatric surgery [24], there is no prospective data showing that weight loss reduces mortality or hard end points, such as CVD (adapted from James et al. [25]).

Drugs Approved by the FDA to Fight Obesity			
Generic name	DEA schedule	Approved use	Year approved
Orlistat	None	Long term	1999
Sibutramine	IV	Long term	1997
Diethylpropion	IV	Short term	1973
Phentermine	IV	Short term	1973
Phendimetrazine	III	Short term	1961
Benzphetamine	III	Short term	1960

FIGURE 15-28. Drugs approved by the FDA to treat obesity. Pharmacotherapy is indicated when lifestyle modification is unsuccessful. Drugs are "added on" rather than replacing lifestyle modification. Do not forget to diagnose and treat sleep apnea or depression *first*. Treating depression with antidepressants that are weight neutral or have modest weight-loss effects can be helpful (e.g., selective serotonin reuptake inhibitors [SSRIs], such as fluoxetine). Also, it is important to treat depression before starting obesity therapy. Unfortunately, the modest weight-loss effects of SSRIs do not appear to be sustained over the long term. When choosing/adjusting antidiabetic therapies, remember that insulin, sulfonylureas, and TZDs cause weight gain. Metformin causes a modest weight loss (1–2 kg) on average. TZDs (i.e., Actos™, Avandia™) are well-known to increase both body fat and, in some patients, fluid retention and congestive heart failure. The effects to increase food intake are probably due to direct actions in the hypothalamus increasing appetite and decreasing satiety. There are only a few drugs that are approved for treating obesity; of these, sympathomimetics have been on the market the longest. These drugs are not approved for long-term use and, because they are controlled substances, are regulated by state laws to short-term use, only 6–8 weeks. Check your state laws carefully before using these drugs. Phentermine is far and away the most prescribed antiobesity drug in the USA. *DEA* drug enforcement agency (adapted from Yanovski and Yanovski [26] see also Padwal [29]).

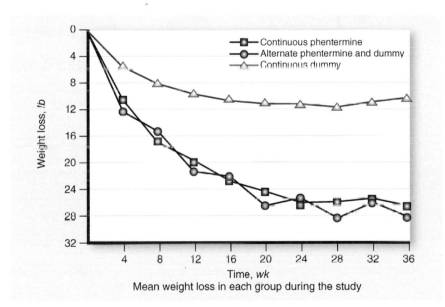

Mean weight loss in each group during the study

FIGURE 15-29. Phentermine. In 1996, there were 11 million prescriptions written for phentermine, and it remains the most-prescribed weight-loss drug. Phentermine is a sympathomimetic that increases energy expenditure and decreases appetite. It is a controlled substance, only approved for short-term use and regulated by state pharmacy boards (adapted from Munro et al. [27]).

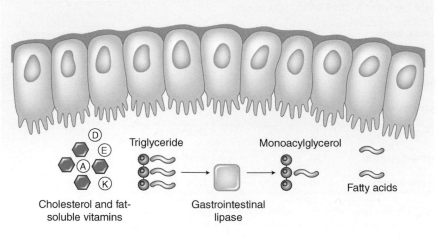

A

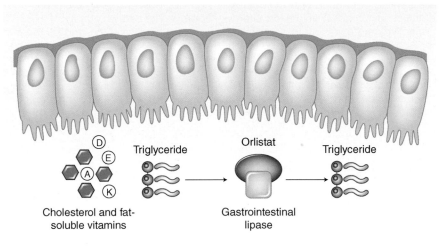

B

FIGURE 15-30. Inhibition of fat absorption by orlistat. Orlistat acts locally within the bowels to prevent the absorption of lipids by inhibiting intestinal lipases. It is associated with local side effects, such as loose bowels, diarrhea, and increased flatulence, but has no systemic side effects. (**A**) Under normal function, the for-mation of micelles in the intestinal lumen allows the absorption of approximately 90% of dietary triglycerides as monoacylglyc-erol and fatty acids; cholesterol and fat-soluble vitamins are absorbed with lipids. (**B**) With orlistat, approximately one-third of dietary triglycerides are excreted unchanged in the stools.

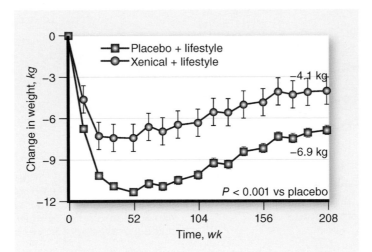

Figure 15-31. Orlistat: Efficacy. Xenical™ (Genentech; San Francisco, CA; orlistat) is a pancreatic lipase inhibitor that produces about 3% body weight loss on average. A reduced-dose version is available OTC under the brand name Alli™ (GlaxoSmithKline; Philadelphia, PA). Xenical™ is safe and an added bonus is data from the Xendos trial, showing that orlistat over 2 years can prevent or delay the development of type 2 diabetes [5]. Side effects include fatty/oily stools in about one-third of treated patients, increased defecation in about 20% of patients, and other similar gastrointestinal-related adverse events should be included in the discussion with patients prior to initiating therapy. Remember, though, that many patients do not experience these effects and that they tend to decrease over time and as patients learn not to consume high-fat foods. The loss of fat-soluble vitamins has been reported and a multivitamin supplement with vitamins A and D is strongly recommended for patients taking Xenical™ or Alli™, as well as for all patients attempting to lose weight. Unfortunately, adding orlistat to sibutramine does not produce additive weight loss. Although orlistat has modest efficacy, the Xendos trial showed that it reduced the conversion of prediabetes to diabetes by 37% [28].

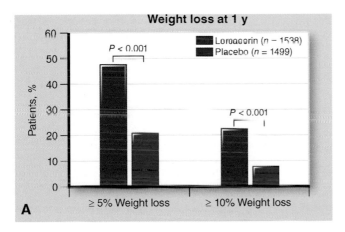

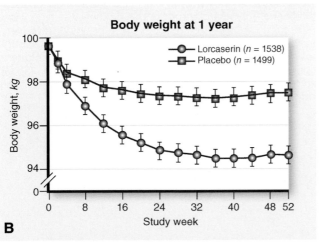

Figure 15-32. Lorcaserin: Efficacy. Lorcaserin is a 5HT2c agonist in the development for treating obesity (adapted from Smith et al. [32]).

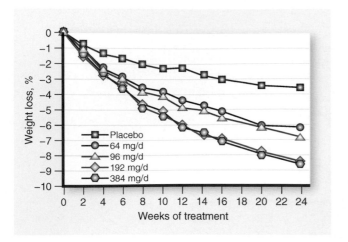

Figure 15-33. Topiramate: Offlabel efficacy. Topiramate is an antiepileptic that reduced body weight through unclear mechanisms. Central nervous system adverse events are common and topiramate is a known teratogen, so caution is warranted (adapted from Bray et al. [33]).

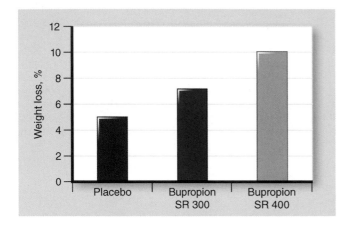

Figure 15-34. Bupropion: Offlabel efficacy. Bupropion has been used for depression and smoking cessation and is also efficacious for weight loss, although not approved for that indication. Major side effects include mood disturbances and seizures. A 24-week computer data is shown here. *SR* sustained release (adapted from Anderson et al. [13]).

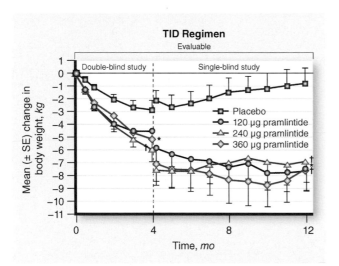

Figure 15-35. Pramlintide: Offlabel efficacy. Amylin is a hormone secreted from the pancreatic β cell along with insulin. Pramlintide is an analogue of amylin that is indicated for glycemic control in type 1 diabetes and in patients with type 2 diabetes taking insulin. It also reduces appetite, increases satiety, and reduces body weight at high doses, probably through activation of specific receptors known to exist in the brainstem. Higher doses may be more effective for obesity [34, 35, 36], although it is not indicated for obesity. *TID* three times daily (adapted from Smith et al. [34]).

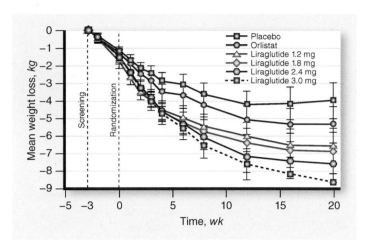

FIGURE 15-36. GLP-1: Offlabel efficacy. Newer injectable agents, like the GLP-1 analogues Byetta™ (Amylin Pharmaceuticals, Inc. and Lilly USA, LLC, San Diego, CA; exenatide), Victoza™ (Novo Nordisk A/S, Princeton, NJ; liraglutide), and the amylin-mimetic Symlin™ (Amylin Pharmaceuticals, San Diego, CA; pramlintide), are drugs approved for treating diabetes; when used as indicated in the package insert, they have modest effects to reduce body weight. GLP-1 agonists, such as exenatide and liraglutide, reduce body weight probably through the activation of GLP-1 receptors in the brainstem and possibly the hypothalamus. Although the effects on body weight are modest in diabetes, this study in obese nondiabetic patients showed good body-weight reduction at doses higher than those necessary for glycemic control (adapted from Astrup et al. [36]).

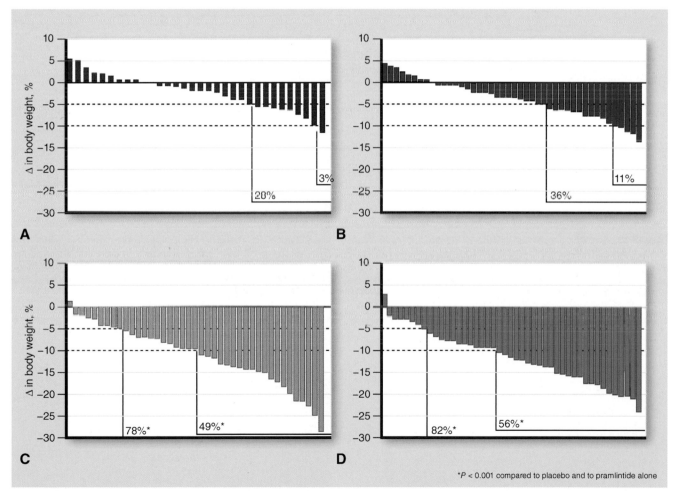

*P < 0.001 compared to placebo and to pramlintide alone

FIGURE 15-37. Pramlintide + phentermine or + sibutramine: Offlabel efficacy. Increasingly, drugs are used in combination to increase efficacy and with a goal to reduce dose and, therefore, side effects. As noted above, pramlintide is effective to reduce body weight. In combination with either sibutramine or phentermine, body weight is reduced even further (adapted from Aronne et al. [37]).

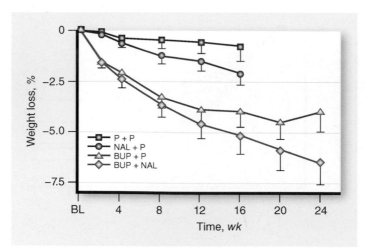

Figure 15-38. Naltrexone (NAL)–bupropion (BUP) in combination for weight loss. In addition to increased efficacy and reduced side effects, some weight-loss drugs are used in combination to produce synergistic effects on body weight. The opioid antagonist NAL has little effect on body weight when used alone, but synergizes when given with BUP. This combination is under evaluation by the FDA. *P* placebo (adapted from Greenway et al. [38]).

Indications for Bariatric Surgery
Indications
1. BMI > 40 kg/m^2 or BMI 35–39.9 kg/m^2 and life-threatening cardiopulmonary disease, severe diabetes, or lifestyle i mpairment
2. Failure to achieve adequate weight loss with nonsurgical treatment
Contraindications
1. History of noncompliance with medical care
2. Certain psychiatric illnesses: personality disorder, uncontrolled depression, suicidal ideation, substance abuse
3. Unlikely to survive surgery

Figure 15-39. Bariatric surgery: Indications. Bariatric surgery is currently the treatment of last resort. As the procedures become refined, there is certainly a pressure downward in terms of the BMI cut points for surgeries. The choice of surgery is beyond the scope of this review, but suffice it to say that the experience of the surgeon has a strong influence on the morbidity and mortality of the procedure; experience is important. Bariatric surgery is currently reserved for the most obese patients and those with established comorbid conditions (adapted from Consensus Development Conference Panel [39]).

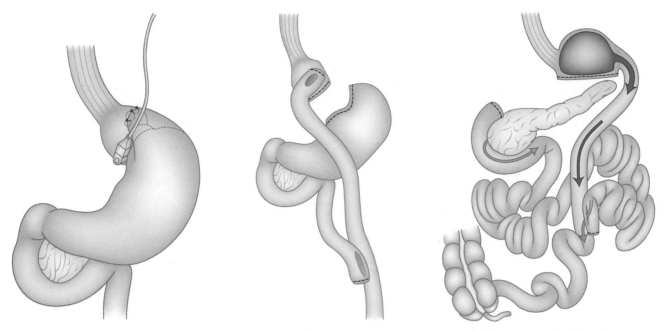

Adjustable gastric banding   **Roux-en-Y gastric bypass**   **Biliopancreatic diversion**

Figure 15-40. Common bariatric surgery procedures. About 220,000 people with morbid obesity in the USA had bariatric surgery in 2009, which represents less than 1% of the eligible population. Roux-en Y and gastric banding are the most common types of the surgery performed in the USA. The risk of death from bariatric surgery is currently about 0.1% and inversely proportional to the experience of the surgeon (adapted from Thaler and Cummings [40]).

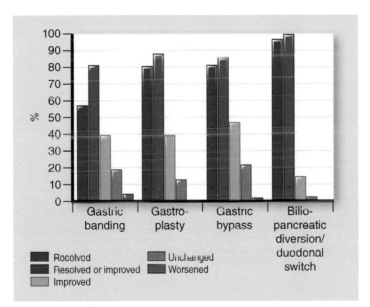

Figure 15-41. Resolution of diabetes after weight-loss surgery. The weight loss produced by bariatric surgery, and possibly other mechanisms, such as increased gut peptide secretion, acts to resolve diabetes in a large portion of patients. Diabetes resolution results in discontinued treatment and diabetes improvement results in reduced treatment (adapted from Buchwald et al. [41]).

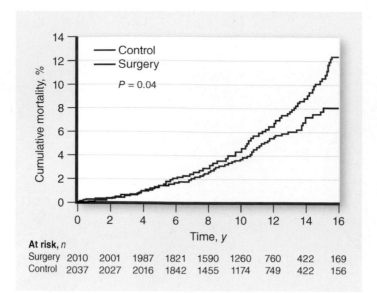

Figure 15-42. Bariatric surgery reduces mortality. Recent data from the Swedish Obese Subjects Study shows that surgery can reduce mortality on a long-term basis. More and more, very obese patients and their doctors are choosing obesity surgery to treat diabetes and other comorbidities leading to the term *metabolic surgery*. In the landmark Swedish Obese Subjects Study, surgery reduced overall mortality and the dominant effect was on CVD. Interestingly, there appeared to be an effect on the development of cancer as well [42] (adapted from Sjöström et al. [24]).

Acknowledgments I would like to acknowledge the two people who taught me the most about obesity therapy, Professors George Bray and Frank Greenway; Corby Martin, who introduced me to the science of behavior modification; and Tim Church, who made exercise science interesting and pertinent to obesity and diabetes.

Resources

The Practical Guide to the Identification, Evaluation, and Treatment of Overweight and Obesity in Adults: Available on the NHLBI Web site at www.nhlbi.nih.gov and http://www.nhlbi.nih.gov/guidelines/obesity/ob_home.htm

References

1. Haslam DW, James WP: Obesity. *Lancet* 2005, 366:1197–1209.

2. Birkmeyer NJ, Dimick JB, Share D: Hospital complication rates with bariatric surgery in Michigan. *JAMA* 2010, 304:435–442.

3. Wang S, Sparks LM, Xie H: Subtyping obesity with microarrays: implications for the diagnosis and treatment of obesity. *Int J Obes (Lond)* 2009, 33:481–489.

4. CDC: Vital signs: state-specific obesity prevalence among adults – United States, 2009. *MMWR*, 59:1–3.

5. Smith SR, Martin C, Katzmarzyk P, *et al.*: Obesity and diabetes: implications for management. In *2009 Educational Review Manual in Endocrinology FOCUS: Diabetes*. Edited by Kendall, DM. New York: Castle Connolly Graduate Medical; 2009.

6. National Institutes of Health: Clinical guidelines on the identification, evaluation, and treatment of overweight and obesity in adults – the evidence report. *Obes Res* 1998, 6(Suppl 2):51S–209S.

7. Gordon-Larsen P, The NS, Adair LS: Longitudinal trends in obesity in the United States from adolescence to the third decade of life. *Obesity (Silver Spring, MD)* 2010, 18:1801–1804.

8. Prospective Studies Collaboration, Whitlock G, Lewington S, *et al.*: Body-mass index and cause-specific mortality in 900 000 adults: collaborative analyses of 57 prospective studies. *Lancet* 2009, 373:1083–1096.

9. Willett WC, Manson JE, Stampfer MJ, *et al.*: Weight, weight change, and coronary heart disease in women. Risk within the 'normal' weight range. *JAMA* 1995, 273:461–465.

10. Sharma AM, Padwal R: Obesity is a sign – over-eating is a symptom: an aetiological framework for the assessment and management of obesity. *Obes Rev* 2010, 11:362–370.

11. Knowler WC, Barrett-Connor E, Fowler SE, *et al.*: Reduction in the incidence of type 2 diabetes with lifestyle intervention or metformin. *N Engl J Med* 2002, 346:393–403.

12. Hamman RF, Wing RR, Edelstein SL, *et al.*: Effect of weight loss with lifestyle intervention on risk of diabetes. *Diabetes Care* 2006, 29:2102–2107.

13. Anderson JW, Greenway FL, Fujioka K, *et al.*: Bupropion SR enhances weight loss: a 48-week double-blind, placebo-controlled trial. *Obes Res* 2002, 10:633–641.

14. Foster GD, Wadden TA, Vogt RA, Brewer G: What is a reasonable weight loss? Patients' expectations and evaluations of obesity treatment outcomes. *J Consult Clin Psychol* 1997, 65:79–85.

15. Sharma AM, Kushner, RF: A proposed clinical staging system for obesity. *Int J Obes (Lond)* 2009, 33:289–295.

16. Hall K: Mechanisms of metabolic fuel selection – modeling human metabolism and body weight change. *IEEE Eng Med Biol Mag* 2010, 29:36–41.

17. Catenacci VA, Ogden LG, Stuht J, *et al.*: Physical activity patterns in the National Weight Control Registry. *Obesity (Silver Spring, MD)* 2008, 16:153–161.

18. Butryn ML, Phelan S, Hill JO, Wing RR: Consistent self-monitoring of weight: a key component of successful weight loss maintenance. *Obesity (Silver Spring, MD)* 2007, 15:3091–3096.

19. Sarwer DB, von Sydow Green A, *et al.*: Behavior therapy for obesity: where are we now? *Curr Opin Endocrinol Diabetes Obes* 2009, 16:347–352.

20. West DS, DiLillo V, Bursac Z, *et al.*: Motivational interviewing improves weight loss in women with type 2 diabetes. *Diabetes Care* 2007, 30:1081–1087.

21. Heymsfield SB, van Mierlo CA, van der Knaap HC , *et al.*: Weight management using a meal replacement strategy: meta and pooling analysis from six studies. *Int J Obes Relat Metab Disord* 2003, 27:537–549.

22. Gupta AK, Smith SR, Greenway FL, Bray GA: Pioglitazone treatment in type 2 diabetes mellitus when combined with portion control diet modifies the metabolic syndrome. *Diabetes Obes Metab* 2009, 11:330–337.

23. Astrup A: Is cardiometabolic risk improved by weight loss drugs? *Lancet* 2010, 376:567–568.

24. Sjöström L, Narbro K, Sjöström CD, *et al.*: Effects of bariatric surgery on mortality in Swedish obese subjects. *N Engl J Med* 2007, 357:741–752.

25. James WP, Caterson ID, Coutinho W, *et al.*: Effect of sibutramine on cardiovascular outcomes in overweight and obese subjects. *N Engl J Med* 2010, 363:905–917.

26. Yanovski SZ, Yanovski JA: Obesity. *N Engl J Med* 2002, 346:591–602.

27. Munro JF, MacCuish AC, Wilson EM, Duncan LJ: Comparison of continuous and intermittent anorectic therapy in obesity. *Br Med J* 1968, 1:352–354.

28. Torgerson JS, Hauptman J, Boldrin MN, Sjöström L: XENical in the prevention of diabetes in obese subjects (XENDOS) study: a randomized study of orlistat as an adjunct to lifestyle changes for the prevention of type 2 diabetes in obese patients. *Diabetes Care* 2004, 27:155–161.

29. Padwal R, Li SK, Lau DC: Long-term pharmacotherapy for overweight and obesity: a systematic review and meta-analysis of randomized controlled trials. *Int J Obes Relat Metab Disord* 2003, 27:1437–1446.

30. Wadden TA, Berkowitz RI, Womble LG, *et al.*: Randomized trial of lifestyle modification and pharmacotherapy for obesity. *N Engl J Med* 2005, 353:2111–2120.

31. Astrup A, Toubro S: When, for whom and how to use sibutramine? *Int J Obes Relat Metab Disord* 2001, 25(Suppl 4):S2–S7.

32. Smith SR, Weissman NJ, Anderson CM, *et al.*: Multicenter, placebo-controlled trial of lorcaserin for weight management. *N Engl J Med* 2010, 363:245–256.

33. Bray GA, Hollander P, Klein S, *et al.*: A 6-month randomized, placebo-controlled, dose-ranging trial of topiramate for weight loss in obesity. *Obes Res* 2003, 11:722–733.

34. Smith SR, Aronne LJ, Burns CM, *et al.*: Sustained weight loss following 12-month pramlintide treatment as an adjunct to lifestyle intervention in obesity. *Diabetes Care* 2008, 31:1816–1823.

35. Smith SR, Blundell JE, Burns C, *et al.*: Pramlintide treatment reduces 24-h caloric intake and meal sizes and improves control of eating in obese subjects: a 6-wk translational research study. *Am J Physiol Endocrinol Metab* 2007, 293:E620–E627.

36. Astrup A, Rössner S, Van Gaal L, *et al.*: Effects of liraglutide in the treatment of obesity: a randomised, double-blind, placebo-controlled study. *Lancet* 2009, 374:1606–1616.

37. Aronne LJ, Halseth AE, Burns CM, *et al.*: Enhanced weight loss following coadministration of pramlintide with sibutramine or phentermine in a multicenter trial. *Obesity (Silver Spring, MD)* 2010, 18:1739–1746.

38. Greenway FL, Dunayevich E, Tollefson G, *et al.*: Comparison of combined bupropion and naltrexone therapy for obesity with monotherapy and placebo. *J Clin Endocrinol Metab* 2009, 94:4898–4906.

39. NIH conference: Gastrointestinal surgery for severe obesity. Consensus Development Conference Panel. *Ann Intern Med* 1991, 115:956–961.

40. Thaler JP, Cummings DE: Minireview: Hormonal and metabolic mechanisms of diabetes remission after gastrointestinal surgery. *Endocrinology* 2009, 150:2518–2525.

41. Buchwald H, Estok R, Fahrbach K, *et al.*: Weight and type 2 diabetes after bariatric surgery: systematic review and meta-analysis. *Am J Med* 2009, 122:248–256 e5.

42. Sjöström L, Gummesson A, Sjöström CD, *et al.*: Effects of bariatric surgery on cancer incidence in obese patients in Sweden (Swedish Obese Subjects Study): a prospective, controlled intervention trial. *Lancet Oncol* 2009, 10:653–662.

16 Reversal of Diabetes: Islet Cell Transplantation

Antonello Pileggi, Rodolfo Alejandro,
and Camillo Ricordi

Chronic hyperglycemia in patients with type 1 diabetes mellitus is frequently associated with progressive complications that can dramatically affect both quality of life and life span [1]. Intensive insulin therapy with tight glycemic control can reduce or delay the risk of diabetes complications [1, 2] and can also be cost-effective [3]. However, the downsides of intensive insulin treatment include the inability to sustain euglycemia throughout the day and the increased frequency of severe (and potentially life-threatening) hypoglycemic episodes [2, 4]. Restoring endocrine function by transplanting islets of Langerhans or the whole pancreas offers the advantage of a more physiological glycemic control over exogenous insulin administration that may also contribute to the reversal of diabetic lesions such as nephropathy, retinopathy, and neuropathy [4–9].

In recent years, a number of centers worldwide have reported on reproducibly improved glucose metabolic control and sustained graft function in patients with type 1 diabetes mellitus after transplantation of allogeneic islet cells [4, 10–13]. This unprecedented success follows the steady progress of this field and the implementation of improved tissue harvesting and preservation methods, progress in cellular isolation and purification technology, and the introduction of safer transplantation techniques, together with the availability of new immunosuppressive agents [11, 13 39].

This chapter provides an overview of the methods for human islet cell isolation, purification, and transplantation and discusses the benefits of islet cell transplantation for the treatment of patients with diabetes.

Infrastructure

Adequate infrastructure and highly qualified personnel with multidisciplinary expertise (endocrinology, transplant surgery, radiology, cell biology, immunology, administrative, and human islet cell processing technologists) are fundamental elements for the success of an islet-transplantation program because they may contribute to achieve the goals of obtaining adequate islet cells from the donor pancreata and assuring appropriate pre- and posttransplant management (i.e., metabolic and immunosuppression) of the recipients.

Islet cell transplantation is regulated in the USA by the Food and Drug Administration (FDA) under the category of *investigational new drug* [40, 41]. The islet cell processing facility should be organized following general manufacture practice (GMP), good laboratory practice (GLP), and good tissue practice (GTP) regulations for clinical trials, along with other FDA regulatory requirements to ensure the highest standards of quality, purity, potency, and safety for medical products for human use. All procedures should be performed under aseptic conditions in class II biological safety cabinets with solutions composed of sterile components. The clean room suite of the clinical islet isolation laboratory should be designed, tested, and certified to meet ISO Class 7 (ISO 14644), should have 24-7 HEPA-filtered air conditioning, and should be dedicated solely to the processing of human islet cells. Access to the facility should be controlled and restricted to authorized personnel. Procedures pertaining to required dirty/clean flow patterns and directions should be enforced by standard operating procedures, training, management, and facility design, with a clean room suite having separate exits for soiled supplies and staff. Both facility and equipments should be inspected periodically by an operations manager and a quality assurance unit to confirm compliance with required standards. Personnel from the GMP facility should receive continuous training and periodical competency assessment should be enforced. In addition to the organization and logistics of the facility, it is essential for the good functioning of the islet cell transplant program to establish a continuous interaction with the organ-procurement organizations and the involvement of medical departments and services, including other transplant programs, radiology, endocrinology, and pathology.

Several successful islet cell transplantation programs have recently been created by establishing collaborations with already well-recognized islet cell processing centers at a distant location where islet cells are isolated and then shipped for transplantation [19, 25, 35, 42–44]. This strategy appears to be very promising because it helps to overcome the timely and costly learning curve to achieve consistent quality and yields. An islet cell processing GMP facility should exist at the distant transplant center where quality control assessment of the islet cells received is performed before transplantation to confirm compliance with product release criteria (i.e., sterility, viability, and potency) [25, 35].

Isolation and Purification of Human Islets

Islets of Langerhans are highly vascularized cellular clusters (*see* Fig. 16.1a) that are scattered throughout the pancreatic gland and are composed of endocrine cells (α cells: glucagon; β cells: insulin; δ cells: somatostatin; pancreatic polypeptide [PP] cells) (*see* Fig. 16.1b). Complex interactions between islet cells and the sur-

rounding environment and within the endocrine islet cell subsets finely regulate glucose metabolism [45]. For this reason, the goal of the isolation and purification procedures is to free the islet cells from the surrounding connective and nonendocrine pancreatic tissue while preserving their integrity.

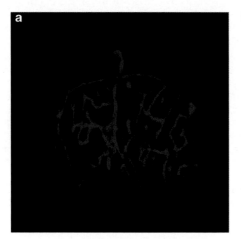
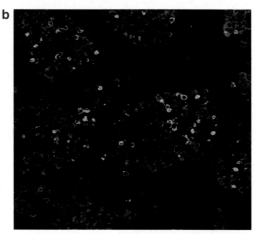

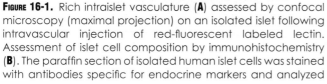

FIGURE 16-1. Rich intraislet vasculature (**A**) assessed by confocal microscopy (maximal projection) on an isolated islet following intravascular injection of red-fluorescent labeled lectin. Assessment of islet cell composition by immunohistochemistry (**B**). The paraffin section of isolated human islet cells was stained with antibodies specific for endocrine markers and analyzed using fluorescence microscopy. Several cell clusters are shown, each composed of endocrine cell subsets that are in close relation to each other. The *red signal* indicates insulin, the *green signal* indicates glucagon, and the *blue signal* indicates 4',6-diamidino-2-phenylindole (DAPI) specific for nuclei (×200 magnification).

Pancreas Procurement

Pancreatic glands for islet cell isolation are obtained from multiorgan cadaveric donors with selection criteria similar to that for solid organ transplantation. Multiple factors, including cerebral death, donor characteristics, warm and cold ischemia, and organ-procurement techniques may affect the outcome (i.e., quality and yields) of islet cell isolations [28, 46–50]. During pancreas recovery for islet cell isolation, extreme care should be taken, as for whole organ transplant, to minimize isch-

emia and preserve organ integrity [28, 49]. After surgical recovery, the pancreas is transported to the cell-processing laboratory into ice-chilled preservation solution, where it generally is processed within 12 h of procurement. An addition of oxygen-carrier moieties to the organ-preservation solution has allowed for extended cold ischemia time and reduced ischemic damage to the pancreatic tissue while also favoring higher islet cell yields after isolation [51, 52].

Digestion of the Pancreatic Gland

Dissociation of the pancreatic tissue is obtained by mechanically enhanced enzymatic digestion [53]. Dissociation enzymes consist of collagenase mixtures, including metalloenzymes that are able to hydrolyze collagen. The availability of purified collagenase or new enzyme blends with low endotoxin contamination and better selectivity for exocrine tissue has contributed to improving the yields and reproducibility of the islet isolation [16]. A key component of the semiautomated digestion process is the dissociation chamber [53], where the digestion of the pancreas takes place.

The chamber is part of a circuit through which the enzymatic solution is circulated by a peristaltic pump (see Fig. 16.2). The chamber consists of two portions separated by a removable stainless steel screen (1) a lower cylindrical portion with inlet ports and an opening for a temperature sensor and (2) an upper conical portion with an outlet at the apex. The temperature of the system is constantly monitored and can be adjusted by the means of a thermostat included in the circuit. After dissecting the pancreas from surrounding tissues (see Fig. 16.3a), the pancreatic duct is cannulated (see Fig. 16.3c) and injected with the enzyme solution either manually (see Fig. 16.3d) or using a peristaltic pump. The gland is then loaded in the chamber in two or more pieces, depending on the temperature of the perfusing collagenase solution. Warm collagenase perfusion does not generally require division of the gland, and separation in multiple pancreatic segments (generally 7–11) is preferred when cold collagenase perfusion is used, to reduce the temperature gradient within the pancreatic tissue after warm solution is recirculating in the chamber. The pancreatic segments (see Fig. 16.3e) are loaded into the chamber (see Fig. 16.3f) along with specially manufactured marbles that serve as digestion enhancers, contributing to the mechanical disruption of the gland. The chamber is then sealed (see Fig. 16.3g) and the circuit filled with enzyme solution without an air–fluid interface to reduce the mechanical stress on the pancreatic tissue and to minimize protein denaturation during the digestion process. The digestion phase begins by increasing the temperature of the circuit for optimal enzymatic activity. The screen retains the gland in the lower portion of the chamber and the marbles enhance the mechanical disruption during controlled amplitude and frequency shaking (see Fig. 16.3g). A combination of enzymatic and mechanical (shaking and flow) actions results in the progressive release of particles from the digesting pancreas that are continuously removed through the screen and, therefore, preserved from further digestion.

During the dissociation phase, critical parameters that may influence the outcome of the isolation are constantly monitored, including temperature, pH, PO_2, PCO_2, bicarbonate concentration, and base excess [54]. The progression of the digestion is also monitored by assessing, under light microscopy, the quality of the digest, the integrity and number of islet cells, and the appearance of acinar tissue on samples collected from the circuit and stained with diphenylthiocarbazone [dithizone (DTZ)] [55]. When numerous free and intact islet cells along with small-sized acinar tissue fragments are observed, the enzymatic activity is sharply inhibited by dilution with serum-enriched cold medium. The pancreatic digest is then concentrated by centrifugation and prepared for the next purification step.

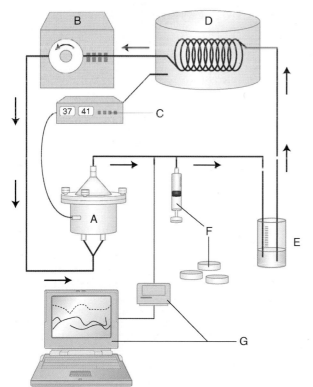

Figure 16-2. Pancreas dissociation circuit. The pancreas is dissociated by mechanically enhanced enzymatic digestion performed using a semiautomated method. The gland is placed in the digestion chamber containing marbles for enhanced mechanical action (A).The circuit is filled with enzyme solution that is circulated (arrows) by a peristaltic pump (B).The temperature of the chamber is monitored (C) and regulated by a thermostat included in the circuit (D). A beaker containing the enzyme solution (E) is used as reservoir and collector of the digest released from the chamber. A sampling port downstream from the chamber (F) allows for the collection of samples for the assessment of the progression of the digestion process. The samples collected are transferred to Petri dishes, stained with DTZ, and assessed by light microscopy. A probe inserted in the circuit and connected to a computer system allows for the continuous collection of multiple parameters (i.e., pH, PO_2, PCO_2) during the digestion process (G).

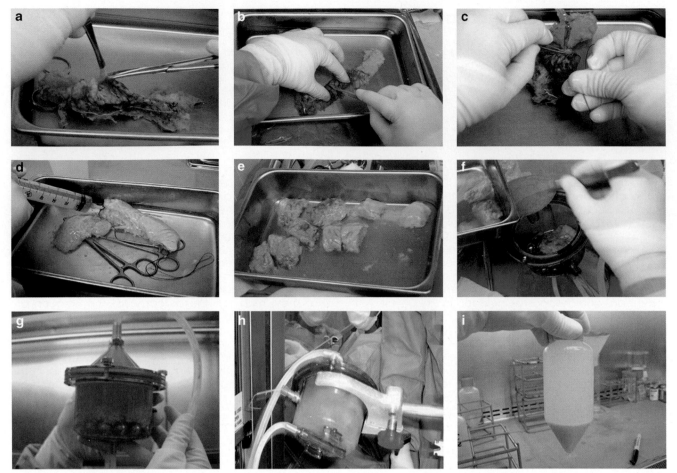

Figure 16-3. Islet cell isolation procedure: preparation of the pancreas. The pancreas is generally obtained en block with spleen and a segment of the duodenum, which are removed on the back table before starting the isolation (**A**). Cleaning also includes the removal of the surrounding adipose and connective tissue, taking great care in preserving the pancreatic capsule integrity to prevent leaking of the enzyme during the distension phase (**B**).The gland is cut into two portions and the pancreatic duct of both portions is then cannulated (**C**) and injected with the enzyme solution, resulting in the distention of the gland (**D**). After distention, the gland is divided into several pieces of equal size (**E**) and transferred into the diges-tion chamber (**F**).The chamber (**G**) consists of a lower cylinder and an upper conical portion separated by a removable stainless steel screen, and it contains hollow stainless steel marbles. The screen retains the pancreas in the lower portion of the chamber and the marbles enhance the mechanical disruption during a manual or automated shaking (**H**). A combination of both enzymatic and mechanical actions lead to the disruption of the tissue and progressive release of small particles, which are removed and preserved from further digestion. After digestion, the pancreatic slurry is concentrated by centrifugation (**I**) and prepared for the next purification step.

Purification of Pancreatic Islet Cell

The purification step is performed to physically separate islet cells from nonendocrine tissue. The goal of the purification step is to minimize the volume of tissue to be implanted in the recipient's portal system to prevent excessive ischemic insult to the liver and elevation of portal pressure, thereby decreasing the potential for procedure-related complications. Islet cell purification is obtained by isopycnic separation, which takes advantage of the differences in density that exist between the endocrine and exocrine tissues [56]. Centrifugation of the pancreatic digest on density gradients allows each tissue to migrate to the gradient of equal density.

Although acinar cells have densities much higher than other cell types, swelling and edema consecutive to the dissociation procedure may alter densities and interfere with the efficiency of the separation, therefore precluding high degrees of purity [56]. The semiautomated separation method uses the COBE 2991 computerized centrifuge system, which consists of a centrifuge bowl that bears a doughnut-shaped bag in which the pellet sediments to the outside and the lower density forms layers to the center (*see* Fig. 16.4) [31, 57, 58]. The centrifuge has a hydraulic system that can apply uniform pressure to the separation bag, allowing for the collection of the fractions starting from the center portion of the bag. The pancreatic digest can be resuspended in preservation solution and loaded on top of the gradient layers. Top loading allows keeping the digested pancreas in the physiological medium for the longest possible time, but it may be associated with increased cell aggregation with acinar tissue migrating to the denser gradient layers, dragging down islet cells from the upper interfaces [56]. It has been suggested that reducing cellular swelling and edema obtained by incubating the slurry in preservation (hyperosmolar) solutions before and during the purification process can significantly improve top-loading efficiency [56]. The use of top-loading and continuous density gradients is currently considered the gold standard because it may allow for higher yields and purity [56]. However, it is a laborious and time-consuming process because numerous fractions are collected and assessed separately. Alternatively, the pancreatic digest can be resuspended in the heaviest density gradient and loaded in the bottom of the bag, generally using discontinuous density gradients [56]. This procedure is faster because only a few fractions are collected and assessed, but it may allow for a lower effective cell load associated with the accumulation of cells at the interfaces, which interferes with the migration-producing cell aggregation [56]. Numerous approaches have been recently proposed to enhance the efficiency of the purification process [31, 59]. The use of an additional purification step (*rescue purification*) on the fraction of pancreatic digest previously undergone to a standard purification step can contribute improving the yield of functional human islet preparations and pancreas utilization for islet transplantation [31].

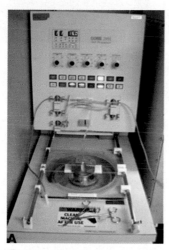 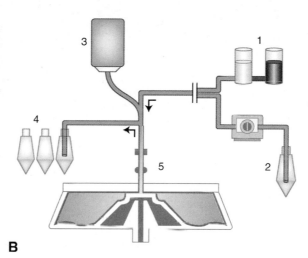

Figure 16-4. Islet cell isolation procedure: purification. Islet cells represent approximately 2% of the total pancreatic tissue. The digested pancreas is centrifuged on isopycnic gradients (separation according to differences in density) using the semiautomated COBE 2991 computerized centrifuge system (**A**). A doughnut-shaped bag is placed in the centrifuge (**B**) and then loaded with either continuous (1) or discontinuous (2) gradients. Continuous gradients are obtained using a gradient mixer (1), followed by top loading of the pancreatic digest in preservation solution using an infusion bag. When using discontinuous gradients, the pancreatic digest is resuspended in the denser gradient and the lower densities are added on top with a peristaltic pump (2). After centrifugation, the hydraulic system of the centrifuge is activated and different fractions are collected separately to assess purity (3).

Pancreatic Islet Cell Assessment and Culture

After purification, islet cells can be transplanted immediately or cultured for a short period before implant [60]. Before transplantation, an assessment of sterility and in vitro function of the islet cell preparation is required for product release. The assessment includes gram staining to exclude bacterial contamination, assessment of endotoxin concentrations (5 EU/mL or greater of final product volume/kg recipient body weight), viability, and potency of the islet cell preparations [11].

Purity and Cell Identity

Islet purity is assessed by DTZ staining to estimate the percentage of endocrine cell clusters in the final preparation [55]. Selective binding of DTZ to the zinc–insulin complex in β-cell granules results in a red staining of the islet cells (*see* Fig. 16.5) that can be observed using light microscopy. Purity of the islet preparation and size distribution of the islet cells is quantified using an ocular micrometer. Islet volume is calculated in islet equivalents (IEQs) using an algorithm, with 1 IEQ equal to a 150-μm islet [61]. Fractions with different degree of purity (generally 30% or greater) can be pooled up to a volume of 10 mL or less to meet the minimal requirement for transplantation of greater than 5,000 IEQ/kg of recipient body weight. An assessment of the cellular composition of final preparation by immunohistopathological techniques can also be used to further characterize the quality of the transplanted tissue [11, 62–64]. The use of immunocytofluorescence methods to evaluate multiple cell subsets in dissociated human islet preparations allows for the high-yield analysis of the proportion of cell subsets present in the cellular product for transplantation (namely, β, α, δ, ductal, and acinar cells, among others; see Fig. 16.5c) [63, 64]. Additionally, when combined with early markers of cell distress or death (i.e., apoptosis, see the next section, Islet Cell Viability), cellular composition may improve the predictive value of product release tests, thereby contributing to better discrimination between optimal and suboptimal cell products [63, 64].

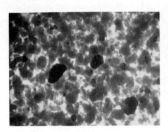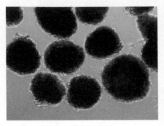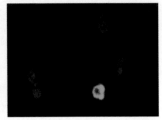

FIGURE 16-5. Assessment of islet cell purity. Islet cells can be recognized by DTZ staining that binds to the zinc present in the secretory granules of the endocrine cells, conferring a characteristic red color to the endocrine cell clusters. After purification, different degrees of islet purity can be obtained, which can be combined before transplantation. An assessment of an islet preparation shows the presence of islet cells with different sizes (*red*) and acinar tissue (*not stained*) (**A**). (**B**) A fraction with higher islet purity. (**C**) Representative immunocytofluorescent staining on dissociated islet cells analyzed by laser scanning cytometry. β (*red*) and α cells (*green*) are detected by the means of specific markers. Nuclei are shown in blue (4',6-diamidino-2-phenylindole, DAPI).

Islet Cell Viability

The viability of islet cell preparations is assessed with the use of fluorescent compounds that are capable of binding to the cell cytoplasm of viable cells [fluorescein diacetate (FDA)] and to nucleic acids by crossing the cell membranes of necrotic cells [propidium iodide (PI)]. Relative percentages of PI-positive over FDA-positive cells allow for a semiquantitative analysis of islet cell viability. Islet preparations with a viability of 70% or above are generally considered suitable for transplantation [11]. Unfortunately, these tests have shown poor predictive value and cannot discriminate between optimal and suboptimal cell products [35, 63, 64]. Several approaches are currently under evaluation to help refine the sensitivity of product-release tests for islet cells. Among these, determining the oxygen consumption rate [65–68] and the quantification of the ratio between adenosine diphosphate and triphosphate [69, 70] as possible measures of islet cell viability have been recently proposed.

Novel methods able to quantify the viability of islet cell subsets and with high discriminative potential may be of assistance in the near future to assess the quality of islet preparation. Indeed, the assessment of islet cell specific viability in dissociated human islets by flow cytometry is showing great promise [63]. The combination of membrane-exclusion fluorescent dyes (i.e., nuclear-binding dyes that can only cross the cell membranes of dead cells) with dyes indicating mitochondrial membrane potential (the reduction of which is associated with early cellular apoptosis) and zinc-binding dyes (to identify β cells) allows for the detection and quantification of β-cell specific viability [63]. The inclusion of additional markers for other cell subsets (i.e., antibodies targeting cell-surface antigens in α and ductal cells, among others) provides further value to these tests [64, 71]. In combination with the cellular composition by high-content immunocytofluorescence techniques, β cell-specific viability has shown great predictive value of in vivo human islet function after transplantation into immunodeficient mice [63] and its value is also being evaluated for clinical outcomes [72].

Islet Potency Assays

Islet cell function can be assessed in vitro by measuring the insulin release during a glucose challenge. This can be performed during a static incubation in which islet cells are exposed to sequential incubations in the presence of low and high glucose concentrations. Insulin output is measured by enzyme-linked immunoassay (ELISA) in the supernatant obtained after each of the incubation steps and the ratio of stimulated insulin (high glucose) release over basal (low glucose) is calculated and expressed as stimulation index (see Fig. 16.6a).

Alternatively, a continuous perfusion method for islet assessment may be used, in which islet cells are exposed to dynamic changes of glucose concentration (*see* Fig. 16.6b).

Measuring insulin output in the perfusate allows estimating the function of isolated islet cells [45, 73, 74]. Transplantation of human islet cells into chemically induced diabetic immunodeficient mice (*see* Fig. 16.7)

allows for the analysis of islet cell potency in vivo in a diabetic environment, measured as the ability to correct diabetes [61, 75]. Immunodeficient mice cannot reject tissues from other strains (allogeneic) or species (xenogeneic, including human) and, therefore, represent an invaluable tool for the study of islet function in the absence of the confounding elements of rejection and autoimmunity.

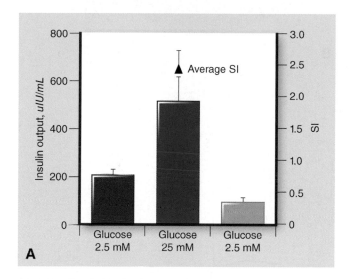

A

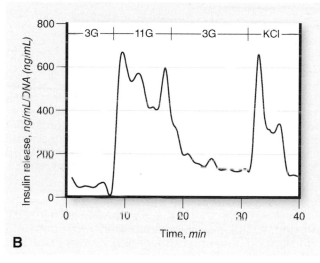

B

FIGURE 16-6. In vitro assessment of islet cell function. The quality of the isolated islet cells can be assessed in vitro by using static or dynamic glucose stimulation. (**A**) Islet aliquots are incubated sequentially in solutions containing low (2.5 mM), high (25 mM), and low (2.5 mM) glucose concentrations, and the amount of insulin released in the media is measured by enzyme-linked immunosorbent assay (*bars*). A stimulation index (SI) can be calculated by dividing the amount of insulin produced during the incubation in high glucose by that produced during the first incubation in low-glucose solution (*black triangle*). (**B**) Dynamic stimulation of islet aliquots is performed in a perfusion apparatus that allows continuously perfusing islets with a buffer containing different concentrations of glucose (3G=3 mM; 11G=11 mM) and with KCl (to obtain depolarization of cell membranes and the release of insulin not via glucose transporter). Perfusates are collected at 1-min intervals and insulin content is measured by ELISA and normalized by DNA content. A representative insulin-release profile from human islets is shown.

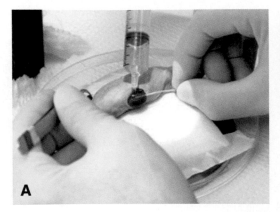

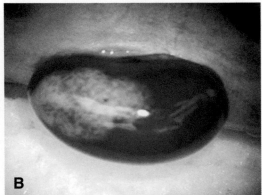

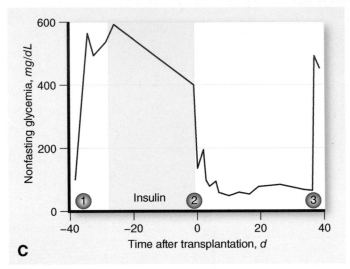

FIGURE 16-7. Assessment of islet cell potency in vivo. In vivo assessment of islet cell function can be performed by the transplantation of aliquots of human islet cells under the kidney capsule of chemically induced diabetic immunodeficient mice. The ability of the islet cells to reverse diabetes in mice is assessed by daily measurements of the blood glucose after transplantation. (**A**) The islet cells are implanted under the kidney capsule by the means of a polyethylene tube. (**B**) An islet cell graft of about 2000 IEQ is implanted under the renal capsule. (**C**) Nonfasting glycemic profile of an immunodeficient mouse transplanted with human islets. Euglycemia is present at baseline (1) before induction of diabetes by administration of the β-cell toxin streptozotocin that results in sustained hyperglycemia requiring insulin therapy (shaded area) until transplantation of human islets (2). After islet transplantation, normalization of nonfasting glycemia is achieved, which can be maintained until removal of the graft-bearing kidney (3), which results in hyperglycemia. The timescale depicts days.

Islet Cell Culture

Islet culture protocols may vary substantially between centers. Islet cells can be cultured after isolation for limited times (2–4 days) before transplantation [60]. Although a relative loss of islet cells may be noticed, the culture may be beneficial to allow recovery from the traumatic isolation process and excluding dead cells from the graft [35, 76]. An invaluable advantage of the culture is the possibility of manipulating the graft before implantation for modulating immunogenicity, inducing upregulation of cytoprotective molecules (using molecular and chemical approaches), or immunoisolation. Additionally, pretransplant culture of the islet cells makes it possible to precondition the recipient by implementing treatments (immunomodulation, immunosuppression, and reduction of inflammation) that may contribute to maximizing both engraftment and survival of the islet cells.

Islet Cell Shipment

The organization of regional islet cell-processing centers that isolate and distribute high-quality islet cell products to remote transplant centers may represent a successful strategy to improve the utilization of cadaveric pancreata while lowering the costs for islet cell preparations, and it may also contribute to maximizing the success rate of clinical islet cell transplantation [19, 25, 35, 42–44, 49]. This strategy has proven quite cost-effective in recent clinical trials, showing that comparable clinical outcomes can be obtained at remote sites receiving islets isolated at regional centers, when compared to the same center performing both islet isolation and transplantation [19, 25].

Optimizing islet shipping protocols is currently underway. Promising results have been reported using gas-permeable bags in which islets are loaded for the transfer between isolation and the transplant center [35]. The ultimate goal is to attain optimal culture conditions (constant temperature and adequate gas exchange) and prevent the packing of islets during the shipment to minimize the loss of functional islet mass (*see* Fig. 16.8).

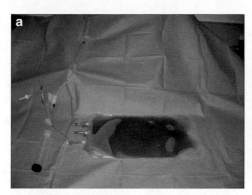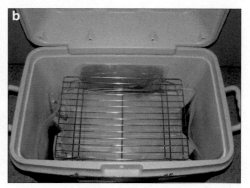

FIGURE 16-8. Shipment of human islets for transplant. (**A**) The islet cell preparation is loaded into a gas-permeable shipping bag using ports that allow a connection with an infusion set. (**B**) The bag is loaded on a rack and transferred to a shipping container containing gel packs and a temperature recorder.

Islet-Transplantation Procedure

The islet cells are infused by gravity using a closed-bag system [14, 77, 78], which allows maintenance in suspension of the final islet product and control of the infusion pressure by adjusting the height of the bag relative to the recipient portal vein (*see* Fig. 16.9a, b). Minimally invasive interventional radiology techniques allow for the catheterization of the portal vein via transhepatic percutaneous access under ultrasound and angiographic guidance (*see* Fig. 16.9d, c). The portal pressure is closely monitored during the infusion via a pressure transducer connected directly to the catheter (*see* Fig. 16.9f). The islet cells are infused under conscious sedation of the patient and the transplant can be performed as an outpatient procedure, repeatable on different occasions. In experienced centers, this approach bears minimal risk and a low incidence of complications [24, 79–81]. The minimally invasive approach is generally performed in nonuremic patients receiving islet transplantation alone (ITA) or in patients bearing a previously transplanted kidney and receiving an islet graft (IAK). For simultaneous islet and kidney (SIK) transplantation and when the percutaneous approach may be contraindicated (i.e., risk of hemorrhage, anatomical abnormalities, lack of experienced interventional radiologist, or patient preference), access to the portal system may be obtained by cannulating a tributary of the portal vein through a laparotomy [14]. Alternative and less-invasive surgical procedures have been explored in the clinical settings, including laparoscopic access through the umbilical vein [82], islet cell implantation between omental layers [83], intramuscular [84–87], and intraperitoneal transplantation (of encapsulated islets) [88].

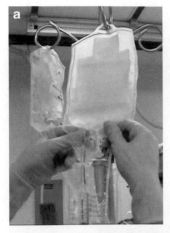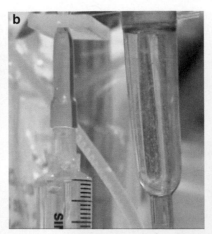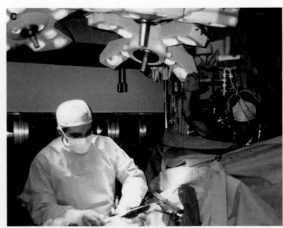

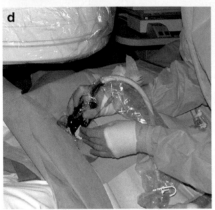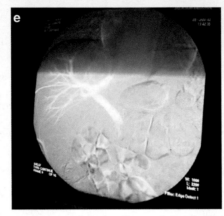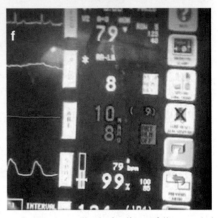

FIGURE 16-9. Intrahepatic islet-transplantation procedure. Isolated islet cells are infused in the portal system of the liver. A transfusion bag containing the islet cells in transplant media (**A**) is connected to a catheter accessing the portal system and is allowed to empty by gravity. The bag is continuously mixed to maintain the islet cells in suspension and prevent aggregation that may result in an increase of portal pressure (**B**). The infusion can be performed using laparotomy to access a tributary of the portal vein (**C**). Percutaneous catheterization of the portal vein can also be performed as an outpatient procedure under neuroleptanalgesia using ultrasound (**D**) and angiographic (**E**) guidance. The portal pressure and vital parameters are constantly monitored during the islet cell infusion (**F**).The implanted islet cells lodge into the hepatic sinusoids of the recipient, where they begin to secrete insulin.

Posttransplant Monitoring

The clinical management of islet graft recipients consists of monitoring graft function and maintaining good levels of immunosuppression to prevent graft loss. During the days after islet cell implant, hematologic and liver function tests are performed to exclude complications related to the transplant procedure. Any adverse events occurring during the trial and related to the procedure or the immunosuppressive treatment are reported to the regulatory boards or agencies.

Graft function can be evaluated using a variety of metabolic tests (see Fig. 16.10) [39, 89–91]. For patients who are euglycemic and free from exogenous insulin after islet cell transplantation, periodic monitoring of glycemic values throughout the day (before and after meals) may assist in evaluating blood glucose excursions and, therefore, assess the performance of implanted islet cells. In patients still requiring exogenous insulin after islet cell transplantation, graft function can be evaluated by comparing daily insulin requirements before and after implantation (see Fig. 16.10), as well as by assessing glycated hemoglobin (see Fig. 16.11). Metabolic tests are performed periodically at follow-up to assess the response of the grafted islet cells to selected secretagogues (defined as mixed meal, glucose, and arginine), consisting in measuring plasma insulin and C-peptide levels at baseline and after challenge (see Fig. 16.12 and 16.13).

The monitoring of graft function is of utmost importance to guide the management of islet cell graft recipients. Notably, predictive tests for the assessment of rejection and recurrence of autoimmunity are currently unavailable, and the implementation of antirejection treatment is generally based on the changes detected in the metabolic function; therefore, only after a measurable mass of transplanted islet cells has been already lost. Additionally, the small size of islet cells (ranging from 100 to 400 μm) and their random distribution throughout the recipient's liver presently limit the possibility of performing a noninvasive imaging assessment of islet grafts during rejection episodes and render biopsies impractical to do so.

Metabolic Monitoring of Islet Graft Function

Standard Tests	Stimulation tests	Indices
Glycated hemoglobin A1c (Hb$_{A1c}$, A1c)	Mixed Meal Tolerance Test	Hypo score
Fasting glycemic values	Intravenous Glucose Tolerance Test	Liability index
Postprandial glycemic values	Intravenous Arginine Stimulation Test	Beta score
Mean Amplitude of Glycemic Excursions		Basal C-peptide/glycemia ratio
Continuous Glucose Monitoring Systems		Homeostasis Model Assessment Beta cell mass
Basal C-peptide		Homeostasis Model Assessment Insulin Resistance
Daily insulin requirements		

FIGURE 16-10. Metabolic monitoring of islet graft function.

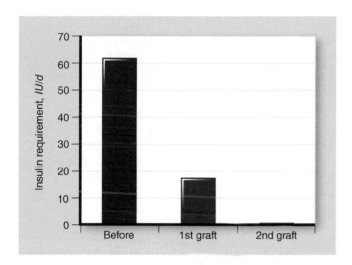

FIGURE 16-11. Reduction of insulin requirements after islet cell transplantation. A remarkable reduction in daily insulin requirements is generally observed after islet cell infusion and insulin independence can be achieved when a sufficient islet cell mass has been implanted. Frequently, transplanted patients require more than one islet preparation (generally two) to achieve insulin independence after transplantation. In general, a reduction of insulin requirements is observed after the first islet infusion and complete independence from exogenous insulin can be observed after the second infusion.

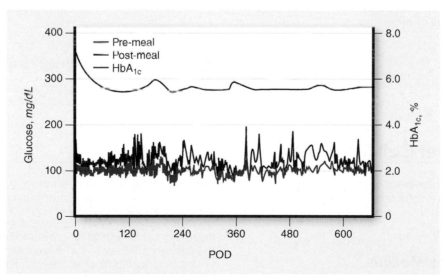

FIGURE 16-12. Stable metabolic control after islet cell transplantation. After islet cell transplantation, improved glucose metabolism can be evidenced as normalization of fasting (*dotted line*) and postprandial (*black line*) glycemic values and the absence of hypoglycemia, even when insulin treatment is still required. The improved metabolic state is also paralleled by normalization of glycated hemoglobin.

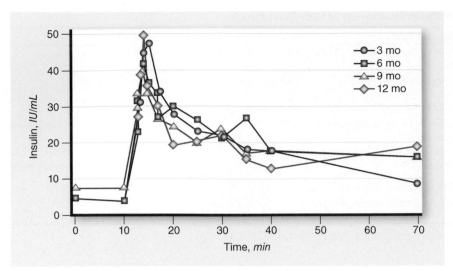

Figure 16-13. Metabolic assessment of islet graft function. Periodic monitoring of graft function with metabolic tests allows assessment of the ability of transplanted islet cells to respond to secretagogues, measured as plasma levels of insulin or C peptides before and during the challenge. The intravenous glucose tolerance test is performed after overnight fasting by injecting a bolus of 50% dextrose (300 mg/kg) and consists of the assessment of plasma insulin at baseline and for a period of 90 min. Adequate insulin secretion in response to a glucose challenge can be obtained in transplanted patients consistently at 3-month intervals between follow-up visits (i.e., 3, 6, 9, and 12 months).

Indications for Islet Cell Transplantation

Allogeneic islet transplantation

Type 1 diabetes mellitus
Insulin-dependence diabetes associated with other metabolic disorders
Cystic fibrosis
Hemochromatosis
Type 2 diabetes mellitus associated with liver cirrhosis
Pancreatectomy-induced diabetes
Abdominal exenteration
Rescue of islet cells from pancreatic grafts explanted for technical complications

Autologous islet cell transplantation

Pancreatectomy-induced diabetes
Chronic pancreatitis
Benign neoplasm
Trauma

Figure 16-14. Indications for islet cell transplantation.

Benefits of Islet Cell Transplantation

Transplantation of pancreatic islets is indicated for a number of conditions to preserve or restore β-cell function (see Fig. 16.14).

Type 1 Diabetes Mellitus

Patients who are unable to control daily glycemic excursions with intensive insulin therapy, with progressive complications and hypoglycemia unawareness, are highly susceptible to severe hypoglycemic events that are frequent and life threatening. Attaining stable metabolic control in these patients is critically important in view of the high mortality recorded in patients who are awaiting a pancreas transplant alone [92]. Medical therapy, unfortunately, cannot attain the desirable therapeutic efficacy for this patient population with unstable type 1 diabetes mellitus. The success of recent clinical trials of allogeneic islet transplantation has opened a new era for the treatment of patients with type 1 diabetes mellitus [4, 10–39, 93]. Transplantation of allogeneic islet cells is currently performed as an ITA procedure in nonuremic patients affected by a brittle form of type 1 diabetes mellitus who, despite strict compliance and intensive insulin therapy, present with severe metabolic lability (mean amplitude of glucose excursions >11.1 mmol/L), progressive secondary diabetes complications, and hypoglycemic unawareness (an absence of autonomic symptoms at glycemic levels <54 mg/dL) [93]. The risks associated with metabolic instability and potentially life-threatening hypoglycemia in patients who lack autonomic symptoms justify the risks of islet cell transplantation and chronic immunosuppression [93]. Insulin independence after ITA is close to 90% at 1-year follow-up, 80% at 2-year follow-up, and 10–60% at 5-year follow-up in most recent clinical trials using a steroid-free immunosuppressive protocol including anti-interleukin-2 antibody induction and maintenance treatment with sirolimus and low doses of tacrolimus [11, 18, 19, 25, 26, 29, 30, 32, 34, 39, 44, 94–99]. Uremic patients can also be transplanted with allogeneic islet cells as either SIK or IAK procedures [23, 37, 100–102]. In recent years, the immunosuppression protocol of patients who are already immunosuppressed for a previously transplanted kidney (recipients of IAK) is generally modified before islet transplantation to avoid the use of drugs potentially toxic for the islet cells while paying great attention to preventing loss of the renal graft [20, 37, 101].

Restoration of β-cell function by islet-transplantation results in significant metabolic changes in the recipients (see Fig. 16.15). A dramatic reduction of insulin requirements can generally be observed after islet cell infusion and sustained independence from exogenous insulin can be achieved when an optimal islet cell mass has been implanted (see Figs. 16.11–16.13). Recent clinical trials have shown that the optimal mass of allogeneic islet cells to achieve insulin independence is quite large (>12,000 islet equivalents per kilogram of body weight) and is generally obtained from more than one islet preparation. In order to reach the critical islet mass needed to restore euglycemia, the implantation of more than one islet cell preparation as sequential or single (a pool of more than one islet cell preparation) infusion can be considered. The need for large islet numbers may be a consequent of multiple factors contributing to the loss of viable insulin-producing cells [103], therefore lowering the yield and quality of islet cells obtained from a cadaveric donor pancreas. Also, nonspecific inflammation generated at the site of implantation may affect the number of islet cells engrafting and functioning after transplantation [103]. The substantial reduction of insulin requirements generally observed after islet cell infusion is paralleled by improved glycemic metabolic control, normalization of glycated hemoglobin (HbA$_{1c}$) (see Fig. 16.12), and the absence of severe hypoglycemic episodes, even when patients are still treated with exogenous insulin due to partial graft function [97, 104, 105]. Islet transplantation is also associated with a significant improvement in the quality of life that parallels the prevention of severe hypoglycemia and restoration of hypoglycemia awareness [37, 106–108]. Notably, improved metabolic control with normalization of HbA$_{1c}$ and an absence of severe hypoglycemia, despite insulin treatment, has been described in recipients of a single islet preparation and with marginal graft function (measurable C-peptide after a mixed-meal test) for more than 13 years [11, 15]. This observation points to the extreme value of islet cell

transplantation in the management of patients with type 1 diabetes. The physiological β-cell response to secretagogues can be partially restored with improved first-phase insulin secretion upon intravenous stimulation and increased overall C-peptide levels following an oral challenge in islet transplant recipients [109, 110]. The abnormal glucagon and epinephrine response to hypoglycemia is partially restored in patients with type 1 diabetes after islet transplantation. Also, normalization of the glycemic thresholds for activation of counterregulatory hormone and symptom responses to hypoglycemia can be observed after transplantation, although the magnitude of such responses remained impaired [111, 112]. It is conceivable that these phenomena may contribute to the improvement of metabolic control and regaining of hypoglycemia awareness after islet transplantation (see Fig. 16.16) [105].

Progressive graft dysfunction has been observed in a proportion of islet transplant recipients treated with steroid-sparing immunosuppression in recent clinical trials [29, 36, 94, 99, 113]. The use of supplemental islet transplants after the development of graft dysfunction has allowed for extending the benefit of the transplant in these patients, but was associated with a similar progressive loss of function over time [29, 114]. The risk of allosensitization of transplant recipients raises some concerns of using islets obtained from multiple donors [115, 116]. The introduction of cytoprotective agents in the management of islet transplant recipients has allowed for improvements in graft performance. The off-label use of the glucagon-like peptide-1 (GLP-1) analog exenatide in islet transplant recipients resulted in insulin independence with a reduced number of islets [117, 118], recovery/improvement of graft function after the onset of dysfunction [119], and improved longevity of insulin independence after the delayed supplemental islet infusion [113]. The effect of exenatide on insulin secretion after islet transplantation has been evaluated [113, 117, 118]. In the presence of exenatide therapy at the time of mixed-meal tolerance (MMT) tests, the increase of blood glucose is reduced and is paralleled by the reduction in glucagon levels, when compared to MTT responses before the initiation of exenatide therapy or when the test is performed after interruption of exenatide therapy (see Fig. 16.17).

Insulin-Requiring Diabetes

Transplantation of allogeneic islet cells may also be considered for the treatment of patients whose diabetes is associated with metabolic disorders, including cystic fibrosis [120] and hemochromatosis [121], who may benefit from an islet cell graft combined with lung or liver transplantation. Allogeneic islet cell transplantation for the treatment of type 2 diabetes secondary to liver cirrhosis has also been reported [122]. Patients with type 2 diabetes may require insulin treatment and develop diabetes-related complications, including diabetic nephropathy. Although transplantation of insulin-producing cells in these patients may be beneficial, characteristic advanced age and obesity represent contraindications due to the increased metabolic demand and the potentially higher morbidity [123].

Transplantation of allogeneic islet cells may also be performed in recipients of multivisceral organs [14]. The use of allogeneic islet transplantation to "rescue" insulin-producing tissue from pancreatic grafts explanted for technical complications has been described [124].

Islet Cell Autotransplantation

Transplantation of autologous islet cells has been performed recently to prevent iatrogenic diabetes and its complications in patients undergoing pancreatectomy for benign conditions [125], including chronic pancreatitis. Chronic pancreatitis leads to diabetes within 5–10 years from onset in 50% of patients, even in the absence of surgery [126], and poor management of diabetes is a main reason for hospital readmission after surgery. Intrahepatic autotransplantation of more than 250,000 islet cells results in normoglycemia and insulin independence in about 70% of patients [125]. The introduction of the automated method for islet cell isolation [53] has resulted in a higher yield and success rate after islet cell autotransplantation [10, 125]. Islet cell autotransplantation after pancreatectomy for trauma or benign neoplasms has been proven a viable option for preserving β-cell function, even for elderly patients [127]. Intramuscular islet autotransplantation has recently been attempted with encouraging results [84, 87].

Benefits of Islet Transplantation

	Readout	Effect of islet transplantation
Metabolic control	Exogenous insulin	Reduction/independence
	Mean Amplitude of Glycemic Excursions	Reduction
	Glycated hemoglobin (1Ac)	Reduction/normalization
	Severe hypoglycemic episodes	Prevention
	Hypoglycemia awareness	Improvement
Quality of life	Fear score (hypoglycemia)	Reduction
	Diabetes quality of life	Improvement
Diabetes complications	Micro- and macro-angiopathy	Improvement
	Cardiovascular and endothelial function	Amelioration
	Acute cardiovascular accidents	Reduction
	Progression of nephropathy	Reduction
	Progression of neuropathy	Stabilization/slower
	Progression of retinopathy	Stabilization/slower

Figure 16-15. Benefits of islet transplantation.

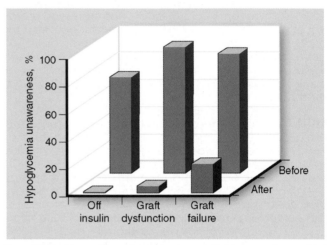

Figure 16-16. Hypoglycemia unawareness is improved upon islet transplantation in patients with unstable type 1 diabetes. When compared to pretransplant data (*before*), the frequency of hypoglycemia unawareness following islet transplantation (*after*) is reduced to zero in all subjects who have a functioning islet graft and insulin independence (off insulin, *n*=8). The proportion of patients with hypoglycemia unawareness increases with graft dysfunction and graft failure, but still is significantly lower than before the transplant, suggesting that the overall benefit of the restoration of islet function with the transplant persists in these patients.

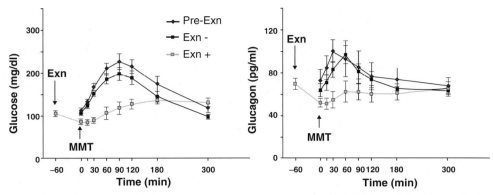

Figure 16-17. Effects of the treatment with the glucagon-like peptide-1 analog exenatide on the function of transplanted human islets during a MMT test. (**A**) A significant reduction of blood glucose occurs after a mixed meal (kinetics at baseline; before exenatide administration) when exenatide is given before ingestion of a meal (exenatide +). (**B**) The reduction of glycemia post-MMT is paralleled by a significant reduction of the abnormal glucagon responses during the MMT test when compared to the response before the initiation of exenatide therapy and when the test was performed without exenatide prior to the test (exenatide –).

Current Challenges and Future Directions

The success rate of islet cell transplantation for the replacement of endocrine function has been steadily improving recently. Numerous challenges need to be addressed to overcome the current limitations and make islet cell transplantation the treatment of choice for a wider number of patients with type 1 diabetes mellitus [4, 103]. Implementation of fair organ allocation rules between whole pancreas and islet cell transplantation programs may contribute to improving both the yield and quality of islet cells obtained from a single cadaveric donor gland and possibly to achieve insulin independence in a higher proportion of recipients by transplanting a single islet cell preparation. Implementation of improved techniques for organ procurement and preservation and for the isolation and purification of human islet cells may allow for the utilization of pancreata from donors who are currently considered to be marginal or following cardiac death, which are currently underused. Insulin-producing cells from xenogeneic donors or those derived from stem cells may represent alternative sources for β-cell replacement because they could provide an unlimited supply of tissue for transplantation [128]. Therapeutic intervention aiming at preserving the mass of transplanted islet cells while promoting engraftment and survival may also be of assistance in reducing the islet cell mass needed for successful islet transplantation. Novel bioengineering approaches show great promise toward overcoming the current limitations of islet transplantation. These include the use of polymers to shield islet cell clusters from immune attack as well as the development of an alternative ectopic bioartificial endocrine pancreas to enhance islet cell engraftment and long-term function. The availability of new immunomodulatory and immunosuppressive drugs with reduced toxicity profiles and higher selectivity for specific immune pathways as well as the promising results of induction of immune tolerance to transplanted tissues in experimental models justify a cautious optimism for their potential clinical applicability in the years to come [129].

Acknowledgments This work was partially supported by the National Institutes of Health (under grants NIDDK 5R01DK25802, 5R01DK56953, 1U01DK70460, 1R21DK076098, 5R01DK059993, 1DP2DK083096, NCRR-ICR5 U42 RR016603, NCRR-GCRC MO1RR16587, NBI 1R01 EB008009, and the Cooperative Study Group for Autoimmune Disease Prevention Formation and History), the Juvenile Diabetes Research Foundation International (under grants 4-2000-946, 4-2000-947, 4-2004-361, and 4-2008-811), the state of Florida, the University of Miami (Interdisciplinary Research Development Initiative), and the Diabetes Research Institute Foundation (http://www.DiabetesResearch.org). A contract for support of this research, sponsored by United States Congressman Bill Young and funded by a special congressional out of the US Navy Bureau of Medicine and Surgery, is presently managed by the Naval Health Research Center, San Diego, CA. The authors alone are responsible for reporting and interpreting these data; the views expressed herein are those of the authors and not necessarily those of the US government.
Additional resources are available from the Clinical Islet Transplant consortium (http://www.citisletstudy.org), Collaborative Islet Transplant Registry (http://www.citregistry.org), United States Department of Health and Human Services (http://www.hhs.gov), Organ Procurement and Transplantation Network (http://www.optn.org), Scientific Registry of Transplant Recipients (http://www.ustransplant.org), Health Resources and Services Administration (http://www.hrsa.gov), and Diabetes Research Institute Foundation (http://www.DiabetesResearch.org).

References

1. LeRoith D, Taylor SI, Olefsky JM: *Diabetes Mellitus: A Fundamental and Clinical Text.* Philadelphia, PA, Lippincott Williams & Wilkins, 2003

2. The effect of intensive treatment of diabetes on the development and progression of long-term complications in insulin-dependent diabetes mellitus. The Diabetes Control and Complications Trial Research Group. *N Engl J Med* 329:977–986, 1993

3. Herman WH, Eastman RC: The effects of treatment on the direct costs of diabetes. *Diabetes Care* 21 Suppl 3:C19-24, 1998

4. Mineo D, Pileggi A, Alejandro R, Ricordi C: Point: steady progress and current challenges in clinical islet transplantation. *Diabetes Care* 32:1563–1569, 2009

5. Del Carro U, Fiorina P, Amadio S, De Toni Franceschini L, Petrelli A, Menini S, Boneschi FM, Ferrari S, Pugliese G, Maffi P, Comi G, Secchi A: Evaluation of polyneuropathy markers in type 1 diabetic kidney transplant patients and effects of islet transplantation: neurophysiological and skin biopsy longitudinal analysis. *Diabetes Care* 30:3063–3069, 2007

6. Fiorina P, Folli F, Bertuzzi F, Maffi P, Finzi G, Venturini M, Socci C, Davalli A, Orsenigo E, Monti L, Falqui L, Uccella S, La Rosa S, Usellini L, Properzi G, Di Carlo V, Del Maschio A, Capella C, Secchi A: Long-term beneficial effect of islet transplantation on diabetic macro-/microangiopathy in type 1 diabetic kidney-transplanted patients. *Diabetes Care* 26:1129–1136, 2003

7. Fiorina P, Folli F, Maffi P, Placidi C, Venturini M, Finzi G, Bertuzzi F, Davalli A, D'Angelo A, Socci C, Gremizzi C, Orsenigo E, La Rosa S, Ponzoni M, Cardillo M, Scalamogna M, Del Maschio A, Capella C, Di Carlo V, Secchi A: Islet transplantation improves vascular diabetic complications in patients with diabetes who underwent kidney transplantation: a comparison between kidney-pancreas and kidney-alone transplantation. *Transplantation* 75:1296–1301, 2003

8. Fiorina P, Folli F, Zerbini G, Maffi P, Gremizzi C, Di Carlo V, Socci C, Bertuzzi F, Kashgarian M, Secchi A: Islet transplantation is associated with improvement of renal function among uremic patients with type I diabetes mellitus and kidney transplants. *J Am Soc Nephrol* 14:2150–2158, 2003

9. Fiorina P, Gremizzi C, Maffi P, Caldara R, Tavano D, Monti L, Socci C, Folli F, Fazio F, Astorri E, Del Maschio A, Secchi A: Islet transplantation is associated with an improvement of cardiovascular function in type 1 diabetic kidney transplant patients. *Diabetes Care* 28:1358–1365, 2005

10. Ricordi C: Islet transplantation: a brave new world. *Diabetes* 52:1595–1603, 2003

11. Pileggi A, Ricordi C, Kenyon NS, Froud T, Baidal DA, Kahn A, Selvaggi G, Alejandro R: Twenty years of clinical islet transplantation at the Diabetes Research Institute--University of Miami. *Clin Transpl*:177–204, 2004

12. Marzorati S, Pileggi A, Ricordi C: Allogeneic islet transplantation. *Expert Opin Biol Ther* 7:1627–1645, 2007

13. Alejandro R, Barton FB, Hering BJ, Wease S: 2008 Update from the Collaborative Islet Transplant Registry. *Transplantation* 86:1783–1788, 2008

14. Tzakis AG, Ricordi C, Alejandro R, Zeng Y, Fung JJ, Todo S, Demetris AJ, Mintz DH, Starzl TE: Pancreatic islet transplantation after upper abdominal exenteration and liver replacement. *Lancet* 336:402–405, 1990

15. Alejandro R, Lehmann R, Ricordi C, Kenyon NS, Angelico MC, Burke G, Esquenazi V, Nery J, Betancourt AE, Kong SS, Miller J, Mintz DH: Long-term function (6 years) of islet allografts in type 1 diabetes. *Diabetes* 46:1983–1989, 1997

16. Linetsky E, Bottino R, Lehmann R, Alejandro R, Inverardi L, Ricordi C: Improved human islet isolation using a new enzyme blend, liberase. *Diabetes* 46:1120–1123, 1997

17. Keymeulen B, Ling Z, Gorus FK, Delvaux G, Bouwens L, Grupping A, Hendrieckx C, Pipeleers-Marichal M, Van Schravendijk C, Salmela K, Pipeleers DG: Implantation of standardized beta-cell grafts in a liver segment of IDDM patients: graft and recipients characteristics in two cases of insulin-independence under maintenance immunosuppression for prior kidney graft. *Diabetologia* 41:452–459, 1998

18. Shapiro AM, Lakey JR, Ryan EA, Korbutt GS, Toth E, Warnock GL, Kneteman NM, Rajotte RV: Islet transplantation in seven patients with type 1 diabetes mellitus using a glucocorticoid-free immunosuppressive regimen. *N Engl J Med* 343:230–238, 2000

19. Goss JA, Schock AP, Brunicardi FC, Goodpastor SE, Garber AJ, Soltes G, Barth M, Froud T, Alejandro R, Ricordi C: Achievement of insulin independence in three consecutive type-1 diabetic patients via pancreatic islet transplantation using islets isolated at a remote islet isolation center. *Transplantation* 74:1761–1766, 2002

20. Toso C, Morel P, Bucher P, Mathe Z, Demuylder-Mischler S, Bosco D, Berney T, Oberholzer J, Shapiro J, Oberholzer J, Philippe J: Insulin independence after conversion to tacrolimus and sirolimus-based immunosuppression in islet-kidney recipients. *Transplantation* 76:1133–1134, 2003

21. Markmann JF, Deng S, Huang X, Desai NM, Velidedeoglu EH, Lui C, Frank A, Markmann E, Palanjian M, Brayman K, Wolf B, Bell E, Vitamaniuk M, Doliba N, Matschinsky F, Barker CF, Naji A: Insulin independence following isolated islet transplantation and single islet infusions. *Ann Surg* 237:741–749; discussion 749–750, 2003

22. Hirshberg B, Rother KI, Digon BJ, 3 rd, Lee J, Gaglia JL, Hines K, Read EJ, Chang R, Wood BJ, Harlan DM: Benefits and risks of solitary islet transplantation for type 1 diabetes using steroid-sparing immunosuppression: the National Institutes of Health experience. *Diabetes Care* 26:3288–3295, 2003

23. Lehmann R, Weber M, Berthold P, Zullig R, Pfammatter T, Moritz W, Madler K, Donath M, Ambuhl P, Demartines N, Clavien And PA, Andreia Spinas G: Successful simultaneous islet-kidney transplantation using a steroid-free immunosuppression: two-year follow-up. *Am J Transplant* 4:1117–1123, 2004

24. Froud T, Yrizarry JM, Alejandro R, Ricordi C: Use of D-STAT to prevent bleeding following percutaneous transhepatic intraportal islet transplantation. *Cell Transplant* 13:55–59, 2004

25. Goss JA, Goodpastor SE, Brunicardi FC, Barth MH, Soltes GD, Garber AJ, Hamilton DJ, Alejandro R, Ricordi C: Development of a human pancreatic islet-transplant program through a collaborative relationship with a remote islet-isolation center. *Transplantation* 77:462–466, 2004

26. Hering BJ, Kandaswamy R, Harmon JV, Ansite JD, Clemmings SM, Sakai T, Paraskevas S, Eckman PM, Sageshima J, Nakano M, Sawada T, Matsumoto I, Zhang HJ, Sutherland DE, Bluestone JA: Transplantation of cultured islets from two-layer preserved pancreases in type 1 diabetes with anti-CD3 antibody. *Am J Transplant* 4:390–401, 2004

27. Goto M, Eich TM, Felldin M, Foss A, Kallen R, Salmela K, Tibell A, Tufveson G, Fujimori K, Engkvist M, Korsgren O: Refinement of the automated method for human islet isolation and presentation of a closed system for in vitro islet culture. *Transplantation* 78:1367–1375, 2004

28. Lee TC, Barshes NR, Brunicardi FC, Alejandro R, Ricordi C, Nguyen L, Goss JA: Procurement of the human pancreas for pancreatic islet transplantation. *Transplantation* 78:481–483, 2004

29. Froud T, Ricordi C, Baidal DA, Hafiz MM, Ponte G, Cure P, Pileggi A, Poggioli R, Ichii H, Khan A, Ferreira JV, Pugliese A, Esquenazi VV, Kenyon NS, Alejandro R: Islet transplantation in type 1 diabetes mellitus using cultured islets and steroid-free immunosuppression: Miami experience. *Am J Transplant* 5:2037–2046, 2005

30. Hering BJ, Kandaswamy R, Ansite JD, Eckman PM, Nakano M, Sawada T, Matsumoto I, Ihm SH, Zhang HJ, Parkey J, Hunter DW,

Sutherland DE: Single-donor, marginal-dose islet transplantation in patients with type 1 diabetes. *Jama* 293:830–835, 2005

31. Ichii H, Pileggi A, Molano RD, Baidal DA, Khan A, Kuroda Y, Inverardi L, Goss JA, Alejandro R, Ricordi C: Rescue purification maximizes the use of human islet preparations for transplantation. *Am J Transplant* 5:21–30, 2005

32. Shapiro AM, Ricordi C, Hering BJ, Auchincloss H, Lindblad R, Robertson RP, Secchi A, Brendel MD, Berney T, Brennan DC, Cagliero E, Alejandro R, Ryan EA, DiMercurio B, Morel P, Polonsky KS, Reems JA, Bretzel RG, Bertuzzi F, Froud T, Kandaswamy R, Sutherland DE, Eisenbarth G, Segal M, Preiksaitis J, Korbutt GS, Barton FB, Viviano L, Seyfert-Margolis V, Bluestone J, Lakey JR: International trial of the Edmonton protocol for islet transplantation. *N Engl J Med* 355:1318–1330, 2006

33. Ichii H, Wang X, Messinger S, Alvarez A, Fraker C, Khan A, Kuroda Y, Inverardi L, Goss JA, Alejandro R, Ricordi C: Improved human islet isolation using nicotinamide. *Am J Transplant* 6:2060–2068, 2006

34. Toso C, Shapiro AM, Bowker S, Dinyari P, Paty B, Ryan EA, Senior P, Johnson JA: Quality of life after islet transplant: impact of the number of islet infusions and metabolic outcome. *Transplantation* 84:664–666, 2007

35. Ichii H, Sakuma Y, Pileggi A, Fraker C, Alvarez A, Montelongo J, Szust J, Khan A, Inverardi L, Naziruddin B, Levy MF, Klintmalm GB, Goss JA, Alejandro R, Ricordi C: Shipment of human islets for transplantation. *Am J Transplant* 7:1010–1020, 2007

36. Froud T, Faradji RN, Pileggi A, Messinger S, Baidal DA, Ponte GM, Cure PE, Monroy K, Mendez A, Selvaggi G, Ricordi C, Alejandro R: The use of exenatide in islet transplant recipients with chronic allograft dysfunction: safety, efficacy, and metabolic effects. *Transplantation* 86:36–45, 2008

37. Cure P, Pileggi A, Froud T, Messinger S, Faradji RN, Baidal DA, Cardani R, Curry A, Poggioli R, Pugliese A, Betancourt A, Esquenazi V, Ciancio G, Selvaggi G, Burke GW, 3rd., Ricordi C, Alejandro R: Improved metabolic control and quality of life in seven patients with type 1 diabetes following islet after kidney transplantation. *Transplantation* 85:801–812, 2008

38. Gangemi A, Salehi P, Hatipoglu B, Martellotto J, Barbaro B, Kuechle JB, Qi M, Wang Y, Pallan P, Owens C, Bui J, West D, Kaplan B, Benedetti E, Oberholzer J: Islet transplantation for brittle type 1 diabetes: the UIC protocol. *Am J Transplant* 8:1250–1261, 2008

39. Vantyghem MC, Kerr-Conte J, Arnalsteen L, Sergent G, Defrance F, Gmyr V, Declerck N, Raverdy V, Vandewalle B, Pigny P, Noel C, Pattou F: Primary graft function, metabolic control and graft survival after islet transplantation. *Diabetes Care*, 2009

40. Weber DJ: FDA regulation of allogeneic islets as a biological product. *Cell Biochem Biophys* 40:19–22, 2004

41. Linetsky E, Ricordi C: Regulatory challenges in manufacturing of pancreatic islets. *Transplant Proc* 40:424–426, 2008

42. Rabkin JM, Olyaei AJ, Orloff SL, Geisler SM, Wahoff DC, Hering BJ, Sutherland DE: Distant processing of pancreas islets for autotransplantation following total pancreatectomy. *Am J Surg* 177:423–427, 1999

43. Benhamou PY, Oberholzer J, Toso C, Kessler L, Penfornis A, Bayle F, Thivolet C, Martin X, Ris F, Badet L, Colin C, Morel P: Human islet transplantation network for the treatment of Type I diabetes: first data from the Swiss-French GRAGIL consortium (1999–2000). Groupe de Recherche Rhin Rhjne Alpes Geneve pour la transplantation d'Ilots de Langerhans. *Diabetologia* 44:859–864, 2001

44. Kempf MC, Andres A, Morel P, Benhamou PY, Bayle F, Kessler L, Badet L, Thivolet C, Penfornis A, Renoult E, Brun JM, Atlan C, Renard E, Colin C, Milliat-Guittard L, Pernin N, Demuylder-Mischler S, Toso C, Bosco D, Berney T: Logistics and transplant coordination activity in the GRAGIL Swiss-French multicenter network of islet transplantation. *Transplantation* 79:1200–1205, 2005

45. Cabrera O, Berman DM, Kenyon NS, Ricordi C, Berggren PO, Caicedo A: The unique cytoarchitecture of human pancreatic islets has implications for islet cell function. *Proc Natl Acad Sci U S A* 103:2334–2339, 2006

46. Contreras JL, Eckstein C, Smyth CA, Sellers MT, Vilatoba M, Bilbao G, Rahemtulla FG, Young CJ, Thompson JA, Chaudry IH, Eckhoff DE: Brain death significantly reduces isolated pancreatic islet yields and functionality in vitro and in vivo after transplantation in rats. *Diabetes* 52:2935–2942, 2003

47. Lakey JR, Warnock GL, Rajotte RV, Suarez-Alamazor ME, Ao Z, Shapiro AM, Kneteman NM: Variables in organ donors that affect the recovery of human islets of Langerhans. *Transplantation* 61:1047–1053, 1996

48. Nano R, Clissi B, Melzi R, Calori G, Maffi P, Antonioli B, Marzorati S, Aldrighetti L, Freschi M, Grochowiecki T, Socci C, Secchi A, Di Carlo V, Bonifacio E, Bertuzzi F: Islet isolation for allotransplantation: variables associated with successful islet yield and graft function. *Diabetologia* 48:906–912, 2005

49. Ponte G, Pileggi A, Messinger S, Alejandro A, Ichii H, Baidal DA, Khan A, Ricordi C, Goss JA, Alejandro R: Toward maximizing the success rate of human islet isolation: Influence of donor and isolation factors. . *Cell Transplant* in press, 2007

50. Pileggi A, Ribeiro MM, Hogan AR, Molano RD, Cobianchi L, Ichii H, Embury J, Inverardi L, Fornoni A, Ricordi C, Pastori RL: Impact of pancreatic cold preservation on rat islet recovery and function. *Transplantation* 87:1442–1450, 2009

51. Kuroda Y, Kawamura T, Suzuki Y, Fujiwara H, Yamamoto K, Saitoh Y: A new, simple method for cold storage of the pancreas using perfluorochemical. *Transplantation* 46:457–460, 1988

52. Fraker CA, Alejandro R, Ricordi C: Use of oxygenated perfluorocarbon toward making every pancreas count. *Transplantation* 74:1811–1812, 2002

53. Ricordi C, Lacy PE, Finke EH, Olack BJ, Scharp DW: Automated method for isolation of human pancreatic islets. *Diabetes* 37:413–420, 1988

54. Fraker C, Montelongo J, Szust J, Khan A, Ricordi C: The use of multiparametric monitoring during islet cell isolation and culture: a potential tool for in-process corrections of critical physiological factors. *Cell Transplant* 13:497–502, 2004

55. Latif ZA, Noel J, Alejandro R: A simple method of staining fresh and cultured islets. *Transplantation* 45:827–830, 1988

56. Ricordi C: *Methods in Cell Transplantation*. Austin, TX, RG Landes, 1995

57. Lake SP, Bassett PD, Larkins A, Revell J, Walczak K, Chamberlain J, Rumford GM, London NJ, Veitch PS, Bell PR, et al.: Large-scale purification of human islets utilizing discontinuous albumin gradient on IBM 2991 cell separator. *Diabetes* 38 Suppl 1:143–145, 1989

58. Alejandro R, Strasser S, Zucker PF, Mintz DH: Isolation of pancreatic islets from dogs. Semiautomated purification on albumin gradients. *Transplantation* 50:207–210, 1990

59. Barbaro B, Salehi P, Wang Y, Qi M, Gangemi A, Kuechle J, Hansen MA, Romagnoli T, Avila J, Benedetti E, Mage R, Oberholzer J: Improved human pancreatic islet purification with the refined UIC-UB density gradient. *Transplantation* 84:1200–1203, 2007

60. Ichii H, Pileggi A, Khan A, C. F, Ricordi C: Culture and Transportation of Islets Between Centers. In *Islet transplantation and beta cell replacement therapy* Shapiro AMJ, Shaw J, Eds. New York, NY, Informa Healthcare, 2007, p. 251–268

61. Ricordi C, Gray DW, Hering BJ, Kaufman DB, Warnock GL, Kneteman NM, Lake SP, London NJ, Socci C, Alejandro R, et al.: Islet isolation assessment in man and large animals. *Acta Diabetol Lat* 27:185–195, 1990

62. Street CN, Lakey JR, Shapiro AM, Imes S, Rajotte RV, Ryan EA, Lyon JG, Kin T, Avila J, Tsujimura T, Korbutt GS: Islet graft assessment in the Edmonton Protocol: implications for predicting long-term clinical outcome. *Diabetes* 53:3107–3114, 2004

63. Ichii H, Inverardi L, Pileggi A, Molano RD, Cabrera O, Caicedo A, Messinger S, Kuroda Y, Berggren PO, Ricordi C: A novel method for the assessment of cellular composition and beta-cell viability in human islet preparations. *Am J Transplant* 5:1635–1645, 2005

64. Ichii H, Miki A, Yamamoto T, Molano RD, Barker S, Mita A, Rodriguez-Diaz R, Klein D, Pastori R, Alejandro R, Inverardi L, Pileggi A, Ricordi C: Characterization of pancreatic ductal cells in human islet preparations. *Lab Invest* 88:1167–1177, 2008

65. Sweet IR, Gilbert M, Scott S, Todorov I, Jensen R, Nair I, Al-Abdullah I, Rawson J, Kandeel F, Ferreri K: Glucose-stimulated increment in oxygen consumption rate as a standardized test of human islet quality. *Am J Transplant* 8:183–192, 2008

66. Sweet IR, Khalil G, Wallen AR, Steedman M, Schenkman KA, Reems JA, Kahn SE, Callis JB: Continuous measurement of oxygen consumption by pancreatic islets. *Diabetes Technol Ther* 4:661–672, 2002

67. Fraker C, Timmins MR, Guarino RD, Haaland PD, Ichii H, Molano D, Pileggi A, Poggioli R, Presnell SC, Inverardi L, Zehtab M, Ricordi C: The use of the BD oxygen biosensor system to assess isolated human islets of langerhans: oxygen consumption as a potential measure of islet potency. *Cell Transplant* 15:745–758, 2006

68. Papas KK, Colton CK, Nelson RA, Rozak PR, Avgoustiniatos ES, Scott WE, 3 rd, Wildey GM, Pisania A, Weir GC, Hering BJ: Human islet oxygen consumption rate and DNA measurements predict diabetes reversal in nude mice. *Am J Transplant* 7:707–713, 2007

69. Sweet IR, Cook DL, DeJulio E, Wallen AR, Khalil G, Callis J, Reems J: Regulation of ATP/ADP in pancreatic islets. *Diabetes* 53:401–409, 2004

70. Goto M, Holgersson J, Kumagai-Braesch M, Korsgren O: The ADP/ATP ratio: A novel predictive assay for quality assessment of isolated pancreatic islets. *Am J Transplant* 6:2483–2487, 2006

71. Gower WR, Moore KD, Burgess M, Alli A, Carter GM, Ichii H, Ricordi C: C-type natriuretic peptide receptor (NPR-C) in human pancreatic alpha cells: Identification, localization and ANP mediated changes in glucagon secretion. *Gastroenterology* 130:A224-A224, 2006

72. Ichii H, Miki A, Mita A, Barker S, Yamamoto T, Sakuma Y, Inverardi L, Alejandro R, Ricordi C: Viable ductal cell mass in human islet preparations correlates with long-term clinical outcomes in islet transplantation. *American Journal of Transplantation* 8:433–433, 2008

73. Sweet IR, Cook DL, Wiseman RW, Greenbaum CJ, Lernmark A, Matsumoto S, Teague JC, Krohn KA: Dynamic perifusion to maintain and assess isolated pancreatic islets. *Diabetes Technol Ther* 4:67–76, 2002

74. Cabrera O, Jacques-Silva M, Berman D, Fachado A, Echeverri F, Poo R, Khan A, Kenyon NS, Ricordi C, Berggren PO, Caicedo A: Automated, High-Throughput Assays for Evaluation of Human Pancreatic Islet Function. *Cell Transplant* 16:1039–1048, 2008

75. Ricordi C, Scharp DW, Lacy PE: Reversal of diabetes in nude mice after transplantation of fresh and 7-day-cultured (24 degrees C) human pancreatic islets. *Transplantation* 45:994–996, 1988

76. Kin T, Senior P, O'Gorman D, Richer B, Salam A, Shapiro AMJ: Risk factors for islet loss during culture prior to transplantation. *Transplant International* 21:1029–1035, 2008

77. Alejandro R, Mintz DH: Experimental and Clinical Methods of Islet Transplantation. In *Transplantation of the Endocrine Pancreas.*, Elsevier Science B.V., 1988, p. 217–223

78. Baidal DA, Froud T, Ferreira JV, Khan A, Alejandro R, Ricordi C: The bag method for islet cell infusion. *Cell Transplant* 12:809–813, 2003

79. Casey JJ, Lakey JR, Ryan EA, Paty BW, Owen R, O'Kelly K, Nanji S, Rajotte RV, Korbutt GS, Bigam D, Kneteman NN, Shapiro AM: Portal venous pressure changes after sequential clinical islet transplantation. *Transplantation* 74:913–915, 2002

80. Goss JA, Soltes G, Goodpastor SE, Barth M, Lam R, Brunicardi FC, Froud T, Alejandro R, Ricordi C: Pancreatic islet transplantation: the radiographic approach. *Transplantation* 76:199–203, 2003

81. Venturini M, Angeli E, Maffi P, Fiorina P, Bertuzzi F, Salvioni M, De Cobelli F, Socci C, Aldrighetti L, Losio C, Di Carlo V, Secchi A, Del Maschio A: Technique, complications, and therapeutic efficacy of percutaneous transplantation of human pancreatic islet cells in type 1 diabetes: the role of US. *Radiology* 234:617–624, 2005

82. Movahedi B, Keymeulen B, Lauwers MH, Goes E, Cools N, Delvaux G: Laparoscopic approach for human islet transplantation into a defined liver segment in type-1 diabetic patients. *Transpl Int* 16:186–190, 2003

83. Casavilla A, Rilo HL, Julian TB, Fontes PA, Starzl TE, Ricordi C: Laparoscopic approach for islet cell transplantation. *Transplant Proc* 24:2800, 1992

84. Weber CJ, Hardy MA, Pi-Sunyer F, Zimmerman E, Reemtsma K: Tissue culture preservation and intramuscular transplantation of pancreatic islets. *Surgery* 84:166–174, 1978

85. Stegall MD, Lafferty KJ, Kam I, Gill RG: Evidence of recurrent autoimmunity in human allogeneic islet transplantation. *Transplantation* 61:1272–1274, 1996

86. Stegall MD: Monitoring human islet allografts using a forearm biopsy site. *Ann Transplant* 2:8–11, 1997

87. Rafael E, Tibell A, Ryden M, Lundgren T, Savendahl L, Borgstrom B, Arnelo U, Isaksson B, Nilsson B, Korsgren O, Permert J: Intramuscular autotransplantation of pancreatic islets in a 7-year-old child: a 2-year follow-up. *Am J Transplant* 8:458–462, 2008

88. Calafiore R, Basta G, Luca G, Lemmi A, Montanucci MP, Calabrese G, Racanicchi L, Mancuso F, Brunetti P: Microencapsulated pancreatic islet allografts into nonimmunosuppressed patients with type 1 diabetes: first two cases. *Diabetes Care* 29:137–138, 2006

89. Baidal D, Faradji RN, Messinger S, Froud T, Monroy K, Ricordi C, Alejandro A: Early metabolic markers of islet allograft dysfunction. *Transplantation* in press, 2009

90. Faradji RN, Monroy K, Messinger S, Pileggi A, Froud T, Baidal DA, Cure PE, Ricordi C, Luzi L, Alejandro R: Simple measures to monitor beta-cell mass and assess islet graft dysfunction. *Am J Transplant* 7:303–308, 2007

91. Geiger MC, Ferreira JV, Hafiz MM, Froud T, Baidal DA, Meneghini LF, Ricordi C, Alejandro R: Evaluation of metabolic control using a continuous subcutaneous glucose monitoring system in patients with type 1 diabetes mellitus who achieved insulin independence after islet cell transplantation. *Cell Transplant* 14:77–84, 2005

92. Gruessner RW, Sutherland DE, Gruessner AC: Mortality assessment for pancreas transplants. *Am J Transplant* 4:2018–2026, 2004

93. Robertson P, Davis C, Larsen J, Stratta R, Sutherland DE: Pancreas transplantation in type 1 diabetes. *Diabetes Care* 27 Suppl 1:S105, 2004

94. Frank A, Deng S, Huang X, Velidedeoglu E, Bae YS, Liu C, Abt P, Stephenson R, Mohiuddin M, Thambipillai T, Markmann E, Palanjian M, Sellers M, Naji A, Barker CF, Markmann JF: Transplantation for type I diabetes: comparison of vascularized whole-organ pancreas with isolated pancreatic islets. *Ann Surg* 240:631–643, 2004

95. Frank AM, Barker CF, Markmann JF: Comparison of whole organ pancreas and isolated islet transplantation for type 1 diabetes. *Adv Surg* 39:137–163, 2005

96. Froud T, Baidal DA, Faradji R, Cure P, Mineo D, Selvaggi G, Kenyon NS, Ricordi C, Alejandro R: Islet transplantation with alemtuzumab induction and calcineurin-free maintenance immunosuppression results in improved short- and long-term outcomes. *Transplantation* 86:1695–1701, 2008

97. Mineo D, Ricordi C, Xu X, Pileggi A, Garcia-Morales R, Khan A, Baidal DA, Han D, Monroy K, Miller J, Pugliese A, Froud T, Inverardi L, Kenyon NS, Alejandro R: Combined islet and hematopoietic stem cell allotransplantation: a clinical pilot trial to induce chimerism and graft tolerance. *Am J Transplant* 8:1262–1274, 2008

98. Ryan EA, Lakey JR, Rajotte RV, Korbutt GS, Kin T, Imes S, Rabinovitch A, Elliott JF, Bigam D, Kneteman NM, Warnock GL, Larsen I, Shapiro AM: Clinical outcomes and insulin secretion after islet transplantation with the Edmonton protocol. *Diabetes* 50:710–719, 2001

99. Ryan EA, Paty BW, Senior PA, Bigam D, Alfadhli E, Kneteman NM, Lakey JR, Shapiro AM: Five-year follow-up after clinical islet transplantation. *Diabetes* 54:2060–2069, 2005

100. Kaufman DB, Baker MS, Chen X, Leventhal JR, Stuart FP: Sequential kidney/islet transplantation using prednisone-free immunosuppression. *Am J Transplant* 2:674–677, 2002

101. Toso C, Baertschiger R, Morel P, Bosco D, Armanet M, Wojtusciszyn A, Badet L, Philippe J, Becker CD, Hadaya K, Majno P, Buhler L, Berney T: Sequential kidney/islet transplantation: efficacy and safety assessment of a steroid-free immunosuppression protocol. *Am J Transplant* 6:1049–1058, 2006

102. Tan J, Yang S, Cai J, Guo J, Huang L, Wu Z, Chen J, Liao L: Simultaneous islet and kidney transplantation in seven patients with type 1 diabetes and end-stage renal disease using a glucocorticoid-free immunosuppressive regimen with alemtuzumab induction. *Diabetes* 57:2666–2671, 2008

103. Pileggi A, Cobianchi L, Inverardi L, Ricordi C: Overcoming the challenges now limiting islet transplantation: a sequential, integrated approach. *Ann N Y Acad Sci* 1079:383–398, 2006

104. Ryan EA, Shandro T, Green K, Paty BW, Senior PA, Bigam D, Shapiro AM, Vantyghem MC: Assessment of the severity of hypoglycemia and glycemic lability in type 1 diabetic subjects undergoing islet transplantation. *Diabetes* 53:955–962, 2004

105. Leitao CB, Tharavanij T, Cure P, Pileggi A, Baidal DA, Ricordi C, Alejandro R: Restoration of hypoglycemia awareness after islet transplantation. *Diabetes Care* 31:2113–2115, 2008

106. Johnson JA, Kotovych M, Ryan EA, Shapiro AM: Reduced fear of hypoglycemia in successful islet transplantation. *Diabetes Care* 27:624–625, 2004

107. Poggioli R, Faradji RN, Ponte G, Betancourt A, Messinger S, Baidal DA, Froud T, Ricordi C, Alejandro R: Quality of life after islet transplantation. *Am J Transplant* 6:371–378, 2006

108. Tharavanij T, Betancourt A, Messinger S, Cure P, Leitao CB, Baidal DA, Froud T, Ricordi C, Alejandro R: Improved long-term health-related quality of life after islet transplantation. *Transplantation* 86:1161–1167, 2008

109. Rickels MR, Naji A, Teff KL: Acute insulin responses to glucose and arginine as predictors of beta-cell secretory capacity in human islet transplantation. *Transplantation* 84:1357–1360, 2007

110. Rickels MR, Schutta MH, Markmann JF, Barker CF, Naji A, Teff KL: {beta}-Cell function following human islet transplantation for type 1 diabetes. *Diabetes* 54:100–106, 2005

111. Paty BW, Ryan EA, Shapiro AM, Lakey JR, Robertson RP: Intrahepatic islet transplantation in type 1 diabetic patients does not restore hypoglycemic hormonal counterregulation or symptom recognition after insulin independence. *Diabetes* 51:3428–3434, 2002

112. Rickels MR, Schutta MH, Mueller R, Markmann JF, Barker CF, Naji A, Teff KL: Islet cell hormonal responses to hypoglycemia after human islet transplantation for type 1 diabetes. *Diabetes* 54:3205–3211, 2005

113. Faradji RN, Tharavanij T, Messinger S, Froud T, Pileggi A, Monroy K, Mineo D, Baidal DA, Cure P, Ponte G, Mendez AJ, Selvaggi G, Ricordi C, Alejandro R: Long-term insulin independence and improvement in insulin secretion after supplemental islet infusion under exenatide and etanercept. *Transplantation* 86:1658–1665, 2008

114. Faradji RN, Froud T, Messinger S, Monroy K, Pileggi A, Mineo D, Tharavanij T, Mendez AJ, Ricordi C, Alejandro R: Long term metabolic effects of exenatide on islet transplant recipients with allograft dysfunction. *Cell Transplant* in press, 2009

115. Campbell PM, Senior PA, Salam A, Labranche K, Bigam DL, Kneteman NM, Imes S, Halpin A, Ryan EA, Shapiro AM: High risk of sensitization after failed islet transplantation. *Am J Transplant* 7:2311–2317, 2007

116. Cardani R, Pileggi A, Ricordi C, Gomez C, Baidal DA, Ponte GG, Mineo D, Faradji RN, Froud T, Ciancio G, Esquenazi V, Burke GW, 3 rd, Selvaggi G, Miller J, Kenyon NS, Alejandro R: Allosensitization of islet allograft recipients. *Transplantation* 84:1413–1427, 2007

117. Gangemi A, Salehi P, Hatipoglu B, Martellotto J, Barbaro B, Kuechle J, Qi M, Wang Y, Pallan P, Owens C, Bui J, West D, Kaplan B, Benedetti E, Oberholzer J: Islet transplantation for brittle type 1 diabetes: the UIC protocol. *Am J Transplant* 8:1250–1261, 2008

118. Ghofaili K, Fung M, Ao Z, Meloche M, Shapiro R, Warnock G, Elahi D, Meneilly G, Thompson D: Effect of exenatide on beta cell function after islet transplantation in type 1 diabetes. *Transplantation* 83:24–28, 2007

119. Froud T, Faradji R, Pileggi A, Messinger S, Baidal D, Ponte G, Cure P, Monroy K, Mendez A, Selvaggi G, Ricordi C, Alejandro R: The use of exenatide in islet transplant recipients with chronic allograft dysfunction: safety, efficacy, and metabolic effects. *Transplantation* 86:36–45, 2008

120. Cretin N, Buhler L, Fournier B, Caulfield A, Oberholzer J, Becker C, Phillippe J, Morel P: Results of human islet allotransplantation in cystic fibrosis and type I diabetic patients. *Transplant Proc* 30:315–316, 1998

121. Brunicardi FC, Atiya A, Stock P, Kenmochi T, Une S, Benhamou PY, Watt PC, Miyamato M, Wanlanabe Y, Nomura Y, et al.: Clinical islet transplantation experience of the University of California Islet Transplant Consortium. *Surgery* 118:967–971; discussion 971–962, 1995

122. Ricordi C, Alejandro R, Angelico MC, Fernandez LA, Nery J, Webb M, Bottino R, Selvaggi G, Khan FA, Karatzas T, Olson L, Mintz DH, Tzakis AG: Human islet allografts in patients with type 2 diabetes undergoing liver transplantation. *Transplantation* 63:473–475, 1997

123. Friedman AL, Friedman EA: Pancreas transplantation for type 2 diabetes at U.S. Transplant centers. *Diabetes Care* 25.1896, 2002

124. Leone JP, Kendall DM, Reinsmoen N, Hering BJ, Sutherland DE: Immediate insulin-independence after retransplantation of islets prepared from an allograft pancreatectomy in a type 1 diabetic patient. *Transplant Proc* 30:319, 1998

125. Wahoff DC, Papalois BE, Najarian JS, Kendall DM, Farney AC, Leone JP, Jessurun J, Dunn DL, Robertson RP, Sutherland DE: Autologous islet transplantation to prevent diabetes after pancreatic resection. *Ann Surg* 222:562–575; discussion 575–569, 1995

126. Robertson RP, Lanz KJ, Sutherland DE, Kendall DM: Prevention of diabetes for up to 13 years by autoislet transplantation after pancreatectomy for chronic pancreatitis. *Diabetes* 50:47–50, 2001

127. Oberholzer J, Mathe Z, Bucher P, Triponez F, Bosco D, Fournier B, Majno P, Philippe J, Morel P: Islet autotransplantation after left pancreatectomy for non-enucleable insulinoma. *Am J Transplant* 3:1302–1307, 2003

128. Ricordi C, Edlund H: Toward a renewable source of pancreatic beta-cells. *Nat Biotechnol* 26:397–398, 2008

129. Ricordi C, Strom TB: Clinical islet transplantation: advances and immunological challenges. *Nat Rev Immunol* 4:259–268, 2004

17

Technology and Diabetes: Insulin Delivery Systems and Glucose Sensing

Bruce W. Bode

Numerous technologic advances have been and continue to be developed in the areas of insulin delivery and glucose sensing. These advances have evolved to allow individuals with diabetes to obtain the best glucose control possible while minimizing the risk of hypoglycemia.

In the area of insulin delivery, there has been dramatic improvement not only in insulin syringes and insulin injection devices (e.g., insulin pens), but also in insulin pump technology. Insulin syringes have evolved from reusable glass syringes with self-sharpening needles in the 1920s to the disposable, multiple-size syringes with 31- to 32-gauge needles currently available. Insulin pens, both disposable and reusable with insulin cartridges, became available in the 1980s and have benefited persons with diabetes with regard to accuracy in dosing and convenience in initiating and implementing both conventional and intensive (basal/bolus) insulin therapies. Continuous, subcutaneous, insulin infusion therapy became available in 1979 and has become the gold standard in basal/bolus therapy, providing persons with diabetes with improved glucose control, with less risk of severe hypoglycemia, as well as a better quality of life. In 2003, the first generation of smart insulin pumps became available. These pumps have software enhancements that help patients calculate their appropriate meal bolus, subtracting active insulin on board as well as reminding patients when to check their blood glucose levels and change their infusion reservoirs. In 2006, the first disposable patch pump became available, allowing the pump user to deliver insulin without pump tubing via a remote controller with a built-in meter.

In the field of glucose testing, blood glucose measurements have gone from being done in the laboratory to patient self-monitoring of blood glucose (SMBG) in the late 1970s and continuous sensing in the interstitial fluid. The accuracy and precision of such measurements have improved dramatically, with a reaction time as short as 5 s for SMBG with some meter systems. The volume of blood required for such measurements has decreased from 15 μL to as little as 0.3 μL with some meter systems. Lancing systems also have evolved from 23- to, most recently, 33 gauge needles. In 1999, retrospective continuous glucose sensing of interstitial fluid was approved, allowing patients to obtain up to 288 glucose measurements per day for up to 72 h. This technology enables clinicians to clearly view patients' glucose patterns and fluctuations, especially nocturnal and after eating. In 2006, real-time continuous glucose sensing of interstitial fluid as an adjunct to SMBG was approved, and now there are three approved real-time continuous glucose monitoring (CGM) systems on the US market: the DexCom Seven (DexCom, San Diego, CA), the MiniMed Paradigm Real-Time Insulin Pump and Continuous Glucose Monitoring System (Medtronic MiniMed, Northridge, CA), and the FreeStyle Navigator (Abbott Diabetes Care, Alameda, CA). In 2009, the Juvenile Diabetes Research Foundation CGM group completed its landmark randomized, controlled, parallel-group study of real-time CGM (RT-CGM) in 450 type 1 diabetes patients. Use of RT-CGM substantially improved glycemic control in adults with type 1 diabetes with a hemoglobin A_{1c} (HbA_{1c}) level $\geq 7.0\%$ without increasing the risk of hypoglycemia [1–5]. Less frequent use limited the effectiveness of CGM in younger age groups; however, if younger patients used RT-CGM six or more times a week, they received the same 0.5% significant lowering in HbA_{1c} as adults. RT-CGM was also beneficial in individuals with type 1 diabetes who had already achieved

J.S. Skyler (ed.), *Atlas of Diabetes: Fourth Edition*,
DOI 10.1007/978-1-4614-1028-7_17, © Springer Science+Business Media, LLC 2012

HbA$_{1c}$ less than 7%; these patients maintained a stable HbA$_{1c}$, with reduced exposure to biochemical hypoglycemia. These benefits in glycemic control were sustained over the course of the 1-year study, with rates of severe hypoglycemia declining during that period. Future research and development must focus on making RT-CGM devices easier to wear and use continuously by younger individuals with type 1 diabetes.

The future looks promising and is not far away. Closed-loop systems incorporating both external and implantable glucose sensors and insulin pumps also are in development, with promising results from phase 1 and 2 trials. Medtronic has launched an insulin pump with a "low suspend" feature that automatically suspends insulin delivery for up to 2 h if the glucose sensor reading is in the low range for more than 15 min, without any patient intervention. Such technologic advances in glucose sensing and insulin delivery will continue at a rapid pace until all persons with diabetes can maintain normal blood glucose levels with no risk of hypoglycemia. Implantable insulin pumps and glucose sensors also are being developed and have shown benefits similar to those of external insulin pumps, with the added benefit of a lower risk of severe hypoglycemia.

Insulin Injection Therapy

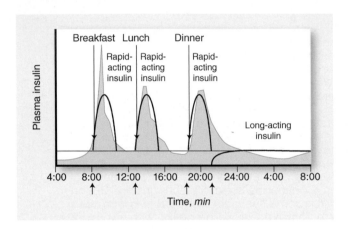

FIGURE 17-1. Basal/bolus treatment program with rapid-acting and long-acting analogues. Insulin is best given in a basal/bolus format, with rapid- or short-acting insulin given before each meal and a long-acting insulin given at bedtime or an intermediate-acting insulin given twice a day. Analogue insulins have the benefit of more predictable absorption with less risk of hypoglycemia.

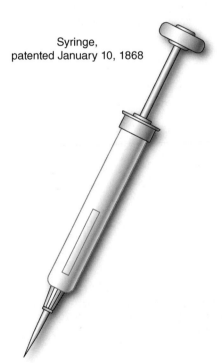

FIGURE 17-2. The earliest picture of the first syringe and needle, patented in 1868. From the 1920s through the 1950s, insulin was given by reusable glass syringes and needles.

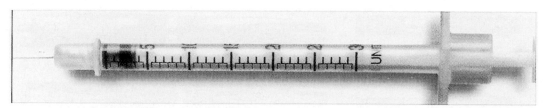

Figure 17-3. Current insulin syringe. Modern syringes are disposable, come in multiple sizes ranging from 0.25 to 1 mL, have 0.5- and 1-U measurements, and have needles that range in size from 29 to 32 gauge.

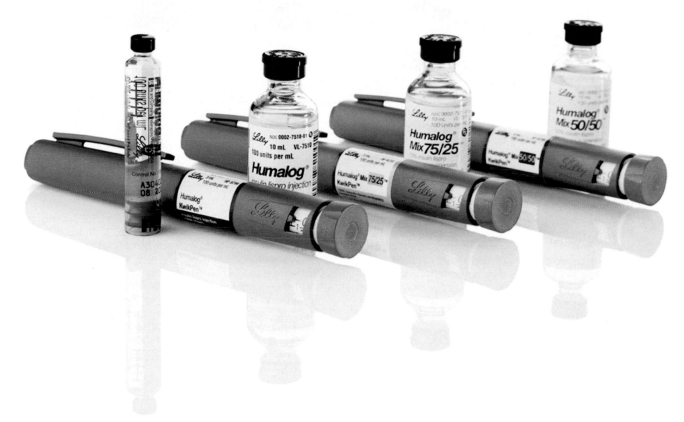

Figure 17-4. Insulin cartridges for reusable and disposable pens. Insulin traditionally was given by vial and syringe. In the 1980s, insulin cartridges for reusable pens were developed, followed by disposable pens. Shown are current Lilly USA (Indianapolis, IN) insulin vials, cartridges, and disposable pens.

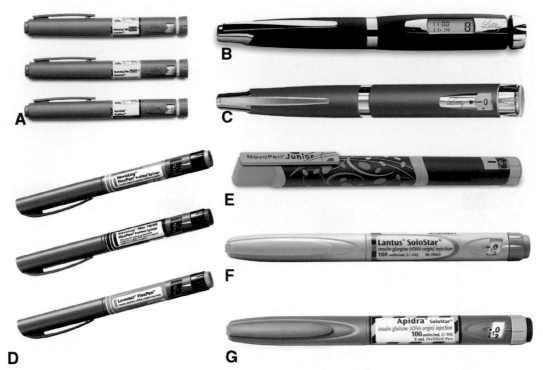

Figure 17-5. Insulin pens. The first insulin pen was developed by Novo Nordisk (Novo Nordisk A/S, Bagsvaerd, Denmark) in 1926, but the first commercial pen was not available until 1985. Since then, numerous pens, both disposable and reusable, have been developed, improving the dosage accuracy and convenience of insulin injection therapy. (**A**) Humalog KwikPen (Lilly USA) is a disposable, prefilled pen containing 3 mL (300 U) of U-100 Humalog, Humalog Mix75/25, and Humalog Mix50/50 insulins, with dosing in 1-U increments up to 60 U. (**B**) HumaPen Memoir (Lilly USA), a reusable pen for use only with Humalog 3-mL insulin cartridges, allows dosing in 1-U increments up to 60 U, with memory recording of the date, time, and amount of

the last 16 doses. (**C**) HumaPen Luxura HD (Lilly USA) is a reusable pen that doses in 0.5-U increments up to 30 U. (**D**) Novo Nordisk FlexPen, a disposable, color-coded, prefilled pen, contains 3 mL (300 U) of U-100 NovoLog, NovoLog Mix 70/30, and Levemir insulins, with dosing in 1-U increments up to 60 U. (**E**) NovoPen Junior (Novo Nordisk A/S) is a reusable pen that doses in 0.5-U increments up to 35 U. (**F**) The Lantus SoloStar (Sanofi-Aventis, Bridgewater, NJ) is a disposable, color-coded, prefilled pen containing 3 mL (300 U) of U-100 Lantus insulin that doses in 1-U increments up to 80 U. (**G**) The Apidra SoloStar (Sanofi-Aventis) is a disposable, color-coded, prefilled pen containing 3 mL (300 U) of U-100 Apidra insulin that doses in 1-U increments up to 80 U.

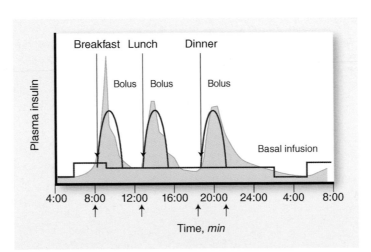

Figure 17-6. Basal/bolus therapy. Insulin pump therapy has been the gold standard for basal/bolus therapy. The basal rate may be varied to cover the dawn phenomenon and exercise, and boluses can be given easily to cover all meals and snacks and may be given over time to cover high-fat meals and slowly absorbing carbohydrates.

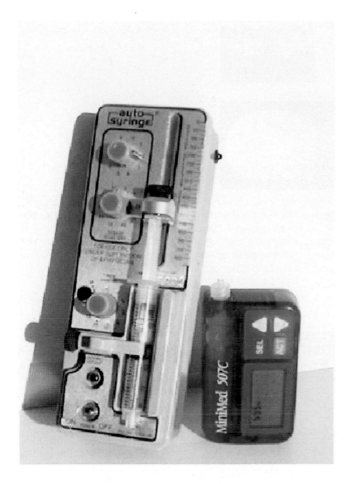

Figure 17-7. Pump therapy: Older versus newer generation. Insulin pump therapy was first approved in the USA in 1979 using the Autosyringe (DEKA, Manchester, NH) 2-C pump, a bulky, rather complicated mechanical syringe. Multiple improvements in size, safety, software enhancements, durability, and ease of programming have been made. Also pictured is the 507-C pump (Medtronic Diabetes), the first downloadable pump, launched in 1998.

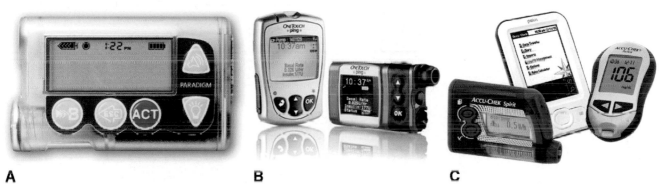

A   B   C

Figure 17-8. Current models of reusable insulin pumps, approved by the US Food and Drug Administration (FDA) for sale in the USA as of September 2009. (**A**) The Medtronic MiniMed Paradigm insulin pump (Medtronic Diabetes). (**B**) The OneTouch Ping glu-cose management system (Animas, West Chester, PA) with the 2020 insulin pump and OneTouch Ping glucose meter-remote. (**C**) Accu-Chek Spirit insulin pump (Roche, Basel, Switzerland) with the Palm device and Accu-Chek glucose meter.

Perpendicular (Sof-set,
Quick-set, Ultraflex, Inset 30)
    Easier insertion
    Prone to kink

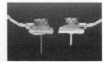

Oblique (Silhouette,
Tender, Comfort)
    More difficult insertion
    Less kinking

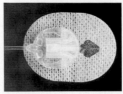

FIGURE 17-9. Insulin pump infusion sets. Perpendicular types (Sof-set [Medtronic MiniMed], Quick-set [Medtronic Diabetes], Ultraflex [DisetronicUSA, Fishers, IN]), and Inset 30 [Animas] are easier to insert but are prone to kinking. Oblique types (Silhouette [Medtronic Diabetes], Tender [DisetronicUSA], and Comfort [Medtronic Diabetes]) are more difficult to insert but are less prone to kinking. The insulin pump and reservoir are connected to the patient via an infusion set, which has either a metal needle or a Teflon catheter at the end. Teflon catheters are inserted with a metal needle inducer and are more comfortable to wear, but they are more prone to kinking. Almost all current sets have a quick-release option to disconnect the pump for showering, sports, and other activities.

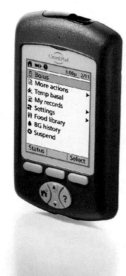

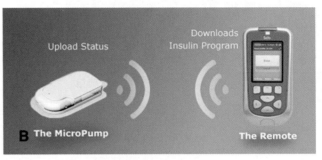

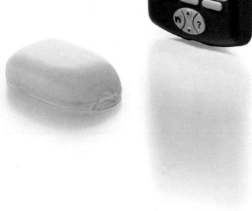

A

FIGURE 17-10. Three insulin patch pumps (free of insulin tubing) approved by the FDA for sale in the USA. (**A**) Insulet's (Bedford, MA) OmniPod insulin management system is a two-part system consisting of a disposable 3-day insulin infusion pod and a personal diabetes manager (PDM). The pod integrates a 200-U insulin reservoir, an angled infusion set, an automated inserter, and a pumping mechanism. The PDM programs the pod and incorporates a blood glucose meter. Development is under way to allow the PDM to receive CGM readings. (**B**) Medingo's (Tampa, FL) Solo MicroPump insulin delivery system is a two-part system consisting of a small insulin pump that holds 200 U of insulin and a remote control device to wirelessly personalize insulin delivery. (**C**) Valeritas (Parsippany, NJ) V-Go, disposable 1-day insulin delivery device, has three different preset basal rates of insulin and discrete on-demand 2-U bolus dosing of insulin.

CURRENT PUMP THERAPY INDICATIONS
Inability to normalize blood glucose
$A_{1c} > 6.5\%$
Glycemic excursions
Dawn phenomenon
Hypoglycemia or hypoglycemia unawareness
Need for flexible treatment regimen (shift work, safety-sensitive job, unpredictable lifestyle)

FIGURE 17-11. Current pump therapy indications. The indications for pump therapy are based on the metabolic advantages of pump therapy: improved glycemic control, better pharmacokinetic delivery of insulin with less hypoglycemia and a lower insulin requirement, and improvement in quality of life. A_{1c}-hemoglobin A_{1c}.

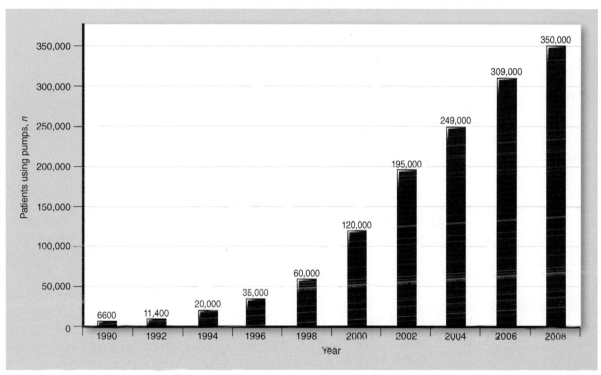

FIGURE 17-12. Pump usage in the USA: Total patients using insulin pumps. Pump therapy increased dramatically in the USA after the 1993 publication of the results of the Diabetes Control and Complications Trial (DCCT), in which more than 40% of patients assigned to the intensive therapy group were using insulin pumps at the end of the trial. Insulin pump therapy continues to grow because of the awareness of the benefits of pump therapy and better pump technology (based on Medtronic internal data/estimates and various reports on pump share by manufacturer).

INSULIN PUMP THERAPY: FACTORS AFFECTING GLYCEMIC CONTROL
Glucose monitoring frequency
A_{1c} = 8.3 – (0.21 × blood glucose per day)
Recording 7.4 vs 7.8
Diet practiced
CHO: 7.2
Fixed: 7.5
WAG: 8.0

Figure 17-13. Insulin pump therapy: Factors that affect glycemic control. Numerous factors may affect glycemic control in patients who use insulin pumps. Most important is the frequency of SMBG. Other factors are recording of blood glucose values and insulin doses, as well as the diet practiced. Carbohydrate counting should be encouraged in all patients. Unfortunately, the "wild-ass guess" (WAG) approach is still commonly practiced. CHO – carbohydrate (adapted from Bode et al. [6] and Davidson et al. [7]).

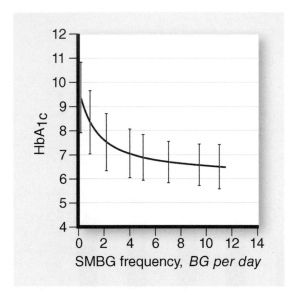

Figure 17-14. Increased SMBG frequency lowers A_{1c}. These data are from 378 patients sorted from a database of 591 pump patients who have a glycemic target of 100 and are C-peptide negative. If one monitors his or her blood glucose (BG) four or more times a day on a pump, his or her mean A_{1c} levels should be ≤7.0%.

INSULIN PUMP FORMULAS
TDD = 0.5 × weight in kg
Basal dose = 0.48 × TDD
CIR = (6 × weight in kg)/TDD (anywhere from 5 to 25 g carbohydrates is covered by 1 U of insulin)
CF = 1700/TDD
Target = 100 mg/dL

Figure 17-15. Insulin pump formulas. These formulas are derived using mathematical modeling from a database of more than 500 pump patients comparing data from patients with hemoglobin A_{1c} levels less than to greater than 7%. The total daily dose (TDD), basal rate, and correction factor (CF) are all correlated with body weight or TDD, whereas the carbohydrate-to-insulin ratio (CIR) is correlated with weight and TDD. The CF is the amount of glucose lowered by 1 U of insulin. The target is the ideal blood glucose level, which may be changed depending on the goal of therapy (80 mg/dL for pregnant women, 100 mg/dL if the patient is male or not pregnant, and 110–120 mg/dL if the patient is at risk for hypoglycemia) (adapted from Davidson et al. [8]).

BOLUS: SOURCE OF ERRORS
"Inability" to count carbohydrates correctly
Lack of knowledge, skill
Lack of time
Too much work
Incorrect use of SMBG number
Incorrect math in calculation
"WAG" estimations

FIGURE 17-16. Bolus: Source of errors. Patients can make several mistakes in dosing for meals, ranging from their inability to count carbohydrates correctly, their inability to calculate their correction bolus appropriately to bring them back to normal blood glucose levels, and their unawareness of their current active insulin on board from their prior insulin bolus. As a result, patients often underestimate their carbohydrates consumed and overcorrect for high postprandial glucose elevations, not taking into account active insulin previously given.

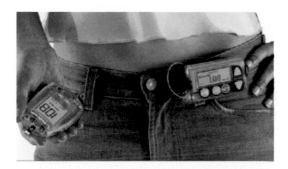

FIGURE 17-17. Smart insulin pumps. Smart insulin pumps have several software enhancements that estimate the appropriate correction bolus based on the current blood glucose minus any active insulin on board from a prior insulin bolus plus the amount of insulin to cover the carbohydrates consumed. Alert reminders also may be set to check blood glucose, take meal boluses, and change the infusion set. For smart insulin pumps to work, it is critical that the basal doses, correction doses, and carbohydrate ratios are accurate. Understanding how to match carbohydrate amounts with insulin is critical. If the target is set too high (>110 mg/dL), glucose will run too high; normal target is 100 mg/dL, and for pregnancy, 80 mg/dL is safe.

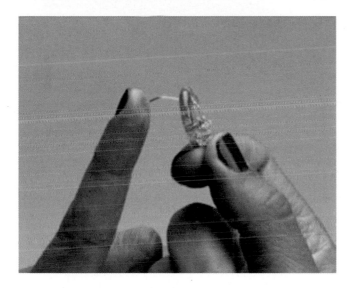

FIGURE 17-18. CGM sensor. The tip of the sensor is a platinum electrode coated with glucose oxidase and covered by a semipermeable membrane. Upon applying voltage to the electrode, ambient glucose and oxygen react, creating a signal that correlates with ambient glucose in the interstitial fluid.

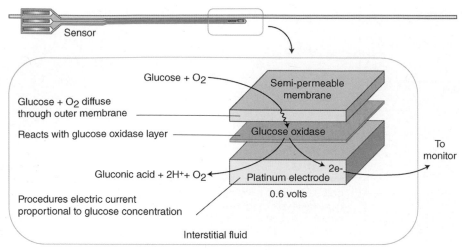

FIGURE 17-19. Method of interstitial glucose sensing by current CGM systems.

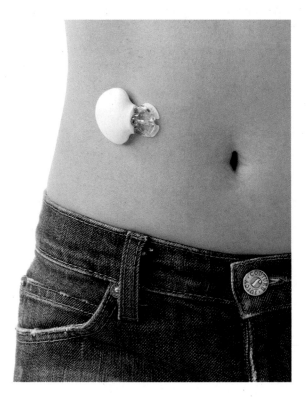

FIGURE 17-20. Medtronic retrospective CGM system (iPro). The iPro includes a reusable MiniLink transmitter and storage device, as well as a disposable glucose sensor. This system records up to 288 glucose readings per day, which is 72 times more information than that provided by the typical four fingerstick measurements. By viewing retrospective blood glucose trends, physicians gain valuable new insights to help them refine diabetes therapy for their patients. Prospective studies have shown improvement in hemoglobin A_{1c} with less hypoglycemia.

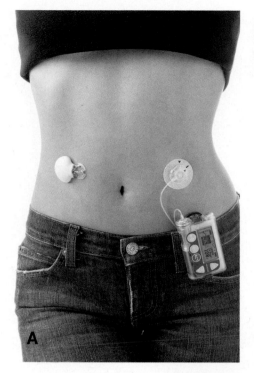
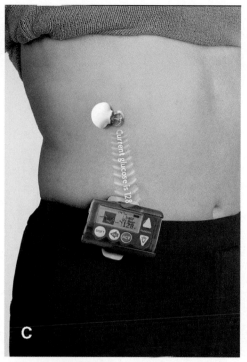
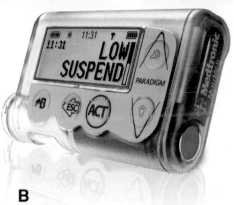

Figure 17-21. (**A**) MiniMed Paradigm real-time insulin pump and CGM system (Medtronic Diabetes). This system includes the reusable MiniLink transmitter and disposable glucose sensor as well as the Paradigm insulin pump. Glucose readings are updated every 5 min and are received by and displayed on the insulin pump, on which the patient can visualize his or her current CGM reading as well as the latest 3- and 24-h CGM graphs. The pump is downloadable into CareLink therapy management software, enabling both the patient and health care professional to visualize the insulin delivery and CGM graphs for further analysis and adjustment of insulin delivery, diet, and other diabetes care behavior. (**B**) Veo Paradigm real-time pump and CCM system (Medtronic Diabetes) with "auto suspend," approved for sale by the European health authorities. In the presence of hypoglycemia detected by CGM for at least 15 min, the pump suspends insulin delivery for up to 2 h. (**C**) Guardian real-time CGM system (Medtronic Diabetes). This system includes the reusable MiniLink transmitter and disposable glucose sensor as well as a receiver that receives and displays glucose readings updated every 5 min. The receiver is downloadable for further analysis of the glucose data by patients and health care providers.

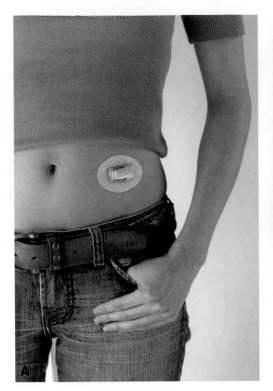

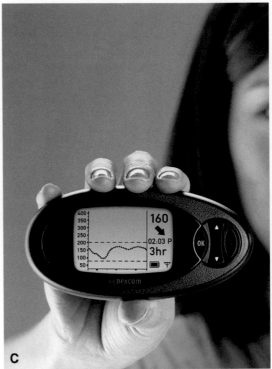

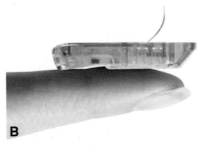

FIGURE 17-22. DexCom Seven Plus CGM system. The DexCom system includes (**A**) a disposable 7-day sensor, (**B**) a small transmitter, and (**C**) a receiver. The system is calibrated every 12 h and displays glucose readings continuously updated every 5 min on the remote receiver. The receiver is downloadable for further analysis of the glucose data by both the patient and health care provider.

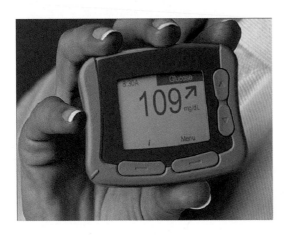

FIGURE 17-23. FreeStyle Navigator CGM (Abbott Laboratories, Abbott Park, IL). The system includes a disposable 5-day sensor, a wireless transmitter, and an integrated glucose monitor used for automatic calibration and display of continuous interstitial glucose readings. The integrated glucose monitor is downloadable for further analysis of the glucose data by both the patient and health care provider.

COMPARISON OF THREE SENSORS			
	Sensor		
Characteristic	**DexCom**	**Medtronic**	**Abbott**
Sensor length, *mm*	13	14	5
Sensor introducer needle, *gauge*	26	22	21
Sensor wear, *d*	≥ 7	≥ 3	≥ 5
Sensor start-up time, *h*	2	2	10
Sensor site(s)	Abdomen	Abdomen	Abdomen, arm
Sensor packaging	4-pack	4- and 10-packs	6-pack
Glucose range, *mg/dL*	40–400	40–400	20–600
Insertion angle	45°	45°	90°

FIGURE 17-24. Comparison matrix of the three sensors (DexCom, Medtronic, and Abbott) listing the specifications of each sensor system (data from Weinzimer et al. [9]).

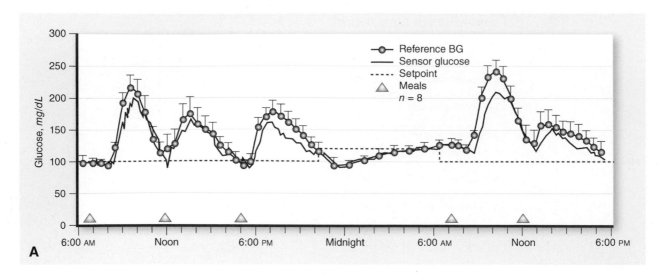

A

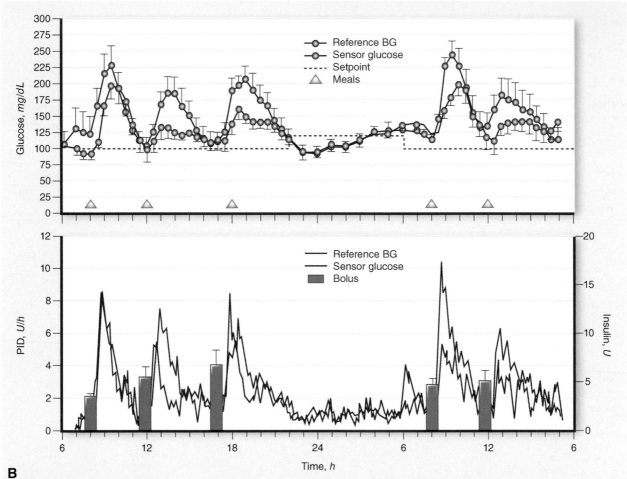

B

Figure 17-25. External artificial pancreas. A future closed-loop system is expected to integrate an external insulin pump and an external CGM system that uses a glucose sensor to record blood sugar readings from interstitial fluid. The external system will be designed to automatically integrate glucose levels and deliver insulin accordingly. This device is not yet cleared by the FDA or European health authorities (from Medtronic Diabetes, with permission).

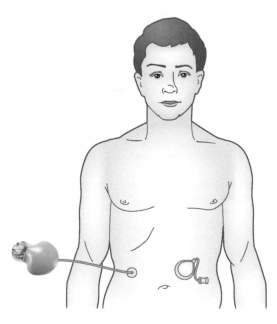

FIGURE 17-26. External artificial pancreas proof-of-concept study. A closed-loop system involving a pump, a glucose sensor, and software was tested in eight individuals with type 1 diabetes. (**A**) CGM readings of a total closed loop with no bolus by a patient. (**B**) CGM readings and insulin levels of a hybrid closed loop with a partial meal bolus given by a patient upon eating. *BG* blood glucose, *PID* physiologic insulin delivery (data from Weinzimer et al. [9]).

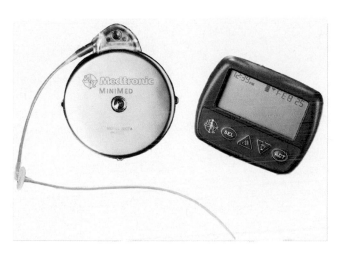

FIGURE 17-27. Implantable insulin pump. Medtronic's implantable insulin pump delivers insulin into the peritoneal cavity, where it is more rapidly and predictably absorbed by the body, with fewer hypoglycemic episodes compared with external pump therapy or multiple daily injections. The pump holds 10 mL of 400-U insulin and needs refilling every 2–4 months. Catheter blockages are the main adverse event. This device is not yet cleared by the FDA; it bears CE approval in Europe (from Medtronic Diabetes, with permission).

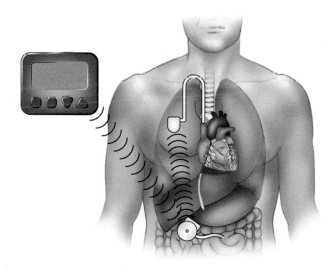

FIGURE 17-28. Implanted artificial pancreas. A future closed-loop system is expected to integrate an implantable insulin pump and an implantable long-term glucose sensor. The implantable sensor is inserted into the superior vena cava, where it is designed to continuously measure glucose levels using an enzyme-based electrode, which detects oxygen consumed in a glucose oxidase reaction. The sensor is designed to be replaced every year through a minor surgical procedure and is connected to an implantable insulin pump by an abdominal lead. This implantable system is designed to automatically record blood glucose levels and deliver insulin to patients with diabetes. This device is not yet cleared by the FDA or European health authorities (from Medtronic Diabetes, with permission).

References

1. JDRF CGM Study Group: JDRF randomized clinical trial to assess the efficacy of real-time continuous glucose monitoring in the management of type 1 diabetes: research design and methods. *Diabetes Technol Ther* 2008, 10:310–321.

2. The Juvenile Diabetes Research Foundation Continuous Glucose Monitoring Study Group; Tamborlane WV, Beck RW, Bode BW, *et al.*: Continuous glucose monitoring and intensive treatment of type 1 diabetes. *N Engl J Med* 2008, 359:1464–1476.

3. Juvenile Diabetes Research Foundation Continuous Glucose Monitoring Study Group: The effect of continuous glucose monitoring in well-controlled type 1 diabetes. *Diabetes Care* 2009, 32:1378–1383.

4. The Juvenile Diabetes Research Foundation Continuous Glucose Monitoring Study Group; Beck RW, Buckingham B, Miller K, *et al.*: Factors predictive of use and of benefit from continuous glucose monitoring in type 1 diabetes. *Diabetes Care* 2009, 32:1947–1953.

5. Juvenile Diabetes Research Foundation Continuous Glucose Monitoring Study Group; Bode B, Beck RW, Xing D, *et al.*: Sustained benefit of continuous glucose monitoring on HbA1c, glucose profiles, and hypoglycemia in adults with type 1 diabetes. *Diabetes Care* 2009, 32:2047–2049.

6. Bode BW, Gross TM, Thornton KR, *et al.*: Continuous glucose monitoring used to adjust diabetes therapy improves glycosylated hemoglobin: a pilot study. *Diabetes Res Clin Pract* 1999, 46:183–190.

7. Davidson P, Hebblewhite H, Steed RD, Bode BW: Analysis: the suboptimal roadmap to the intensive therapy target. *Diabetes Technol Ther* 2004, 6:17–19.

8. Davidson P, Hebblewhite H, Steed RD, Bode BW: Analysis of guidelines for basal-bolus insulin dosing: basal insulin, correction factor, and carbohydrate-to-insulin ratio. *Endocr Pract* 2008, 14:1095–1101.

9. Weinzimer SA, Steil GM, Swan KL, *et al.*: Fully automated closed-loop insulin delivery versus semiautomated hybrid control in pediatric patients with type 1 diabetes using the artificial pancreas. *Diabetes Care* 2008, 31:934–939.

18

Newer Diabetes Medications

Jay S. Skyler

Before 1995, the only approved medications in the USA for the treatment of diabetes hyperglycemia were various insulin preparations and a number of sulfonylureas. Previously, the Food and Drug Administration (FDA) removed the biguanide phenformin from the market in 1977 due to its potential to induce fatal lactic acidosis. However, although almost every other country in the world was marketing metformin (which made its initial appearance in the 1950s), the patent for the drug had long since expired, leaving companies with little motivation to go through the registration process to bring metformin to the US market due to the immense possibility of generic copying.

With the passage of the Hatch–Waxman Act in the early 1980s, a new chemical entity registered in the USA would have 5 years of market exclusivity after its launch. This led to the implementation of appropriate clinical trials, which were needed for the introduction of metformin (Glucophage; Bristol-Myers Squibb, New York) to the USA in May 1995, thus expanding the therapeutic options for diabetes management. Metformin was greeted by diabetes specialists with much enthusiasm due to its nearly 40-year track record throughout the rest of the world. The availability of metformin led to the appreciation that medications with complementary mechanisms of action (e.g., sulfonylureas plus metformin) could facilitate the attainment of better glycemic control.

The mid-1990s also saw the launch of the first rapid-acting insulin analogue, insulin lispro (Humalog; Eli Lilly, Indianapolis, IN); a second rapid-acting insulin analogue, insulin aspart (Novolog; Novo Nordisk, Princeton, NJ); and (much later) insulin glulisine (Apidra; Sanofi-Aventis US, Bridgewater, NJ). These so-called designer insulins more closely matched the physiologic insulin profile with meals. However, the use of these rapid-acting analogues highlighted the need for a more physiologic basal insulin replacement. This need was achieved with the development of basal insulin analogues, such as insulin glargine (Lantus; Sanofi-Aventis, Bridgewater, NJ) in 2001 and insulin detemir (Levemir; Novo Nordisk, Princeton, NJ) in 2006. Thus, insulin therapy has changed dramatically over the past two decades.

Major changes in diabetes management have been facilitated by the development of several new classes of therapeutic agents that have a variety of mechanisms of action, therefore markedly onhancing therapeutic options. The late 1990s saw the introduction of three classes, the first of which was the thiazolidinediones (TZDs), also referred to as glitazones or proliferator-activated receptor γ activators. The earliest TZD, troglitazone (Rezulin; Pfizer, New York), was subsequently withdrawn from the market due to hepatic toxicity. This drug was followed by two other TZDs – rosiglitazone (Avandia; GlaxoSmithKline, Philadelphia, PA) and pioglitazone (Actos; Takeda, Deerfield, IL). Rosiglitazone has been embroiled in controversy and recently has had its use markedly restricted by regulatory agencies. The second class of therapeutic agents was the a-glucosidase inhibitors, including acarbose (Precose; Bayer, Pittsburgh, PA: Glucobay; Bayer, Pittsburgh, PA: Glucor; Bayer Santé, Cede, France: and Rebose), miglitol (Glyset; Pfizer, New York), and voglibose (Basen; Takeda, Deerfield, IL; Voglib and Volix: Ranbaxy Laboratories, Gurgaon, India). The third class, glinides (sometimes, inappropriately called "meglitinides"), includes repaglinide (Prandin; Novo Nordisk, Princeton, NJ) and nateglinide (Starlix; Novartis, Basel, Switzerland). These classes are discussed in other chapters, particularly Chap. 8.

J.S. Skyler (ed.), *Atlas of Diabetes: Fourth Edition*,
DOI 10.1007/978-1-4614-1028-7_18, © Springer Science+Business Media, LLC 2012

Since 2005, there has been an explosion of new classes of therapeutic agents. All of the agents discussed in this chapter belong in one of the following therapeutic classes: (1) incretin mimetics, (2) incretin enhancers, (3) dopamine agonists, (4) bile acid sequestrants, (5) amylin mimetics, (6) inhaled insulins, and (7) inhibitors of renal glucose reabsorption. This chapter addresses the agents that have been approved since 2005 or that are pending approval at the FDA in 2011.

Incretin Effects

The "incretin effect" describes the fact that the insulin secretory response to oral glucose consumption is greater than the response to a similar glucose challenge given intravenously. The incretin effect is mediated by the gut hormones glucagon-like peptide-1 (GLP-1) and glucose-dependent insulinotropic peptide (GIP). There are a multitude of biological effects of GLP-1, particularly related to glucose metabolism, which are depicted in Fig. 18.1. The incretin effect is depicted in Fig. 18.2. The effect is reduced in type 2 diabetes, as shown in Fig. 18.3. In large part, this may be due to reduced postprandial GLP-1 concentrations in both type 2 diabetes and impaired glucose tolerance (IGT) (see Fig. 18.4).

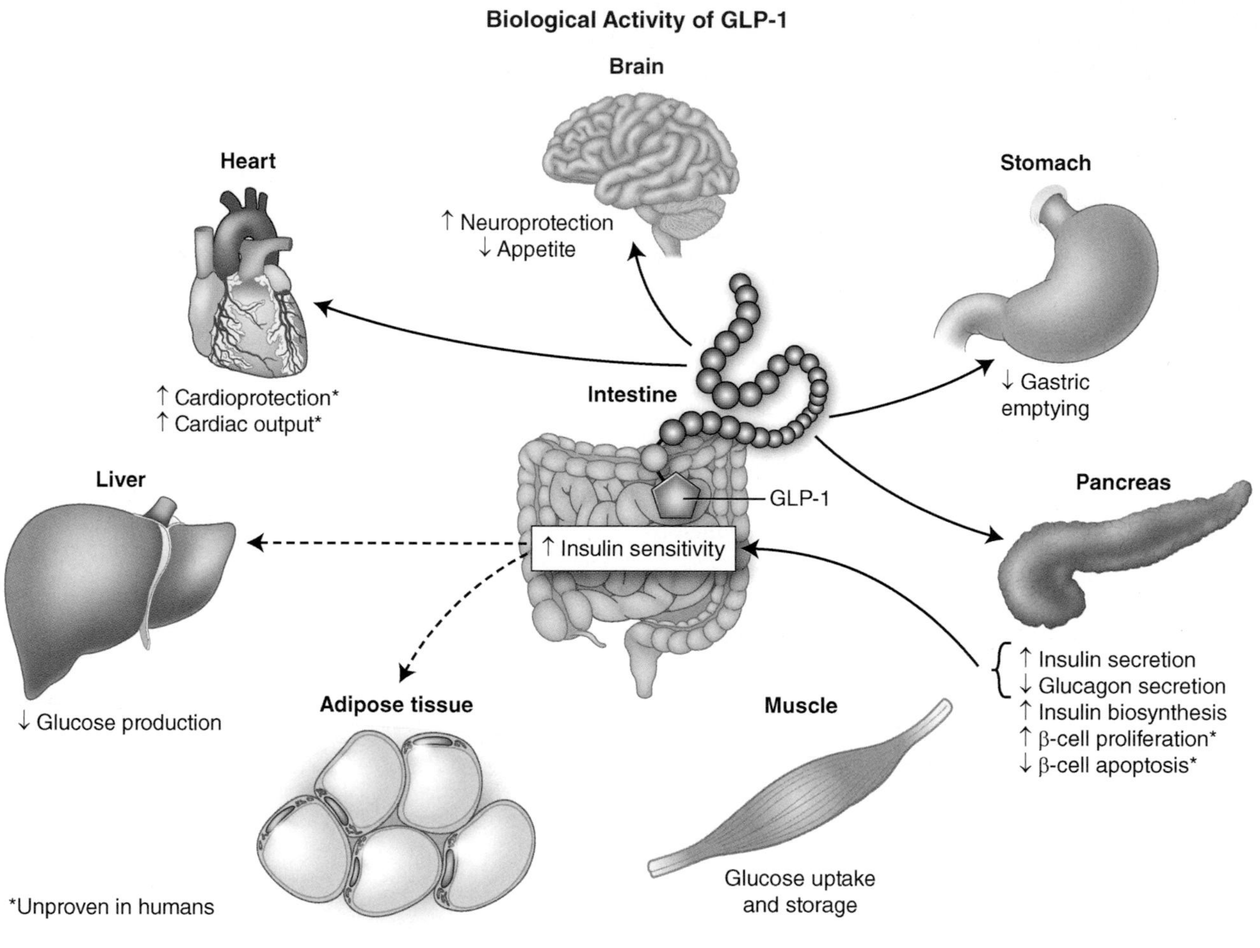

Biological Activity of GLP-1

Brain
↑ Neuroprotection
↓ Appetite

Heart
↑ Cardioprotection*
↑ Cardiac output*

Stomach
↓ Gastric emptying

Intestine

Liver
↓ Glucose production

—GLP-1

↑ Insulin sensitivity

Pancreas
↑ Insulin secretion
↓ Glucagon secretion
↑ Insulin biosynthesis
↑ β-cell proliferation*
↓ β-cell apoptosis*

Adipose tissue

Muscle
Glucose uptake and storage

*Unproven in humans

Figure 18-1. Plethora of biologic activity of glucagon-like peptide-1 (GLP-1). There is a range of effects on multiple aspects of glucose homeostasis, as well as direct effects on the heart, as shown here (adapted from Baggio and Drucker [1]).

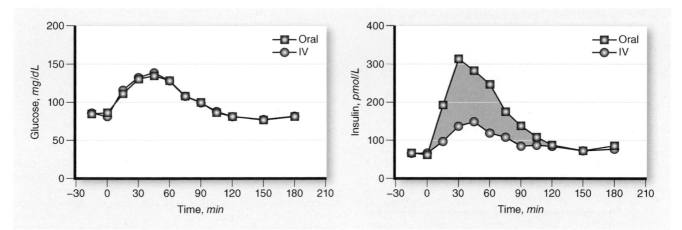

Figure 18-2. Measurement of the incretin effect: Oral glucose tolerance test and matched intravenous (IV) infusion. Superimposed glucose and insulin profiles during IV and oral glucose administration are shown. As the second step in measuring the incretin effect, glucose is infused intravenously at a variable rate to reproduce the arterial glucose profile observed after the 50-g oral glucose load. The difference between the insulin curves during the oral and IV glucose loads is attributed to nonglycemic β-cell stimuli and taken as a measure of the "incretin effect" (adapted from Nauck et al. [2]).

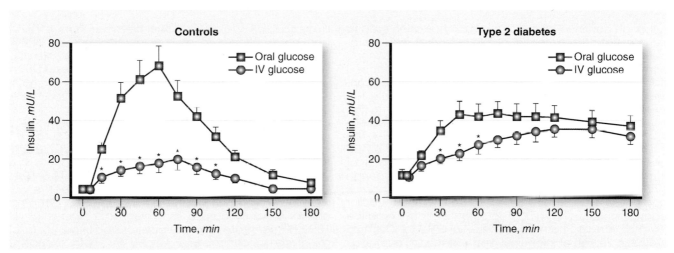

Figure 18-3. Incretin effect on insulin. The incretin effect describes the enhanced secretion of insulin observed following energy (usually, glucose) ingestion via the enteral vs. parenteral routes. The incretin effect is diminished in human subjects with type 2 diabetes. *IV* Intravenous (adapted from Nauck et al. [3]).

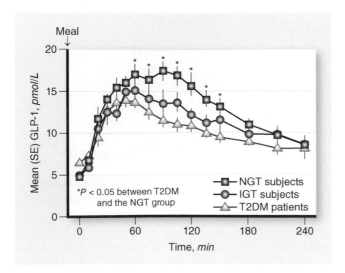

Figure 18-4. Postprandial glucagon-like peptide-1 (GLP-1) concentrations are reduced in subjects with type 2 diabetes and impaired glucose tolerance (IGT). The top line represents GLP-1 concentrations in subjects with normal glucose tolerance (NGT). GLP-1 concentrations are statistically significantly reduced in patients with type 2 diabetes compared to NGT subjects. *T2DM* type 2 diabetes mellitus (adapted from Toft-Nielsen et al. [4]).

Incretin Mimetics

Although continuous infusion of GLP-1 has been used to demonstrate the potential of this hormone as a therapeutic agent, the rapid degradation of the hormone from its active to inactive form by dipeptidyl peptidase-4 (DPP-4) has precluded the clinical use of GLP-1, as continuous infusion was deemed by most to be both too expensive and impractical. This finding has led to the development of GLP-1 receptor agonists as incretin mimetics. These agents are not degraded by DPP-4. The first of these agents to come to clinical usage is based on the peptide exendin-4. Exendin-4 is a component of the secretions of the salivary gland of the lizard *Heloderma suspectum* (Gila monster), has some sequence homology to GLP-1, has been shown to be a GLP-1 receptor agonist, and thus has glucoregulatory effects. Exenatide (Byetta; Amylin Pharmaceuticals, San Diego, CA) is a synthetic version of exendin-4 and was the first marketed insulin mimetic. It is generally prescribed as twice-daily injections. A long-acting version, exenatide QW (once weekly) (Bydureon; Amylin Pharmaceuticals, San Diego, CA), is pending regulatory approval. Lixisenatide, an analogue of exendin-4, is also in development. In addition to incretin mimetics built on an excedin-4 backbone,

a number of analogues have been built on a GLP-1 backbone, altered to escape degradation by DPP-4. The first of these is liraglutide (Victoza; Novo Nordisk, Princeton, NJ), which has been modified to resist DPP-4 degradation and also has a fatty acid tail to prolong its half-life. It is currently marketed. There also are several GLP-1 analogues still in development – taspoglutide, albiglutide (Syncria; Glaxo Smith Kline, Philadelphia, PA), and dulaglutide (Eli Lilly, Indianapolis, IN). Figure 18.5 summarizes all of these incretin mimetics or GLP-1 receptor agonists.

Collectively, the studies depicted in Figs. 18.6–18.10 demonstrate that exenatide (Byetta) is an effective glucose-lowering agent in which improvement in glycemic control is accompanied by weight loss. Figures 18.11–18.13 demonstrate similar effects for liraglutide (Victoza) on glycemic control with weight loss. Both exenatide (Byetta) and liraglutide (Victoza) are currently marketed.

The effects of the GLP-1 receptor agonists still in development are shown for exenatide QW (Bydureon) in Figs. 18.14–18.16, taspoglutide in Fig. 18.17, lixisenatide in Fig. 18.18, albiglutide in Fig. 18.19, and dulaglutide in Fig. 18.20.

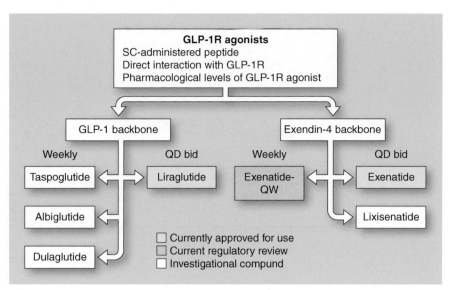

FIGURE 18-5. Glucagon-like peptide-1 receptor (GLP-1R) agonists. There are multiple GLP-1R agonists in clinical use or in clinical development. bid – twice a day; QD – daily; *SC* subcutaneous.

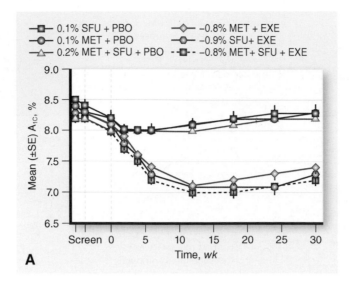

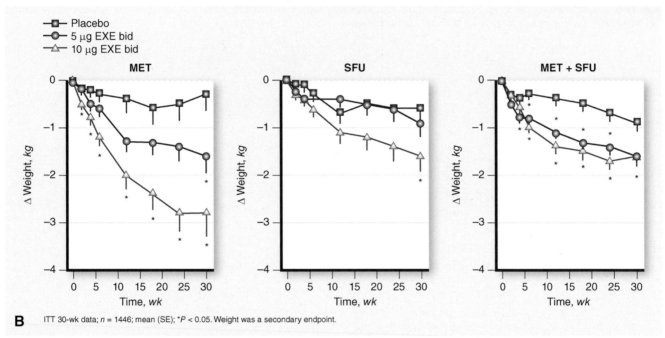

ITT 30-wk data; *n* = 1446; mean (SE); *P < 0.05. Weight was a secondary endpoint.

Figure 18-6. Exenatide (EXE) effects. (**A**) EXE (10 µg) used twice daily resulted in the lowering of A_{1c} in three trials used for registration. These trials compared exenatide to placebo (PBO) and were used as add-on therapy in patients treated with sulfonylureas (SFU), metformin (MET), or both. (**B**) EXE (both 10 and 5 µg) used twice daily resulted in progressive reductions in body weight in three trials used for registration. These trials compared EXE to PBO and were used as add-on therapy in patients treated with SFU, MET, or both. *bid* – twice a day, *ANOVA* analysis of variance, *ITT* intention to treat (adapted from DeFronzo et al. [5], Buse et al. [6], and Kendall et al. [7]).

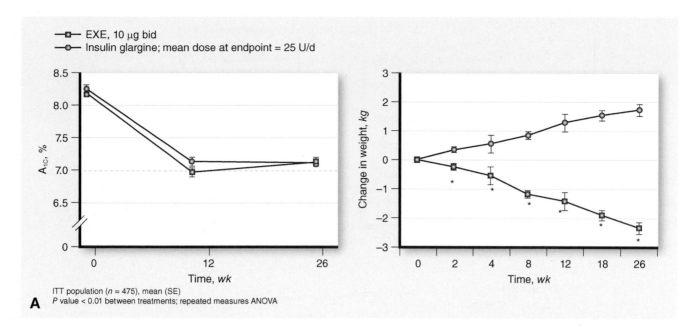

ITT population (n = 475), mean (SE)

A P value < 0.01 between treatments; repeated measures ANOVA

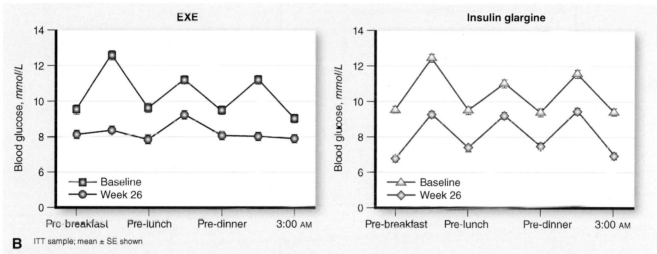

B ITT sample; mean ± SE shown

FIGURE 18-7. Exenatide (FXE) trials vs. insulin glargine (**A**) and glargine (**D**). (**A**) FXE (10 μg) used twice daily resulted in lowering of A_{1c} and a reduction in body weight, whereas insulin glargine resulted in an equal lowering of A_{1c} but an increase in body weight. (**B**) Glucose profiles at baseline and study end, demonstrating reductions principally in fasting glucose in the insulin glargine group and in postprandial glucose excursions in the EXE (twice a day [bid]) group. *ANOVA* analysis of variance, *ITT* intention to treat (adapted from Heine et al. [8]).

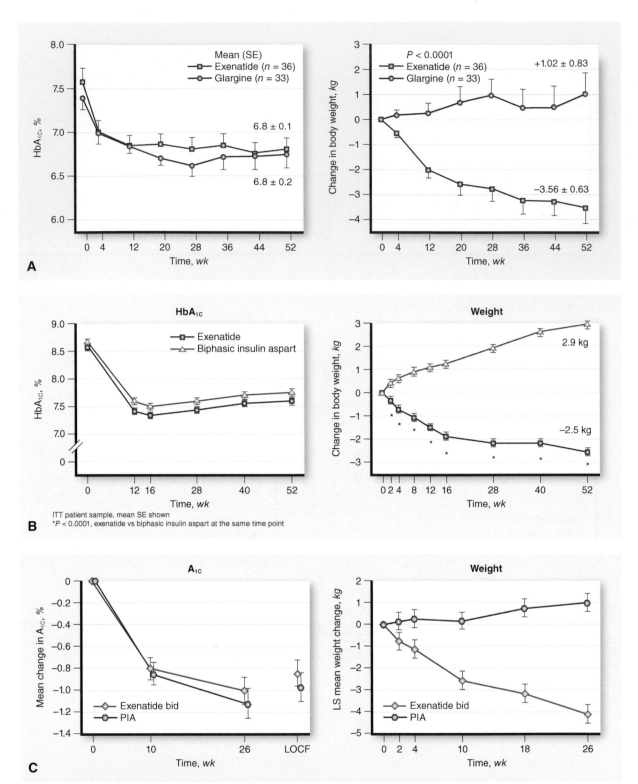

Figure 18-8. Exenatide vs. glargine (**A**), biphasic aspart (**B**), and prandial insulin aspart (PIA) (**C**). (**A**) In one longer study, exenatide (10 μg) used twice daily (bid) resulted in lowering of A₁c and a reduction in body weight, whereas insulin glargine resulted in equal lowering of A₁c but a modest increase in body weight. (**B**) In another study, exenatide (10 μg) used twice daily resulted in lowering of A_{1c} and a reduction in body weight, whereas biphasic insulin aspart 70/30, also used twice daily, resulted in equal lowering of A_{1c} but an increase in body weight. *HbA1c* hemoglobin A_{1c}; *ITT* intention to treat; *LOCF* last observation carried forward [(**A**) adapted from Bunck et al. [9], (**B**) adapted from Nauck et al. [10], and (**C**) adapted from Gallwitz et al. [11]].

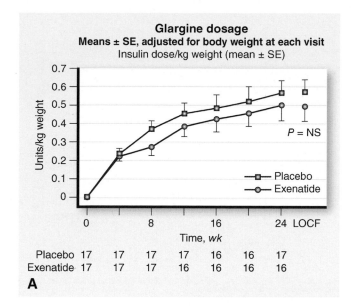

Glargine dosage
Means ± SE, adjusted for body weight at each visit
Insulin dose/kg weight (mean ± SE)

P = NS

Placebo	17	17	17	17	16	16	17
Exenatide	17	17	17	16	16	16	16

A

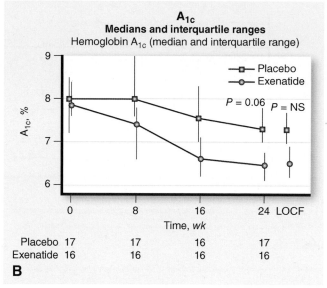

A₁c
Medians and interquartile ranges
Hemoglobin A₁c (median and interquartile range)

P = 0.06   *P* = NS

Placebo	17	17	16	17
Exenatide	16	16	16	16

B

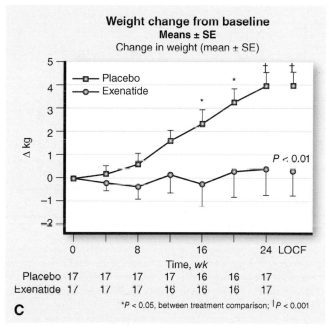

Weight change from baseline
Means ± SE
Change in weight (mean ± SE)

P < 0.01

Placebo	17	17	17	17	16	16	17
Exenatide	17	17	17	16	16	16	17

*P < 0.05, between treatment comparison; †P < 0.001

C

Figure 10-9. Mexelin study results: Metformin plus exenatide or placebo each added to titrated basal insulin. This study evaluated the efficacy of adding exenatide in patients who are being treated with a combination of metformin and basal insulin as insulin glargine. The insulin dose was titrated upward based on fasting plasma glucose (**A**) and A₁c improvement (**B**). Weight remained stable in the exenatide group but was increased with insulin dose titration in the placebo group (**C**). *LOCF* last observation carried forward [(**A–C**) adapted from Riddle et al. [12]].

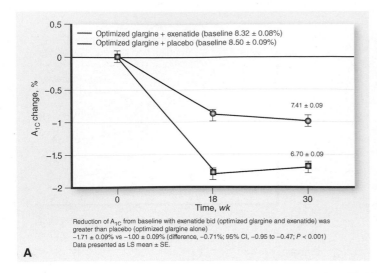

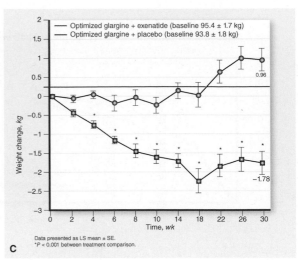

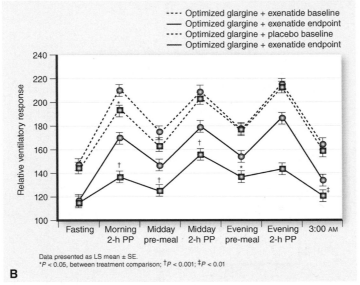

FIGURE 18-10. Add-on exenatide to insulin glargine-treated type 2 diabetes patients A_{1c} change from baseline. In this study, exenatide was added to optimized insulin glargine. There was greater lowering of A_{1c} in the exenatide group (**A**). The addition of exenatide resulted in greater lowering of postprandial glucose levels (**B**). There was weight reduction in the exenatide group (**C**). bid – twice a day; *LS* least squares [(**A–C**) adapted from Buse et al. [13]].

FIGURE 18-11. Efficacy of liraglutide. The liraglutide effect and action in diabetes (LEAD) trials evaluated liraglutide in a variety of settings in type 2 diabetes, either as monotherapy in LEAD-3 vs. glimepiride, in combination with metformin (MET) in LEAD-2 vs. both placebo and glimepiride, in combination with sulfonylurea (SFU) in LEAD-1 vs. both placebo and rosiglitazone, in combination with both metformin and a thiazolidinedione (TZD) in LEAD-4 vs. placebo, in combination with metformin and a sulfonylurea in LEAD-5 vs. placebo and insulin glargine, and in LEAD-6 vs. exenatide. A study in combination with metformin was also done, comparing liraglutide to sitagliptin. (**A**) A_{1c} changes in this series of studies are shown, most of which included two doses of liraglutide: 1.2 and 1.8 mg daily. (**B**) Changes in fasting plasma glucose in the LEAD studies are shown. (**C**) Changes in body weight in the LEAD studies are shown. *ADA* American Diabetes Association; *HbA1c* hemoglobin A_{1c}; *OAD* oral antidiabetic. [(**A, C**) adapted from Garber et al. [14], Nauck et al. [15], Marre et al. [16], Zinman et al. [17], Russell-Jones et al. [18], and Pratley et al. [20]; (**B**) adapted from Garber et al. [14], Nauck et al. [15], Marre et al. [16], Zinman et al. [17], Russell-Jones et al. [18], and Buse et al. [19]].

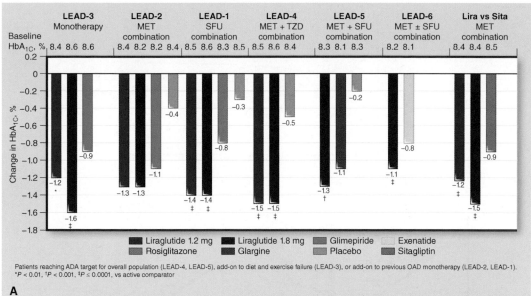

Patients reaching ADA target for overall population (LEAD-4, LEAD-5), add-on to diet and exercise failure (LEAD-3), or add-on to previous OAD monotherapy (LEAD-2, LEAD-1).
*$P < 0.01$, †$P < 0.001$, ‡$P \leq 0.0001$, vs active comparator

A

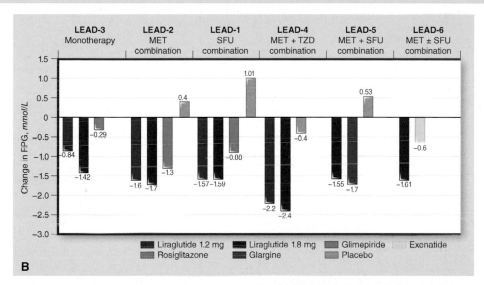

B

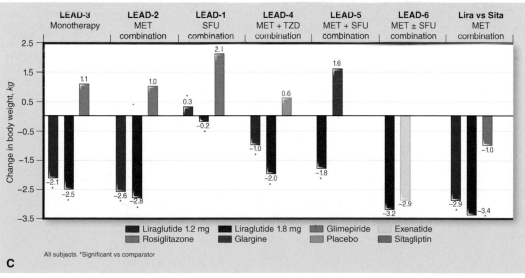

All subjects. *Significant vs comparator

C

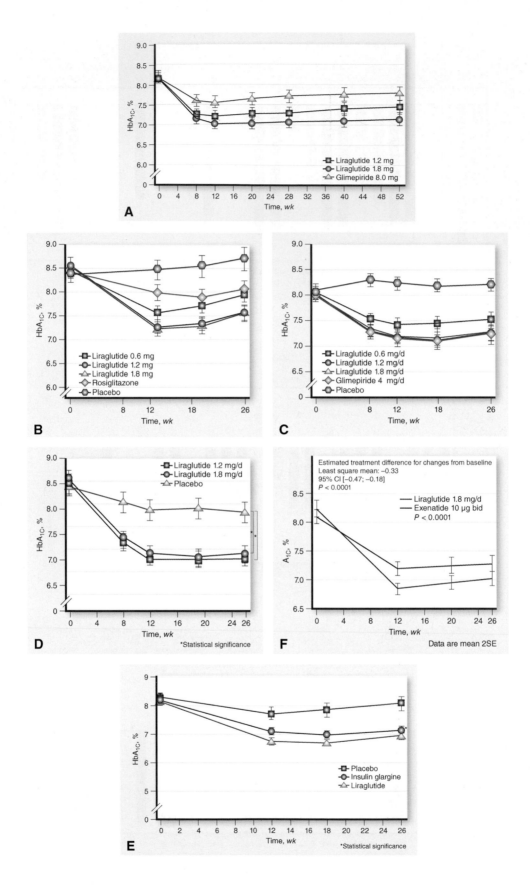

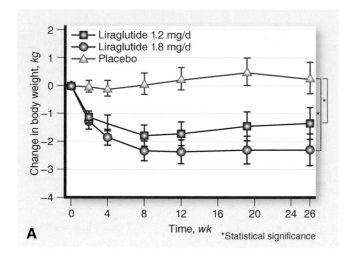

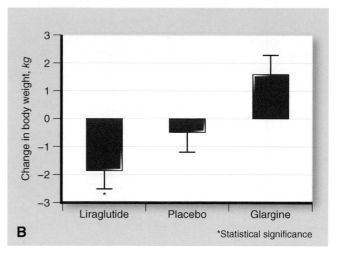

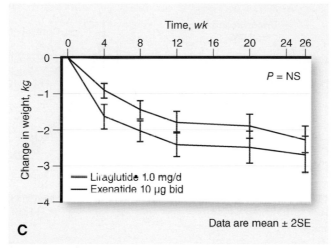

Figure 18-13. Liraglutide: Liraglutide effect and action in diabetes (LEAD) trial results. (**A**) Changes in body weight over time in LEAD-4, a trial on background metformin and rosiglitazone comparing liraglutide with placebo, are shown. (**B**) Changes in body weight in LEAD-5, a trial on background metformin and sulfonylurea comparing liraglutide with both placebo and insulin glargine, are shown. (**C**) Changes in A_{1c} over time in LEAD-5, a trial on background metformin and sulfonylurea comparing liraglutide with exenatide, are shown. bid – twice a day [(**A**) adapted from Zinman et al. [17]; (**B**) adapted from Russell-Jones et al. [18]; (**C**) adapted from Buse et al. [19]].

Figure 18-12. A_{1c} change over time: Liraglutide effect and action in diabetes (LEAD) trial results. (**A**) Changes in A_{1c} over time in LEAD-3, a monotherapy trial comparing liraglutide and glimepiride. (**B**) Changes in A_{1c} over time in LEAD-1, a trial on background sulfonylurea, comparing liraglutide with both placebo and rosiglitazone. (**C**) Changes in A_{1c} over time in LEAD-2, a trial on background metformin, comparing liraglutide with both placebo and glimepiride. (**D**) Changes in A_{1c} over time in LEAD-4, a trial on background metformin and rosiglitazone, comparing liraglutide with placebo. (**E**) Changes in A_{1c} over time in LEAD-5, a trial on background metformin and sulfonylurea, comparing liraglutide with both placebo and insulin glargine. (**F**) Changes in A_{1c} over time in LEAD-6, a trial on background metformin and sulfonylurea, comparing liraglutide with exenatide. *HbA1c* hemoglobin A_{1c}; bid twice a day [(**A**) adapted from Garber et al. [14]; (**B**) adapted from Marre et al. [16]; (**C**) adapted from Nauck et al. [15]; (**D**) adapted from Zinman et al. [17]; (**E**) adapted from Russell-Jones et al. [18]; (**F**) adapted from Buse et al. [19]].

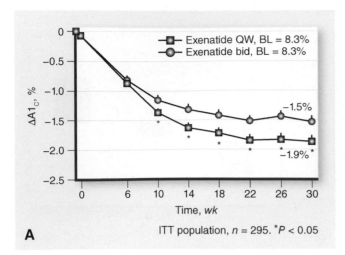

A

ITT population, *n* = 295. *P < 0.05

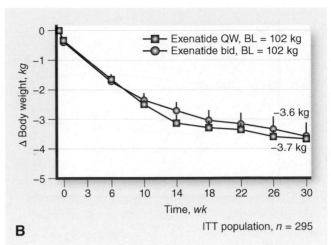

B

ITT population, *n* = 295

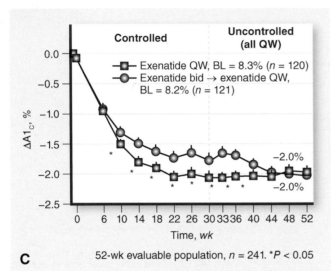

C

52-wk evaluable population, *n* = 241. *P < 0.05

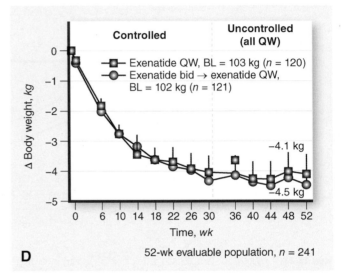

D

52-wk evaluable population, *n* = 241

Figure 18-14. Results of the diabetes therapy utilization: Researching changes in A$_{1c}$, weight, and other factors through intervention with exenatide once weekly (DURATION-1) trial, which compared exenatide once weekly (QW) with exenatide twice daily (bid). Changes in A$_{1c}$ (**A**) and body weight (**B**) over time are shown. Changes in A$_{1c}$ (**C**) and body weight (**D**) over time in an extension of DURATION-1 are shown, in which subjects previously treated with exenatide twice daily were subsequently converted to exenatide once weekly. *BL* baseline; *ITT* intention to treat [(**A**, **B**) adapted from Drucker et al. [21]; (**C**, **D**) adapted from Buse et al. [22]].

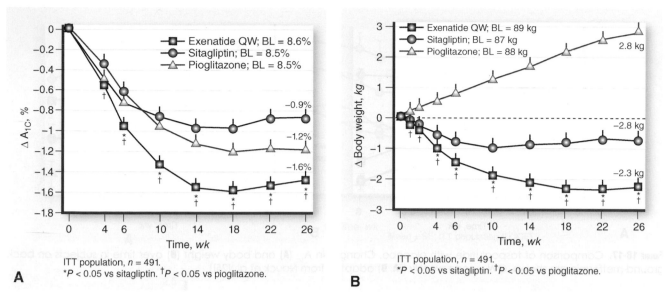

A

ITT population, n = 491.
*P < 0.05 vs sitagliptin. †P < 0.05 vs pioglitazone.

B

ITT population, n = 491.
*P < 0.05 vs sitagliptin. †P < 0.05 vs pioglitazone.

Figure 18-15. Results of DURATION-2, a trial comparing exenatide once weekly (QW) with sitagliptin and pioglitazone. Changes in A_{1c} (**A**) and body weight (**B**) over time are shown. *ITT* intention to treat; *BL* baseline [(**A**, **B**) adapted from Bergenstal et al. [23]].

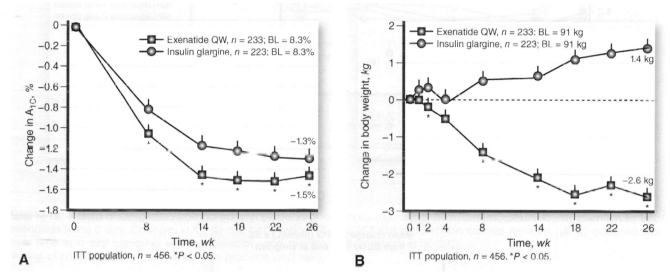

A ITT population, n = 456. *P < 0.05.

B ITT population, n = 456. *P < 0.05.

Figure 18-16. Results of DURATION-3, a trial comparing exenatide once weekly (QW) with insulin glargine. Changes in A_{1c} (**A**) and body weight (**B**) over time are shown. *BL* baseline [(**A**, **B**) adapted from Diamant et al. [24]].

Incretin Enhancers

As previously noted, the rapid degradation of GLP-1 by DPP-4, converting it from its active form to an inactive form, has precluded the clinical use of GLP-1. The sequence of secretion and rapid degradation of GLP-1 is schematically depicted in Fig. 18.21a. The inhibition of DPP-4 increases levels of the active form of GLP-1, as schematically depicted in Fig. 18.21b. This increase has led to the pharmacological approach of developing incretin enhancers by using DPP-4 inhibitors (also known as *gliptins*). The chemical structures of several DPP-4 inhibitors are shown in Fig. 18.21c. The DPP-4 inhibitors work by blocking inactivation of the incretins, thus serving to prolong the circulation of the active forms both of GLP-1 and GIP, as shown in Fig. 18.22a. As a consequence, there also is a reduction in plasma glucagon levels (see Fig. 18.22b) and an improvement in glucose profiles throughout the day (see Fig. 18.22c).

The first DPP-4 inhibitor to be approved was sitagliptin (Januvia; Merck, Whitehouse Station, NJ). Figures 18.23–18.26 demonstrate the glycemic effects of sitagliptin (Januvia). Similar effects are shown for vildagliptin (Galvus and Zomelis; Novartis, Basel, Switzerland), which is not available in the USA, in Figs. 18.27 and 18.28. The glycemic effects of saxagliptin (Onglyza; Bristol-Myers Squibb; New York) are shown in Figs. 18.29 and 18.30. Alogliptin (Nesina; Takeda, Deerfield, IL) is another DPP-4 inhibitor in development; its glycemic effects are shown in Figs. 18.31 and 18.32. Another DPP-4 inhibitor is linagliptin (Trajenta; Boehringer Ingelheim, Ridgefield, CT), the effects of which are shown in Figs. 18.33 and 18.34.

There also are combination products of a DPP-4 plus metformin. These include sitagliptin plus metformin (Janumet; Merck), vildagliptin plus metformin (Eucreas; Novartis), and saxagliptin plus metformin (Kombiglyze XR; AstraZeneca; Wilmington, DE). These are quite logical combinations since DPP-4s and metformin have complementary mechanisms of action and most usage of DPP-4s is likely to be in combination with metformin. Alogliptin is being developed in combination with metformin and in combination with pioglitazone.

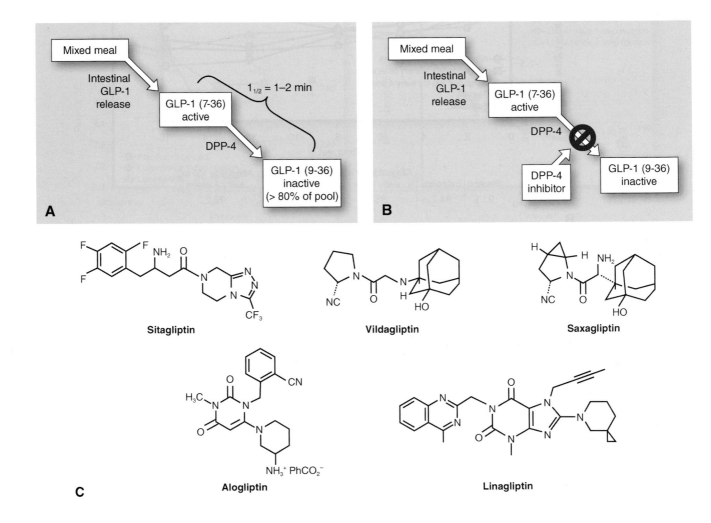

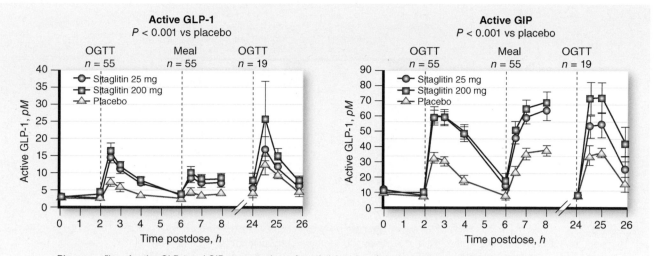

Active GLP-1
P < 0.001 vs placebo

Active GIP
P < 0.001 vs placebo

Plasma profiles of active GLP-1 and GIP concentrations after administration of single oral doses of sitaglitin 25 or 200 mg or placebo and OGTTS at 2 and 24 h postdose and a standardized meal at 6 h postdose. Data are expressed as geometric mean ± SE.

A

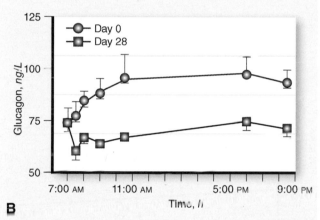

B

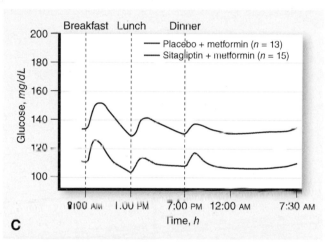

C

Figure 18-22. Impact of DPP-4 inhibition. (**A**) The impact of DPP-4 inhibition on circulating levels of the active incretins, GLP-1 and GIP, is illustrated with sitagliptin. (**B**) The impact of DPP-4 inhibition on the circulating plasma glucagon profile, illustrated with vildagliptin, used 100 mg twice daily for 28 days. These results suggest that one of the mechanisms by which DPP-4 inhibitors improve glycemic control may be reduced glucagon levels. (**C**) The impact of DPP-4 inhibition on 24-h glucose profile is illustrated with sitagliptin. Glucose levels were reduced throughout the day during both the postprandial and fasting periods. *OGTT* oral glucose tolerance test. [(**A**) adapted from Herman et al. [31]; (**B**) adapted from Mari et al. [32]; (**C**) adapted from Brazdy et al. [33]].

Figure 18-21. GLP-1 secretion and inactivation. Much interest has developed in the incretins as potential therapeutic agents for treatment of type 2 diabetes. However, problems have occurred with the administration of native GLP-1 and glucose-dependent insulinotropic peptide. Although a continuous infusion of GLP-1 has been used to demonstrate the potential of this hormone as a therapeutic agent, the rapid degradation of the hormone from its active to inactive form by DPP-4 has precluded the clinical use of GLP-1: continuous infusion was deemed expensive and impractical. (**A**) The sequence of secretion and rapid degradation of GLP-1 is shown. (**B**) The inhibition of DPP-4 to increase active GLP-1 prolongs the duration of circulating GLP-1 and, as a consequence, DPP-4 inhibitors that prevent the inactivation of the incretins (both GLP-1 and GIP) have been developed as pharmacologic agents, as shown. (**C**) The chemical structures of several DPP-4 inhibitors are shown [(**A**, **B**) adapted from Drucker [29]; (**C**) adapted from Deacon [30]].

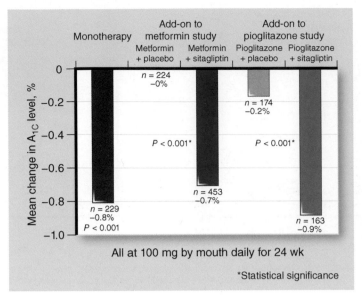

Figure 18-23. Changes in A$_{1c}$ in three sitagliptin studies: The first as monotherapy, the second adding sitagliptin (vs. placebo) to metformin, and the third adding sitagliptin (vs. placebo) to pioglitazone (adapted from Aschner et al. [34], Charbonnel et al. [35], and Rosenstock et al. [36]).

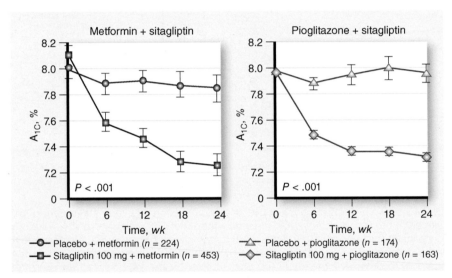

Figure 18-24. Changes in A$_{1c}$ over time in two trials, one adding sitagliptin (vs. placebo) to metformin and the other adding sitagliptin (vs. placebo) to pioglitazone (adapted from Charbonnel et al. [35] and Rosenstock et al. [36]).

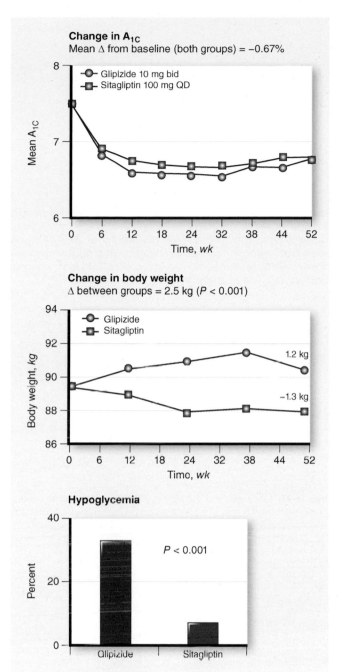

Change in A$_{1C}$
Mean Δ from baseline (both groups) = −0.67%

Change in body weight
Δ between groups = 2.5 kg (*P* < 0.001)

Hypoglycemia

FIGURE 18-25. Changes in A$_{1c}$, body weight, and the frequency of hypoglycemia in a study comparing the addition of either sitagliptin or glipizide in patients who are already on metformin. The hypoglycemia rates were significantly different and there were 22 episodes of severe hypoglycemia with glipizide while only two with sitagliptin. bid – twice a day; QD – daily (adapted from Nauck et al. [37]).

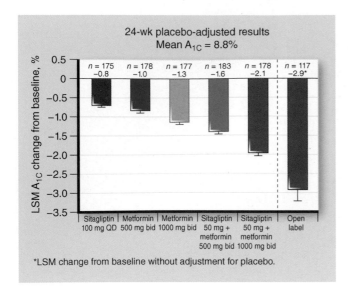

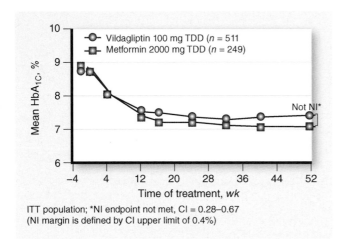

Figure 18-26. Results of a study in which initial pharmacologic therapy was with metformin, sitagliptin, or a combination of the two. Data shown are A_{1c} reductions over 24 weeks, an open-label extension of the combination of sitagliptin and the higher metformin dose. bid – twice a day; *LSM* least squares method; QD – daily (adapted from Goldstein et al. [38]).

Figure 18-27. Changes in A_{1c} over time in a trial comparing vildagliptin and metformin as monotherapy. *CI* confidence interval; *HbA1c* hemoglobin A_{1c}; *NI* noninferiority; *TDD* total daily dose (adapted from Schweizer et al. [39]).

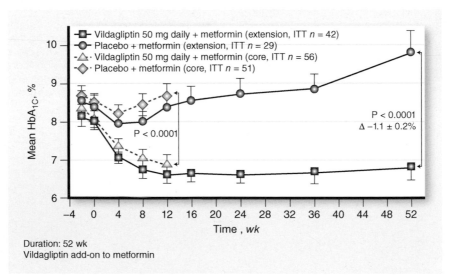

Figure 18-28. Changes in A_{1c} over time in which vildagliptin was added in subjects who were already treated with metformin. The initial 12-week period was a double-blind, placebo-controlled study. The 12-week core study was followed by a 40-week extension that allowed a comparison of the efficacy of vildagliptin with that of placebo over 1 year. *n* refers to the intention-to-treat (ITT) population. *HbA1c* hemoglobin A_{1c} (adapted from Ahrén et al. [40]).

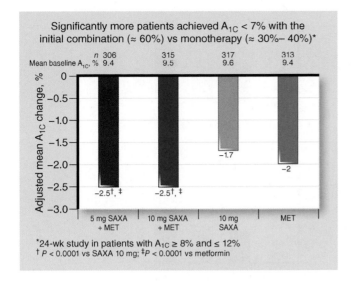

Figure 18-29. A$_{1c}$ change with initial saxagliptin and metformin vs. monotherapy. A study in which initial pharmacologic therapy was with metformin, saxagliptin, or a combination of the two. Data shown are A$_{1c}$ reductions over 24 weeks. *MET* metformin; *SAXA* saxagliptin (adapted from Jadzinsky et al. [41]).

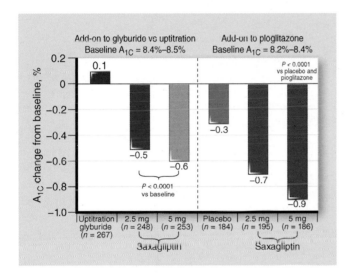

Figure 18-30. Add-on efficacy of saxagliptin: Change in A$_{1c}$ at 24 weeks. The change in A$_{1c}$ in two trials, one adding saxagliptin to glyburide (in which the control group had an uptitration of glyburide) and the other adding saxagliptin (vs. placebo) to pioglitazone, is shown (adapted from Chacra et al. [42] and Hollander [43]).

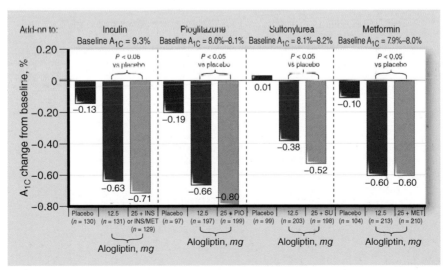

Figure 18-31. Alogliptin in combination therapy: Change in A$_{1c}$ at 26 weeks. Changes in A$_{1c}$ in four trials are shown, all comparing alogliptin to placebo (PBO). The first adds alogliptin to insulin, the second adds alogliptin to pioglitazone, the third adds alo- gliptin to glyburide, and the fourth adds alogliptin to metformin. *INS* insulin; *MET* metformin; *PIO* pioglitazone; *PBO* placebo (adapted from Rosenstock et al. [44], Pratley et al. [45, 46], and Nauck et al. [47]).

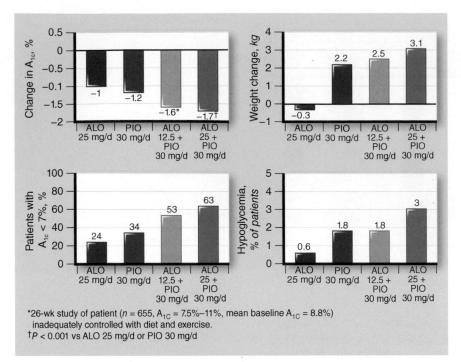

*26-wk study of patient (n = 655, A$_{1C}$ = 7.5%–11%, mean baseline A$_{1C}$ = 8.8%) inadequately controlled with diet and exercise.

†P < 0.001 vs ALO 25 mg/d or PIO 30 mg/d

FIGURE 18-32. Initial combination therapy with alogliptin and pioglitazone. A study in which initial pharmacologic therapy was with alogliptin, pioglitazone, or a combination of the two drugs. Data shown are A$_{1c}$ reductions over 26 weeks, weight change over 26 weeks, the proportion of subjects achieving A$_{1c}$ less than 7%, and the proportion of patients having hypoglycemia. *ALO* alogliptin; *PIO* pioglitazone (adapted from Rosenstock et al. [48]).

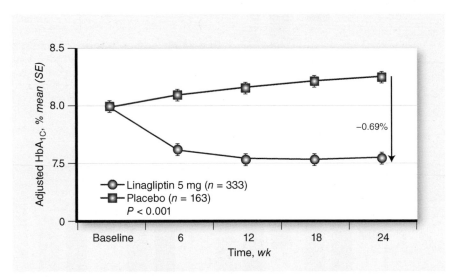

FIGURE 18-33. Linagliptin monotherapy trial. Changes in A$_{1c}$ over time in a trial are shown, comparing linagliptin (as monotherapy) and placebo. *HbA1c* hemoglobin A$_{1c}$ (adapted from Del Prato et al. [49]).

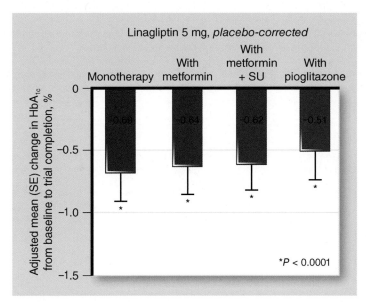

Figure 18-34. Linagliptin clinical research program: Consistent hemoglobin A~1c~ (HbA~1c~) reductions. The change in A~1c~ in four trials is shown. All trials compared linagliptin to placebo; one studied linagliptin as monotherapy, the second studied adding linagliptin to metformin, the third studied adding linagliptin to the combination of metformin and sulfonylurea (SU), and the fourth studied adding linagliptin to pioglitazone (adapted from Del Prato et al. [49], Taskinen et al. [50], Owens et al. [51], and Gomis et al. [52]).

Dopamine Agonists

Bromocriptine, an ergot derivative, is a dopamine receptor agonist. Bromocriptine-QR (Cycloset; VeroScience, Tiverton, RI) is one of the newest oral medications to receive approval by the FDA. Although the mechanism of action by which bromocriptine QR improves glycemic control in humans is not fully understood, it is presumed to exert its actions on the central nervous system. Figure 18.35 summarizes the proposed mechanism of action of bromocriptine-QR. The glyce-mic effects of bromocriptine-QR (Cycloset) are depicted in Figs. 18.36 and 18.37. One of the most interesting things about bromocriptine-QR is the results of a safety study that included more than 3,000 patients with type 2 diabetes who received either bromocriptine QR or placebo. The cardiovascular outcomes of that study are depicted in Fig. 18.38; these results demonstrate a reduction in cardiovascular events in the bromocriptine-QR group.

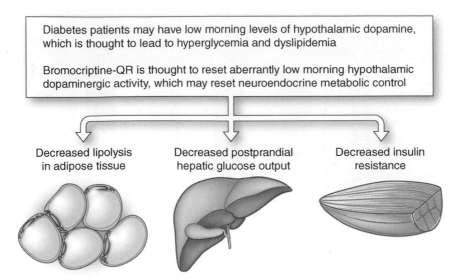

Diabetes patients may have low morning levels of hypothalamic dopamine, which is thought to lead to hyperglycemia and dyslipidemia

Bromocriptine-QR is thought to reset aberrantly low morning hypothalamic dopaminergic activity, which may reset neuroendocrine metabolic control

Decreased lipolysis in adipose tissue

Decreased postprandial hepatic glucose output

Decreased insulin resistance

FIGURE 18-35. Bromocriptine-QR: Proposed mechanism of action. Low hypothalamic dopamine release, particularly at the suprachiasmatic nuclei (SCN), is coupled with elevated norepinephrine and serotonin release at the ventromedial hypothalamus (VMH) and each is a characteristic neurophysiological feature of diabetes. This hypothalamic alteration potentiates increases in circulating glucose, free fatty acids, and triglycerides, which in turn contribute to insulin resistance in the liver and muscle and β-cell dysfunction via lipotoxicity and glucotoxicity. In an animal model of type 2 diabetes, timed-pulse bromocriptine-QR increased SCN (and elsewhere in the central nervous system) the dopaminergic tone and decreased the VMH norepinephrine and serotonin release in insulin-resistant animal models. These neurophysiological activities are believed to represent a target-response system responsible for the subsequent multiple downstream biochemical effects of timed Cycloset administration in peripheral tissues, such as adipose tissue and the liver (adapted from Meier and Cincotta [53]).

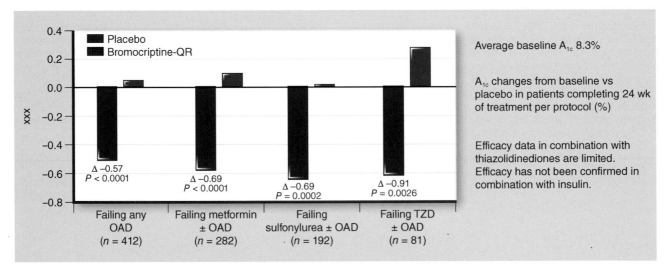

Average baseline A_{1c} 8.3%

A_{1c} changes from baseline vs placebo in patients completing 24 wk of treatment per protocol (%)

Efficacy data in combination with thiazolidinediones are limited. Efficacy has not been confirmed in combination with insulin.

FIGURE 18-36. Bromocriptine-QR: Evaluation of A_{1c} reduction. The change in A_{1c} among subjects with a baseline $A_{1c} \geq 7.5\%$, who are taking one or two oral diabetes medications and complete 24 weeks of therapy with bromocriptine-QR (vs. placebo), is shown. Subgroups were defined as: (1) all subjects on one or two oral antidiabetics (OADs) of any type (n, bromocriptine-QR = 261, placebo = 151); (2) subjects on metformin and another OAD (n, bromocriptine-QR = 181, placebo = 101); (3) subjects on sulfonylurea and/or another OAD (n, bromocriptine-QR = 76, placebo = 106); and (4) subjects on thiazolidinediones and/or OAD. TZD thiazolidinediones (adapted from Scranton et al. [54] and Cincotta et al. [55]).

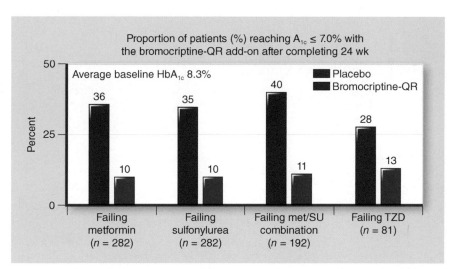

FIGURE 18-37. Bromocriptine-QR: Percent reaching the A_{1c} goal of less than or equal to 7 after 24 weeks. For the subset of patients with baseline A_{1c} greater than 7.5%, the proportion of those who reach an A_{1c} target of less than 7% compared to a placebo in the subset of patients on metformin, sulfonylureas (SU), both metformin (met) and sulfonylureas, or thiazolidinediones (TZDs) is shown. *HbA1c* hemoglobin A_{1c} (adapted from Scranton et al. [54] and Cincotta et al. [55]).

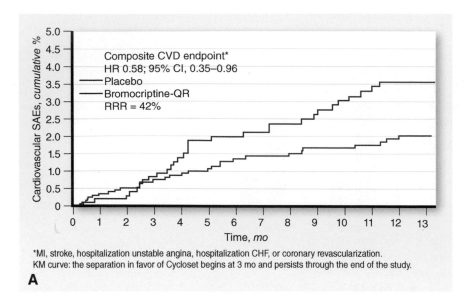

*MI, stroke, hospitalization unstable angina, hospitalization CHF, or coronary revascularization.
KM curve: the separation in favor of Cycloset begins at 3 mo and persists through the end of the study.

A

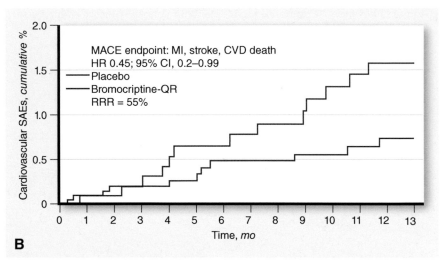

B

Figure 18-38. Bromocriptine-QR Safety Trial results: Percent composite cardiovascular disease (CVD) end point (**A**) and post hoc analysis of cumulative percent the major adverse cardiac event (MACE) end point (**B**). (**A**) These data are from a safety study involving 3,095 patients with type 2 diabetes randomized 2:1 to bromocriptine-QR or placebo. The cumulative frequency of prespecified composite cardiovascular events (defined as myocardial infarction [MI], stroke, coronary revascularization, or hospitalization for either unstable angina or congestive heart failure) is shown. There is a 42% relative risk reduction (RRR) in the bromocriptine-QR group. (**B**) In the safety study, the cumulative frequency of a post hoc analysis of a composite cardiovascular end point (defined as MI, stroke, or CVD death) is depicted. There is a 55% RRR in the bromocriptine-QR group. *CHF* chronic heart failure; *SAE* serious adverse event (adapted from Gaziano et al. [56]).

Bile Acid Sequestrants

Bile acid sequestrants have long been used in the treatment of lipid elevations, with lowering of low-density lipoprotein-cholesterol (LDL-C). For cholesterol lowering, these agents work by binding bile acids, particularly glycocholic acid, in the intestines to form a product that is excreted. One bile acid sequestrant, colesevelam (Welchol; Daiichi-Sankyo, Tokyo, Japan), has also been approved for the treatment of type 2 diabetes, although its mechanism of action for glucose lowering is unknown. The effects of colesevelam (Welchol) on both glucose and LDL-C in patients with type 2 diabetes are shown in Fig. 18.39.

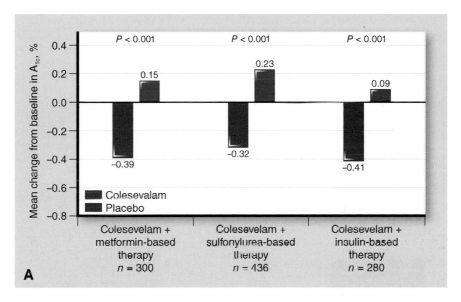

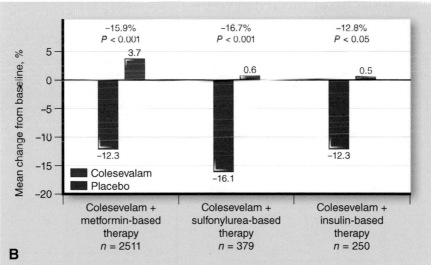

Figure 18-39. Colesevelam effects. In a series of three studies to assess the glucose-lowering effects of colesevelam added to metformin-, sulfonylurea-, or insulin-based therapy, colesevelam consistently produced significant reductions in A$_{1c}$ (**A**) and low-density lipoprotein-cholesterol (LDL-C) (**B**) compared with placebo. (**A**) In this figure, colesevelam's ability to facilitate glycemic control in patients with type 2 diabetes is shown. This figure compares the placebo-adjusted change in A$_{1c}$ with the three treatment regimens. (**B**) The effect of colesevelam added to antidiabetic therapy is shown. This figure compares the placebo-adjusted change in LDL-C for the three treatment regimens (adapted from Fonseca et al. [57]).

Amylin Mimetics

The hormone amylin was first isolated and characterized at Oxford University from amyloid deposits in the islets of Langerhans and was reported in 1987. Amylin is colocalized with insulin in secretory granules within pancreatic islet β cells (as depicted in Fig. 18.40a) and is cosecreted with insulin (as depicted in Fig. 18.40b). Pramlintide (Symlin; Amylin Pharmaceuticals, San Diego, CA) is a human amylin analogue specifically engineered with three proline substitutions to overcome the tendency of human amylin to self-aggregate. The prandial administration of pramlintide in addition to prandial insulin improves prandial glycemic control, regardless of whether the prandial insulin is a regular or rapid-acting insulin analogue (see Fig. 18.41). The clinical effects in both type 2 and type 1 diabetes are depicted in Figs. 18.42 and 18.43 while Fig. 18.44 shows the data from a recent study comparing prandial pramlintide with prandial insulin in patients with type 2 diabetes being treated with a basal insulin.

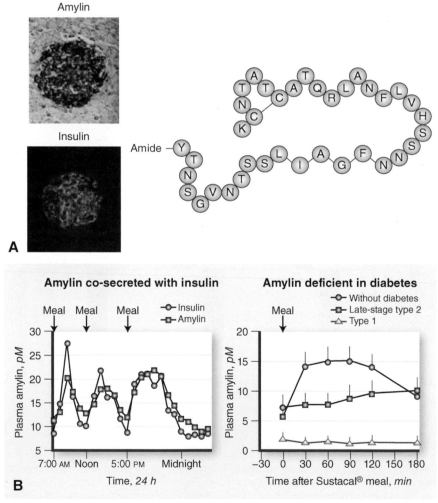

FIGURE 18-40. Amylin: The "other" β-cell hormone. (A) Amylin, a 37-amino acid peptide, is colocalized with insulin in secretory granules within pancreatic islet β cells and is cosecreted with insulin. Also shown is the amino acid sequence of human amylin. (B) Amylin is cosecreted with insulin in healthy individuals (*left panel*) and has a secretory pattern similar to that of insulin in patients with type 1 and type 2 diabetes [(B) adapted from Kruger et al. [59]].

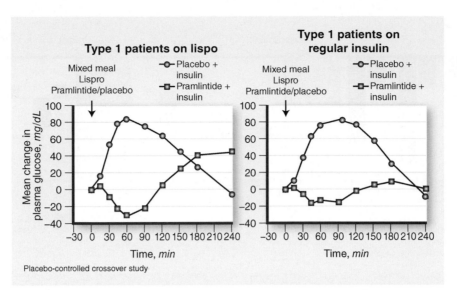

FIGURE 18-41. Addition of pramlintide to insulin. The addition of the amylin analogue pramlintide to insulin improves postprandial glucose control. The prandial administration of pramlintide in addition to prandial insulin improves prandial glycemic control, regardless of whether the prandial insulin is regular or a rapid-acting insulin analogue (adapted from Weyer et al. [60]).

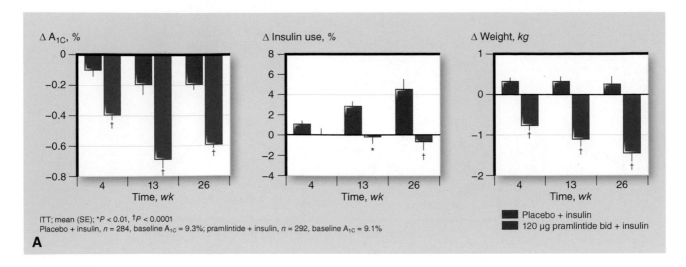

Figure 18-42. Pramlintide clinical effects: Type 1 and type 2 diabetes combined pivotal trials. (**A**) Shown is data from a post hoc analysis of pooled data from patients with type 2 diabetes who received 120 μg pramlintide twice a day (bid) in pivotal trials, showing that pramlintide-treated subjects had an overall reduction in A_{1c} with less insulin used, as well as a reduction in weight compared with placebo. (**B**) Shown is data from a post hoc analysis of pooled data from patients

with type 1 diabetes who received 30 or 60 μg pramlintide three or four times a day in pivotal trials, showing that pramlintide-treated subjects had an overall reduction in A_{1c} with less insulin used, as well as a reduction in weight compared with placebo. However, in the pivotal trials included in the analysis, no titration of insulin doses occurred. *ITT* intention to treat; qid – four times a day; tid – three times a day (adapted from Edelman et al. [61]).

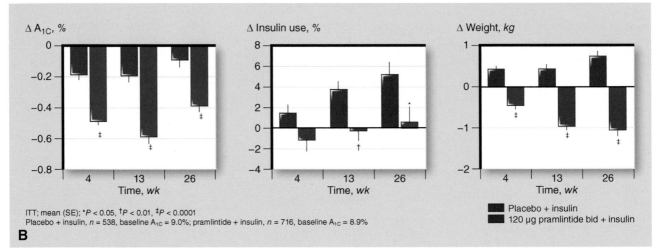

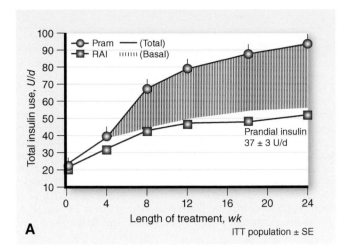

A

ITT population ± SE

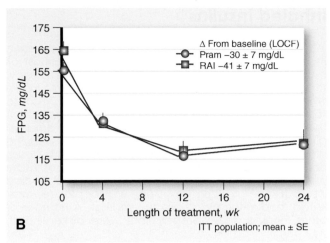

B

ITT population; mean ± SE

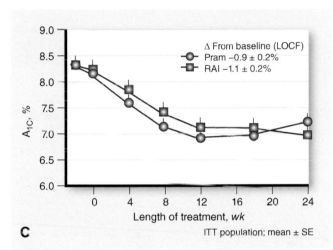

C

ITT population; mean ± SE

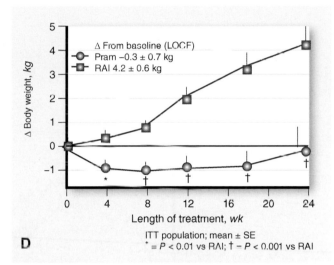

D

ITT population; mean ± SE
* = P < 0.01 vs RAI; † = P < 0.001 vs RAI

FIGURE 18-44. Pramlintide (Pram) vs. rapid-acting insulin, each added to titrated basal insulin: **(A)** insulin doses, **(B)** fasting plasma glucose (FPG), **(C)** A₁ᴄ, and **(D)** weight. **(A)** In this study, 113 subjects were randomized 1:1 to pramlintide or rapid-acting insulin (RAI). In both groups, basal insulin was titrated to achieve a fasting plasma glucose of 70–100 mg/dl. Oral diabetes medication was continued. This panel shows total insulin use during the study. Basal insulin doses were similar in both groups. **(B)** Shows that there was a similar decrement on fasting plasma glucose in both groups and **(C)** shows that there was a similar decrement on A₁ᴄ in both groups. **(D)** Shows that there was a weight gain in the rapid-acting insulin analogue group, but not in the pramlintide group. Fewer patients reported mild to moderate hypoglycemia with pramlintide, but more reported nausea. There was no severe hypoglycemia in either group. *ITT* intention to treat; *LOCF* last observation carried forward (adapted from Riddle et al. [63]).

FIGURE 18-43. Pramlintide clinical effects: Type 1 diabetes dose-titration study. Shown are results from a randomized placebo-controlled trial in 295 subjects with type 1 diabetes on intensive insulin therapy, randomized to pramlintide (dose escalation for 4 weeks followed by a fixed dose of 30 or 60 μg) or placebo, with an initial 30–50% dose reduction of preprandial insulin. The study was designed to achieve equivalent glycemic control. The pramlintide group did so with weight loss while the placebo group, adjusting insulin, gained weight (adapted from Edelman et al. [62]).

Inhaled Insulins

In type 2 diabetes, a progressive decline in pancreatic β-cell function occurs such that, ultimately, almost all patients progress to the need for insulin therapy. Unfortunately, many patients do not advance to insulin when needed, despite poor glycemic control. Because some patients (and health care providers) are reluctant to initiate insulin injections, a movement to develop alternate routes of insulin delivery has begun. Since the alveolar surface area of the lung is 100–140 m² and is only one cell in thickness, pulmonary delivery of insulin has emerged as a therapeutic option. One inhaled insulin (Exubera; Pfizer, New York) was approved, marketed, and withdrawn from the market. A number of other inhaled insulin preparations were discontinued.

Figure 18.45 depicts the pharmacodynamics time-action profiles of several inhaled insulin preparations in comparison to a subcutaneous injection of rapid-acting insulin lispro. It can be seen that the upstroke of most is similar to that of lispro but with a longer tail. The exception is the very rapid-acting insulin from MannKind, Technosphere insulin (Afrezza; MannKind, Valencia, CA), which is pending regulatory approval. Its ultra-rapid profile (see Fig. 18.46) may provide a unique advantage in limiting postprandial glucose elevations while its shorter duration of action may limit both hypoglycemia and weight gain. The clinical effects of Technosphere insulin (Afrezza) are shown in Fig. 18.47 while the Afrezza inhaler is shown in Fig. 18.48.

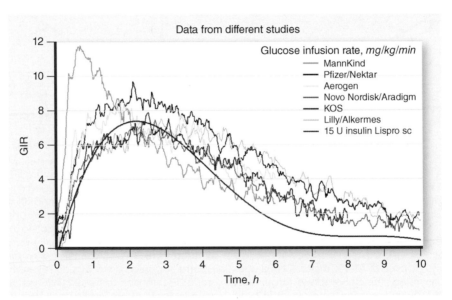

FIGURE 18-45. Time-action profiles of inhaled insulin. Inhaled insulin is a suitable prandial insulin. This figure shows the pharmacodynamics time-action profiles of several inhaled insulin preparations in comparison to a subcutaneous injection of rapid-acting insulin, lispro. It can be seen that the upstroke of most is similar to that of lispro but with a longer tail. The exception is the very rapid-acting insulin from MannKind (adapted from Heinemann et al. [64]).

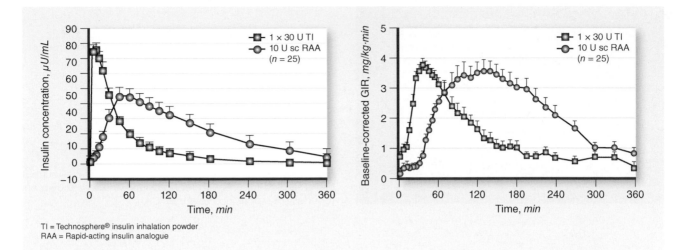

TI = Technosphere® insulin inhalation powder
RAA = Rapid-acting insulin analogue

Figure 18-46. Technosphere insulin inhalation powder (Afrezza; MannKind, Valencia, CA). This figure shows a comparison of the pharmacokinetics and pharmacodynamics of single insulin doses of Technosphere insulin powder and subcutaneous insulin lispro in subjects with type 1 diabetes utilizing a glucose clamp. In the left panel, the peak plasma insulin concentrations measured after Technosphere insulin inhalation were observed at 10 min, whereas the peak lispro concentrations following subcutaneous injection occurred at 60 min. In the right panel, the pharmacokinetic differences translate into the need for a more rapid glucose infusion for Technosphere with a median T_{max} of 35 min and for lispro a corresponding glucose response peak at 110 min. [65].

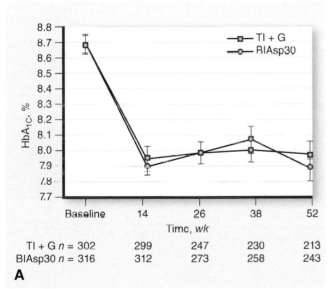

| TI + G n = | 302 | 299 | 247 | 230 | 213 |
| BIAsp30 n = | 316 | 312 | 273 | 258 | 243 |

A

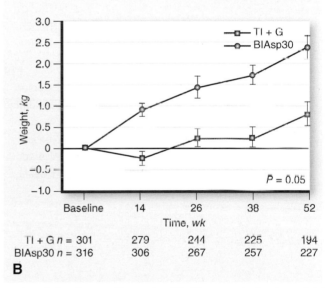

| TI + G n = | 301 | 279 | 244 | 225 | 194 |
| BIAsp30 n = | 316 | 306 | 267 | 257 | 227 |

B

Figure 18-47. Mean hemoglobin A_{1c} (HbA$_{1c}$) (**A**) and change from baseline (**B**) in the intention-to-treat population. (**A**) Changes in A$_{1c}$ over time in a study comparing prandial inhaled insulin (plus subcutaneous, basal insulin glargine [G]) with twice-daily, subcutaneous, biphasic insulin aspart (BIAsp) 70/30 in subjects with type 2 diabetes are shown. The reduction from baseline in A$_{1c}$ was comparable between groups and sustained over 52 weeks. (**B**) Changes in body weight over time in a study comparing prandial inhaled insulin (plus subcutaneous basal insulin G) with twice-daily, subcutaneous, biphasic insulin aspart 70/30 in subjects with type 2 diabetes are shown. There was less weight gain in the inhaled insulin group. *TI* Technosphere insulin (adapted from Rosenstock et al. [66]).

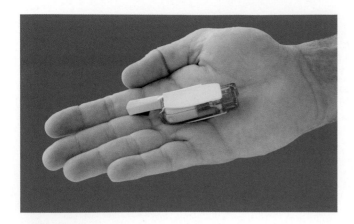

Figure 18-48. Technosphere insulin inhaler. The inhaler currently being studied for use with Technosphere insulin is shown here (courtesy of MannKind, Valencia, CA).

Inhibitors of Renal Glucose Reabsorption

The concept of inhibiting renal glucose reabsorption has been studied for more than 150 years (see Fig. 18.49). Normally, glucose is filtered by the glomerulus in the kidney, and in the proximal tubule virtually all filtered glucose is reabsorbed back into the circulation through the sodium–glucose transporter-2 (SGLT-2). In the face of hyperglycemia, the capacity for glucose reabsorption may be exceeded and glycosuria may result. With the use of an inhibitor of SGLT-2, glycosuria can be increased while hyperglycemia is reduced, as less glucose is reabsorbed. This process is depicted in Fig. 18.50. No SGLT-2 inhibitors are yet approved, but data have been reported for dapagliflozin, canagliflozin, and BI-10773, as depicted in Figs. 18.51–18.53.

Phlorizin

1835	Petersen	Isolated apple bark
1886	von Mering	Glycosuric effect
1903	Stiles	Renal actions (rat)
1933	Chassis	Renal actions (human)
1962	Alvarado	Glucose transport (gut)
1987	Rossetti	Antidiabetic effect (rat)

B

Phlorizin

Figure 18-49. Phlorizin. Phlorizin, a natural inhibitor of sodium–glucose transport, was first isolated from apple bark by Petersen in 1835. It was extensively studied over the next 150 years. In the late 1980s, Rossetti and DeFronzo demonstrated in rodents with diabetes that using phlorizin to lower glucose by causing glycosuria resulted in an improvement of both insulin secretion and insulin action, and in so doing established the concept of glucose toxicity (adapted from Bailey [67]).

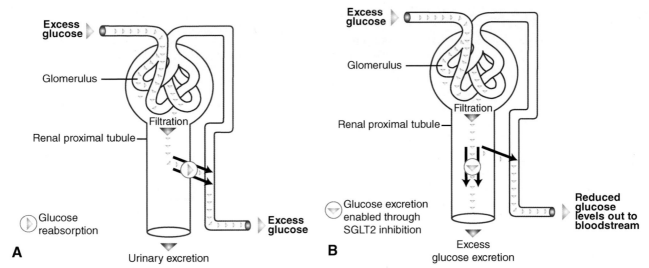

Figure 18-50. Renal glucose handling (**A**) and rationale for sodium–glucose transporter-2 (SGLT-2) in type 2 diabetes (**B**). (**A**) In healthy individuals, glucose is filtered by the glomerulus in the kidney and, in the proximal tubule, virtually all filtered glucose is reabsorbed back into the circulation. (**B**) In type 2 diabetes, the use of an SGLT-2 inhibitor results in blocking the reabsorption of glucose in the proximal tubule, thus increasing glycosuria, with consequent reduction in hyperglycemia (adapted from Bailey [67]).

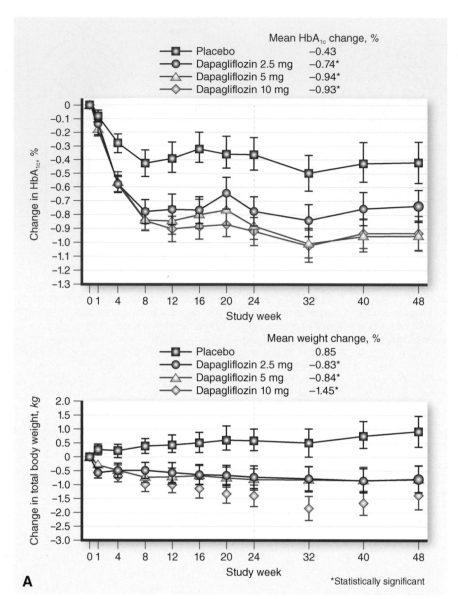

Mean HbA$_{1c}$ change, %
Placebo   −0.43
Dapagliflozin 2.5 mg   −0.74*
Dapagliflozin 5 mg   −0.94*
Dapagliflozin 10 mg   −0.93*

Mean weight change, %
Placebo   0.85
Dapagliflozin 2.5 mg   −0.83*
Dapagliflozin 5 mg   −0.84*
Dapagliflozin 10 mg   −1.45*

*Statistically significant

A

FIGURE 18-51. Dapagliflozin add-on to insulin study results. (**A**) Shown are changes in A$_{1c}$ and body weight over time in a dose-ranging study of the sodium–glucose transporter-2 (SGLT-2) inhibitor dapagliflozin (vs. placebo) in patients with type 2 diabetes already treated with insulin. (**B**) Adverse events in a study of the SGLT-2 inhibitor dapagliflozin (vs. placebo) in patients with type 2 diabetes already treated with insulin are shown. The concern is that with increasing glycosuria there may be an excess of urinary tract infections or genital infections. *HbA1c* hemoglobin A$_{1c}$ (adapted from Wilding et al. [68]).

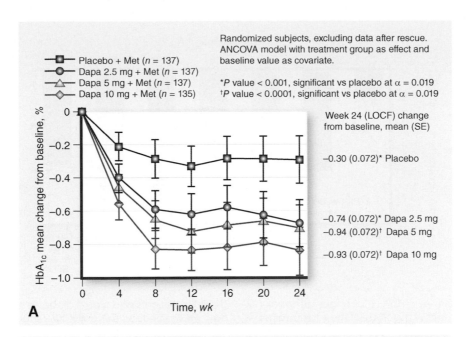

Randomized subjects, excluding data after rescue.
ANCOVA model with treatment group as effect and
baseline value as covariate.

*P value < 0.001, significant vs placebo at α = 0.019
†P value < 0.0001, significant vs placebo at α = 0.019

Legend:
- Placebo + Met (n = 137)
- Dapa 2.5 mg + Met (n = 137)
- Dapa 5 mg + Met (n = 137)
- Dapa 10 mg + Met (n = 135)

Week 24 (LOCF) change
from baseline, mean (SE)

−0.30 (0.072)* Placebo

−0.74 (0.072)* Dapa 2.5 mg
−0.94 (0.072)† Dapa 5 mg
−0.93 (0.072)† Dapa 10 mg

A

	Week 24 (LOCF)* change from baseline		Week 24 (LOCF)† % subjects with decreased body weight	
	kg (SE)	% Δ (SE)	≥ 5%	≥ 10%
Placebo	−0.89 (0.24)	−1.02 (0.29)	5.9%	0%
Dapa 2.5	−2.21 (0.24)‡	−2.66 (0.28)	24.1%	1.5%
Dapa 5	−3.04 (0.24)‡	−3.66 (0.28)	25.5%	3.6%
Dapa 10	−2.86 (0.24)‡	−3.43 (0.28)	27.8%	3.0%

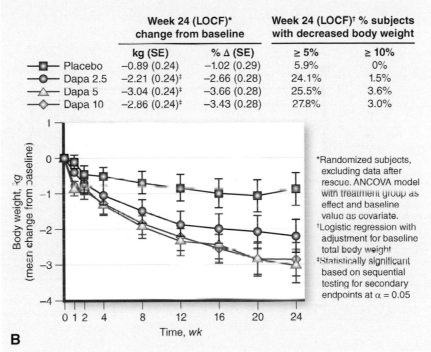

*Randomized subjects,
excluding data after
rescue. ANCOVA model
with treatment group as
effect and baseline
value as covariate.
†Logistic regression with
adjustment for baseline
total body weight
‡Statistically significant
based on sequential
testing for secondary
endpoints at α = 0.05

B

FIGURE 18-52. Dapagliflozin (Dapa) added to metformin. (**A**) Changes in A$_{1c}$ over time in a dose-ranging study of the sodium–glucose transporter-2 (SGLT-2) inhibitor dapagliflozin (vs. placebo) in patients with type 2 diabetes treated with metformin (Met) are shown (1° end point). (**B**) Changes in body weight over time in a dose-ranging study of the SGLT-2 inhibitor Dapa (vs. placebo) in patients with type 2 diabetes treated with Met are shown (2° end point). *ANCOVA* analysis of covariance; *HbA1c* hemoglobin A$_{1c}$; *LOCF* last observation carried forward (adapted from Bailey et al. [69]).

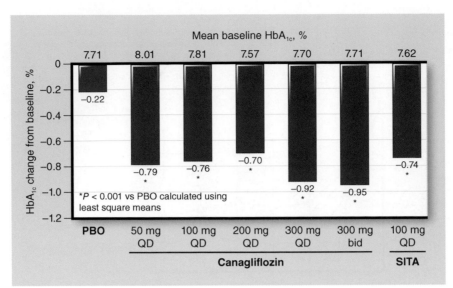

Figure 18-53. Hemoglobin A$_{1c}$ (HbA$_{1c}$) changes at week 12. Changes in A$_{1c}$ in a dose-ranging study of the sodium–glucose transporter-2 inhibitor canagliflozin (vs. both placebo and sita-gliptin) in patients with type 2 diabetes are shown. *bid* twice a day; *PBO* placebo; *QD* daily; *SITA* sitagliptin (adapted from Rosenstock et al. [70]).

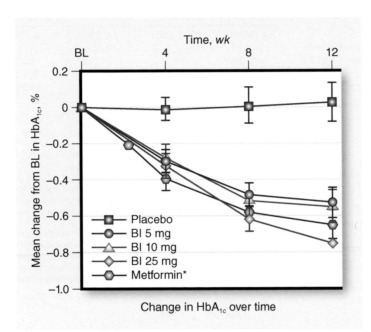

Figure 18-54. BI-10773: Mean nonadjusted change in hemoglobin (HbA$_{1c}$) from baseline over time. Changes in A$_{1c}$ over time in a dose-ranging study of the sodium–glucose transporter-2 inhibitor BI-10773 (vs. both placebo and metformin) in patients with type 2 diabetes are shown. *BL* baseline (adapted from Ferrannini et al. [71]).

Conclusion

The development of many new classes of medications for the treatment of type 2 diabetes has dramatically expanded the therapeutic options available to clinicians. Because they work on different pathways, their use in combination offers the potential of better controlling glycemia while using lower doses that avoid side effects. It has been a rapid explosion that is changing the management of the disease.

References

1. Baggio LL, Drucker DJ: Biology of incretins: GLP-1 and GIP. *Gastroenterology*. 2007, 132:2131–2157.

2. Nauck MA, Homberger E, Siegel EG, *et al.*: Incretin effects of increasing glucose loads in man calculated from venous insulin and C-peptide responses. *J Clin Endocrinol Metab* 1986, 63:492–498.

3. Nauck M, Stockmann F, Ebert R, Creutzfeldt W: Reduced incretin effect in type 2 (non-insulin-dependent) diabetes. *Diabetologia* 1986, 29:46–52.

4. Toft-Nielsen MB, Damholt MB, Madsbad S, *et al.*: Determinants of the impaired secretion of glucagon-like peptide-1 in type 2 diabetic patients. *J Clin Endocrinol Metab* 2001, 86:3717–3723.

5. DeFronzo RA, Ratner RE, Han J, *et al.*: Effects of exenatide (exendin-4) on glycemic control and weight over 30 weeks in metformin-treated patients with type 2 diabetes. *Diabetes Care* 2005, 28:1092–1100.

6. Buse JB, Henry RR, Han J, *et al.*: Effects of exenatide (exendin-4) on glycemic control over 30 weeks in sulfonylurea-treated patients with type 2 diabetes. *Diabetes Care* 2004, 27:2628–2635.

7. Kendall DM, Riddle MC, Rosenstock J, *et al.*: Effects of exenatide (exendin-4) on glycemic control over 30 weeks in patients with type 2 diabetes treated with metformin and a sulfonylurea. *Diabetes Care* 2005, 28:1083–1091.

8. Heine RJ, Van Gaal LF, Johns D, *et al.*: Exenatide versus insulin glargine in patients with suboptimally controlled type 2 diabetes: a randomized trial. *Ann Int Med* 2005, 143:559–569.

9. Bunck MC, Diamant M, Cornér A, *et al.*: One-year treatment with exenatide improves beta-cell function, compared with insulin glargine, in metformin-treated type 2 diabetic patients: a randomized, controlled, trial. *Diabetes Care* 2009, 32:762–768.

10. Nauck MA, Duran S, Kim D, *et al.*: A comparison of twice-daily exenatide and biphasic insulin aspart in patients with type 2 diabetes who were suboptimally controlled with sulfonylurea and metformin: a non-inferiority study. *Diabetologia* 2007, 50:259–267.

11. Gallwitz B, Böhmer M, Segiet T, *et al.*: Exenatide vs. insulin aspart in patients with type 2 diabetes: results of a randomised, open-label study. *Diabetologia* 2010, 53(Suppl 2): 862.

12. Riddle M, Ahmann A, Basu A, *et al.*: Metformin + exenatide + basal insulin vs metformin + placebo + basal insulin: reaching A1c <6.5% without weight-gain or serious hypoglycemia. *American Diabetes Association Annual Scientific Sessions 2010*, late-breaking abstract , poster 18-LB.

13. Buse JB, Bergenstal RM, Glass LC, *et al.*: Use of twice-daily exenatide in basal insulin–treated patients with type 2 diabetes. *Ann Intern Med* 2011, 154:103–112.

14. Garber A, Henry R, Gracia-Hernandez PA, *et al.*: Liraglutide versus glimepiride monotherapy for type 2 diabetes (LEAD-3 Mono): a randomized, 52-week, phase III, double-blind, parallel-treatment trial. *Lancet* 2009, 373:473–481.

15. Nauck M, Frid A, Hermansen K, *et al.*: Efficacy and safety comparison of liraglutide, glimepiride, and placebo, all in combination with metformin, in type 2 diabetes. The LEAD-2 Study. *Diabetes Care* 2009, 32:84–90.

16. Marre M, Shaw J, Brandle M, *et al.*: Liraglutide, a once-daily human analogue, added to a sulfonylurea over 26 weeks produces greater improvements in glycaemic and weight control compared with adding rosiglitazone or placebo in subjects with type 2 diabetes (LEAD-1 SU). *Diabet Med* 2009, 26:268–278.

17. Zinman B, Gerich J, Buse JB, *et al.*: Efficacy and safety of human glucagon-like peptide-1 analog liraglutide in combination with metformin and thiazolidinedione in patients with type 2 diabetes (LEAD-4 Met + TZD). *Diabetes Care* 2009, 32:1224–1230.

18. Russell-Jones D, Vaag A, Schmitz O, *et al.*: Liraglutide versus insulin glargine and placebo in combination with metformin and sulfonylurea therapy in type 2 diabetes mellitus (LEAD-5 met + SU): a randomized controlled trial. *Diabetologia* 2009, 52:2046–2055.

19. Buse JB, Rosenstock J, Sesti G, *et al.*: Liraglutide once a day versus exenatide twice a day for type 2 diabetes: a 26-week randomized, parallel-group, multinational, open-label trial (LEAD-6). *Lancet* 2009, 374:39–47.

20. Pratley RE, Nauck M, Bailey T, *et al.*: Liraglutide versus sitagliptin for patients with type 2 diabetes who did not have adequate glycaemic control with metformin: a 26-week, randomised, parallel-group, open-label trial. *Lancet* 2010, 375:1447–1456.

21. Drucker DJ, Buse JB, Taylor K, *et al.*: Exenatide once weekly versus twice daily for the treatment of type 2 diabetes: a randomised, open-label, non-inferiority study. *Lancet* 2008, 372:1240–1250.

22. Buse JB, Drucker DJ, Taylor KL, *et al.*: DURATION 1: exenatide once weekly produces sustained glycemic control and weight loss over 52 weeks. *Diabetes Care* 2010, 33:1255–1261.

23. Bergenstal RM, Wysham C, MacConell L, *et al.*: Efficacy and safety of exenatide once weekly versus sitagliptin or pioglitazone as an adjunct to metformin for treatment of type 2 diabetes (DURATION-2): a randomised trial. *Lancet* 2010, 376:431–439.

24. Diamant M, Van Gaal L, Stranks S, *et al.*: Once weekly exenatide compared with insulin glargine titrated to target in patients with type 2 diabetes (DURATION-3): an open-label randomised trial. *Lancet* 2010, 375:2234–2243.

25. Nauck MA, Ratner RE, Kapitza C, *et al.*: Treatment with the human once-weekly glucagon-like peptide-1 analog taspoglutide in combination with metformin improves glycemic control and lowers body weight in patients with type 2 diabetes inadequately controlled with metformin alone: a double-blind placebo-controlled study. *Diabetes Care* 2009, 32:1237–1243.

26. Gerich JE, Fonseca VA, Alvarado-Ruiz R, *et al.*: Monotherapy with GLP-1 receptor agonist, Lixisenatide, significantly improves glycaemic control in type 2 diabetic patients. *Diabetologia* 2010, 53(Suppl 2):abstract 830.

27. Rosenstock J, Reusch J, Bush M, *et al.*: Potential of albiglutide, a long-acting GLP-1 receptor agonist, in type 2 diabetes: a randomized controlled trial exploring weekly, biweekly, and monthly dosing. *Diabetes Care* 2009, 32:1880–1886.

28. Umpierrez G, Blevins T, Rosenstock J, *et al.*: The effect of LY2189265 (GLP-1 analogue) once weekly on HbA1c and beta cell function in uncontrolled type 2 diabetes mellitus: the EGO study analysis. *Diabetologia* 2009, 52(Suppl 1):abstract OP-22.

29. Drucker DJ: Enhancing incretin action for the treatment of type 2 diabetes. *Diabetes Care* 2003, 26:2929–2940.

30. Deacon CF: Dipeptidyl peptidase-4 inhibitors in the treatment of type 2 diabetes: a comparative review. *Diabetes Obes Metab* 2011, 13:7–18.

31. Herman GA, Bergman A, Stevens C, *et al.*: Effect of single oral doses of sitagliptin, a dipeptidyl peptidase-4 inhibitor, on incretin and plasma glucose levels after an oral glucose tolerance test in patients with type 2 diabetes. *J Clin Endocrinol Metab* 2006, 91:4612–4619.

32. Mari A, Sallas WM, He YL, *et al.*: Vildagliptin, a dipeptidyl peptidase-IV inhibitor, improves model-assessed beta-cell function in patients with type 2 diabetes. *J Clin Endocrinol Metab* 2005, 90:4888–4894.

33. Brazdg R, Xu L, Dalla Man C, *et al.*: Effect of adding sitagliptin, a dipeptidyl peptidase-4 inhibitor, to metformin on 24-h glycaemic control and beta-cell function in patients with type 2 diabetes. *Diabetes Obes Metab* 2007, 9:186–193.

34. Aschner P, Kipnes MS, Lunceford JK, *et al.*: Effect of the dipeptidyl peptidase-4 inhibitor sitagliptin as monotherapy on glycemic control in patients with type 2 diabetes. *Diabetes Care* 2006, 29:2632–2637.

35. Charbonnel B, Karasik A, Liu J, *et al.*: Efficacy and safety of the dipeptidyl peptidase-4 inhibitor sitagliptin added to ongoing metformin therapy in patients with type 2 diabetes inadequately controlled with metformin alone. *Diabetes Care* 2006, 29:2638–2643.

36. Rosenstock J, Brazg R, Andryuk PJ, *et al.*: Efficacy and safety of the dipeptidyl peptidase-4 inhibitor sitagliptin added to ongoing pioglitazone therapy in patients with type 2 diabetes: a 24-week, multicenter, randomized, double-blind, placebo-controlled, parallel-group study. *Clin Ther* 2006, 28:1556–1568.

37. Nauck MA, Meininger G, Sheng D, *et al.*: Efficacy and safety of the dipeptidyl peptidase-4 inhibitor, sitagliptin, compared with the sulfonylurea, glipizide, in patients with type 2 diabetes inadequately controlled on metformin alone: a randomized, double-blind, non-inferiority trial. *Diabetes Obes Metab* 2007, 9:194–205.

38. Goldstein BJ, Feinglos MN, Lunceford JK, *et al.*: Effect of initial combination therapy with sitagliptin, a dipeptidyl peptidase-4 inhibitor, and metformin on glycemic control in patients with type 2 diabetes. *Diabetes Care* 2007, 30:1979–1987.

39. Schweizer A, Couturier A, Foley JE, Dejager S: Comparison between vildagliptin and metformin to sustain reductions in HbA(1c) over 1 year in drug-naïve patients with type 2 diabetes. *Diabet Med* 2007, 24:955–961.

40. Ahrén B, Gomis R, Standl E, *et al.*: Twelve- and 52-week efficacy of the dipeptidase IV inhibitor LAF237 in metformin-treated patients with type 2 diabetes. *Diabetes Care* 2004, 27:2874–2880.

41. Jadzinsky M, Pfützner A, Paz-Pacheco E, *et al.*: Saxagliptin given in combination with metformin as initial therapy improves glycaemic control in patients with type 2 diabetes compared with either monotherapy: a randomized controlled trial. *Diabetes Obes Metab* 2009, 11:611–622.

42. Chacra AR, Tan GH, Apanovitch A, *et al.*: Saxagliptin added to a submaximal dose of sulphonylurea improves glycaemic control compared with uptitration of sulphonylurea in patients with type 2 diabetes: a randomised controlled trial. *Int J Clin Pract* 2009, 63:1395–1406.

43. Hollander P: Saxagliptin added to a thiazolidinedione improves glycemic control in patients with type 2 diabetes and inadequate control on thiazolidinedione alone. *J Clin Endocrinol Metab* 2009, 94:4810–4819.

44. Rosenstock J, Rendell MS, Gross JL, *et al.*: Alogliptin added to insulin therapy in patients with type 2 diabetes reduces HbA(1C) without causing weight gain or increased hypoglycaemia. *Diabetes Obes Metab* 2009, 11:1145–1152.

45. Pratley RE, Reusch JE, Fleck PR, *et al.*: Efficacy and safety of the dipeptidyl peptidase-4 inhibitor alogliptin added to pioglitazone in patients with type 2 diabetes: a randomized, double-blind, placebo-controlled study. *Curr Med Res Opin* 2009, 25:2361–2371.

46. Pratley RE, Kipnes MS, Fleck PR, *et al.*: Efficacy and safety of the dipeptidyl peptidase-4 inhibitor alogliptin in patients with type 2 diabetes inadequately controlled by glyburide monotherapy. *Diabetes Obes Metab* 2009, 11:167–176.

47. Nauck MA, Ellis GC, Fleck PR, *et al.*: Efficacy and safety of adding the dipeptidyl peptidase-4 inhibitor alogliptin to metformin therapy in patients with type 2 diabetes inadequately controlled with metformin monotherapy: a multicentre, randomised, double-blind, placebo-controlled study. *Int J Clin Pract* 2009, 63:46–55.

48. Rosenstock J, Inzucchi SE, Seufert J, *et al.*: Initial combination therapy with alogliptin and pioglitazone in drug-naïve patients with type 2 diabetes. *Diabetes Care* 2010, 33:2406–2408.

49. Del Prato S, Barnett AH, Huisman H, *et al.*: Effect of linagliptin monotherapy on glycaemic control and markers of b-cell function in patients with inadequately controlled type 2 diabetes: a randomised controlled trial. *Diabetes Obes Metab* 2011, 13:[Epub ahead of print] 3 Dec 2010.

50. Taskinen MR, Rosenstock J, Tamminen I, *et al.*: Safety and efficacy of linagliptin as add-on therapy to metformin in patients with type 2 diabetes: a randomized, double-blind, placebo-controlled study. *Diabetes Obes Metab* 2011, 13:65–74.

51. Owens DR, Swallow R, Jones P, *et al.*: Linagliptin improves glycemic control in type 2 diabetes patients inadequately controlled by metformin and sulfonylurea without weight gain or hypoglycemia. *Diabetes* 2010, 59(Suppl 1):abstract 548-P.

52. Gomis R, Espadero RM, Jones R, *et al.*: Efficacy and safety of initial combination therapy with linagliptin and pioglitazone in patients with inadequately controlled type 2 diabetes. *Diabetes* 2010, 59(Suppl 1):abstract 551-P.

53. Meier AH, Cincotta A: Circadian rhythms regulate the expression of the thrifty genotype/phenotype. *Diabetes Rev* 1996, 4:464–487.

54. Scranton RE, Farwell W, Ezrokhi M, *et al.*: Quick release bromocriptine (Cycloset™) improves glycaemic control in patients with diabetes failing metformin/sulfonylurea combination therapy. *Diabetologia* 2008, 51(Suppl 1):abstract 930.

55. Cincotta AH, Gaziano JM, Ezrokhi M, Scranton R: Cycloset (quick-release bromocriptine mesylate), a novel centrally acting treatment for type 2 diabetes. *Diabetologia* 2008, 51(Suppl 1):abstract 39.

56. Gaziano JM, Cincotta AH, O'Connor CM, *et al.*: Randomized clinical trial of quick release-bromocriptine among patients with type 2 diabetes on overall safety and cardiovascular outcomes. *Diabetes Care* 2010, 33:1503–1508.

57. Fonseca VA, Handelsman Y, Staels B: Colesevelam lowers glucose and lipid levels in type 2 diabetes: the clinical evidence. *Diabetes Obes Metab* 2010, 12:384–392.

58. Unger RH, Foster DW: Diabetes mellitus. In *Williams Textbook of Endocrinology*, edn. 8. Edited by Wilson JD and Foster DW. Philadelphia: WB Saunders; 1992:1273–1275.

59. Kruger DF, Gatcomb PM, Owen SK: Clinical implications of amylin and amylin deficiency. *Diabetes Educ* 1999, 25:389–397.

60. Weyer C, Gottlieb A, Kim DD, *et al.*: Pramlintide reduces post-prandial glucose excursions when added to regular insulin or insulin lispro in subjects with type 1 diabetes. *Diabetes Care* 2003, 26:3074–3079.

61. Edelman SV, Darsow T, Frias JP: Pramlintide in the treatment of diabetes. *Int J Clin Pract* 2006, 60:1647–1653.

62. Edelman S, Garg S, Frias J, *et al.*: A double-blind, placebo-controlled trial assessing pramlintide treatment in the setting of intensive insulin therapy in type 1 diabetes. *Diabetes Care* 2006, 29:2189–2195.

63. Riddle M, Pencek R, Charenkavanich S, *et al.*: Randomized comparison of pramlintide or mealtime insulin added to basal insulin treatment for patients with type 2 diabetes. *Diabetes Care* 2009, 32:1577–1582.

64. Heinemann L, Heise T: Current status of the development of inhaled insulin. *Br J Diabetes Vasc Dis* 2004, 4:295–301.

65. Potocka E, Cassidy JP, Haworth P, *et al.*: Pharmacokinetic characterization of the novel pulmonary delivery excipient fumaryl diketopiperazine. *J Diabetes Sci Technol* 2010, 4:1164–1173.

66. Rosenstock J, Lorber DL, Gnudi L, *et al.*: Prandial inhaled insulin plus basal insulin glargine versus twice daily biaspart insulin for type 2 diabetes: a multicentre randomised trial. *Lancet* 2010, 375:2244–2253.

67. Bailey CJ: Renal glucose reabsorption inhibitors to treat diabetes. *Trends Pharmacol Sci* 2011, 32:[Epub ahead of print] 4 Jan 2011.

68. Wilding JP, Norwood P, T'joen C, *et al.*: A study of dapagliflozin in patients with type 2 diabetes receiving high doses of insulin plus insulin sensitizers: applicability of a novel insulin-independent treatment. *Diabetes Care* 2009, 32:1656–1662.

69. Bailey CJ, Gross JL, Pieters A, *et al.*: Effect of dapagliflozin in patients with type 2 diabetes who have inadequate glycaemic control with metformin: a randomised, double-blind, placebo-controlled trial. *Lancet* 2010, 375:2223–2233.

70. Rosenstock J, Arbit D, Usiskin K, *et al.*: Canagliflozin, an inhibitor of sodium glucose co-transporter 2 (SGLT2), improves glycemic control and lowers body weight in subjects with type 2 diabetes (T2D) on metformin. *Diabetes* 2010, 59(Suppl 1):abstract 77-OR.

71. Ferrannini E, Seman LJ, Seewaldt-Becker E, *et al.* The potent and highly selective sodium-glucose co-cransporter (SGLT-2) inhibitor BI 10773 is safe and efficacious as monotherapy in patients with type 2 diabetes mellitus. *Diabetologia* 2010, 53(Suppl 2):abstract 877.

Index

J.S. Skyler (ed.), *Atlas of Diabetes: Fourth Edition*,
DOI 10.1007/978-1-4614-1028-7, © Springer Science+Business Media, LLC 2012

Printed in the United States of America